Neurogenic Disorders of Language and Cognition

Neurogenic Disorders of Language and Cognition

Evidence-Based Clinical Practice

SECOND EDITION

Laura L. Murray

Heather M. Clark

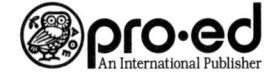

8700 Shoal Creek Boulevard
Austin, Texas 78757-6897
800/897-3202   Fax 800/397-7633
www.proedinc.com

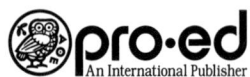

© 2015, 2006 by PRO-ED, Inc.
8700 Shoal Creek Boulevard
Austin, Texas 78757-6897
800/897-3202   Fax 800/397-7633
www.proedinc.com

All rights reserved. Except as indicated below, no part of the material protected by this copyright notice may be reproduced or used in any form or by any means, electronic or mechanical, including photocopying, recording, or by any information storage and retrieval system, without prior written permission of the copyright owner.

This product includes a DVD with reproducible pages.

Limited Photocopy License

PRO-ED, Inc. grants to individual purchasers of this material nonassignable permission to reproduce the reproducible forms on the DVD. This license is limited to you, the individual purchaser, for use with your clients. This license does not grant the right to reproduce these materials for resale, redistribution, or any other purposes (including but not limited to books, pamphlets, articles, video- or audio- recordings, Web sites, and handouts or slides for lectures or workshops). Permission to reproduce these materials for these and other purposes must be obtained in writing from the Permissions Department of PRO-ED, Inc.

Library of Congress Cataloging-in-Publication Data

Murray, Laura L., author.
  Neurogenic disorders of language and cognition : evidence-based clinical practice / by Laura L. Murray and Heather M. Clark.— 2nd ed.
    p. cm.
  Preceded by Neurogenic disorders of language : theory driven clinical practice / Laura L. Murray, Heather M. Clark. 2006.
  Includes bibliographical references.
  ISBN 978-1-4164-0585-6
  I. Clark, Heather M., author. II. Title. [DNLM: 1. Language Disorders—diagnosis.   2. Language Disorders—therapy.   3. Brain Diseases—complications.   4. Cognition Disorders—diagnosis.   5. Cognition Disorders—therapy.   6. Evidence-Based Medicine—methods.
WL 340.2] RC423
616.85'5—dc23
                                                                2013035668

Art Director: Jason Crosier
Designer: Lissa Hattersley
This book is designed in Minion and Neutra Text.

Printed in the United States of America
1 2 3 4 5 6 7 8 9 10   23 22 21 20 19 18 17 16 15 14

To those friends and family who over the years have said, "Yes, you can"—
I think you might be right.
—*Laura Murray*

To the countless individuals with neurogenic communication disorders I have been privileged to serve. Your wisdom and insight inspire my clinical practice, scholarship, and philosophy.
—*Heather Clark*

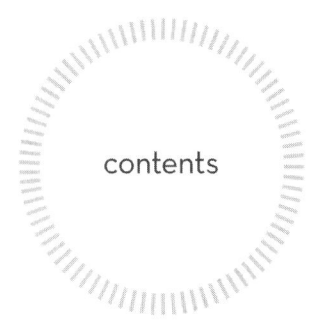

contents

DVD Contents ix

Preface xi

Acknowledgments xv

CHAPTER 1
Introduction: Models and Concepts 1

CHAPTER 2
Overview of Neurogenic Language and Cognitive Disorders 35

CHAPTER 3
Neuropathology of Neurogenic Language and Cognitive Disorders 79

CHAPTER 4
A General Model of Assessment 115

CHAPTER 5
Identifying Complicating Conditions 147

CHAPTER 6
Assessment of Body Structure and Function: Quantifying and Qualifying Linguistic Disorders 165

CHAPTER 7
Assessment of Body Structure and Function: Quantifying and Qualifying Cognitive Disorders 225

CHAPTER 8
Assessment of Activity, Participation, and Quality of Life 273

CHAPTER 9
Remediation of Body Structure and Function: Behavioral Approaches for Linguistic Disorders 299

CHAPTER 10
Remediation of Body Structure and Function: Behavioral Approaches for Cognitive Disorders   357

CHAPTER 11
Remediation of Body Structure and Function: Pharmacotherapy Approaches   395

CHAPTER 12
Remediation of Activity and Participation: Approaches for Linguistic and Cognitive Disorders   411

CHAPTER 13
The Context of Care: Legislative and Economic Influences   469

Glossary   493

References   513

Index   601

About the Authors   641

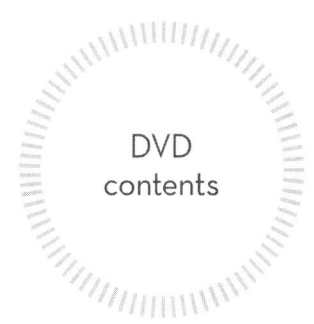

DVD contents

PATIENT 1: DESCRIPTION
Video: 1

PATIENT 2: DESCRIPTION
Videos: 2a, 2b, and 2c

PATIENT 3: DESCRIPTION
Videos: 3a, 3b, and 3c

PATIENT 4: DESCRIPTION
Video: 4

PATIENT 5: DESCRIPTION
Video: 5

PATIENT 6: DESCRIPTION
Videos: 6a, 6b, 6c, and 6d

PATIENT 7: DESCRIPTION
Video: 7

PATIENT 8: DESCRIPTION
Videos: 8a, 8b, 8c, 8d, 8e, 8f, 8g, 8h, 8i, 8j, 8k, 8l, and 8m
Picture 8n

PATIENT 9: DESCRIPTION
Videos: 9a, 9b, 9c, 9d, 9e, 9f, 9g, and 9h
Picture 9i

PATIENT 10: DESCRIPTION
Videos: 10a, 10b, 10c, 10d, 10e, 10f, 10g, 10h, 10i, 10j, 10k, 10l, 10m, 10n, 10o, 10p, 10q, and 10r
Picture 10s

PATIENT 11: DESCRIPTION
Videos: 11a, 11b, 11c, and 11d

CASE HISTORY OR PATIENT INTAKE FORM (FIGURE 6.1)

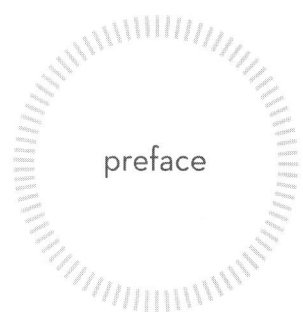

preface

In the United States and worldwide, brain damage due to stroke, traumatic brain injury (TBI), progressive neurological disease, and other etiologies is extremely common. Each year in the United States, approximately 1.7 million individuals will suffer a TBI (Faul, Xu, Wald, & Coronado, 2010); over 66,000 will be diagnosed with a brain tumor (American Brain Tumor Association, 2012); 795,000 will have a stroke (Roger et al., 2011); and well over 6 million are living with a progressive disorder such as Alzheimer's disease, Parkinson's disease, or multiple sclerosis (e.g., Alzheimer's Association, 2012; Wright Willis, Evanoff, Lian, Criswel, & Racette, 2010). Neurogenic language and cognitive disorders are common consequences of these forms of brain damage and disease.

The purpose of this book is to provide a thorough review of neurogenic language and cognitive disorders for speech-language pathology students, clinicians, and researchers, as well as those in related health-care disciplines (such as occupational therapy, neuropsychology, physiatry, and nursing), who provide services to the above patient populations. Several features of this book, in terms of both content and organization, make it a valuable resource, regardless of the reader's degree of experience with neurogenic language and cognitive disorders. First, a number of neurogenic language and cognitive disorders are systematically described, including aphasia and cognitive-communicative disorders associated with right hemisphere brain damage, TBI, and dementing diseases such as frontotemporal lobar degeneration and Alzheimer's or Parkinson's disease. Second, traditional descriptions of neurogenic language disorders are expanded upon by discussing both the linguistic and cognitive bases of these disorders, and by including a thorough review of cognitive assessment and treatment approaches. Third, both theoretical and applied clinical issues are highlighted throughout the book, with a special emphasis on the World Health Organization's (WHO, 2001) International Classification of Functioning, Disability, and Health (ICF) as a guiding framework for understanding and managing neurogenic language and cognitive disorders. Fourth, our description of treatment procedures includes evidence-based reviews of not only more traditional behavioral protocols (e.g., melodic intonation therapy; spaced retrieval), but also pharmacotherapy and alternative therapies (e.g., relaxation therapy) for neurogenic language and/or cognitive disorders. Accordingly, this book will serve not only as a comprehensive textbook for university courses that must cover a range of neurogenic language and cognitive disorders, but also as an up-to-date reference for both researchers and clinicians looking to expand their knowledge base.

On an editorial note, readers will note that throughout the book we use the term "patients" to refer to individuals who have been diagnosed with a neurogenic language or cognitive disorder. We acknowledge that there is a move in both research and clinical practice to replace terms that denote impairment with more neutral language (e.g., using "individuals" or "adults" instead of "patients"); however, in those sections of the book in which discussions focus on both patients and caregivers, the text became too cumbersome and confusing when trying to use neutral terminology for all individuals being discussed. Therefore, for clarity purposes, we elected to use the term "patients."

Organization of This Text

Several frameworks have been adopted to organize the material in this book. First, the ICF classification system is used to highlight the importance of addressing neurogenic language and cognitive disorders in terms of not only linguistic and cognitive symptoms (i.e., ICF levels of body structure and function) but also the effects of these symptoms on patients' daily personal, social, education, and/or vocational endeavors. Likewise, the ICF system acknowledges the influence of contextual factors (e.g., supportive vs. deleterious environmental variables) on the severity of and recovery from neurogenic language and cognitive disorders. Second, a language-processing model is followed to organize and allow in-depth descriptions of procedures for assessing and treating linguistic aspects of neurogenic language and cognitive disorders. Lastly, because neurogenic disorders commonly cause both linguistic and cognitive symptoms, rather than discussing assessment and treatment with respect to separate neurogenic language or cognitive disorders (e.g., aphasia, dementia), we separated management approaches in terms of those appropriate for addressing linguistic problems and those appropriate for addressing cognitive problems.

The first three chapters of this book review constructs and conditions essential to managing neurogenic language and cognitive disorders. In Chapter 1, constructs pertaining to the book's organizational frameworks (e.g., the ICF classification system) are introduced and explained. In Chapters 2 and 3, impairments and activity limitations associated with neurogenic language and cognitive disorders, including those associated with aphasia, right hemisphere brain damage, TBI, or dementia, and common etiologies of these are described.

The next five chapters pertain to diagnostic issues. First, Chapter 4 provides an overview of the assessment process, then Chapters 5 through 8 review procedures for identifying complicating conditions and for evaluating the linguistic symptoms; cognitive abilities; and daily communication activity, participation, and quality of life of patients with neurogenic language and cognitive disorders.

The next four chapters offer a discussion of treating neurogenic language and cognitive disorders. Management strategies targeting underlying impairments in linguistic and cognitive processing are explored in Chapters 9 and 10, respectively, and pharmacological treatment approaches are summarized in Chapter 11. These chapters are followed by a consideration of procedures suitable for targeting activity and participation restrictions, in Chapter 12.

Finally, in recognition that managing neurogenic language and cognitive disorders does not take place in a vacuum but rather takes place within the larger health-care culture and under certain policies, Chapter 13 provides an overview of the U.S. health-care system, exploring the influences of legislative and economic variables on the assessment and treatment of neurogenic language and cognitive disorders. Chapter 13 concludes with an exploration of how the management of neurogenic language and cognitive disorders may evolve in the coming decades.

Features

Within each chapter, the reader will find a number of special features. These features were designed to augment the reader's experience and to help the reader successfully navigate the content. Special features include:

- *Learning Objectives*: Each chapter begins with a carefully constructed list of its main concepts. These can be used as a framework for what to expect, as well as a review and study aid.
- *Key Terms*: Also setting the tone for each chapter is a list of its key terms. Definitions for each of these terms can be found in the Glossary. Readers can scan the terms as an orientation to the chapter's terminology, as well as use them as review and study aids.
- *Video Samples*: Callouts to video clips, as well as samples of patients' writing, are included in most chapters. These samples illustrate a number of neurogenic language and cognitive disorders, as well as assessment and treatment procedures reviewed throughout the book.
- *Sidebars*: Sidebars are included throughout to place information in the real-life context of clinical practice. Directly related to the chapter, sidebars provide models for applying the theoretical concepts in clinical settings with clients.
- *Summaries*: Each chapter concludes with a summary that pulls everything together and provides solid footing for moving on to subsequent chapters.
- *Discussion Questions*: For each chapter, discussion questions have been provided. Such questions may serve to promote readers' application of the material reviewed in each chapter, as well as to assist instructors in leading class discussions pertaining to the book's content.
- *Comprehensive References*: The book provides a highly comprehensive, up-to-date, relevant list of references for readers looking for further information on the topics covered.

Given the prevalence of neurogenic language and cognitive disorders, there is an ongoing need to identify effective and efficient means by which to manage them. By reviewing the current literature and highlighting areas in need of additional investigation, it is our hope that this book will spur further theoretical and clinical interest in understanding, assessing, and treating neurogenic language and cognitive disorders, and thus in turn will result in improved outcomes for those patients and caregivers directly affected by neurogenic language and cognitive disorders.

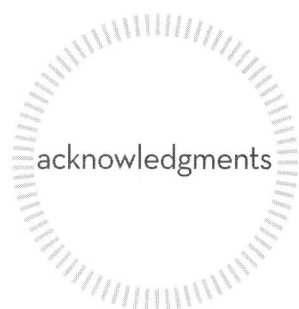

acknowledgments

This revision represents a major accomplishment for us that could not have come to fruition without the assistance and support of our new publisher, PRO-ED. We are indebted to our past and current mentors and colleagues, whose support, research, and feedback concerning the first edition of this book not only influenced the contents and format of this revision but also continue to inspire our own research, clinical, and teaching endeavors. And finally, and most importantly, we are most grateful to our families, especially Dylan and Norman, for their continued encouragement and patience. They are no doubt as relieved as we are that this book is finally finished.

Introduction: Models and Concepts

chapter 1

Learning Objectives

After reading this chapter, you should be able to:

- Discuss the International Classification of Function, Disability, and Health (ICF) and its application to the study and management of neurogenic language and cognitive disorders
- Discuss the components of evidence-based practice and strategies for incorporating consideration of best available evidence in assessment and treatment decisions
- Identify and describe the linguistic processes (body functions) that support language comprehension and production
- Identify and describe the components of attention, memory, and executive functioning (body functioning) and their contribution to communication
- Identify the neuroanatomy (body structures) that supports language, attention, memory, and executive functioning

Key Terms

- activities and participation
- attention
- body function
- body structure
- cognition
- cognitive flexibility
- communication
- contextual factors
- critical appraisal
- critical thinking
- effectiveness
- efficacy
- efficiency
- environmental factors
- evidence-based practice (EBP)
- executive functioning
- inhibition
- International Classification of Functioning, Disability, and Health (ICF)
- language
- memory
- metacognitive abilities
- organization
- outcome
- outcome evaluation
- personal factors
- planning
- practice-based evidence
- problem solving
- prospective memory
- repetition
- self-monitoring

Introduction

As adults, most of us have progressed through our lives giving only passing notice to our ability to communicate. We listen, speak, read, and write—often without effort—and we expect other adults to experience similar ease in their communication with us. We know, however, that even otherwise healthy adults can experience illnesses or accidents that suddenly impact their communication or cognition in both subtle and dramatic ways. Likewise, as we age, we become more susceptible to a number of chronic diseases that may progressively and irreversibly limit our communication abilities, as well as our thinking or cognitive skills. Adult neurogenic language and cognitive disorders arise when these illnesses, accidents, or progressive diseases cause brain damage and, in turn, that brain damage negatively impacts the communicative and possibly cognitive well-being of the affected individual. Accordingly, speech-language pathologists serving adults must be familiar with the variety of medical conditions that can produce neurogenic language and cognitive disorders. Additionally, they must possess the knowledge and skills necessary not only to evaluate how these accidents or diseases are affecting the communicative and cognitive functioning of their patients, but also to design and implement treatments that will remediate or stabilize the negative effects of these conditions. This book provides students, as well as practicing clinicians and researchers, with a comprehensive review of the concepts and procedures germane to managing neurogenic language and cognitive disorders.

Guiding Framework

Throughout this text, a number of theoretical models addressing the characterization, assessment, and treatment of neurogenic language and cognitive disorders will be presented. These models often explain relationships among areas of impairment, inform differential diagnosis, and direct selection of treatment targets and strategies. Consistent with the American Speech-Language-Hearing Association (ASHA, 2007) Scope of Practice for Speech-Language Pathology, we have chosen the World Health Organization (WHO, 2001) **International Classification of Functioning, Disability, and Health (ICF)** as a guiding framework for this text. Although the specific terms adopted by the ICF differ from those introduced in the original International Classification of Impairment, Disability, and Handicap (ICIDH; WHO, 1980), the key concepts of the ICIDH have been maintained in the revised ICF.

The ICF includes a system for describing the impact of disease or injury on the body and its functions, as well as patients' ability to complete tasks or activities relevant to their personal, social, educational, and/or vocational pursuits (see Figure 1-1). The ICF constructs of **body structure** and **body function** are closely related, describing the integrity of tissues and organs, along with the functions they perform. This level of description parallels the construct of **impairment** described in the ICIDH and traditionally has been a primary focus of medical assessment, as well as medical/surgical interventions. The categories of body structure particularly relevant to communication and cognition are *structures of the nervous system; structures of the eye, ear, and related structures; structures involved in voice and speech;* and additional *musculoskeletal structures related to movement* (e.g., muscles). Similarly, the body functions of *mental functions, sensory functions, voice and speech functions,* and *neuromusculoskeletal and movement-related functions* contribute to communication and cognitive behaviors. With respect to language and cognition, as well as neurogenic language and cognitive disorders specifi-

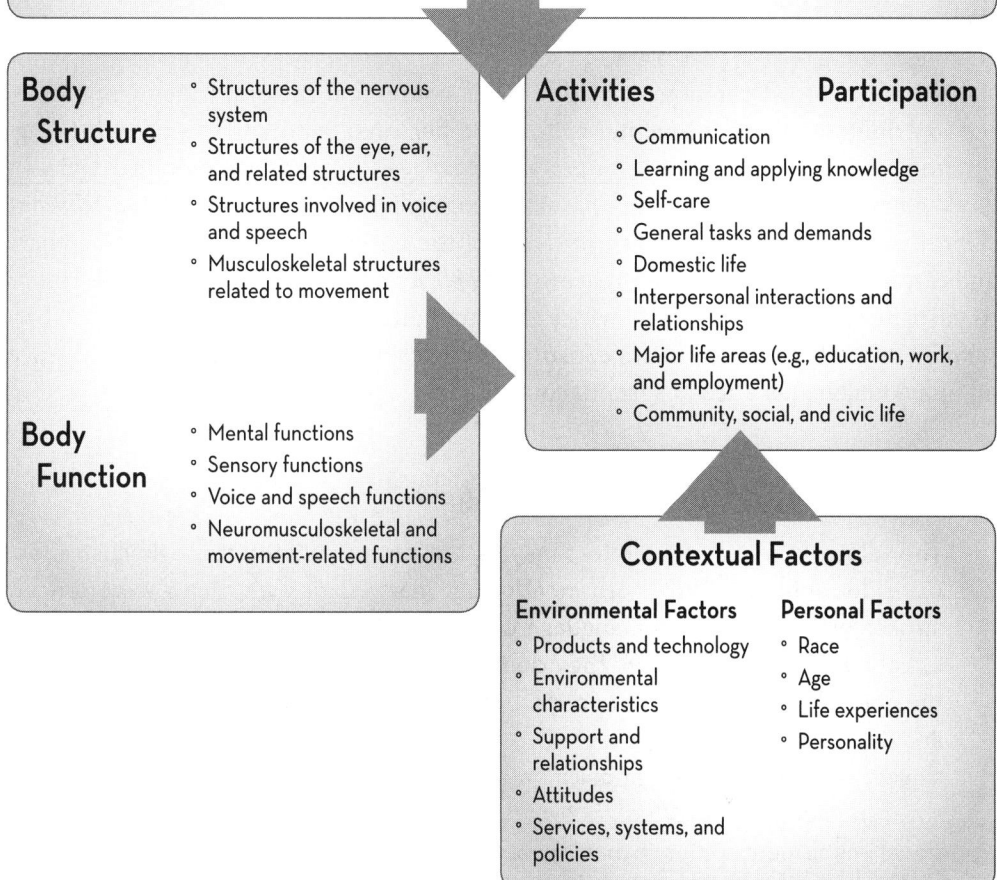

Figure 1-1. Components of the International Classification of Functioning, Disability, and Health (ICF; WHO, 2001).

cally, *the structures of the nervous system* and a number of the *specific mental functions* (e.g., attention, memory, the mental functions of language) are of primary interest.

The ICF also incorporates the construct of **activities and participation**, which highlights the ability of the individual to use language to communicate and cognition to function in a variety of contexts. Although the ICF combines activities and participation in a single classification construct, the ICIDH terms of "**disability**" and "**handicap**" are roughly synonymous with activities and participation, respectively. Within the area of activities and participation, a primary construct of interest to the discussion of neurogenic language and cognitive disorders is *communication,* which involves receiving and producing spoken, nonverbal, formal sign language, and/or written messages. Within this category, the ICF also includes descriptions of conversation and the use of communication devices. Additional categories potentially influenced by the presence of neurogenic language and cognitive disorders are *learning and applying knowledge, self-care, general tasks and demands, domestic life, interpersonal interactions and relationships, major life areas* (e.g., education, work, employment), and *community, social, and civic life.*

The final broad component of the ICF is **contextual factors,** which emphasizes the contribution of **environmental factors** and **personal factors** to overall well-being. Environmental factors include *products of technology* (e.g., assistive mobility devices), *environmental characteristics* (e.g., physical geography, lighting), *support and relationships* (e.g., family, care providers), *attitudes* of the individual and of family members and care providers, and *services, systems, and policies* relating to the individual's ability to participate fully in desired activities. An individual's *race, age, life experiences, personality*, and other characteristics constitute the personal factors that further influence an individual's experience of a health condition.

The ICF Applied

The value of the ICF descriptors may be better appreciated through illustration. Consider John and Bob, both men in their early sixties who have experienced strokes with resulting mild language disorders. With respect to underlying *body structure* and *body function*, they demonstrate similar structural impairments of the central nervous system and disruption in the mental functions of receptive and expressive language, potentially leading to the prediction that each would be similarly affected by their impairments.

A number of *contextual factors*, however, influence the effects of these functional impairments on each man's communicative *activity*. John has a college education and, as a vice president for an international corporation, has considerable experience communicating in a variety of settings using flexible linguistic styles. Thus, he readily compensates for his new language disorder, and his communication impairment is judged to be quite mild by his friends and family. Nonetheless, John expresses frustration that he experiences occasional anomia (i.e., word retrieval difficulty), particularly in high-pressure communication situations.

Bob, on the other hand, is a small-business owner in a rural community. His communication partners generally are limited to family and community members. Although his impairment is equal to John's, Bob does not spontaneously compensate, and his communication impairments are notable during conversations and other interactions.

The ICF also provides a way to characterize the impact of a neurogenic language disorder on John's and Bob's lives (*activities and participation*). Considering again contextual factors, Bob has a generally patient, laid-back personality and does not express great frustration with his language symptoms (*individual attitude*). Bob's communication partners are quite familiar with his typical conversation topics, which facilitates successful communication in spite of the presence of linguistic breakdowns. Moreover, the dialect in Bob's geographic region is characterized by a relatively slow speech rate and precise articulation, which facilitate Bob's comprehension. Ultimately, Bob's neurogenic language disorder has little impact on his participation in activities he enjoyed prior to his stroke.

In contrast, both John's professional and leisure activities (e.g., leading group Bible studies, traveling) involve diverse communication contexts, most of which are demanding and relatively unaccommodating to reduced communicative efficiency (*attitudes of colleagues, strangers*); thus, John expresses greater concern that his language disorder will significantly impact his participation in desired activities. Fortunately, a number of additional contextual factors will facilitate John's participation: Electronic communication options (*products of technology*) are available to John, and he is willing to utilize them (*individual attitude*). He lives in a metropolitan area with a wealth of community resources, and he has already made contact with an appropriate support group (*support and relationships*). Finally, John has access to sufficient economic resources and quality health care (*services, systems, and policies*) to assist with necessary adaptations to maximize participation.

It is clear that the nature of the neurogenic language disorder, which is the same for both men, does not tell the whole story. Only by considering the impact of the neurogenic language disorder on communicative effectiveness in real-life contexts, the implications on life *activities and participation*, and the *contextual factors* influencing the impact of the disorder can we gain a more complete understanding of the patient's needs.

Readers familiar with the ICF may note that the overview provided here differs slightly from most descriptions included in other speech-language pathology (SLP) literature. Specifically, it is common for the SLP literature to discuss **body structure** and **body function** as a single construct (i.e., **impairment**) and to separate the construct of **activities and participation** into two distinct constructs: (1) **activity** and (2) **participation**. When the concepts are separated in this way, the term "**activity**" relates to the patient's ability to complete specific tasks (e.g., speak, write, comprehend gestures, activate short-term recall), whereas "**participation**" addresses the impact of impairments and activity limitations on the patient's ability to participate in desired life activities and social roles. This minimal modification of the published ICF framework is useful to clinicians managing neurogenic language and cognitive disorders because it underscores the value of considering the nature of underlying language and cognitive impairments and the resulting communication and cognitive limitations, as well as the impact of these deficits on life participation and quality of life.

In their original or modified form, the ICF constructs provide a framework for describing the myriad characteristics possible in neurogenic language and cognitive disorders, planning assessment and treatment strategies, and measuring outcomes (see Hopper, 2007; Larkins, 2007; and Simmons-Mackie & Kagan, 2007, for additional reviews). The ICF recognizes the importance of multidisciplinary involvement throughout the care process and emphasizes the value of full participation by the patient and family members in the planning and implementing of care plans.

This text is organized to explicitly acknowledge the ICF framework. In the current chapter, the various **body structures** and **body functions** contributing to language behaviors are reviewed. Chapter 2 expands the discussion of body structure and function with a thorough description of the nature of various neurogenic language and cognitive disorders. The chapters addressing assessment and treatment are organized with respect to underlying impairments, functional communication and cognition (i.e., *activity*), *participation*, and quality of life. Similarly, the discussion of treatment is structured such that strategies addressing underlying impairments, functional communication and cognition, and quality of life are considered. Finally, issues surrounding *contextual factors* are incorporated throughout the discussions of both assessment and treatment.

Evidence-Based Practice[1]

The title of this text—*Neurogenic Disorders of Language and Cognition: Evidence-Based Clinical Practice*—highlights the importance of *evidence* in guiding clinical decision-making. A commonly cited definition of **evidence-based practice (EBP)** is "the conscientious, explicit, and judicious use of current best evidence in making decisions about the care of individual patients" (Sackett, Rosenberg, Gray, Haynes, & Richardson, 1996, p. 71). The goal of EBP extends beyond the use of scientific evidence, seeking also to integrate clinical expertise, patient values, and the best available evidence into the clinical decision-making process (ASHA, 2005). We have developed this textbook with EBP as a central guiding principle. With that in mind, we will review the key concepts of EBP and discuss resources that facilitate EBP.

Overview and Philosophy of EBP

Guyatt and colleagues (2008) proposed two basic tenets that underlie effective EBP. The first tenet posits a *hierarchy of evidence*, recognizing that varying research designs provide weaker or stronger evidence. Specific criteria for evaluating evidence differ somewhat according to the type of clinical decision to be made (ASHA, 2004a). Consequently, there are numerous published evidence hierarchies or classifications for each type of clinical question; further discussion and examples will be presented below.

---

[1]Portions of this section of Chapter 1 were taken from a chapter in the original edition of this textbook contributed by William H. Irwin.

The second principle, *evidence is never enough,* implies that there are other important factors to consider when making clinical decisions. This simple but powerful statement suggests that clinical decisions about patient care must take into account both the best available external evidence and clinical expertise; this includes the skills necessary for "more thoughtful identification and compassionate use of individual patients' predicaments, rights, and preferences in making clinical decisions about their care" (Sackett, Richardson, Rosenberg, & Haynes, 1997, p. 2). In addition to patient considerations, clinical and societal values are brought to bear in the decision-making process. Considering and evaluating these numerous and varying sources of information to arrive at a clinical decision requires **critical thinking** (Jenicek, Croskerry, & Hitchcock, 2011). The application of critical thinking is fundamental to effective clinical practice, but it is particularly critical to each of the steps of EBP (Sackett, Strauss, Richardson, Rosenberg, & Haynes, 2000): question formulation, searching for evidence, critical appraisal of the evidence, using the results of the critical appraisal in clinical practice, and performance evaluation.

The five critical steps of EBP include the following:

1. Convert the need for information into an answerable question.
2. Identify the best evidence with which to answer that question.
3. Critically appraise the evidence.
4. Apply the results of this appraisal in clinical practice.
5. Evaluate your performance.

The first step, formulating a question, requires a focus on a specific aspect of practice. S. Reilly (2004a) suggested that "one of the most useful tools for developing clinical questions is the PECOT approach to question-framing (P = patient/population group; E = exposure or intervention if about therapy; C = control or comparison; O = outcome(s); and T = time-frame)" (p. 114). For example, we may ask the question, "Has stimulation treatment been shown to improve the spoken language production of patients with chronic aphasia?" In this case, P = patients with aphasia, E = stimulation treatment, C = patients with aphasia who do not receive stimulation treatment, O = improved spoken productions, and T = in the chronic phase of recovery. Narrowing the question in this way to a specific focus on these aspects of a clinical question greatly facilitates performing Step 2, identifying relevant evidence.

The astute evidence-based practitioner knows where and how to look for the evidence, if it is to be found. For example, searchable electronic databases such as those in Table 1-1 include research citations relevant to neurogenic language and other communication disorders, as well as neurogenic cognitive disorders. Journal articles, book chapters, texts, instrument manuals, and bibliographies provide other, though less efficient, means of locating evidence. With the advent of online discussion forums, and email contact information listed in journal articles, the experts are often accessible for questions and/or requests for relevant references and, in most cases, are enthusiastic about helping. Don't underestimate the value of this approach; in some cases, the expert's opinion may constitute the current best evidence!

TABLE 1-1
Electronic Indexes in Which Neurogenic Language and Cognitive Disorders Research Citations May Be Found

INDEX	DESCRIPTION	ACCESS URL
CINAHL	Database serving nursing and allied health disciplines	www.cinahl.com
Cochrane	Database with emphasis on evidence-based reviews	www.cochrane.org
Dissertation Abstracts Online	Indexed doctoral dissertations across disciplines	http://library.dialog.com/bluesheets/html/bl0035.html
EMBASE	Database serving biomedical and pharmacological disciplines	www.embase.com
The Evidence-Based Review of Moderate to Severe Acquired Brain Injury (ABIEBR)	Index of literature for rehabilitation or rehabilitation-related interventions for brain injury	www.abiebr.com
PsycBITE	Database of cognitive and psycho-behavioral/emotional treatment research studies; can search database via various variables (e.g., age group, study design, cognitive or psychobehavioral disorder)	www.psycbite.com
PsycINFO®	Abstract database of psychological literature	www.apa.org/pubs/databases/psycinfo/index.aspx
PubMed	Comprehensive biomedical database provided by the National Library of Medicine	www.ncbi.nlm.nih.gov/sites/pubmed
Social Science Citation Index®	Index of science and technical journals	http://thomsonreuters.com/social-sciences-citation-index/
Science Direct	Comprehensive scientific database offering journal articles and book chapters	www.sciencedirect.com
Scopus	Simplifies identifying articles that have cited a specific author or work	www.elsevier.com/online-tools/scopus
SpeechBITE	Database of speech and language treatment research studies; can search database via multiple variables (e.g., author, study design, speech or language disorder)	www.speechbite.com

Note. Many of these indexes may be accessed through university or health-center libraries at no cost.

EBP Applied to Diagnostic Questions

At present, EBP principles have been adopted most widely with respect to treatment, even though they apply to diagnostic issues as well. Although a detailed discussion of EBP concepts unique to assessment is beyond the scope of this chapter, the following illustration highlights how the process may be applied to diagnosing neurogenic language and cognitive disorders.

Imagine we receive a referral for a patient who had a single left hemisphere stroke two weeks ago. Our own clinical experience may lead us to predict that a patient with this lesion site will exhibit aphasia (an acquired language disorder that involves difficulty understanding and producing spoken and written language), and we can further support this prediction with EBP. For example, a prospective study determined that in a group of 106 consecutively admitted stroke patients, 34% were diagnosed as having aphasia in the acute phase (Kauhanen et al., 2000). Thus, with only this knowledge and no additional data from the patient, 34% is a good estimate of the probability that this patient has aphasia. After conducting a brief initial interview, we may further suspect that the patient has mild aphasia. If we are considering using a formal test to determine whether the patient indeed has aphasia, we may want to know how well a specific formal test assists in diagnosing mild aphasia. A literature search reveals a study that applied EBP in determining the importance of selected formal tests for diagnosing mild aphasia (K. B. Ross & Wertz, 2004). Using the process and these empirical data, we determine that the ASHA FACS-Communication Dimensions score provides a 96% probability of correctly diagnosing mild aphasia, providing ample evidence to support using this tool.

Although additional issues must be considered when using EBP to answer diagnostic questions (e.g., whether the evidence employed independent, blind administration of a gold standard or included a large sample of patients), it is clear that the basic principles of identifying and critically evaluating available evidence will help inform assessment as well as treatment decisions.

Critical appraisal is the process of deciding whether a specific piece of evidence can help in answering the clinical question. One aspect of this process is considering the nature of the **outcomes** described in the study being appraised. For example, using the ICF framework, clinical outcomes regarding treatment effects might rely upon measuring changes at the body structure or body function, activity, and/or participation level. Furthermore, treatment outcomes may relate to treatment **efficacy** research or treatment **effectiveness** research (Robey, 2004). "Efficacy," according to the Office of Technology Assessment (OTA; 1978), is "[t]he probability of benefit to individuals in a defined population from a medical technology applied for a given medical problem under ideal conditions of use" (p. 16). Evidence of treatment efficacy indicates the *potential* maximum benefit of a particular treatment administered under ideal conditions and may not be equivalent to the actual benefits of treatment in clinical practice. In contrast, OTA (1978) specified that "evidence of treatment effectiveness establishes the value of a particular treatment protocol for effecting beneficial change under the conditions of routine clinical practice" (p. 6). Ideally, research to establish a treatment's effectiveness is conducted after that treatment's efficacy has been established (Robey, 2004; Robey & Schultz, 1998; Wertz & Irwin, 2001). **Efficiency** implies high productivity: a maximum effect for the effort expended. For example, a treatment determined to be efficacious and effective might be compared with another treatment to determine which results in the better or more *efficient* outcome.

Another component of critical appraisal is determining the level of evidence provided by research findings. Levels-of-evidence rating scales offer structured hierarchies, from strongest to weakest, for rating the strength or quality of scientific evidence. Although specific scales vary with respect to the code assigned a given level of evidence, there is general agreement regarding the type of studies that provide weakest versus strongest evidence. For example, the system proposed by the Oxford Centre for Evidence-Based Medicine (OCEBM Levels of Evidence Working Group, 2011), which includes five levels, rates systematic reviews of randomized controlled trials (RCTs) as providing the highest level of evidence (rated *1*) and expert opinion based on mechanism-based reasoning providing the lowest level of evidence (rated *5*).

Inferring strength of evidence from study design alone, however, may be problematic; other factors that influence evidence quality must be adequately considered. For example, sample size, recruitment bias, losses to follow-up, atypical patient groups, and other threats to internal and external validity do not affect ratings on many scales. Likewise, results from a single RCT with a small sample size do not necessarily provide more convincing evidence than do consistent results with high precision from numerous high-quality trials with nonrandomized designs (Galante, Gazzi, & Caffarra, 2011; Guyatt, Sinclair, Cook, & Glasziou, 1999; Whyte, Gordon, Nash, & Gonzalez Rothi, 2009). Finally, there remains controversy regarding what design should be considered the gold standard for behavioral intervention research (Galante et al., 2011; Tucker & Reed, 2008; Whyte et al., 2009): Although RCTs work well for drug intervention studies, concerns over the suitability for establishing the effectiveness and efficiency of behavioral interventions have been raised (e.g., poor generalization power; problems in identifying appropriate activities for the control or placebo group). Therefore, critical evidence appraisal must extend beyond study design to include additional issues concerning validity, importance, and usefulness.

ASHA and EBP

Clinicians may wonder how the policy statements issued by ASHA relate to EBP. In fact, many principles of EBP are typically incorporated into the development of Practice Guidelines, which recommend procedures for specific areas of practice based on research findings and expert opinion. Moreover, ASHA's National Center for Evidence-Based Practice has produced a number of systematic reviews of the literature (see Figure 1-2) to assist clinicians in their efforts to both locate and appraise relevant evidence.

Given the vastness of the potential literature to be searched and the time and effort involved in critical appraisal of individual studies, these aspects of the EBP process may seem overwhelming. Fortunately, the EBP framework accomodates considering preprocessed evidence in which evidence validity and importance have already been critically appraised. Researchers and clinicians in the area of neurogenic communication and cognitive disorders are leading the way in their efforts to preprocess the evidence. Critical appraisal must also be applied to preprocessed evidence, and guidelines are available to assist in this process (e.g., Ciliska, Cullum, & Marks, 2001; Manchikanti, Singh, Smith, & Hirsch, 2009). Nonetheless, systematic reviews and meta-analyses can be very useful, in that much of the time-consuming work of searching for and obtaining the evidence and evaluating its validity and importance has been performed according to specific criteria to ensure its quality.

Once the appropriate evidence has been identified and critically appraised, the clinician has to make a decision about whether and how to use the clinical procedure under consideration. Moreover, critical thinking must be employed to determine whether adaptations to the techniques are desirable or even unavoidable. It is not inappropriate to adapt techniques; however, the clinician must acknowledge that the evidence upon which the clinical decision was initially made to select the technique is necessarily weakened.

It is helpful to consider an additional step in the EBP process, that of **outcome evaluation**. Using empirical methods to track clinical progress provides an additional source of evidence to support future clinical decisions. The practice of collecting objective data from clinical practices is one component of **practice-based evidence** (Horn, Gassaway, Pentz, & James, 2010). Objective treatment data can be generated from individual patients using a single-subject research design (for a comprehensive introduction, see Byiers, Reichle, & Symons, 2012), patient and caregiver satisfaction questionnaires, and consistent and reliable data collection during treatment administration.

The concepts inherent to EBP and the ICF framework are complementary and are most powerful when practiced in concert. To appreciate the patient's values and priorities in the clinical decision process, we are helped by considering the contextual factors unique to him or her. The clinical expertise contributed by each clinician is frequently developed from an observation of the benefits of a technique not only at the level of body function but also with respect to activity and participation. These observations are strengthened if conducted with the objectivity inherent to practice-based evidence.

- **The Academy of Neurologic Communication Disorders & Sciences: Evidence-Based Practice Guidelines for the Management of Communication Disorders in Neurologically Impaired Individuals (www.ancds.org)**

  This resource is home to the EBP project initiated to improve the quality of services to individuals with neurologic communication disorders by helping clinicians make decisions using guidelines based on research evidence. Practice guidelines are provided in the following areas related to the management of neurogenic language and cognitive disorders.

    o Dementia
      Simulated presence therapy
      Reminiscence therapy
      Spaced retrieval therapy
      Cognitive stimulation
      Educating caregivers
      Computer-assisted cognitive interventions
      Montessori-based interventions

    o TBI
      Standardized and nonstandardized assessment
      Behavioral and social interventions disorders
      Group intervention
      External memory aids
      Direct attention training

    o Aphasia (available through http://aphasiatx.arizona.edu/)
      Lexical retrieval
      Syntax
      Speech production
      Reading and writing
      Alternative communication strategies

- **Agency for Healthcare Research and Quality (AHRQ): Evidence-Based Practice Centers (www.ahcpr.gov/clinic/epcix.htm)**

  The AHRQ's Evidence-Based Practice Centers develop evidence reports and technology assessments on topics relevant to clinical, social science/behavioral, economic, and other health-care organization and delivery issues—specifically those that are common, expensive, and/or significant for the Medicare and Medicaid populations.

- **ASHA: EBP Resources**

    Overview and processes: www.asha.org/members/ebp/
    Compendium of EBP guidelines and systematic reviews: www.asha.org/members/ebp/compendium/
    Evidence maps: www.ncepmaps.org/
    Systematic reviews: www.asha.org/members/ebp/EBSRs.htm
    Intensity of treatment and constraint-induced language therapy
    Treatment for bilingual individuals with aphasia

- **The Cochrane Library (www.thecochranelibrary.com)**

  A source of reliable and up-to-date information on the effects of interventions in health care. Published on a quarterly basis, The Cochrane Library is designed to provide information and evidence to support decisions taken in health care and to inform those receiving care. The Cochrane Library consists of a regularly updated collection of evidence-based medicine databases. (www.cochrane.org/reviews/clibintro.htm)

Figure 1-2. Annotated list of selected EBP resources. (Many of these sources include preprocessed evidence to help the clinician both identify and critically appraise treatment evidence.)

> - **Centre for Evidence-Based Medicine at the University of Toronto Health Network (www.ktclearinghouse.ca/cebm)**
>
>   An EBP center with the goal of helping to develop, disseminate, and evaluate resources that can be used to practice and teach EBP for undergraduate, postgraduate, and continuing education for health-care professionals from a variety of clinical disciplines. Among the resources available are glossaries, tutorials, syllabi, and other resources for teaching EBP; a list of evidence resources; worksheets; calculators; appraisal checklists; and numerous links to other EBP resources.
>
> - **The Oxford Centre for Evidence-Based Medicine (www.cebm.net)**
>
>   An extensive resource center designed to promote evidence-based health care and provide support and resources to all practitioners. Among the resources available are glossaries, tutorials, tips for searching for evidence, a list of critically appraised topics, and numerous links to other EBP resources.
>
> - **PsycBITE (www.psycbite.com)**
>
>   PsycBITE is a database that catalogues studies of cognitive, behavioral, and other treatments for psychological problems and issues occurring as a consequence of acquired brain impairment (ABI). These studies are rated for their methodological quality, evaluating various aspects of scientific rigor.
>
> - **speechBITE (www.speechbite.com)**
>
>   An EBP initiated between the University of Sydney and Speech Pathology Australia. The database provides citations and abstracts for studies describing outcomes of interventions for communication disorders. Sources are rated for methodological quality and level of evidence.
>
> - **Users' Guides to the Medical Literature: A Manual for Evidence-Based Clinical Practice (2nd Edition) (www.jamaevidence.com/resource/520)**
>
>   A comprehensive resource for EBP. Accompanying resources include critical appraisal worksheets, question wizards, and education guides.

Figure 1-2. (*continued*)

It is our goal with this text to provide students and clinicians with numerous models of how the ICF and EBP can inform effective clinical practice.

Language and Cognition (Body Structure and Body Function)

Before reviewing specific diseases or language or cognitive disorders, familiarity with and understanding of fundamental concepts such as *communication*, *language*, and *cognition* are essential. Therefore, in this section we provide explicit definitions of each of these terms and discuss the relationships among communication, language, and cognition. Then, we present more detailed information about the myriad linguistic and cognitive processes that support communication and other aspects of daily functioning.

Communication, defined as an exchange of ideas, is a fundamental human behavior. Even infants communicate their needs (primarily via crying), and as children age and develop, communication is enhanced by the development of speech, language, and sophisticated nonverbal communication skills. For adults, a primary communication tool is language. **Language** may be defined as a shared code for representing concepts through the use of symbols and rule-based combinations of symbols (Owens, Metz, & Haas, 2007). Language can manifest in various modalities, including spoken (e.g., listening, speaking), written (e.g., reading, writing), or nonverbal/gestural (e.g., facial expressions, conventional gestures, formal sign language). Regardless of the modality used to convey linguistic messages, language involves symbols (e.g., sounds, letters, words, signs) that convey meanings that may vary according to how they are combined, sequenced, or both. For example, the word "can" in the phrases "the can held tomatoes" and "she will can the tomatoes" describes an object in the first phrase and an action in the second phrase. Moreover, the meaning of identical linguistic messages may be influenced by the communicative context, as is illustrated by idioms and other figures of speech (e.g., "We had better *get on the ball* and fix that leak").

Although the term "language" is typically used as a noun, it may be more accurate to think about language as a verb, in the sense that using language to communicate involves the execution of complex mental processes. In effect, humans "do" language. The following sections will underscore the highly active nature of language functions by providing an overview of not only the specific processes comprising language but also the additional cognitive processes that support language.

Components of Language and Cognitive Processing

Cognition encompasses all processes by which we transform, condense, elaborate, store, retrieve, and exploit sensory information, and thus allows us to cope with and process incoming information so that we can understand and interact with our environment (Guilford & Hoepfner, 1971; Neisser, 1967). Accordingly, *language* is considered a part of cognition and shares an intimate relationship with other cognitive functions, such as *attention*, *memory*, and *executive functioning*. Language, attention, memory, and executive functioning are similar in that all are considered multidimensional and consist of various subcomponents. Additionally, language and other cognitive processes are linked in terms of function, architecture, and neurophysiological circuitry. That is, language, attention, memory, and executive functioning are subserved by many overlapping neural structures and pathways, and thus, when damage to one of these neural structures or pathways results in a neurogenic language disorder, it will, in addition to affecting language, typically compromise several other cognitive functions. Therefore, having a good understanding of these cognitive functions and their subcomponents is germane to appropriate management of neurogenic language disorders.

It is important to note that in many models of cognition, *perception* is included as a germane component (e.g., Rosen & Viskontas, 2008); that is, perceptual abilities are fundamental to processing and interpreting incoming sensory information (Guilford & Hoepfner, 1971; Neisser, 1967). Likewise, patients with neurogenic language and cognitive disorders frequently have concomitant perceptual symptoms (see Chapters 2 and 3 for a description of these symptoms and Chapter 5 for a listing of tools for identifying perceptual problems). However, the nature and strength of the relationship between perception and cognition have not been as firmly established as those between other abilities, such as attention or memory (e.g., Pylyshyn, 1999). Likewise, because the in-depth assessment and treatment of perceptual disorders fall outside the professional purview of speech-language pathology, the primary audience target of this text, we have elected not to include a comprehensive description of theoretical or clinical aspects of perception and its disorders.

Components of Language Processing

As illustrated in Figure 1-3, language is composed of several linguistic representation stores and operations. Collectively, these various linguistic processes function to support language comprehension, production, or both in one or more language modalities. Because neurogenic language disorders may be a product of impaired access to or functioning of one or a combination of these language subcomponents, assessment and treatment of neurogenic language disorders will depend on clinicians' familiarity with each of these functions within the linguistic system.

Phonological and Orthographic Processing. Understanding phonological and orthographic processes is essential to the management of neurogenic language disorders in which production, comprehension, or both of spoken or written language, respectively, has been compromised. The phonological system encompasses both the set of sounds (i.e., phonemes) in one's language and the rules necessary to order and combine those sounds into words (Alexander & Hillis, 2008; Owens, 2012). It consists of two subsystems: (1) a segmental subsystem, which relates to our processing of distinctive sound elements or phonemes within syllables or words, and (2) a suprasegmental subsystem, which encompasses abilities such as processing of intonation (i.e., modulation of vocal pitch to indicate grammatical segmentation or complexity or emotional status), stress (i.e., accentuation of a certain sound or syllable to assist with determining word or utterance meaning), and pauses (Blumstein, 1998).

Phonological processes contribute at several levels to our understanding and production of spoken language (Alexander & Hillis, 2008; Goodglass, 1998; R. Martin, 2003). For instance, the following processes depicted in Figure 1-3 involve manipulation and interpretation of phonological information: (1) the auditory phonological analysis that allows discrimination of the incoming speech signal into words, syllables, and sounds, and determination of suprasegmental characteristics (e.g., stressed vs. unstressed syllables), despite different speech accents; (2) the phonological input buffer that provides temporary storage of spoken stimuli while they are being processed or prepared for processing; (3) the phonological input lexicon that represents our library of spoken words that have been previously heard; (4) the acoustic-phonological conversion that allows translating what is heard directly into individual phonemes, a process needed to repeat aloud unfamiliar words; (5) the phonological output lexicon that represents our library of spoken words that have been previously produced; and (6) the

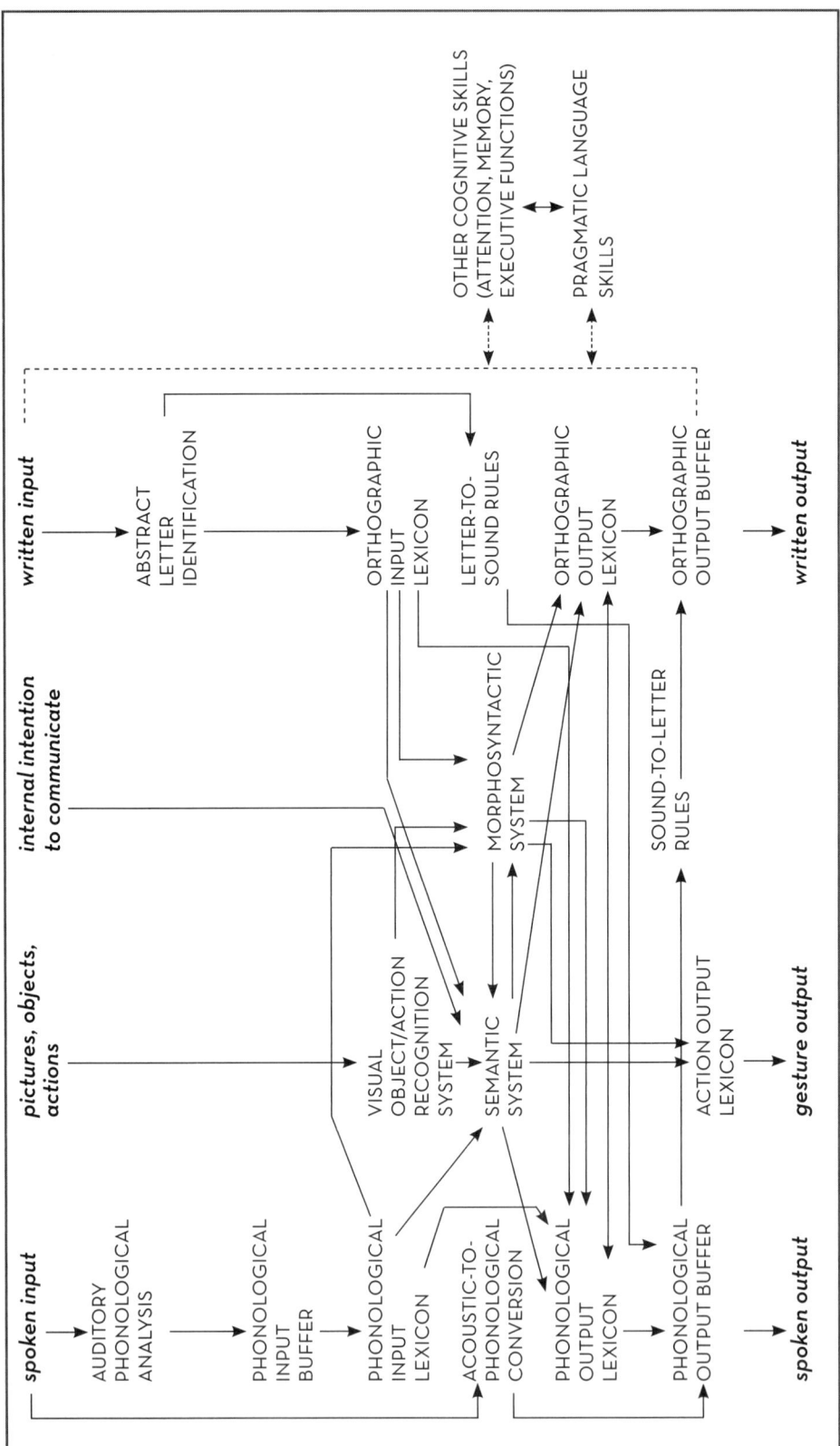

Figure 1-3. Model of linguistic processing. Dashed line indicates that pragmatic language and other cognitive skills may exert an influence across most levels of linguistic processing. *Note.* From "Psycholinguistic assessments of language processing in aphasia (PALPA): An introduction," by J. Kay, R. Lesser, and M. Coltheart, 1996, *Aphasiology, 10,* p. 172. Copyright 1996 by Taylor & Francis, Ltd., http://www.informaworld.com. Adapted with permission.

phonological output buffer that temporarily stores the phonemes of a given word while the motor speech plans for producing that word are being instigated. Phonological processes also are interconnected with several orthographic processes, as described in the next paragraph.

The orthographic system functions to facilitate processing of graphemes, which are individual letters or letter clusters that represent a single phoneme (e.g., "c," "k," and "ck" are graphemes for the sound/phoneme /k/; Kay, Lesser, & Coltheart, 1996; R. Martin, 2003). For reading, orthographic processes are engaged to convert graphemes into phonemes (i.e., letter-to-sound translation). Alternately, for writing, this aspect of the linguistic system functions to identify and arrange graphemes into words. In the model of linguistic processing represented in Figure 1-3, orthographic processing contributes to the following: (1) abstract letter identification that fosters visual recognition of letters written in various fonts or formats (e.g., cursive vs. printed letters, upper- vs. lowercase); (2) the orthographic input lexicon that stores the letter strings that correspond to our vocabulary of written words; (3) letter-to-sound rules that are used to translate graphemes into phonemes on a letter-by-letter basis, particularly when reading unfamiliar words; (4) sound-to-letter rules that are used to translate individual phonemes into graphemes, as when spelling unfamiliar words; (5) the orthographic output lexicon that stores spellings of written vocabulary we have previously used; and (6) the orthographic output buffer that temporarily holds word spellings while a word is being written or prepared to be written.

Lexical–Semantic Processing. Production and understanding of language content or meaning are products of processing at the lexical–semantic level. The term "lexical" is typically used to refer to representations or processes related to word forms in the various language modalities (e.g., writing, spoken language), whereas "semantic" refers to the concepts that these word forms represent (Alexander & Hillis, 2008; R. Martin, 2003; Owens, 2012). In the model of linguistic processing shown in Figure 1-3, lexical–semantic processing relies upon the phonological input and output lexicons that store previously heard or produced spoken word forms, the orthographic input and output lexicons that store previously read or written word forms, and the semantic system that consists of the network of information we have acquired pertaining to objects, actions, people, attributes, experiences, and relationships, including superordinate, coordinate, and subordinate associations. Although most linguistic models (like the one depicted in Figure 1-3) propose an amodal semantic system in which one system provides meaning to all stimuli or ideas regardless of their input (e.g., picture, written word) or output (e.g., gesture, drawing, spoken word), contrasting models (e.g., Shallice, 1988) have been put forward in which separate semantic stores are available for different input and/ or output modalities.

Morphosyntactic Processing. Both morphological and syntactic language functions contribute to providing structure to linguistic input and output. More specifically, morphology encompasses the rule system that mediates assembling word forms from the basic elements of meaning (i.e., morphemes), and syntax consists of the set of rules that govern ordering words into sentences (Caplan, 1993; Owens, 2012). For example, in English, words can be formed by affixing derivational or inflectional morphemes. Derivational morphemes change words into different word classes (e.g., "slow," an adjective, into "slowly," an adverb), whereas inflectional morphemes provide information about syntactic relationships (e.g., subject-verb agreement of "talk" in the sentence "The child talks."). Our syntactic abilities allow us to produce and understand a variety of sentence types, including those with canonical word order (i.e., subject-verb-object order, as in active and conjoined sentences) or noncanonical word order (e.g., passive sentences with the less common object-verb-subject order).

Pragmatics and Discourse Processing. Pragmatics encompasses the system of rules and knowledge that directs our use and interpretation of language in social settings (Bates, 1976; Cutica, Bucciarelli, & Bara, 2006; Prutting, 1979). Our pragmatic abilities allow us to adjust our language output and interpretations to different communication partners (e.g., familiar vs. unfamiliar partner; person of authority vs. peer) and contexts or environments (e.g., at supper at home vs. during a church service; one-on-one vs. group setting; a happy vs. sad occasion). Pragmatics also includes our ability to use language for a variety of functions or intents (sometimes called "speech acts"), such as requesting, stating, greeting, asserting, and protesting (Cutica et al., 2006; Dore, 1974; Lucas, 1980). These intents may be directly or indirectly expressed and comprehended through current, previous, and/or subsequent verbal output, as well as nonverbal cues such as facial expressions and gestures.

To be successful language users, we also must acquire a set of discourse rules that regulate our participation in conversation and other discourse genres (e.g., narration or storytelling, procedural discourse; Le, Coelho, Mozeiko, & Grafman, 2011; Prutting & Kirchner, 1987; Stein & Glenn, 1979). For instance, conversational rules guide our turn-taking, topic selection, maintenance, and switching or termination, and use of repair or revision strategies (e.g., **repetition**, elaboration, simplification). Likewise, narrative rules govern how to construct story episodes (i.e., must include a setting, an initiating event, an action, and an outcome) and organize them. Collectively, adherence to these rules should result in successful discourse, which according to Grice (1975) is achieved when (1) a sufficient amount of information is provided by the message sender, (2) the information is truthful, (3) appropriate and relevant vocabulary is used, and (4) information is shared in a concise manner to prevent ambivalence and obscurity.

Components of Cognitive Processing

In addition to an understanding of language, clinicians working with patients who have neurogenic disorders must have appropriate insight into the structure and function of other cognitive skills, as these too may be compromised and additionally contribute to their patients' communication difficulties. In fact, in certain patient populations (e.g., individuals with certain forms of dementia), the primary impairment is at the level of these cognitive functions, and communication problems are essentially a byproduct of these cognitive versus linguistic deficits (Bayles, 2003; Griffin et al., 2006; McDonald, 2000). Additionally, deficits in cognitive functions such as attention, memory, and executive functioning can influence rehabilitation outcomes because of their effect on learning, whether related to the reacquisition of skills or the acquisition of compensatory strategies (Evans, Wilson, Needham, & Brentnall, 2003; L. Murray, 2004a; Nicholas, Sinotte, & Helm-Estabrooks, 2011; Purdy & Koch, 2006), and consequently negatively impact maintenance and generalization of treatment effects (Fish, Manly, Emslie, Evans, & Wilson, 2009; Yeung & Law, 2010). Accordingly, an understanding of the cognitive functions of attention, memory, and executive functioning and their subcomponents is essential to providing appropriate management of not only neurogenic cognitive disorders but also neurogenic language disorders.

Attention. It has yet to be resolved whether **attention** can be adequately defined by just one theoretical conceptualization. For example, many researchers describe attention as a capacity-limited system (e.g., L. Murray, 2012b; L. Murray & Kean, 2004), whereas others view it as a cognitive bottleneck (e.g., Shuster, 2004). In capacity or resource models, attention is proposed to consist of (1) one or several finite pools (i.e., limited capacity) of attentional or processing resources, and (2) a governing system that manages distribution of these attentional resources to one or more activities (Kahneman, 1973; D. A. Norman & Shallice, 1986). According to capacity models, performance on a given task will suffer if an individual does not have access to a sufficient amount of attentional resources (i.e., capacity problem) and/or allots resources in an inefficient or inappropriate manner (i.e., allocation problem). For instance, if a lady was watching television and knitting at the same time, the quality of her knitting might suffer if she was very tired (i.e., had insufficient attention resources to split between watching television and knitting) or if she was paying more attention to the television program than to her knitting (i.e., inappropriate division of sufficient attention resources). In bottleneck or structural models of attention, an inescapable bottleneck is hypothesized to underlie limits on our attentional capabilities. That is, the time required to select a response is the restricting factor (i.e., bottleneck) that results in performance breakdowns, particularly when we attempt to complete two or more activities simultaneously (Pashler, 1994a, 1994b). In the previous example of the lady watching television and knitting, bottleneck theories would predict that the lady's knitting quality or her ability to follow her television program would primarily decline when she had to make a change in her knitting behavior (e.g., switch to a new type of knitting stitch, start a new row) because at that point she would need to select a new "knitting" response. Accordingly, her attention abilities at that point would switch from accomplishing two tasks at once (i.e., watching television and knitting) to completing just one task (i.e., hopefully, knitting) because of the bottleneck in our attentional system (i.e., in this example, the time needed to select a knitting behavior).

Although the debate over the adequacy of these two models of attention continues, researchers do agree that attention is multidimensional, and several attention functions have been identified (Kahneman, 1973; Raz, 2006; Van Zomeren & Brouwer, 1994;

Yantis, 2008). One of the more basic functions is **sustained attention,** sometimes also called "vigilance," which refers to our ability to maintain attention and, thus, consistent performance over long periods of time. **Focused** or **selective attention** allows us to concentrate on and prioritize certain features of our external or internal environment in the presence of competing features or stimuli. **Divided attention** represents the more complex attentional skill of attending to and completing more than one task, or simultaneously attending to and processing multiple stimuli. **Attention switching** is also considered by several researchers to represent a separate attention function; this aspect of attention facilitates moving attentional focus from one task or stimulus to another. Examples of how these attention functions support our performance of daily activities are provided in Table 1-2.

Memory. The cognitive function of **memory** allows us to store, retain, and subsequently retrieve processed information (Davachi & Dobbins, 2008; Squire, 1987). Memory is viewed as a multifaceted system consisting of various memory stores and processes that are essential to depositing and recovering information from these stores. A common framework used to conceptualize memory stores and functions divides memory into long-term memory and short-term, or working, memory capabilities, each of which can be further separated into different types of memory skills (see Figure 1-4).

Long-Term Memory. Two forms of long-term memory, declarative and nondeclarative, have been identified. **Declarative memory** holds information that can be stored and accessed explicitly, intentionally, or consciously and can be thought of as our "knowledge base" (Sohlberg & Mateer, 2001, p. 168). It is often subdivided into **semantic** and

TABLE 1-2
Activities That Exemplify Various Aspects of Attention

ATTENTION FUNCTION	ACTIVITY
Sustained attention/vigilance	• Watching the ticker at the bottom of the television screen to determine if your child's school has been closed or delayed due to bad weather • Looking for whales on a whale-watching boat trip
Focused/selective attention	• Studying for a test in your dormitory room while your roommate is talking and laughing on the telephone with her boyfriend • Participating in a one-on-one conversation during your office's annual holiday party
Divided attention	• Driving and talking on your cell phone • Listening to a lecture and taking notes on that lecture
Attention switching	• Preparing two different dishes for a meal in which you alternate completing steps of each recipe • Switching between helping your child complete his homework and completing your own work

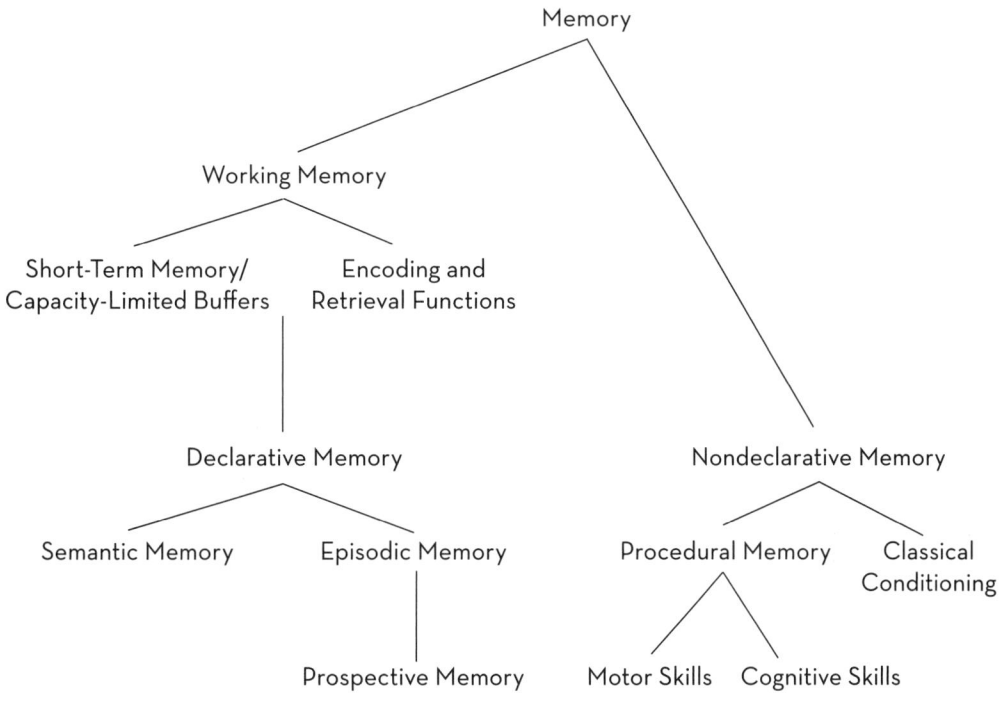

Figure 1-4. Components of memory.

episodic memory stores (Davachi & Dobbins, 2008; Markowitsch, 1998; Winocur & Moscovitch, 2011). Whereas semantic memory holds context-independent, factual memories (e.g., state capitals, names of U.S. presidents, physics formulae, word definitions), episodic memory contains context-dependent memories and thus represents our autobiographical memory store (e.g., your first date, what you ate for breakfast this morning, where you were when you heard about the September 11, 2001, terrorist attacks). Episodic memory also includes storage of information and tasks you need to recall or perform, respectively, in the future; such types of episodic memories are referred to as prospective memories (R. G. Knight, Titov, & Crawford, 2006; Sohlberg & Mateer, 2001). **Prospective memory** encompasses information or tasks you need to recall at a future time (e.g., remembering to pay a bill by a certain date, remembering to take a medication at a certain time) or when a future event occurs (e.g., remembering to get a phone number from a friend the next time you see that friend, remembering to buy stamps the next time you're at the post office).

Importantly, semantic and episodic declarative memory subsystems are related and may influence each other (D. Greenberg & Verfaellie, 2010; Winocur & Moscovitch, 2011). For example, many memories initially stored as episodic memories may over time be consolidated within semantic memory. For example, when you were first learning information pertaining to the U.S. Civil War, you might have tied that information to who taught you the information, what class covered the information, and what information was covered in which lecture. Over time, however, this contextual information can fade, and now you may just remember certain facts about this war.

In contrast to declarative memories, **nondeclarative memories** are implicit in that they can be evoked and, in some cases, stored unconsciously or unintentionally (Henke, 2010; Knowlton & Foerde, 2008; Schacter, 1992). For example, **procedural memory** is a form of nondeclarative, long-term memory that holds your memory for motor skills (e.g., typing, fingering for a musical instrument) and cognitive skills (e.g., arithmetic operations) that are habitual, often require little effort to recall, and typically represent a rigid or inseparable memory representation (e.g., to recall the last three digits of your social security number, you likely need to first recall your entire social security number). Classical conditioning (i.e., stimulus-response learning) is also accomplished via our nondeclarative memory system. Declarative and nondeclarative memory systems are not completely distinct (Henke, 2010). For instance, some declarative memories, over time, may become procedural. Take, for example, when we first learn how to tie our shoes: The steps to complete this task may be stored in semantic or episodic memory; after a few months, however, this skill becomes automatic and may then become a procedural memory.

In patient populations, long-term memory (both declarative and nondeclarative forms) also may be subdivided into anterograde versus retrograde memory (Markowitsch, 1998; Vakil, 2005). **Anterograde memories** are those long-term memories that are stored after brain damage has occurred, or after the onset of the neurological disease process. In contrast, **retrograde memories** are those that were acquired prior to brain damage or neurological disease onset. For example, in the case of a patient with dementia due to Alzheimer's disease, in the earlier stages of the disease, this patient may primarily have problems with anterograde memories, such as where he left the car keys when he got home from work or the names of some new neighbors. As the disease progresses, this patient also experiences difficulties recalling retrograde memories, such as what year he graduated from college, the capital city of the state in which he lives, or how to operate a power tool that he has owned for many years.

Short-Term and Working Memory. **Short-term memory** is our transient store of information, which for most people is limited to retaining seven, plus or minus two, pieces of information for a short time span of a few minutes (Baddeley, 2007; N. Martin & Reilly, 2012). In recent memory models, short-term memory has been replaced or encompassed by working memory. **Working memory** extends the function of short-term memory not only by temporarily storing information, but also by concurrently processing or manipulating that information (Baddeley, 2007; A. R. A. Conway, Cowan, Bunting, Therriault, & Minkoff, 2002; Cowan, 2010). Working memory is often conceptualized as consisting of several short-term, capacity-limited buffers or stores, and an executive component that supervises information storage and manipulation within the buffers. Whereas the number and nature of short-term buffers vary across models (e.g., Crosson, 2000 vs. Baddeley, 2003; see also Cowan, 2010, for a review), at least two storage systems are frequently proposed, a visuospatial sketchpad and a phonological buffer or loop dedicated to processing visuospatial and verbal-acoustic information, respectively. Working memory's executive system is domain-free and capacity-limited and therefore is similar to the governing system described in some attention models (e.g., D. A. Norman & Shallice, 1986). Furthermore, the executive component of working memory is proposed to manage sustaining target goals or information in a highly active state, particularly in the presence of distraction (Cowan, 2010; Engle, 2002; Kane, Bleckley, Conway, & Engle, 2001), and thus is also similar to inhibition, a cognitive function typically categorized as an executive function (see the "Executive Functioning" section of this chapter that follows).

Storage and Retrieval Memory Functions. Another important aspect of memory pertains to the functions responsible for helping keep information active in working memory, storing information into long-term memory, and subsequently retrieving information from long-term memory (Davachi & Dobbins, 2008; H. C. Ellis & Hunt, 1993; Gamino, Chapman, & Cook, 2009). Accordingly, storage and retrieval strategies are akin to learning and remembering, respectively. **Encoding** functions such as association, rehearsal, categorization, chunking, and verbal mediation are used to maintain information in working memory, as well as to transfer that information to long-term memory stores. More specifically, *encoding* refers to our ability to construct internal representations of incoming information or to associate that information with previously stored memories. For example, the encoding strategy of association might be used to help remember the name of a business associate, Harry, because the business associate has round glasses, like those of Harry Potter. Strategies that involve more deliberate and deeper encoding of the to-be-learned material (e.g., semantic association) are more likely to be associated with more durable long-term memory storage as compared to strategies that involve more shallow manipulation of the to-be-remembered material (e.g., rote rehearsal; Nyberg, 2002).

Retrieval functions are essential to transferring information from long-term storage to consciousness. This transfer involves searching among activated memories for those that are most accurate and appropriate to the situation. Like encoding, a number of strategies can be used to facilitate memory retrieval; these include alphabet search (e.g., when trying to recall an individual's name, you start at the letter *A* to see if that helps cue recall of the correct name; if *A* does not work, you move on to *B*, and so on) and retracing or re-creating the events or contexts in which the information was stored (e.g., retracing your trip to the mall to recall in which store you saw a product on sale and what the sale price of that item was). Retrieval skills can be evaluated by comparing an individual's speed and accuracy of recall when completing recognition tasks (e.g., multiple choice or true/false questions) versus free recall tasks (e.g., open-ended requests or questions such as "List the first 10 presidents of the United States" or "Who visited you yesterday?"). Because of the additional context information inherent in recognition tasks (i.e., the additional context will help activate the appropriate memories), it is normal for people to demonstrate superior recognition versus free recall performance.

Like components of long-term memory, encoding and retrieval can be more conscious, deliberate, and effortful in nature (similar to declarative long-term memory) or less conscious, repetitive, and thus more automatic in nature (similar to nondeclarative memory; Henke, 2010; Schacter & Buckner, 1998). This distinction will prove important to keep in mind when language and cognitive treatments are discussed in Chapters 9 and 10, as some treatment approaches require patients to exploit relatively effortful and intentional learning and retrieval strategies (e.g., Treatment of Underlying Forms, Goal Management Training), whereas others utilize relatively effortless and less intentional learning and retrieval strategies (e.g., spaced retrieval, vanishing cues).

Executive Functioning. Executive functioning refers to the set of high-level, interrelated, supervisory cognitive abilities responsible for generating, selecting, planning, and monitoring goal-directed and adaptive responses that in turn initiate and sustain completion of independent, purposeful, and/or novel behavior (Alvarez & Emory, 2006; R. Chan, Shum, Toulopoulou, & Chen, 2008; Miyake, Emersob, & Friedman, 2000). Executive functions recruit, coordinate, and integrate more basic cognitive skills and their products, and thus are key to facilitating efficient completion of complex tasks and abstract interpretation of incoming stimuli. In some models, self-regulation, or **metacognitive abilities** (i.e., being able to think and talk about one's own memory abilities, language abilities, or overall cognitive functioning), are viewed as essential components of executive functioning, as such abilities are involved in goal-directed behaviors, the process of decision making, and behavioral and cognitive adaptability or flexibility (Chan et al., 2008; Kennedy et al., 2008). Because of the complicated nature of these cognitive processes, theoretical models of executive functioning are not yet well specified, including how many or which cognitive functions should be considered "executive" (R. Chan et al., 2008; Constantinidou, Werthmeier, Tsanadis, Evans, & Paul, 2012; Miyake et al., 2000; L. Murray & Ramage, 2000). Likewise, there is variation in the nomenclature used to identify specific executive functions. Accordingly, the executive domains described below should not be considered the only possible set of executive functions, and differences are possible between the names we use to label these executive functions and those encountered in other textbooks or research articles.

There are several executive functions that we rely upon to succeed in completing our daily activities. Particularly important executive processes include (1) **planning,** which allows us to devise strategies and sequence the steps of those strategies to achieve intended goals throughout our day; (2) **organization,** or the ability to structure or categorize incoming information, as well as our own responses; (3) **inhibition,** which refers to our ability to regulate and repress automatic, routine, potent, or extraneous processing or responding; (4) **cognitive flexibility,** which allows us to change, shift, or adapt our behavior in the event of failure or the instruction to do so; (5) **problem solving,** which includes problem identification, as well as generation, selection, and implementation of solutions; and (6) **self-monitoring,** or our ability to appraise and adjust our performance and behavior on the basis of environmental feedback, our knowledge of task difficulty, and our awareness of our own strengths and weaknesses. Again, it is important to keep in mind that additional domains of executive functioning may exist and that cognitive processes within these domains may overlap.

Model of Linguistic Processing

There are several reasons for including and discussing the model of linguistic processing shown in Figure 1-3. First, as previously mentioned, it depicts the multidimensional nature of linguistic processing by illustrating not only the various linguistic functions involved in comprehending and producing language across verbal, written, and gestural modalities, but also the relationships among these functions. Second, the model also demonstrates that other cognitive functions—such as attention, memory, and executive functioning, as well as higher-level language skills that fall under the realm of pragmatics and discourse skills—influence each other and are interrelated with phonological, orthographic, action, semantic, and morphosyntactic processes. Third, this model can serve as a guide for assessing and treating neurogenic language disorders by helping clinicians identify which language behaviors or symptoms are dependent on which linguistic or cognitive processes. For example, a patient who has difficulty matching printed names of objects to pictures of those objects, but who has adequate visual abilities, has good auditory comprehension (indicating that problems at the semantic level are unlikely), and can still read aloud (indicating that problems with abstract letter identification and use of letter-to-sound rules are unlikely) might be hypothesized to have a breakdown at the level of the orthographic input lexicon. Further examples of what language symptoms might occur following interruption at certain linguistic levels of this model are provided in our discussion of aphasia (see the "Aphasia" section in Chapter 2).

Neural Bases of Language and Cognition (Body Structure)

It is commonly understood that the brain plays a critical role in the functioning of the entire body. Moreover, specific neural areas are proposed to be primarily responsible for specific functions or behaviors. The following section overviews our current understanding of the neural bases of the linguistic and cognitive processes reviewed above. Although we have attempted to summarize the vast literature addressing relevant brain–behavior relationships, readers are cautioned that methods for investigating the function of various brain areas, while sophisticated, have not yet been perfected, nor have all studies revealed the same findings.

Do We Really Know What the Brain Does?

The idea that specific parts of the brain are responsible for specific functions has been around only since the early 1800s, with the earliest theorists being ostracized for their radical speculations (see Roth & Heilman, 2000, for a review). Fortunately, a number of scientists considered the notion worthy of study, and many methods for examining brain–behavior relationships have evolved, each with unique advantages and limitations. A general familiarity with these methods will be helpful to clinicians as they interpret studies examining brain–behavior relationships.

One of the earliest techniques for studying localization of brain function, and one that is still used today, is the **lesion method.** In this method, scientists note changes in behavior following brain injury and/or disease, and by deduction attribute the control of those behaviors to the injured neural area. In the early days of this science, identifying specific sites of brain injury was usually accomplished at autopsy, as no other means of visualizing the brain were possible except on the rare occasions when individuals survived a penetrating brain injury (Damasio, 1995). Presently, however, the lesion method capitalizes on imaging techniques such as **computerized tomography (CT scans)** and **magnetic resonance imaging** (**MRI**; see Table 4-5 in Chapter 4), which allow scientists to identify brain lesions in live patients.

A criticism of many lesion studies is their failure to incorporate behavioral measures thorough or sensitive enough to characterize impaired behaviors (D. Caplan, 1981; Knopman & Rubens, 1986). Moreover, some authors (e.g., Rorden & Karnath, 2004) have questioned whether it is appropriate to infer normal brain function from disruptions in function when the brain is damaged. That is, it may be that injury alters brain function to such an extent that examining brain–behavior relationships after brain injury does not provide an accurate picture of brain–behavior relationships typical of neurologically healthy individuals.

These criticisms notwithstanding, a variation of the lesion method was developed in the late 1950s, when scientists discovered that temporary brain "lesions" could be produced by applying electrical stimulation to the brain. Applying **cortical stimulation** to patients undergoing brain surgery as a treatment for epilepsy, Penfield and Roberts (1959) were the first to describe its effects on behavior. More recently, studies using this method have "mapped" various communication functions, such as naming (Ojemann & Whitaker, 1978); use of sign language (Mateer, Polen, Ojemann, & Wyler, 1982; Mateer, Rapport, & Kettrick, 1984); and memory, syntax, and phonology (Ojemann & Mateer, 1979). A related technology is **transcranial magnetic stimulation,** which alters the function of cortical neurons by using magnetic fields (e.g., Chrysikou & Hamilton, 2011; Floel et al., 2004; Roux et al., 2004). Although both of these methods hold promise for advancing our understanding of brain functions, a key limitation is that stimulation results are not clearly interpretable. For example, studies often involve very small samples of behavior, frequently targeting only one stimulus type or response mode. Thus, a negative response (i.e., stimulation did not disrupt performance on a task) could indicate that the neural site was not active during the task, but does not rule out that the site would be active at different levels of task complexity or other variations of task parameters. Similarly, positive responses are difficult to interpret. First, a stimulated neural site may be relevant to processes targeted by the experimental task, but it may also be active for many other processes not targeted during the experiment. Further, due to the connectivity and conductivity of neurons, stimulation of one cortical site can elicit responses in neurons far from the stimulation site (Chrysikou & Hamilton, 2011; Ojemann & Whitaker, 1978); therefore, it may be unclear if the task disruption was related to the directly or indirectly stimulated neurons.

Whereas both lesion and stimulation studies require inferring brain function based on *disruptions* of typical function, other methods instead attempt to measure the activity of specific brain areas during *normal* functioning. **Electroencephalography (EEG),** which measures electrical activity in the brain, and **magnetoencephalography (MEG),** which measures the magnetic fields generated by electrical activity of the brain, are closely related technologies and allow for gross localization of brain activity. **Functional magnetic resonance imaging (fMRI)**, a variation of the more well-known imaging technique of MRI, provides images of changes in blood oxygenation within the brain. Because oxygenation changes are hypothesized to occur in response to neural activity, fMRI images have been used to identify brain areas that are active during specific cognitive and linguistic tasks (Krasuski, Horwitz, & Rumsey, 1996). Related imaging technologies, **positron emission tomography (PET)** and **single photon emission computed tomography (SPECT),** utilize injected radioactive isotopes to track blood flow in the brain, which, again, is thought to reflect neural activity (Demonet, Thierry, & Cardebat, 2005).

A notable limitation is common to each of these methods of measuring brain activity. Because most tasks are proposed to involve a number of cognitive processes (e.g., reaching for a pencil involves the visual system, the attention system, the motor and sensory systems, etc.), it is anticipated that many areas of the brain are active during such tasks. Thus, even when neural activity is detected, it may be difficult to isolate the brain activity associated with discrete mental functions.

In summary, although many technologies have been developed to study brain function, as of yet, no one tool reveals the whole story of brain–behavior relationships. When two or more tools are combined in a single experiment, however, (e.g., Dogil, Frese, Haider, Rohm, & Wokurek, 2004), or as a number of independent investigations report similar findings, the nature of brain–behavior relationships will become clearer. Nonetheless, given the limitations of the current methods, it is likely that our current understanding of how various brain areas contribute to language and cognition is at best incomplete and potentially even inaccurate. Thus, clinicians may wish to use lesion information to predict likely areas of impairment, but should not rule out the possibility of disruptions to other linguistic and cognitive functions.

Neural Bases of Language

It is widely accepted that the left, or dominant, hemisphere plays the primary role in language function for most individuals, even those who are left-handed. Within the left hemisphere, a number of specific brain areas have been associated with unique language functions (see Figure 1-5).

Broca's area, located in the inferior lateral frontal lobe, is generally proposed to play a primary role in language expression, regardless of output modality (e.g., speaking, writing, subvocalizing). With respect to specific linguistic processes, activation of Broca's area has been associated with maintenance of phonological representations, production of speech sounds, and syntactic processing (Alexander & Hillis, 2008; Beeson, Rapcsak, et al., 2003; Friederici, 2011; Hillis, 2008). Additional anterior regions of both frontal lobes have been implicated in the more complex aspects of language processing that support pragmatic and discourse skills (Alexander, 2006; Alexander & Hillis, 2008).

The area of the brain linked to language comprehension is **Wernicke's area,** which is located in the posterior aspects of the superior temporal lobe. Because comprehension involves processing of phonologic, semantic, and morphosyntactic structures, it is not surprising that activation of Wernicke's area is associated with these linguistic processes (Alexander & Hillis, 2008; Friederici, 2011; Hillis, 2008). The **supramarginal**

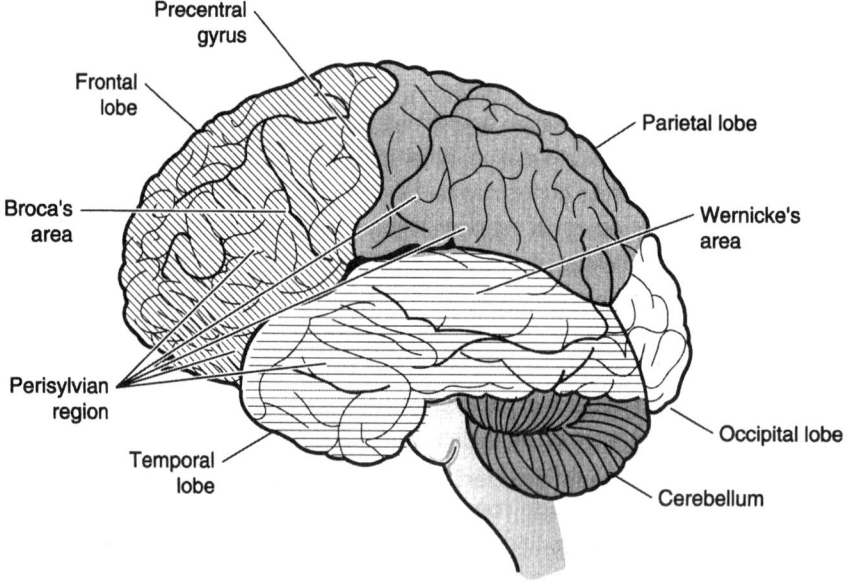

Figure 1-5. Left hemisphere of the brain. Broca's area in the frontal lobe and Wernicke's area in the temporal lobe are both located in the perisylvian region of the left hemisphere. Other areas important to language processing include the supramarginal and angular gyri. Dorsolateral prefrontal regions of both frontal lobes have been associated with high-level cognitive abilities, including executive functioning.

gyrus and **angular gyrus** within the parietal lobe also have been found to contribute to comprehending written language (Hillis, 2008); these gyri also contribute to production of written language (Beeson, Rapcsak, et al., 2003; Hillis, 2008). Activation in the cortical areas surrounding Broca's and Wernicke's areas, often termed **association areas** (e.g., temporal association area, parietal association area), is also common during language processing.

> ### The Naming Power of Discovery
>
> Two regions of the brain—Broca's area and Wernicke's area—are named after the physician scientists who studied patients experiencing disruptions to their language abilities. Paul Broca and Carl Wernicke were pioneers in the thorough description of language impairments associated with damage to the left hemisphere, with Broca's area being associated with skills relating to language expression and Wernicke's area with language comprehension abilities.

In addition to these cortical areas (gray matter), bundles of axons (white matter) connecting cortical areas—known as "association fibers"—function in language processing. The **superior longitudinal fasciculus** connects the frontal cortex with the parietal, temporal, and occipital cortices, and contains the **arcuate fasciculus,** which connects Wernicke's and Broca's areas. Accordingly, these fiber tracts play a critical role in the communication process by integrating receptive and expressive language processes.

Although the cerebral cortex is considered a primary contributor to our communication abilities, it is likely that select subcortical structures also function in language processing. Evidence for subcortical involvement comes primarily from studies describing patients with aphasia who demonstrated lesions in the **thalamus, basal ganglia,** and/or **internal capsule** (e.g., De Witte, Engelborghs, De Deyn, & Marien, 2008; De Witte et al., 2011; Yang, Zhao, Wang, Chen, & Zhang, 2008; see Radanovic & Scaff, 2003, for a review). The precise contribution of these subcortical structures (depicted in Figure 1-6) continues to be debated. The thalamus has been proposed to play a crucial role in verbal memory and executive functions and thus may influence both expressive and receptive language modalities (De Witte et al., 2011; Metter et al., 1983). Some researchers have theorized that the basal ganglia and surrounding white matter regulate the initiation of the motor production of language formulated by cortical structures (Crosson, 1985) or may serve to connect cortical structures (Alexander, Naeser, & Palumbo, 1987). More recent studies, however, have offered strong evidence that lesions involving the basal ganglia impact language functioning only when accompanied by reduced blood flow to cortical sites (Alexander & Hillis, 2008; Hillis et al., 2004; Radanovic & Scaff, 2003), leading researchers to question the direct role of the basal ganglia in language processing.

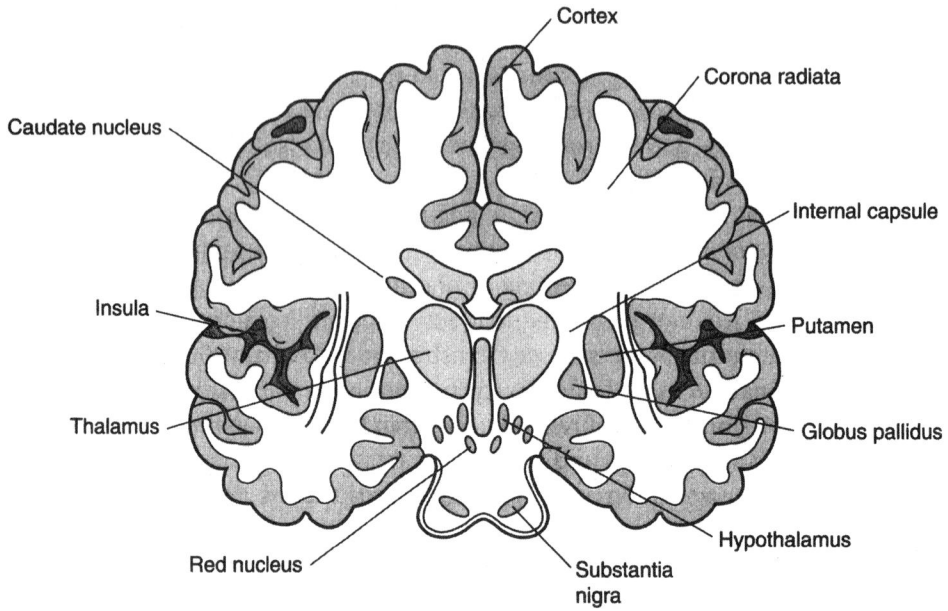

Figure 1-6. Subcortical structures viewed in the coronal plane. The thalamus, basal ganglia, and internal capsule may play a role in language processing. The thalamus and basal ganglia have also been associated with other cognitive functions, including certain attention, memory, and executive function abilities.

Neural Bases of Cognition

Many of the neural structures and pathways upon which language functions rely also subserve one or more cognitive processes. Given that it is well beyond the scope of this book to examine all neural areas and circuits that support cognition, our review will highlight only those structures with well-established contributions to attention, memory, and/or executive functioning, and that are highly vulnerable to the forms of brain damage that result in neurogenic language disorders.

Neural Bases of Attention

Given that numerous neural structures and pathways located in a spectrum of cortical and subcortical regions have been found to support one or more attentional processes, it is not surprising that attention deficits are common among patients with neurogenic language or cognitive disorders, even those with very little permanent brain damage (e.g., L. Murray, 2012b; Saunders & Summers, 2011). To help provide a framework by which to organize these various neural contributions, Filley (2002) has proposed two neural networks of attention: a diffuse network that supports primarily more basic attention functions (e.g., arousal, sustained and focused attention), and a right hemisphere network that mediates attention allocation to focal spatial stimuli. Important neural structures and pathways within the diffuse network include the thalamus, white matter connections between the thalamus and cortical areas of both cerebral hemispheres, lateral and medial aspects of both frontal lobes, and the cerebellum (Filley, 2002; Highnman & Bleile, 2011; Rosen & Viskontas, 2008; Yantis, 2008). There are some distinctions between the right and left frontal lobes' contributions to this diffuse attention network: The right frontal lobe appears more dominant for sustained attention, whereas the left prefrontal cortex plays a fundamental role in functions such as attention switching (Coull, 1998; Dreher & Grafman, 2003; Rosen & Viskontas, 2008). The right posterior parietal cortex, prefrontal cortex, cingulate gyrus (particularly the anterior portion), and subcortical structures (such as the thalamus and basal ganglia) are important components of the right hemisphere attention network (Filley, 2002; Raz, 2006; Rosen & Viskontas, 2008; Yantis, 2008). Those structures that are more anteriorly located within the right hemisphere contribute to complex spatial attention functions, whereas more posteriorly located structures support more basic spatial attention abilities, such as stimulus scanning and selection (Coull, 1998; Filley, 2002). Several of the neural structures that participate in attention functioning are depicted in Figures 1-5 and 1-6.

Neural Bases of Memory

Many neural regions help support the variety of memory stores and functions essential to our overall memory abilities. For example, several aspects of memory, including the application of encoding and retrieval memory strategies and working memory, rely on frontal lobe functioning (Crosson, 2000; Nyberg, 2002; Osaka et al., 2004; Winocur & Moscovitch, 2011). More specifically, research indicates that working memory's phonological buffer relies upon Broca's area, left supplemental motor and premotor areas, the visuospatial buffer on the right premotor cortex, and the executive component on the anterior cingulate gyrus and dorsolateral prefrontal areas of both hemispheres (see Figures 1-5 and 1-7). Additionally, subcortical structures such as the thalamus and basal ganglia, as well their connections with these frontal lobe regions, contribute to working memory, with a hypothesized specialization for preserving the temporal order of information being temporarily held in working memory buffers (Crosson, 2000; Kubat-Silman, Dagenbach, & Absher, 2002). The cerebellum too may help support certain aspects of working memory (Highnman & Bleile, 2011; Ravizza et al., 2006).

Long-term memory relies on both cortical regions and deeper brain structures (Davachi & Dobbins, 2008; Rosen & Viskontas, 2008; Winocur & Moscovitch, 2011). For instance, the hippocampus, located deep within the temporal lobe, and medial regions of the temporal lobe have been implicated in a number of memory functions, including declarative memory (particularly episodic memory) and anterograde memory (see Figure 1-7). In contrast, semantic memories appear to be stored in modality (e.g., auditory concepts within the temporal cortex; visual concepts within parieto-occipital regions) and domain-specific regions (e.g., word meanings within the temporoparietal cortex) of the cortex. Finally, subcortical areas such as the caudate nucleus and other basal ganglia structures illustrated in Figure 1-6, as well as the cerebellum, are germane to procedural memory (Highnman & Bleile, 2011; Winocur & Moscovitch, 2011). It is always important to keep in mind that these subcortical regions maintain

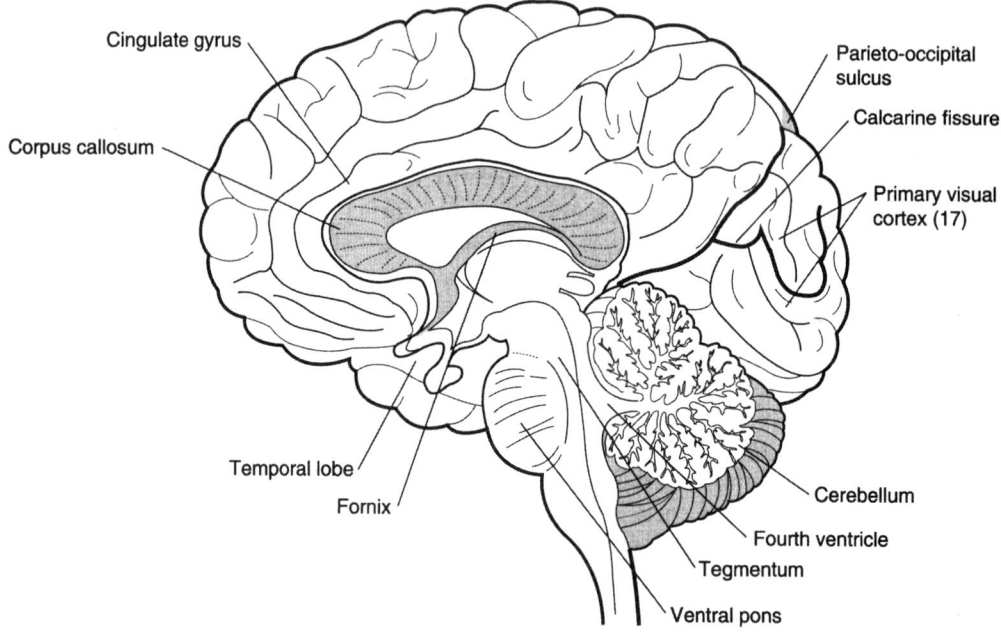

Figure 1-7. A sagital view of the right hemisphere. Attention functions have been related to the cingulate gyrus. Several deep structures, such as the fornix, may play a role in certain memory abilities.

communication with the many cortical structures that subserve memory, so that damage to the neural pathways that connect cortical and subcortical regions also can result in a variety of memory problems.

Neural Bases of Executive Functioning

Research consistently indicates that executive functioning is primarily achieved, although not completely, by frontal lobe areas (Alvarez & Emory, 2006; Mitchell, 2008; Rosen & Viskontas, 2008; Stuss, 2011). Furthermore, within the frontal lobes, different regions have been found to support different executive functions. For example, inferior regions of the frontal lobes (i.e., orbitofrontal areas) have been associated with inhibition and self-regulation; superior regions (i.e., dorsolateral prefrontal cortex) are more involved with problem solving and reasoning, planning, and cognitive flexibility; medial regions (e.g., anterior cingulate gyrus) have been implicated in initiation, motivation, and mental-state inferencing; and the frontal poles that encompass the most anterior portions of the frontal lobes appear to support some of the most complex executive functions, such as self-awareness (see Figure 1-5).

In addition to the frontal lobes, however, other brain areas appear to contribute to executive functioning; that is, more distributed neural networks support our executive functions (Alvarez & Emory, 2006; Constantinidou et al., 2012). For example, findings from lesion and imaging studies indicate that neural structures such as the cerebellum, caudate, putamen, and certain components of the limbic system also support aspects of executive functioning (Alvarez & Emory, 2006; Highnman & Bleile, 2011; Montoya, Price, Menear, & Lepage, 2006). Likewise, pathways to and from the frontal lobes, in particular those connecting to subcortical structures such as the basal ganglia and thalamus, participate in executive function abilities (Alvarez & Emory, 2006; Constantinidou et al., 2012; Delano-Wood et al., 2009; Stuss, 2011).

Summary and Looking Ahead

It is helpful to approach any area of study from a framework that will serve to highlight relationships among concepts and guide the development of clinical management strategies. In this beginning chapter, we introduced the WHO's (2001) ICF classification system as the guiding framework for our examination of neurogenic language and cognitive disorders. With the review of the body structures and body functions supporting language and cognition as a foundation, Chapter 2 explores the nature of impairments and activity limitations resulting from damage to relevant body structures and/or disruption of relevant body functions. The discussion of concepts foundational to managing neurogenic language and cognitive disorders is continued in Chapter 3, as the etiologies of these disorders are explored. The concepts explored in these introductory chapters inform both assessment and treatment of neurogenic language and cognitive disorders, as will become clear in the remaining chapters.

An overview of the assessment process is provided in Chapter 4, followed by detailed descriptions of the strategies, methods, and tools employed in screening for confounding conditions (Chapter 5) and in assessing linguistic and cognitive impairments in Chapters 6 and 7, respectively. Consistent with the ICF framework, Chapter 8 explores the assessment of functional cognition and communication (i.e., activity) and participation, as well as examines the evaluation of quality of life, a construct not represented in the ICF model but clearly related to the concept of life participation.

Management strategies targeting underlying impairments in linguistic and cognitive processing are explored in Chapters 9 and 10, respectively, and pharmacological treatment approaches are summarized in Chapter 11. These chapters are followed by a discussion of procedures suitable for targeting functional cognition and communication and participation in Chapter 12.

Finally, in recognition that managing neurogenic language and cognitive disorders does not take place in a vacuum, but rather is framed within the larger health-care culture and policies, Chapter 13 provides an overview of the U.S. health-care system, exploring the influences of this system on our assessment and treatment of neurogenic language and cognitive disorders. Chapter 13 concludes with an exploration of how our management of neurogenic language and cognitive disorders may evolve in the coming decades.

So that this book may serve as a rich resource of clinical and research ideas, a comprehensive and diverse set of assessment procedures and treatment approaches are covered, some that can be applied to neurogenic language and cognitive disorders in general and others that are specific to aphasia, cognitive-communicative disorders associated with right hemisphere brain damage or traumatic brain injury, or dementia. It is our hope that by reviewing the theoretical and applied material in this book, readers will acquire the conceptual background essential to managing adult neurogenic language and cognitive disorders in a variety of health-care and research settings.

Discussion Questions

1. What are some aspects of your own activity and participation that would be affected if you experienced a sudden change in cognitive or language function? What environmental and personal factors would positively or negatively influence the impact of these impairments on your activities and participation?
2. Consider a decision that many individuals make regularly: whether to use a pain reliever or what type of pain reliever to use. Discuss how evidence-based practice could inform this decision. As a consumer, do you hold particular values that would influence your decision (e.g., Should pain relievers be taken for any severity of pain? Are nonprescription medications more acceptable than prescription medications? Are nonpharmaceutical methods more acceptable than medications?)? Does your health-care provider express a professional opinion about those same questions? Could you identify relevant evidence to inform a specific decision (e.g., Should you take Medication A for pain related to muscle strain?)? Do you think evidence-based practice principles are useful for these types of decisions?
3. What is the relationship between cognitive and language processing? Given the interdependence of many cognitive and language processes, why is it important to distinguish unique components of function?

Overview of Neurogenic Language and Cognitive Disorders

chapter 2

Learning Objectives

After reading this chapter, you should be able to:

- Define *aphasia* and describe the language impairments characteristic of aphasia
- Identify and describe aphasia types based on the connectionist model of aphasia
- Describe the nature of impairments in attention, memory, and executive functioning typical of right hemisphere brain damage (RHD)
- Discuss the impact of the cognitive impairments in RHD on communication
- Describe the nature of impairments in attention, memory, and executive functioning typical of traumatic brain injury (TBI)
- Discuss the impact of the cognitive impairments in TBI on communication
- Describe the nature of impairments in attention, memory, and executive functioning typical of dementia
- Discuss the impact of the cognitive impairments in dementia on communication
- Compare and contrast the language impairments of aphasia, RHD, TBI, and dementia

Key Terms

- agrammatism
- agraphia
- alexia
- Alzheimer's disease (AD)
- anomia
- anomic aphasia
- anosognosia
- aphasia
- coma
- conduction aphasia
- dementia
- fluency
- jargon
- mild cognitive impairment (MCI)
- minimally conscious state
- neglect syndrome
- paragrammatism
- paraphasia
- post-traumatic amnesia (PTA)
- primary progressive aphasia
- pure word deafness
- social cognition
- subcortical aphasia
- Theory of Mind
- traumatic brain injury (TBI)

Introduction

This chapter describes a number of neurogenic language and cognitive disorders with which patients in a variety of health-care settings may present, highlighting how disruptions to specific linguistic and cognitive processes affect these patients' communication abilities. Readers may find that the model of linguistic and cognitive processing included in Chapter 1 (see Figure 1-3) will aid their understanding of the various linguistic and cognitive symptoms associated with neurogenic language disorders, such as aphasia, cognitive-communicative disorders subsequent to right hemisphere brain damage (RHD) or traumatic brain injury (TBI), and dementia.

Aphasia

Although the term "**aphasia**" literally means "without speech," a number of specific definitions have been developed to capture more accurately the nature and features of this neurogenic language disorder (see Rosenbek, LaPointe, & Wertz, 1989, for a review). In general, aphasia refers to a disruption in using and understanding language following neurological injury or disease (Brookshire, 2007; Sinanovic, Mrkonjic, Zukic, Vidovic, & Imamovic, 2011) that is not related to general intellectual decline or sensorimotor deficits (Darley, 1982); any language modality may be affected, including speaking, listening, writing, and reading. Accordingly, a diagnosis of aphasia is typically not applied to patients with communication disorders related to traumatic brain injury, nondominant or right hemisphere brain damage, or a dementing disease, because in these cases deficits in cognitive domains other than language (i.e., attention, memory, and/or executive functioning) often are the primary bases of these patients' communicative difficulties.

Many Americans will develop aphasia each year. Code and Petheram (2011) recently reviewed the prevalence literature and noted that .1 to .4% of the general population in multiple countries presents with aphasia. It is estimated that 20 to 40% of stroke patients will, at least acutely, be aphasic (Berthier, 2005; Sinanovic, Mrkonjic, Zukic, Vidovic, & Imamovic, 2011), and the American Heart Association (Roger et al., 2011) reported that by 6 months, approximately 20% of ischemic stroke survivors (see Chapter 3 for a definition of "ischemic stroke") who are age 65 years or older will still present with aphasia. Given that these data are based predominantly on aphasia due to stroke, these numbers most likely underestimate the number of individuals experiencing aphasia.

Symptoms of Aphasia

Aphasia is frequently characterized by impairments in a number of linguistic processes. The types of behavioral deficits resulting from these impairments, however, are usually grouped into disruptions of comprehension, speech fluency, naming, and repetition. Examples of the various aphasic behaviors are provided in Table 2-1. Additionally, gestural communication, pragmatic or social language, and nonlinguistic cognitive profiles associated with aphasia are reviewed.

Comprehension

Disruption in language comprehension, in both spoken and written modalities, is common in aphasia, although the severity of comprehension deficits varies greatly across patients (see the included DVD: Patients 3a, 3c, 10b, 10e). Comprehension deficits can arise

TABLE 2-1
Examples of Speech Production Characteristics in Aphasia

SPEECH BEHAVIOR	EXAMPLE	COMMON UNDERLYING IMPAIRMENT(S)
Anomic pause	"Can you hand me the … er … remote?"	• Semantic representation • Lexical access • Phonologic representation • Phonologic processing
Semantic paraphasia	"Can you hand me the TV?"	• Semantic representation • Lexical access
Phonemic paraphasia	"Can you hand me the rebote?"	• Phonologic representation • Phonologic processing
Anomic circumlocution	"Can you hand me the … other there … the clicker … for the TV?"	• Semantic representation • Lexical access • Phonologic representation • Phonologic processing
Neologism	"Can you hand me the jazzlepam?"	• Semantic representation • Lexical access • Phonologic representation • Phonologic processing
Jargon	"Griss me the jazzlepam."	• Semantic representation • Lexical access • Phonologic representation • Phonologic processing
Agrammatism	"You … uh … remote?"	• Morphosyntactic processing
Paragrammatism/ Empty speech	"Fast the jazzleman on the choose."	• Semantic representation • Lexical access • Morphosyntactic processing

from impairments to any of the linguistic processes contributing to assigning meaning to linguistic messages (e.g., phonological analysis, semantic processing, morphosyntactic parsing; see also Figure 1-3). Because the behavioral manifestations of auditory and reading comprehension deficits are often the same regardless of the underlying impairment (i.e., the patient fails to understand what is said or read), careful assessment is usually necessary to identify which specific linguistic impairment or combination of impairments is contributing to comprehension breakdowns (see Chapter 6). Additionally, several stimulus factors may facilitate or impede comprehension (in individuals who do, as well as those who do not, have aphasia) and thus should be considered when evaluating and remediating aphasia. Such factors include syntactic complexity, stimulus length, word familiarity and frequency, stimulus presentation rate, degree of concreteness or abstractness, and presence or absence of contextual cues.

Speech Fluency

The term "fluency" is often used to describe aspects of speech production affecting rate, rhythm, and ease of speech output. Disruptions to these features of speech fluency are called "disfluencies" and are associated with speech disorders, such as stuttering. With respect to the speech production of patients with aphasia, **fluency** refers primarily to phrase length (Rosenbek et al., 1989) but may also incorporate characteristics of melodic line, articulatory agility or effort, speech rate, and grammatical form (Alexander & Hillis, 2008; Goodglass, Kaplan, & Barresi, 2001). Patients with aphasia-related fluency difficulties, referred to as "nonfluent output," produce effortful, halting speech (i.e., many pauses) that is limited to short phrases and is often spoken at a slow rate with nominal melodic contour (see included DVD: Patients 5, 6, 10g). In contrast, patients with fluent speech generally produce speech without apparent effort, even in the presence of sound, word, or grammatical errors, and sound "normal" in terms of their phrase length and intonation (see included DVD: Patients 1, 3, 4, 7).

A phenomenon sometimes associated with nonfluent speech is **agrammatism** (also previously referred to as "telegraphic speech"), in which patients produce short utterances that consist primarily of content words (e.g., nouns, verbs, adjectives, adverbs) and that lack or use a restricted diversity of function words (e.g., articles, conjunctions, pronouns). Syntax is also compromised, appearing simplified, incomplete, or restricted in terms of the types of grammatical forms used (see included DVD: Patients 5, 10g). Agrammatism is hypothesized to reflect impairments in morphosyntactic processing and may also be characterized by morphologically simplified word forms (e.g., omitted plural endings and/or tense markers) (Caramazza & Berndt, 1985; Goodglass, 1993).

Another speech characteristic proposed to reflect disrupted morphosyntactic processing is **paragrammatism**, which describes speech that incorporates atypical syntax (Goodglass, 1993; Goodglass et al., 2001; see included DVD: Patient 3b). Whereas a patient exhibiting agrammatism may omit syntactic elements, a patient with paragrammatism may substitute inappropriate morphosyntactic elements (e.g., using a verb where a noun should be). The concept of paragrammatism has been called into question (e.g., G. A. Davis, 2007) because careful study of paragrammatic speech has failed to reveal syntactic errors that vary significantly from those observed in agrammatic speech (see Heeschen & Kolk, 1988, for review). Additionally, because the presence of paragrammatism often results in a marked reduction or misuse of content words important for communicating meaning, the term "**empty speech**" may be appropriately used to describe fluent speech lacking in information content.

It is important to note that patients' written output is often similar to their spoken output. Thus, patients' written language might also be characterized as agrammatic or paragrammatic. For example, Figure 2-1 shows a writing sample from a patient with chronic nonfluent aphasia that is an excellent example of agrammatic writing.

Naming

A ubiquitous characteristic of aphasia is **anomia**, or difficulty recalling the names of people, objects, locations, and actions (see included DVD: Patients 1, 3b, 4, 5, 8g, 9b). Anomia may be manifest by a variety of behaviors, including delayed naming resulting in excessive pausing (see included DVD: Patient 6d), no responses, and errors in naming referred to as **paraphasias**. There are a number of types of paraphasias (see Table 2-2),

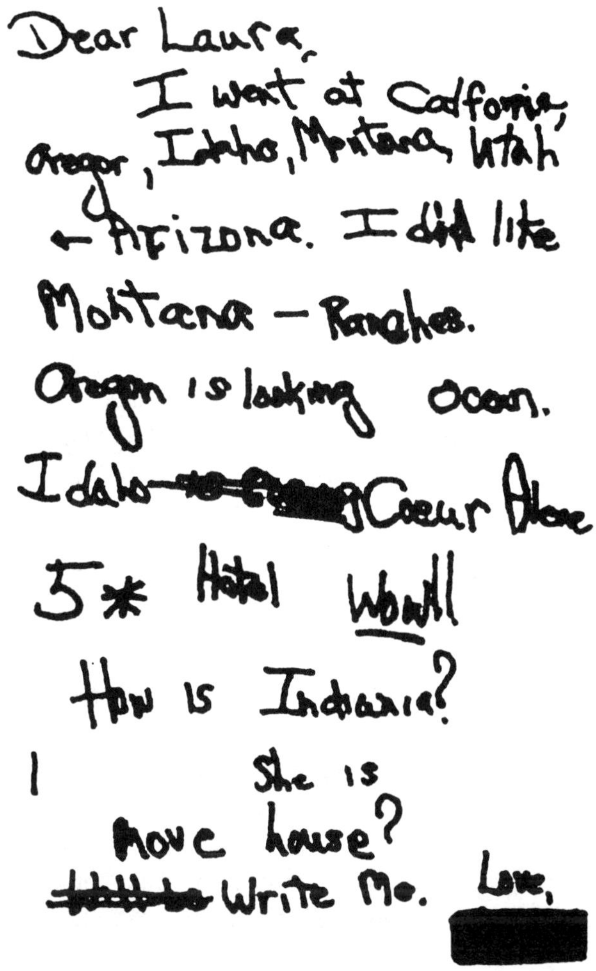

Figure 2-1. Example of agrammatic writing from a patient with primary progressive aphasia. See the "Other Aphasia Types" section of this chapter for a description of primary progressive aphasia.

including (a) **phonemic, graphemic, or literal paraphasia**, which contains substitutions, additions, omissions, and/or rearrangements of target word phonemes (see included DVD: Patients 4, 5, 9g, 10r); (b) **semantic paraphasia**, which is the substitution of a word that is semantically related to the target word (see included DVD: Patients 3b, 9d, 11a, 11b); (c) **random paraphasia**, which is the substitution of a word that lacks apparent semantic relations to the target word; (d) **circumlocution**, which involves the use of a description or definition for the target word (see included DVD: Patients 1, 4, 8g); (e) **neologism**, which involves the use of a nonsense versus a target word (see included DVD: Patients 10f, 10r); (f) **indefinite substitution**, which involves the use of a nonspecific word or description for the target word (see included DVD: Patients 3a, 3b, 4, 8a, 8g, 8h, 8l); and (g) **stereotypy**, which is a restricted form, single word, or phrase that may be produced involuntarily, may or may not be propositional, and appears frequently in the patient's speech. Patients with severe anomia may produce entire sentences in which all content words (and in some cases even functor words) are replaced with neologisms—a phenomenon known as **jargon**.

TABLE 2-2
Examples of Types of Paraphasias or Word Retrieval Errors

PARAPHASIA TYPE	EXAMPLES
Phonemic, graphemic, or literal paraphasia	• "Bloomton" for "Bloomington" • "moustain" for "mountain"
Semantic paraphasia	• "divan" for "chair" • "nurse" for "doctor"
Random paraphasia	• "sleepy" for "purple" • "singing" for "jogging"
Circumlocution	• "When you get out the cake and blow off the candles" for "birthday"
Indefinite substitution	• "them" for "the neighbors" • "stuff" for "money"
Neologism	• "wimber" for "quickly" • "tarndis" for "forty"
Stereotypy	• "September" for "cat," "hello," and "I'm fine"

Impairments in several linguistic processes may produce anomia in patients' speech, writing, or both (see Figure 1-3). For example, degraded semantic representations may cause increased processing time as the appropriate concepts are accessed. Disrupted lexical access may result in pauses, circumlocutions, or word choice errors (i.e., semantic paraphasias). Finally, impairments to any of the various levels of phonological processing may result in anomic behaviors, particularly sound errors (i.e., phonemic paraphasias; see Table 2-1).

Repetition

Another speech behavior impacted by aphasia is **repetition** (see included DVD: Patients 8f, 9g, 10f, 10l). When asked to repeat words or phrases, some patients with aphasia will produce verbal output that is similar to their productions during spontaneous or elicited speech (e.g., agrammatic, paraphasic). Interestingly, other patients with aphasia will demonstrate repetition ability that is either much more or much less impaired than other spoken productions. Repetition without processing for meaning is proposed to involve a specific set of decoding and encoding processes (e.g., acoustic-to-phonologic conversion; see Figure 1-3) that may be disrupted to a different degree than other linguistic processing functions. Impairments in certain cognitive functions, such as short-term memory deficits, may also negatively affect repetition ability (Alexander & Hillis, 2008; R. C. Martin & Allen, 2008).

Disruptions in Written Language

As indicated previously, the language impairments of aphasia extend to written as well as spoken modalities. Disruption in comprehending written language is termed **alexia** or *acquired dyslexia* (see included DVD: Patients 10, 11). As noted above, a number of underlying impairments may result in comprehension deficits, including difficulty decoding written forms (e.g., identifying letters or converting graphemes to phonemes), as well as disruptions in semantic or morphosyntactic processing (see Figure 1-3). Accordingly, a number of different types of alexia have been identified (Beeson & Henry, 2008; Hillis, 2008; Sinanovic et al., 2011). Table 2-3 reviews some alexia types and their symptoms.

Agraphia, or *acquired dysgraphia*, refers to impaired written expression and may be manifest by the same characteristics described for spoken expression (e.g., agrammatic), as well as by difficulty in phoneme-to-grapheme conversion (e.g., writing to dictation) and production of specific allographs (e.g., printed letters, cursive handwriting; Beeson & Henry, 2008; Hillis, 2008; Sinanovic et al., 2011). Like alexia, several types of agraphia have been forwarded, each associated with different underlying deficits (see Table 2-3). It is important to keep in mind that some individuals with aphasia will be attempting to write with either a parietic, dominant hand or a nondominant hand. Consequently, some errors and compromised legibility might reflect motoric issues. For example, M. Whurr and Lorch (1991) found that written language ability could be improved in one of their aphasic patients by treating motor issues, and Hansen and McNeil (1986) reported that the writing of healthy adults was less legible when they wrote with their nondominant versus dominant hand.

Gestural Communication

Patients with aphasia may display difficulties with gestural communication, although these are typically of a lesser degree compared to the linguistic problems described above (Christopoulou & Bonvillian, 1985; Rose, 2006). Gestural communication includes a number of skills, such as gesticulating, which involves spontaneous hand and arm movements that co-occur with speech (e.g., a speaker putting both hands out in front of himself when saying "The snake was at least a foot long"), and pantomiming, which involves hand and arm movements to demonstrate concepts in the absence of speech (for a review of gesture types, theoretical models, and the role of gesture in speech production, see Rose, 2006). Deficits in gesture comprehension, production, or both may co-occur with aphasia, with these deficits arising from one or a number of possible underlying problems, including degraded semantic representations (see Figure 1-3), limb apraxia (see Chapter 5), and sensorimotor issues (e.g., hemiparesis). Gestural communication may also be, however, an area of strength for some patients with aphasia (Carlomagno, Pandolfi, Martini, Di Iasi, & Cristilli, 2005; Rose, 2006); for example, Carlomagno and colleagues (2005) observed that their participants with anomic aphasia used more gestures than their non-aphasic peers, and that this increased use of gesture was associated with increased communicative effectiveness.

Pragmatic Abilities

Despite the above difficulties in producing and comprehending language, it has long been acknowledged that pragmatic language abilities remain an area of strength for most patients with aphasia. That is, they are often still able to get their message across, even in the face of significant speaking, listening, reading, and writing impairments (see included DVD: Patient 3b). In fact, many patients with aphasia use their relatively

TABLE 2-3
Examples of Types of Alexia and Agraphia and Their Symptoms

TYPE OF ACQUIRED READING OR WRITING DISORDER	PROPOSED PRIMARY UNDERLYING DEFICIT(S)	SYMPTOMS
Deep alexia	Difficulties with grapheme–phoneme conversion and semantic system	• Greater difficulty reading: ~ Low- vs. high-frequency words ~ Low- vs. high-imageable words ~ Nonwords ~ Functors vs. content words • Semantic errors
Letter-by-letter reading	Difficulties accessing orthographic input lexicon	• Greater difficulty reading long vs. short words • Utilize letter-by-letter strategy (i.e., name each letter in the word)
Surface alexia	Difficulties within orthographic output lexicon and/or semantic lexicon system or phonologic output	• Greater difficulty reading: ~ Irregularly spelled words ~ Homophones • Phonological errors • Utilize grapheme–phoneme conversion strategy • Can read nonwords
Deep agraphia	Difficulties with phoneme–grapheme conversion and semantic system	• Greater difficulty spelling: ~ Low- vs. high-frequency words ~ Low- vs. high-imageable words ~ Nonwords ~ Functors vs. content words • Semantic errors
Surface agraphia	Difficulties within orthographic output lexicon	• Greater difficulty spelling: ~ Irregularly spelled words ~ Homophones • Utilize phoneme–grapheme conversion strategy • Can spell nonwords
Graphemic buffer agraphia	Difficulties maintaining information in the graphemic buffer	• Greater difficulty spelling long vs. short words

preserved pragmatic skills to compensate for their deficits in other components of language (Hengst, Frame, Neuman-Stritzel, & Gannaway, 2005; Simmons-Mackie, Kingston, & Schultz, 2004). For instance, Simmons-Mackie and colleagues (2004) noted that patients with aphasia will "train" others to act as their "spokesperson" during daily communication interactions.

Concomitant Cognitive Symptoms

Although clearly linguistic problems are the most prominent symptoms observed in and typically reported by patients with aphasia, a growing body of research indicates that aphasia is often accompanied by deficits in cognition that extend beyond language processing. Given that there is overlap in the lesion locations that commonly produce aphasia and the neural regions that support nonlinguistic cognitive functions (see Chapter 1), it should be anticipated that patients with a variety of aphasia types and severities might present with impairments of one or several of these nonlinguistic cognitive abilities. Indeed, aphasia is commonly accompanied by problems of attention, memory, and executive functioning, and according to some researchers, these latter cognitive problems may not only contribute to or exaggerate the language difficulties of patients with aphasia but also impede patients' recovery of language abilities, their acquisition of compensatory strategies, or both (Kalbe, Reinhold, Brand, Markowitsch, & Kessler, 2005; Lambon Ralph, Snell, Fillengham, Conroy, & Sage, 2010; L. Murray, 2004a; Nicholas et al., 2011; Yeung & Law, 2010).

Attention Problems. The results of previous investigations indicate that no, one, some, or all aspect(s) of attention might be impaired in patients with aphasia (see L. Murray, 1999, 2002a, for reviews). More specifically, compared to their healthy age-matched peers, patients with aphasia, and more broadly patients with left hemisphere damage, have been found to be less accurate, slower, or both on sustained attention, attention switching, and focused and divided attention tasks (Barker-Collo et al., 2009, Barker-Collo, Feigin, Lawes, Parag, & Senior, 2010; Hula, McNeil, & Sung, 2007; Laures, 2005; L. Murray, 2012b). Furthermore, these performance differences between aphasic and non-aphasic adults are evident regardless of whether the attention tasks have relatively high or low linguistic demands or are in the auditory or visual modality.

Patients with aphasia also may display neglect, an attention deficit more frequently associated with right hemisphere brain damage (for a more detailed description of neglect, see the "Right Hemisphere Disorders" section of this chapter). It is estimated that between 15 and 65% of patients who suffer left hemisphere brain damage will present with right-sided neglect or impaired attention to information presented on the right side of the body (Barker-Collo et al., 2010; Kerkhoff, 2000; Wee & Hopman, 2008). Although symptoms of visual neglect are easiest to observe (e.g., failing to eat food on the right side of the plate; omitting words on the right side of the page when reading aloud), neglect can affect processing of and responding to information presented in other modalities as well (e.g., failing to attend to sounds presented to their right ear; failing to notice that their eyeglasses are not sitting properly on their right ear). Even though both research and clinical practice have most frequently focused on neglect subsequent to nondominant hemisphere brain damage, a study by Wee and Hopman (2008) evaluating neglect among consecutive-stroke patients admitted for inpatient rehabilitation identified that (a) neglect regularly co-occurred with aphasia and (b) the clinical consequences for right and left neglect were comparable (e.g., longer stays in rehabilitation, fewer home discharges).

Memory Problems. As with attention, most (if not all) facets of memory appear vulnerable in patients with aphasia. For example, Visser-Keizer, Meyboom-de Jong,

Deelman, Berg, and Gerritsen (2002) interviewed stroke survivors and their caregivers about troublesome stroke-related symptoms and found that more than half of the left hemisphere stroke study participants (close to half of whom had aphasia) and their partners reported memory impairments following their stroke.

With respect to the various memory functions, short-term and working memory problems appear to coincide frequently with aphasia. These memory impairments have been identified when patients with aphasia complete tasks that involve the temporary storage and subsequent recall of verbal (Baldo & Dronkers, 2006; Mayer & Murray, 2013; Sung et al., 2009), episodic (Yasuda, Nakamura, & Beckman, 2000), auditory-nonverbal (Gordon, 1983), or visuospatial (Christensen & Wright, 2010; Fucetola, Connor, Strube, & Corbetta, 2009; Mayer & Murray, 2013) information. Further, difficulties with the buffers, executive component, or both have been observed when evaluating the working memory skills of patients with aphasia (Baldo & Dronkers, 2006; Martin & Allen, 2008; see also Chapter 1 for a description of working memory).

Although only a limited number of studies have evaluated long-term memory subsequent to aphasia onset, initial findings suggest that getting verbal or visual information into or out of long-term memory stores is difficult for many patients with aphasia (Burgio & Basso, 1997; Della Barba, Frasson, Mantovan, Gallo, & Denes, 1996; Vukovic, Vuksanovic, & Vukovic, 2008). Further investigations are necessary, however, to determine which patients are at greatest risk for concomitant long-term memory deficits, as the current research has produced disparate findings with respect to the influence of lesion location and aphasia variables (i.e., aphasia type and severity) on long-term memory status.

I Got Married When?

Although few empirical studies have described the long-term memory deficits of patients with aphasia, our clinical experiences suggest that these deficits frequently co-occur with aphasia. As an example, a gentleman in our university aphasia support group recounted that subsequent to his stroke, he had noticed that he had forgotten certain events that had occurred prior to his stroke. Of particular concern to him and his wife was that he no longer recalled memories pertaining to his wedding (e.g., when it took place, where it took place, who attended). With respect to the types of long-term memory described in Chapter 1, this gentleman was experiencing impaired recall of episodic memories.

Executive Function Problems. Researchers have been interested in evaluating the executive function abilities of patients with aphasia for many decades. Whereas initial studies (e.g., Kertesz & McCabe, 1975) were driven by the quest to determine if aphasia compromised intelligence, the impetus of more recent research (e.g., Nicholas et al., 2011) has been to establish whether the influential negative relationship between the presence of executive function impairments and rehabilitation and functional outcomes observed in other neurogenic patient populations (e.g., Struchen et al., 2008a) also applies to patients with aphasia. Findings from most aphasia studies indicate that these patients are at risk for deficits in a variety of executive domains, including problem solving and reasoning, planning, organization, inhibition, self-monitoring, and cognitive flexibility (Fucetola et al., 2009; Keil & Kaszniak, 2002; Purdy, 2002; Vukovic et al., 2008), and that such deficits are associated with poorer language recovery or treatment outcomes (Lesniak, Bak, Czepiel, Seniow, & Czlonkowska, 2008; Nicholas et al., 2011; Purdy & Koch, 2006). There is little consensus, however, on whether a significant relationship exists between presence of executive function problems and aphasia type or severity, or lesion size or location (e.g., Kalbe et al., 2005, vs. Helm-Estabrooks, 2002). Accordingly, future research is needed to determine whether any language, medical, or demographic variables might help clinicians identify which patients with aphasia are at greatest risk for these high-level cognitive impairments.

Explanations of Aphasia

Although descriptions of the behavioral characteristics of aphasia are largely agreed upon, several differing views exist regarding the pattern of characteristics necessary to warrant the label of aphasia. One notion is that aphasia reflects a generalized impairment of all language functions, such that the term "aphasia" applies only to individuals who exhibit deficits across modalities and linguistic functions (Darley, 1982; Schuell & Jenkins, 1959). Other researchers have argued that the term "aphasia" can and should be additionally applied to selective impairments of specific language functions (e.g., naming, reading; Caplan & Utman, 1992; Caramazza & Miceli, 1991; Caramazza, Papagno, & Ruml, 2000; Damasio, 1981; Goodglass et al., 2001; Ni et al., 2000). Contributing to the debate regarding behavioral criteria for the diagnosis of aphasia is a lack of consensus about the precise nature of the impairments underlying aphasia.

A first area of disagreement is whether underlying language skills, processes, or representations are lost as a result of the brain damage causing the aphasia (i.e., **loss of language competence**; Goodglass, 1993; Grodzinsky, 1984; Lichtheim, 1885), or instead whether aphasia reflects disrupted access to or execution of intact language structures (i.e., **disrupted language performance**; Friederici & Frazier, 1992; McNeil, Odell, & Tseng, 1991; Schuell, Jenkins, & Jimenese-Pabon, 1964). Evidence often cited to support viewing aphasia as disrupted language performance is the observation that patients with aphasia are often able to demonstrate specific language skills that are thought to be impaired (lost) when certain conditions are modified (e.g., change in response modality, enhanced contextual cues, reduced task complexity). Proponents argue that if a skill can be demonstrated under *any* circumstances, then underlying linguistic competence must exist (McNeil et al., 1991).

Theorists also disagree about which specific processes are disrupted in aphasia (see Hallowell & Chapey, 2008, for a review). Early characterizations of aphasia suggested a *reduced ability to use language propositionally* (i.e., with the intent to communicate a specific meaning; H. H. Jackson, 1878). This view accounts for the observation that many patients with aphasia may successfully use nonpropositional language (e.g., rote recitation, automatic greetings). Subsequently, Goldstein and Scheerer (1948) suggested that aphasia results from an *impaired ability to form abstractions,* a skill required to manipulate linguistic symbols. More recently, a prominent explanation for aphasia has arisen out of the fields of psycholinguistics and cognitive neuropsychology, and specifies that *disruptions to specific linguistic processes,* either individually or in concert, result in predictable language performance breakdowns (Caplan & Utman, 1992; Caramazza et al., 2000; Damasio, 1981). Finally, the language characteristics of aphasia also have been characterized as either a *disruption of the cognitive processes supporting language* or *reduced access to or inefficient allocation of cognitive resources to the mental processes relevant to language* (McNeil et al., 1991; L. Murray, 2000a; L. Murray & Kean, 2004).

Classification Systems for Aphasia

As indicated previously, patients with aphasia may demonstrate varying degrees of impairment in the areas of comprehension, speech fluency, naming, and repetition, as well as across modalities. Researchers who subscribe to a unidimensional view of aphasia (e.g., Darley, 1982; Schuell et al., 1964) consider these variations in behavioral manifestations as just that: *variations* in the presentation of a uniform disorder, and all patients with aphasia are diagnosed with aphasia (without adjectives; Rosenbek et al., 1989). Other researchers, and likewise clinicians, however, find it helpful to assign different designations for the various patterns of aphasic behaviors; thus a number of aphasia classification systems have evolved.

Dichotomous Classification Systems

One of the more common ways of classifying aphasia subtypes is according to speech fluency. Patients with **nonfluent aphasia** typically exhibit speech characterized by utterances of four words or fewer, often produced haltingly and with great effort and compromised grammar (Alexander & Hillis, 2008; Sinanovic et al., 2011). In contrast, patients with **fluent aphasia** demonstrate an ease of speech production, with melodic line, rhythm, rate, and flow similar to those of non-aphasic speakers. This classification system does not, however, address other language characteristics, in that patients with either fluent or nonfluent aphasia may demonstrate impaired comprehension, naming, and/or repetition. These overlapping symptoms are no doubt responsible for the difficulty and unreliability that have been associated with attempting to classify patients into one of these two aphasia categories (J. K. Gordon, 1998).

Patients with aphasia also have been classified according to degree of comprehension deficit. The term "**receptive aphasia**" has been used to describe the language characteristics of significantly impaired auditory and written comprehension, whereas "**expressive aphasia**" denotes relatively spared language comprehension but compromised language output abilities. Similar to the fluent/nonfluent dichotomy, however, the labels of *expressive* or *receptive aphasia* do not imply a specific level of impairment in speech fluency, naming, or repetition. Additionally, these terms are slight misnomers, given that patients who might be classified as having receptive aphasia typically have expressive deficits as well.

Although the two dichotomies described above are based solely on behavioral characteristics, researchers have proposed that each of these aphasia types can be associated with specific lesion sites (e.g., Goodglass, 1981). For example, both nonfluent and expressive forms of aphasia have historically been associated with relatively anterior lesions (e.g., damage to Broca's area or surrounding frontal association areas). In contrast, fluent and receptive forms of aphasia are traditionally associated with relatively posterior lesions (e.g., damage to Wernicke's area or surrounding temporal and parietal association areas). However, lesion and imaging studies (e.g., Binder et al., 1997; Kang et al., 2010; Metter et al., 1989; Z. Yang, Zhao, Wang, Chen, & Zhang, 2008) have revealed a number of exceptions to this lesion pattern, potentially reflecting, at least in part, that behavioral characteristics (e.g., severity, fluency) change over the course of recovery even when the lesion is static.

Connectionist Classification System

The classification system adopted by commonly used aphasia diagnostic batteries—the *Boston Diagnostic Aphasia Examination–Third Edition* (Goodglass et al., 2001) and the *Western Aphasia Battery–Revised* (Kertesz, 2006; see Chapter 6)—and thus used most frequently by professionals serving patients with aphasia, is a system that incorporates both behavioral characteristics and neuroanatomical correlates of the observed behaviors. This system is often termed the "connectionist" model because of the inherent assumption that the various aphasic subtypes reflect disruption of specific brain centers or to the connections between these centers (see Table 2-4).

Conduction Today, Broca's Tomorrow

Even though the connectionist classification system remains popular among clinicians and researchers, it is important to keep in mind that the validity and reliability of these aphasia types have yet to be established. For example, Mr. Duncan attended our university clinic for individual and support group services for many years and completed the *Western Aphasia Battery* (WAB), an aphasia battery that yields a connectionist aphasia type, several times as we monitored his progress. Interestingly, he regularly fluctuated between Broca's and conduction aphasia across those repeated administrations of the WAB. Our clinical impression was that Mr. Duncan's aphasia type was more a reflection of his level of fatigue rather than the location of his brain lesion or the integrity of his language abilities: If he was tired, speaking was much more effortful for him, resulting in nonfluent output, and thus his WAB subtest scores were more consistent with Broca's aphasia. Further discussion of the pros and cons of aphasia classification systems is provided in Chapter 6.

TABLE 2-4
Connectionist Aphasia Types

APHASIA TYPE	PREDICTED SITE OF LESION	COMPREHENSION	FLUENCY	NAMING	REPETITION
Broca's	Broca's area	Mild to moderately impaired	Nonfluent	Impaired	Similar to spontaneous speech
Wernicke's	Wernicke's area	Moderately to severely impaired	Fluent	Impaired	Similar to spontaneous speech
Global	Anterior and posterior left hemisphere	Moderately to severely impaired	Nonfluent	Impaired	Similar to spontaneous speech
Transcortical motor	Anterior or superior to Broca's area	Mild to moderately impaired	Nonfluent	Impaired	Less impaired than spontaneous speech
Transcortical sensory	Posterior temporal lobe extending into the occipital lobe	Moderately to severely impaired	Fluent	Impaired	Less impaired than spontaneous speech
Transcortical mixed (Isolation)	Anterior and posterior association areas in the left hemisphere	Moderately to severely impaired	Nonfluent	Impaired	Less impaired than spontaneous speech
Conduction	Left arcuate fasciculus and/or supramarginal gyrus in the inferior parietal lobe	Mild to moderately impaired	Fluent	Impaired	More impaired than spontaneous speech
Anomic	Anywhere in the left hemisphere	Normal to mildly impaired	Fluent	Impaired	Similar to spontaneous speech

Broca's aphasia, named for physician Paul Broca, who first described this behavior pattern and the brain lesion responsible for it, is characterized by nonfluent language output and relatively spared language comprehension compared to output fluency difficulties (i.e., these patients may have comprehension problems, but they are not as prominent as their output difficulties). As might be deduced from the name, aphasias of this type are thought to result from damage to Broca's area, but also may be associated with lesions in surrounding frontal lobe areas, the white matter beneath the frontal cortex, and the insula (Jodzio, Gasecki, Drumm, Lass, & Nyka, 2003; Kang et al., 2010; Yang et al., 2008; see included DVD: Patient 5).

Often considered the aphasia type in greatest contrast to Broca's aphasia is **Wernicke's aphasia,** which is characterized by marked comprehension, naming, and repetition impairments. Language output in Wernicke's aphasia, though fluent, typically contains many paraphasias, and is often described as "empty speech," reflecting the paucity of information that is communicated. Although exceptions are not uncommon (e.g., Binder et al., 1997; Kang et al., 2010), Wernicke's aphasia is usually associated with lesions to Wernicke's area and other regions within or near the posterior superior temporal lobe (Jodzio et al., 2003; Yang et al., 2008).

The aphasia type marked by significant impairments in all language modalities and functions (i.e., comprehension, speech fluency, naming, and repetition) is **global aphasia.** As might be expected from the breadth of impairments, global aphasia typically results from large lesions affecting both anterior and posterior language centers (Jodzio et al., 2003; Yang et al., 2008), although exceptions have been noted (Vignolo, Boccardi, & Caverni, 1986). Global aphasia has been reported to be the most common type of aphasia among acute stroke patients (Sinanovic et al., 2011). Keep in mind that by some definitions, all forms of aphasia are global (affecting all modalities), so a high prevalence of global aphasia would not be unexpected (Darley, 1982; Schuell & Jenkins, 1959). In practice, however, the term "global aphasia" is most typically applied when the individual demonstrates pronounced deficits across all modalities without relative strengths in either comprehension or ease of verbal expression.

Each of the aphasias described above (Broca's, Wernicke's, and global) is characterized by repetition that is similar to spontaneous speech with respect to fluency, presence of paraphasic errors, morphosyntactic accuracy, and so forth. The following three aphasia types are similar to these hallmark aphasia types, with the exception that repetition is much less impaired than would be predicted from spontaneous speech. **Transcortical motor aphasia** is similar to Broca's aphasia with respect to speech fluency, comprehension, and naming. When patients with transcortical motor aphasia are asked to repeat phrases and sentences, however, their spoken output is generally more fluent and contains fewer errors than their spontaneous verbal output. Lesions resulting in transcortical motor aphasia are usually anterior or superior to Broca's area (Alexander & Hillis, 2008; Sinanovic et al., 2011) and are hypothesized to reflect a disconnection between Broca's area and the supplemental motor area (Freedman, Alexander, & Naeser, 1984). Subcortical lesions involving the caudate or thalamus have also been observed to produce transcortical motor aphasia (Yang et al., 2008).

Similar to Wernicke's aphasia, **transcortical sensory aphasia** is characterized by poor comprehension and fluent speech. Repetition tends to be more preserved than spontaneous speech, which typically contains many paraphasias and neologisms. Lesions resulting from disrupted blood supply to the posterior cerebral artery that affect the inferior temporal lobe and parts of the occipital lobe are typically associated with transcortical sensory aphasia (Alexander & Hillis, 2008; Sinanovic et al., 2011), although basal ganglia lesions have also been reported to produce this aphasia type (Yang et al., 2008).

The final transcortical aphasia type is **transcortical mixed aphasia**, also known as **isolation aphasia**. Similar to global aphasia, patients with isolation aphasia exhibit notable impairments in comprehension, speech fluency, and naming, but retain the ability to repeat at a level not predicted by the severity of their other language deficits. As might be anticipated, isolation aphasia tends to be associated with large lesions involving both anterior and posterior language association or watershed areas (Sinanovic et al., 2011; Yang et al., 2008), such as those that result from hypoxic-ischemic brain injuries (e.g., cardiac arrest, carbon monoxide poisoning; see Chapter 3 for a description of hypoxic-ischemic brain injury).

In contrast to the aphasia types characterized by preserved repetition ability, **conduction aphasia** is notable for disproportionately severe deficits during repetition. Patients with conduction aphasia tend to have relatively good comprehension and fluent speech, with mild to moderate naming deficits. However, when they are asked to repeat, their speech may become more nonfluent, or paraphasias may become more prominent than is observed during their spontaneous speech. The lesion sites traditionally associated with conduction aphasia are the left arcuate fasciculus, the supramarginal gyrus in the inferior parietal lobe, or both (Jodzio et al., 2003; Yang et al., 2008).

The final classic connectionist aphasia type is **anomic aphasia**. Patients with anomic aphasia exhibit a relatively isolated impairment of naming, with fluent speech and good comprehension. Although some patients may demonstrate anomic aphasia early postonset, other patients' impairments will evolve via spontaneous recovery and language treatment into anomic aphasia (Pedersen, Vinter, & Olsen, 2004; Sinanovic et al., 2011); consequently, anomic aphasia is the most common aphasia type in the chronic stages of recovery (see included DVD: Patients 1, 4, 7). Unlike the other aphasia types, which have been associated with lesions to specific brain structures or pathways, anomic aphasia can result from brain damage to various cortical and subcortical regions (Alexander & Hillis, 2008; Yang et al., 2008).

Other Aphasia Types

Although not necessarily included in the traditional aphasia classification systems, additional aphasia types have been identified. **Subcortical aphasia**, referring to aphasia resulting from damage to noncortical sites (e.g., thalamus, basal ganglia), has been reported by a number of researchers (Jodzio et al., 2003; Kang et al., 2010; Pedersen et al., 2004; Radanovic & Scaff, 2003). Although the behavioral descriptions of subcortical aphasia are quite varied (see Hillis et al., 2004, for a review), they may overlap with those for any other type of aphasia, with anomic aphasia being most frequently observed following subcortical lesions (Kang et al., 2010; Pedersen et al., 2004). As discussed in Chapter 1, the direct role of subcortical structures in language function and related aphasias has been called into question by recent studies demonstrating that language disruptions associated with subcortical lesions can be explained by reduced oxygenation to relevant cortical sites (e.g., Hillis et al., 2004). Nonetheless, clinicians should be aware that patients with subcortical lesions may demonstrate aphasia and that the nature of their aphasia may not be predictable from their lesion site.

Crossed aphasia describes aphasia resulting from lesions to the hemisphere non-dominant for language (i.e., the right hemisphere for most people). Because even most left-handed individuals are left hemisphere dominant for language, crossed aphasia is quite rare (Zangwill, 1967), with estimates that less than 3% of right-handed patients with aphasia will present with crossed aphasia (Coppens, Hungerford, Yamaguchi, & Yamadori, 2002; De Witte et al., 2008; Marien, Paghera, De Deyn, & Vignolo, 2004). Similar to subcortical aphasias, the pattern of language impairment in crossed aphasia is quite variable. Moreover, crossed aphasia may result from lesions to a number of right hemisphere sites. Interestingly, the language characteristics of crossed aphasia may co-occur with not only deficits that frequently accompany aphasia due to dominant left hemisphere damage (e.g., oral or constructional apraxia) but also the cognitive-communicative deficits (e.g., neglect) more commonly associated with right hemisphere lesions.

Occasionally, the term "**pure aphasia**" is used to denote apparently isolated impairments of specific language functions. For example, patients who demonstrate reading difficulties in the absence of any other language impairment are said to demonstrate **pure alexia,** or word blindness (Barton, 2011; Hillis, 2008; Sinanovic et al., 2011). Similarly, **pure agraphia** refers to isolated impairments of writing (Hillis, 2008; Luzzi & Piccirilli, 2003; Sakurai, Asami, & Mannen, 2010), and **pure word deafness** describes profound auditory comprehension deficits without evidence of impairment in other language functions (e.g., speaking, reading) (Polster & Rose, 1998; Rosen & Viskontas, 2008; Wee & Menard, 1999). Such isolated linguistic impairments are uncommon (Alexander & Hillis, 2008; Hillis, 2008), and as indicated previously, some authors would not consider isolated impairments indicative of aphasia. Nonetheless, such impairments are likely to be identified and managed in ways similar to those employed for the more typical aphasias.

When individuals who use two or more languages acquire aphasia, a diagnosis of **bilingual** or **multilingual aphasia**, respectively, may be given (for reviews, see Lorenzen & Murray, 2008b; P. Roberts, 2008). There are a number of unique variables to consider when dealing with patients who have bilingual or multilingual aphasia. For example, although most patients experience similar degrees of impairment and recovery in their languages (i.e., parallel recovery pattern), some will display other patterns, such as better recovery in one language versus the other (i.e., differential recovery pattern), recovery in only one language (i.e., selective recovery), or gains in one language while the other language gets worse (i.e., antagonistic recovery). Furthermore, in addition to the aphasic characteristics described above (e.g., anomia, comprehension difficulties), patients with bilingual or multilingual aphasia may acquire a translation disorder, such as only being able to translate in one direction (i.e., paradoxical translation), translating when translation was not requested or required (i.e., spontaneous translation), or having difficulties with the translation process (i.e., impaired translation).

The final aphasia type to be described is unique primarily with respect to etiology. Whereas aphasia most frequently results from acute neurological injury (e.g., strokes; see Chapter 3), it also may be a symptom of progressive disease. Aphasia of this type is called **primary progressive aphasia (PPA)** and is generally associated with left hemisphere pathology (Gorno-Tempini et al., 2011; Ogar, 2010). Although in many patients with PPA the cause of their progressive language problems is not known, pathology associated with dementing diseases such as Alzheimer's, Pick's, and frontotemporal lobar degeneration (for a description of these dementing diseases, see Chapter 3) has been identified in cases that have gone to autopsy (Gorno-Tempini et al., 2011; Grossman et al., 2007; Grossman et al., 2008; Kertesz, 2010). Patients with PPA may demonstrate a range of impairments in comprehension, naming, speech fluency, and reading and writing skills (Gorno-Tempini et al., 2011; Ogar, 2010). Nevertheless, three PPA subtypes have been identified: progressive nonfluent aphasia (see included DVD: Patients 6, 10), a fluent form called "semantic dementia," and logopenic progressive aphasia; characteristics of each of these forms of PPA are listed in Table 2-5. It is important to keep in mind that not all patients with PPA will have symptom profiles that fit into one of these three subtypes, with some presenting with an isolated, progressive symptom (e.g., anomia) and others with a mixed symptom profile.

Unlike aphasia resulting from acute brain injury, which is generally expected to improve over time, the deficits associated with PPA continue to progress. In fact, one of the original diagnostic criteria for PPA was that patients had to show a relatively isolated decline of language abilities for at least two years (Weintraub, Rubin, & Mesulam, 1990). Careful assessment will generally reveal that at least initially, broader intellect, including memory and executive functions, and the ability to complete daily activities independently are relatively spared, often for many, many years (e.g., L. Murray, 1998). Over time, however, patients with PPA do develop concomitant cognitive symptoms (e.g., Banks & Weintraub, 2008) and will typically eventually be diagnosed with dementia.

Right Hemisphere Disorders

In contrast to the primarily linguistically based symptoms of patients with aphasia, the communication difficulties of patients who have suffered right hemisphere brain damage (RHD) are for the most part a product of concomitant cognitive deficits (Lehman Blake, 2007; Lindell, 2006; McDonald, 2000; Surian & Siegal, 2001). For this reason, the

TABLE 2-5
Types of Primary Progressive Aphasia (PPA)

PPA TYPE	SYMPTOMS	PRIMARY LOCATION OF NEURAL DEGENERATION
Progressive non-fluent aphasia	• Nonfluent, agrammatic output • Motor speech issues (apraxia of speech, dysarthria) • Impaired comprehension of complex grammatical constructions • Impaired word retrieval, with greater difficulty with verbs vs. nouns	Left posterior fronto-insular region
Semantic dementia	• Fluent output • Impaired single-word comprehension, typically with greater difficulty with low- vs. high-frequency vocabulary • Impaired word retrieval, with frequent semantic paraphasias • Impaired semantic/conceptual representations • Surface dyslexia or dysgraphia	Anterior temporal lobe bilaterally, but more involvement in the left hemisphere
Logopenic progressive	• Slow and halting/nonfluent output • Impaired phrase and sentence repetition • Impaired word retrieval, with frequent phonemic paraphasias • Reduced auditory-verbal short-term memory	Left temporoparietal junction

term "cognitive-communicative disorders" is often used when referring to the types of communicative symptoms observed following RHD. An ever-increasing research base indicates that patients with RHD can vary significantly in terms of the nature and severity of their cognitive-communicative disorder (Cote, Payer, Giroux, & Joanette, 2007; Sherratt & Bryan, 2012; Tompkins, 2012). This heterogeneity no doubt arises from the variety of deficits, including impairments of perception, attention, memory, executive functioning, and certain aspects of language that may directly or indirectly influence these patients' communicative abilities.

Despite progress in understanding the types of cognitive-communicative disorders associated with RHD, limited data exist to help predict the frequency with which these disorders may occur. Whereas early estimates and small sample studies suggested that approximately 50% of RHD patients should be expected to present with some form of cognitive-communicative disorder (e.g., E. Benton & Bryan, 1996), Lehman Blake, Duffy, Myers, and Tompkins (2002) more recently reported that 96% of the RHD patients identified in their review of an inpatient hospital's medical charts had been diagnosed with at least one type of cognitive-communicative symptom. The specific symptom(s) with which a given patient presents will depend on which neural structures and pathways within the right hemisphere were compromised by the brain damage. Therefore, clinicians must keep in mind that it is unlikely that all RHD patients will display all of the following impairments.

Perceptual Problems

Deficits in perceiving either visual or auditory information frequently occur following RHD (Lehman Blake et al., 2002; Rosen & Viskontas, 2008; Vignolo, 2003). An understanding of these perceptual problems is necessary given that they may be the underlying basis of some language symptoms (McDonald, 2000; Nicholson et al., 2003; Peper & Irle, 1997). For instance, problems with pitch discrimination may contribute to the prosody-processing difficulties that are sometimes observed following RHD. Likewise, complex visuospatial discrimination and integration problems may result in a variety of communicative symptoms, such as a decreased ability to profit from nonverbal cues (e.g., patients are unable to discriminate the facial expressions of their communicative partners), inappropriate proxemics (e.g., patients with depth-perception problems may get too close to their communicative partners), poor writing legibility, or naming errors and illogical verbal output (e.g., a patient's narrative sample does not match with the picture stimulus because of his inability to perceive the items and events depicted in the picture). A list of possible perceptual problems associated with RHD is provided in Table 2-6, and further information about several of these deficits is provided later in this book (see Chapter 4).

Attention Problems

Attention is one of the most commonly impaired cognitive functions subsequent to RHD (Lehman Blake et al., 2002). All aspects of attention, including sustained attention, focused attention, attention switching, and divided attention, may be compromised (Barker-Collo et al., 2009, 2010; Gerritsen, Berg, Deelman, Visser-Keizer, & Meyboom-de Jong, 2003; Rosen & Viskontas, 2008). These attention problems are important to qualify and quantify, as they may be the source of several communicative symptoms (L. Murray, 2000a; Sherratt & Bryan, 2012). For instance, pragmatic and discourse problems such as poor eye contact, difficulty in understanding lengthy conversations, and inadequate topic maintenance may be byproducts of decreased sustained attention abilities, rather than impairments of higher-level language abilities.

Neglect Syndrome

Without question, the most frequently studied attention symptoms associated with RHD are collectively referred to as **neglect syndrome.** Generally, "neglect" refers to a set of attention problems in which patients are slow or inaccurate at reporting, reacting to, orienting to, or seeking out stimuli that are presented contralateral to the side

TABLE 2-6
Visual and Auditory Perceptual and Related Disorders That May Occur Subsequent to Onset of RHD, TBI, and Certain Dementing Diseases

DISORDER	DEFINITION/ DESCRIPTION	EXAMPLES OF BEHAVIORS RESULTING FROM VISUAL OR AUDITORY PROBLEMS
Topographical disorientation	Difficulty orienting to the immediate location	Problems following directions to find a product in a store not because of comprehension problems, but because of problems orienting in the store
Impaired figure-ground perception	Difficulty finding visual target amid background	Problems finding communication partner at a party with lots of guests and decorations
Difficulties judging depth and distance		Standing too close or too far when speaking with someone
Geographic disorientation	Difficulty understanding one's general location	Apparent confabulation when the patient is asked about where he or she is or was (e.g., "I ate dinner in North Dakota last night" when actually is in Indiana)
Prosopagnosia*	Facial recognition deficits	Failing to greet familiar communication partners because the patient does not visually recognize the partners
Visual agnosia*	Unable to recognize or apply meaning to what is seen	Inability to label objects or pictures without information in another modality (e.g., auditory, tactile)
Achromatopsia	Color perception deficit in which the patient sees in grayscale or colors are dull	Misperception of objects, resulting in naming errors (e.g., picture of an orange is named "ball")
Impaired visual closure	Difficulties recognizing incomplete visual stimuli	Failing to greet a familiar communication partner who in the winter was wearing a scarf to keep his face warm
Simultanagnosia*	Inability to integrate the visual details of a scene	Being able to describe details of a social event he or she saw (e.g., many women, presents) but unable to report what type of social event it was (e.g., baby shower)
Sound localization deficits	Inability to determine from where a sound has been generated	Responding to the wrong communication partner in a group conversation
Auditory agnosia*	Unable to recognize or apply meaning to auditory stimuli	Unable to recognize and therefore respond appropriately to environmental sounds (e.g., checks to see who is at the door when the phone rings)
Impaired pitch discrimination	Difficulties identifying pitch changes or whether pitches are the same or different	Difficulty determining the emotional intonation of the communication partner

(continues)

TABLE 2-6 (continued)

DISORDER	DEFINITION/ DESCRIPTION	EXAMPLES OF BEHAVIORS RESULTING FROM VISUAL OR AUDITORY PROBLEMS
Impaired loudness discrimination	Difficulties identifying loudness changes or whether two sounds are similar or different in terms of loudness	Difficulty determining which words in the utterance of a communication partner have been stressed

*Agnosias (i.e., problems applying meaning to what is being seen or heard) most frequently occur following bilateral brain damage, but also have been periodically reported following unilateral RHD (Rosen & Viskontas, 2008).

of their brain damage (Cherney, 2002; Kortte & Hillis, 2011; Robertson & Halligan, 1999). Therefore, if patients with RHD present with neglect, they will have difficulty attending to information presented on their left side. Although neglect is most obvious when it affects patients' attention to visual information or stimulation, it also may negatively influence information processing in other modalities (e.g., auditory, tactile, olfactory). Whereas estimates of neglect prevalence following RHD vary, most suggest that 30 to over 50% of RHD patients will display one or more neglect symptoms (Kortte & Hillis, 2011; Lehman Blake et al., 2002; Sinanovic, 2010; Vallar, 2007). Research indicates that neglect also can occur in patients with left hemisphere brain damage, but that neglect associated with RHD is more severe and enduring (Robertson & Halligan, 1999; Sinanovic, 2010). Researchers have hypothesized that neglect is more debilitating following RHD because of the right hemisphere's relative dominance for allocating attention within both hemispaces (Mesulam, 1981); in contrast, the left hemisphere may contribute to distributing and directing attention within the right hemispace, but if it is damaged, the right hemisphere can compensate and continue to support attention to the right hemispace. Because of the frequency with which this attention deficit may occur, because it can be a persistent symptom, and because several studies have found neglect to be a particularly influential negative prognostic indicator of functional outcome (de Haan, Nys, & van Zandvoort, 2006; Kortte & Hillis, 2011; Wee & Hopman, 2008), understanding the variety of symptoms that contribute to the syndrome of neglect is essential to managing patients with RHD.

One of the most overt neglect symptoms is **hemi-inattention,** which includes problems such as (a) poor response to or report of stimuli presented contralaterally in the absence of sensory impairments or (b) poor performance of tasks or activities in the contralateral hemispace that cannot be attributed to motor impairments (Cherney, 2002; Kortte & Hillis, 2011; Vallar, 2007). When this symptom occurs in the visual modality, several other terms may be applied, including "hemispatial neglect," "visuospatial neglect," or "unilateral spatial neglect." Symptoms such as omitting details from the left side of their drawings (see Figure 2-2), failing to brush the teeth on the left side of their mouths, leaving their left shoelace untied, and bumping into furniture that is on their left side are also considered a product of hemi-inattention. These

Figure 2-2. Example of a freehand drawing of a butterfly from a patient with left visuospatial neglect subsequent to a right hemisphere stroke.

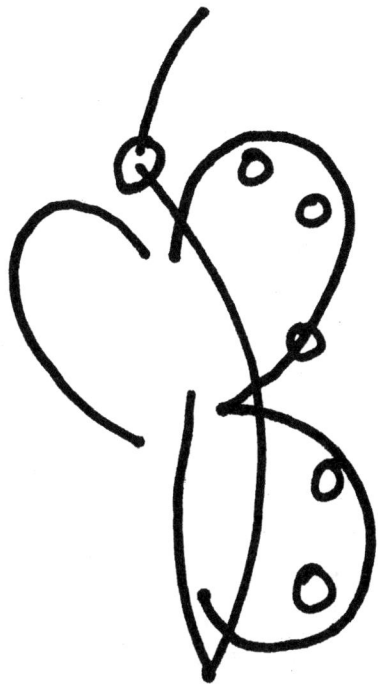

behaviors are considered to have an attentional basis because neither sensory nor motor impairments can explain their occurrence (e.g., patients are not failing to brush the teeth on the left side of their mouths because of hemiparesis or apraxia), and when you draw patients' attention to the information or task on their neglected side, they are able to process the information or complete the task.

Another obvious symptom of neglect is **hemiakinesia,** which is also sometimes referred to as "hemihypokinesia," "motor extinction," "motor impersistence," or "motor neglect." Patients with hemiakinesia underuse or in some cases never use the left side of their body, even in the absence of hemiparesis. Signs of hemiakinesia include poor balance because postural muscles on the left side of the body are not being fully exploited, failing to evade painful stimuli, difficulties completing bilateral tasks (e.g., problems buttoning a shirt or putting hair in a ponytail), and minimal exploration of the left hemispace with the left hand or limb when an activity necessitates this exploration.

Other neglect symptoms are not as obvious. For instance, "sensory extinction to simultaneous stimulation" refers to the phenomenon in which patients with neglect fail to report being stimulated on their left side when stimulation was presented bilaterally. For example, if the examiner touches the right and left sides of the RHD patient's back, the patient would report only being touched on the right side. Interestingly, this symptom often persists even after hemi-inattention has recovered.

Another less noticeable symptom is **allesthesia.** This term is applied when RHD patients report being stimulated on their right side when they were actually stimulated on their left side. For instance, the clinician might enter an RHD patient's hospital room from the left side and then greet the patient from that left side. If the patient has allesthesia, she will look to her right to respond to the clinician.

The presence of neglect will have significant effects on RHD patients' language abilities. For example, patients with visual hemi-inattention may have reading difficulties related to not attending to the left side of words or the left side of the page. When these types of reading problems occur, patients may be diagnosed with **neglect dyslexia.** Similarly, **neglect dygraphia** refers to writing problems related to neglect. Signs that neglect is affecting writing include failing to cross or dot letters (e.g., "t," "f," "x," "i," "j"), leaving a large left side margin that increases in width as patients' writing progresses down the page, and displaying a right upward slant to their writing as they progress from the left to the right side of the page.

Memory Problems

RHD frequently produces a variety of memory impairments (Lehman Blake et al., 2002; Tompkins, 2012). Traditionally, RHD has been associated with impaired temporary (as well as long-term) recall of nonverbal more so than verbal material (de Haan et al., 2006; Rosen & Viskontas, 2008; Vallar, 2007). That is, patients with RHD might be expected to have difficulty encoding and remembering one or more of the following: (a) visual information (e.g., complex designs, faces, and facial expressions; spatial locations and routes); (b) auditory information (e.g., the rhythm or tune of a song); or (c) information presented in other sensory modalities (e.g., olfaction). Additionally, RHD patients, particularly those with frontal lobe lesions, may display problems remembering the temporal order of the to-be-recalled nonverbal information (e.g., they forget the sequence in which a series of faces was shown) or under what circumstances they encoded the information (i.e., source memory deficit) (Buklina, 2003).

Although nonverbal memory problems have been traditionally associated with RHD and verbal memory problems with left hemisphere damage (Rosen & Viskontas, 2008), researchers have more recently found that encoding and subsequent recall of verbal information may be additionally compromised following RHD (Culbertson, Tanner, Peck, & Hopper, 1998; A. S. Halper, Cherney, Drimmer, & Chang, 1996; L. Murray, 2004b). For example, Tompkins, Bloise, Timko, and Baumgaertner (1994) found that their study participants with RHD performed an auditory-verbal working memory task more poorly than their non–brain-damaged study participants. Furthermore, the working memory performances of the RHD participants correlated with their performances of a discourse comprehension task that involved resolving contextual discrepancies or revising linguistic inferences. Recent studies have also documented that difficulties recalling autobiographical events stored prior to the onset of brain damage are more common following RHD, particularly temporal lobe damage, than left hemisphere damage (Batchelor, Thompson, & Miller, 2008; Buccione, Fadda, Serra, Caltagirone, & Carlesimo, 2008) and that learning new skills appears more dependent on the right versus left hemisphere (Schutz, 2005). Accordingly, the memory problems of RHD patients need to be identified given their potential to interfere with discourse and other communicative and cognitive abilities, the rehabilitation process, or both.

Executive Functioning Problems

A growing literature has documented that executive skills such as planning, problem solving, cognitive flexibility, and inhibition will be compromised in at least some patients with RHD, particularly those with damage to their frontal lobe or to connections between their right frontal lobe and subcortical structures such as the thalamus (Champagne-Lavau & Joanette, 2009; de Haan et al., 2006; Godefroy et al., 2010; Lehman Blake et al., 2002; Zinn, Bosworth, Hoenig, & Swartzwelder, 2007). A particularly problematic RHD symptom related to executive dysfunctioning is **anosognosia**, or an impaired awareness or denial of one's own deficits (Jehkonen, Laihosalo, & Kettunen, 2006; Sinanovic, 2010). Several forms of anosognosia are possible (Starkstein, Jorge, & Robinson, 2010). The term "verbal asomatognosia" (also sometimes called "somatognosia") is used when patients deny ownership of their limb or limbs contralateral to the side of their brain lesion. If patients admit they are experiencing symptoms subsequent to the onset of their brain damage, but appear unconcerned or show nominal emotional response about these symptoms, they may be diagnosed with "anosodiaphoria."

Anosognosia in its various forms is common in RHD patients, particularly those with neglect (Jehkonen et al., 2006; Kortte & Hillis, 2011; Sinanovic, 2010) and those who are of an older age and have experienced prior brain damage (Starkstein et al., 2010). Sinanovic (2010) reported that across prior studies, anosognosia was reported to occur in approximately 30 to 85% of patients who suffer RHD versus less than 20% among those with left hemisphere damage. Patients may be unaware of just one symptom, several symptoms, or all of their symptoms, although it is more common for patients to have limited awareness of their cognitive rather than motor or sensory impairments. Like neglect, anosognosia is a negative prognostic indicator (Jehkonen et al., 2006; Kortte & Hillis, 2011; Starkstein et al., 2010). Accordingly, diagnosing anosognosia is imperative, as patients who are unaware of their deficits or who cannot appreciate the consequences of their deficits will not understand the need for treatment, will not be motivated to apply whatever strategies are suggested if they attend treatment, or may place themselves in physical or emotional jeopardy by attempting activities that are beyond their current ability level.

Communication Symptoms

Generally, the communicative problems of patients with RHD might be viewed as the inverse of those described for patients with aphasia: Whereas aphasia is associated with impaired phonological, lexical-semantic, and morphosyntactic processing, but relatively preserved pragmatic abilities, RHD is associated with relatively intact phonological, lexical-semantic, and morphosyntactic processing, but compromised pragmatic skills. That is, patients with RHD are typically capable of communicating on superficial levels but may experience breakdowns in more complex, less structured, abstract, and sophisticated communicative situations. This means that in acute-care settings, the communicative problems of patients with RHD may not be obvious (Benton & Bryan, 1996). Instead, only when these patients return to their home, work, or other more demanding and unpredictable environments and communicative activities may their communicative difficulties be fully realized by the patients themselves or by their caregivers.

Lexical-Semantic Abilities

Before describing the types of pragmatic and related discourse problems associated with RHD, it is important to evaluate research pertaining to lexical–semantic abilities following RHD. Some studies suggest deficits at this level of language processing, particularly in terms of processing subordinate, distant or weakly associated, or context-discordant word meanings (Cote et al., 2007; Lindell, 2006; Tompkins, Fassbinder, Scharp, & Meigh, 2008; Tompkins, Scharp, Meigh, & Fassbinder, 2008). The lexical–semantic comprehension and production difficulties of RHD patients may also reflect problems in perception or other areas of cognition rather than in lexical–semantic processes per se (Fassbinder & Tompkins, 2001; Hough, DeMarco, & Schmitzer, 1997; Tompkins, 2012). For instance, problems with visuoperceptual discrimination may result in inaccurate completion of confrontation naming tasks. Attention problems also may contribute to apparent lexical–semantic breakdowns, as several studies have indicated that patients with RHD display more difficulties with word finding under more complex attention conditions (e.g., L. Murray, 2000a). Additionally, the patient's native language may influence whether deficits at the lexical–semantic level will be present following RHD. For example, patients with RHD who speak and write Chinese display similar levels of word finding difficulties as their peers with left hemisphere damage because the neural representation of Chinese is more bilateral compared to other languages (e.g., English) (Cheung, Cheung, & Chan, 2004).

Pragmatic and Discourse Symptoms

Clinicians are most likely to observe communicative problems at the pragmatic and discourse levels of language processing in their patients with RHD. In terms of comprehension, impairments with one or more of the following have been reported (Champagne-Lavau & Joanette, 2009; Cheang & Pell, 2006; Cote et al., 2007; Cutica et al., 2006; G. Schmidt, Kranjec, Cardillo, & Chatterjee, 2010; Tompkins, 2008, 2012; Tompkins, Scharp, Meigh, & Fassbinder, 2008):

- *Appreciating humor:* For example, some, but not all, patients with RHD are less accurate than their non–brain-damaged peers at picking an ending to a short narrative to make a joke.
- *Comprehending nonliteral language:* This would include understanding indirect speech acts, idioms, sarcasm, proverbs, irony, metaphors, and other forms of figurative language, particularly if the speech act or figurative language form is unconventional or less common.
- *Being sensitive to and interpreting cues related to communicative context, intent, and partners:* This would include processing of extralinguistic aspects of communication (e.g., body gestures, distance and positioning of communication partner[s], facial expressions).

- *Resolving lexical ambiguity based on previous world knowledge and/or current communicative content and context:* As an example, the utterance "John won the race" could be interpreted as John won a *speed* race or a *political* race, and thus, the listener might use his or her prior knowledge of John or, if the listener didn't know John, synthesize other content and contextual cues to determine which was the correct interpretation.
- *Inferencing, which involves garnering information that is not explicitly provided, or revising preliminary inferences:* For example, determining a character's motive when reading a murder mystery and then shifting one's view of that character after a twist in the plot would involve both inferencing and revision of inferencing.
- *Differentiating between relevant versus irrelevant information, which is necessary for accurate interpretation:* For instance, when listening to a lecture, understanding the main points requires determining what might be tangents versus central ideas.
- *Identifying the moral or theme of a story or recognizing the gist of a conversation:* This would involve several of the above skills, such as inferencing, being sensitive to and synthesizing contextual cues, and differentiating between relevant and irrelevant details.

In terms of language expression, the informativeness and efficiency of the spoken and written output of patients with RHD may be negatively affected. More specifically, their discourse production may be characterized by one or more of the following deficits (Cote et al., 2007; Hird & Kirsner, 2003; Lehman Blake, 2007; Marini, Caltagirone, & Nocentini, 2005; Rousseaux, Daveluy, & Koslowski, 2010; Sherratt & Bryan, 2012; Tompkins, 2012):

- Inefficient organization and summarization of information that can lead to compromised discourse coherence (i.e., flow of meaning across utterances)
- Inclusion of tangential or irrelevant details (e.g., off-topic remarks, digressions from the topic or story, unnecessary embellishment or elaboration)
- Output paucity (i.e., taciturn) or excess (i.e., verbose), both of which negatively affect informativeness
- Impaired use of extralinguistic communication cues (e.g., flat facial affect; inadequate eye contact; inappropriate, infrequent, or excessive use of gestures)
- Problems with discourse cohesion (i.e., flow within and between utterances), such as unclear pronoun referencing or restricted use or diversity of conjunctions
- Confabulation or inclusion of fabricated verbal material
- Inaccurate or incomplete discourse macrostructure (e.g., failing to introduce a conversational topic, using an incomplete or incorrect sequence of story episodes, describing the steps of a procedure in an inappropriate order)
- Egocentric or overpersonalized output (e.g., injecting personal information or opinions that are inappropriate for the communicative context)

- Impaired topic management (e.g., introducing fewer or inappropriate topics, switching topics too frequently or not frequently enough, failing to terminate a topic properly)

All of the above comprehension and production symptoms are exacerbated as the cognitive demands of the communicative task or context increase. For example, for many patients with RHD, nominal discourse comprehension or production problems would be expected when they are conversing in a typical one-on-one situation with a familiar partner about a common and straightforward topic. In contrast, these same patients might be predicted to demonstrate conversational difficulties in a group discussion with unfamiliar communicative partners when the conversational topic is unusual and the communicative setting is novel.

Possible Sources of Pragmatic and Discourse Symptoms. Research has focused on determining processing deficits that might underlie pragmatic and discourse-level comprehension and production problems associated with RHD (for a more comprehensive review, see Tompkins, 2012). For example, several investigators have suggested that other cognitive deficits (e.g., attention, working memory) cause or contribute to the pragmatic and discourse impairments of patients with RHD (Griffin et al., 2006; Lehman Blake, 2003; Martin & McDonald, 2003). For instance, sustained and focused attention deficits may interfere with the ability of patients with RHD to process and select relevant contextual cues, which in turn may result in misinterpretation of their conversational partners' discourse output, inappropriate selection of their own conversational content or style, or both.

Another hypothesis is that patients with RHD have difficulties suppressing word meanings or discourse interpretations that are irrelevant or incompatible with the communicative context (Fassbinder & Tompkins, 2001; Tompkins, 2012; Tompkins, Fassbinder, Blake, Baumgaertner, & Jayaram, 2004; Tompkins, Lehman Blake, Baumgaertner, & Fassbinder, 2001; Tomkins, Fassbinder, et al., 2008). Inefficient or inappropriate suppression may be particularly problematic in contexts in which patients must make revisions to their preliminary interpretations of the linguistic stimuli, as is necessary when understanding jokes or following complex story plots. That is, empirical studies have documented that patients with RHD can often generate multiple interpretations of ambiguous utterances such as "My uncle fell off the bank" (i.e., the river bank vs. place of finance), but within a discourse comprehension task, are slow to reject the interpretation that doesn't fit the discourse context (e.g., "My uncle fell off the bank. He shouldn't have gone fishing when it was wet and slippery from rain"). Such deficits could affect not only their understanding of discordant or ambiguous information but also their verbal output choices (Kennedy, 2000). For example, failure to suppress certain discourse or vocabulary options might result in including irrelevant information or inappropriate word selections.

Other researchers have suggested that compromised social cognition or Theory of Mind abilities may be responsible for the pragmatic and discourse problems associated with RHD (Brownell, Griffin, Winner, Friedman, & Happe, 2000; Champagne-Lavau & Joanette, 2009; Griffin et al., 2006; Happé, Brownell, & Winner, 1999). **Social cognition** encompasses our knowledge of social rules and conventions, and guides our interpretation of others' social actions, as well as generation of our own social actions and responses (Eslinger, Moore, Anderson, & Grossman, 2011; McDonald, 2012). Similarly, **Theory of Mind**, a construct more frequently encountered in the child development literature, refers to our ability to appreciate that other people may have knowledge and beliefs that differ from ours (Brownell et al., 2000; Martin & McDonald, 2003). Although prior research indicated that patients with RHD have difficulties on causal inference tasks that involve construing a character's motives (e.g., Happé et al., 1999), more recent work by Tompkins, Scharp, Fassbinder, and colleagues (2008) suggested that difficulties dealing with complex stimuli—regardless of whether they involved social inferencing—(rather than Theory of Mind deficits) could account for the performance pattern of RHD patients. Indeed, other researchers have noted that broader, perhaps domain-general problems with complex, executive abilities (e.g., inferencing, integration, awareness) may be an alternate or additional source of the social inferencing and pragmatic problems following onset of RHD, as well as other neurogenic disorders (Champagne-Lavau & Joanette, 2009; Eslinger et al., 2011; Martin & McDonald, 2003; Tompkins, 2012).

Further investigation of factors that contribute to the variety of pragmatic and discourse symptoms observed following RHD is needed (Lehman Blake, 2007; McDonald, 2000; Tompkins, 2012; Tompkins, Scharp, Fassbinder et al., 2008); the findings of such research will be essential to helping clinicians identify and subsequently treat patients with RHD who are most at risk for these high-level language difficulties that have the potential to severely restrict resumption of social and vocational relationships and activities.

Here's Some Bad News... and Here's Some MORE Bad News

When learning about neurogenic language and cognitive disorders, it is useful to consider impairments individually to appreciate how they uniquely impact communicative function. In reality, however, patients frequently present with a combination of neurogenic language and cognitive disorders. Consider Mrs. Kelsey, who was diagnosed with frontotemporal dementia (see Chapter 3 for a description of this type of dementia) following a 12-month decline in cognitive and communicative function. Not long after this diagnosis, she experienced a left middle cerebral artery stroke, resulting in significant aphasia. Her history of cognitive impairment complicated the diagnostic and rehabilitative processes. Not only did the clinician have to discriminate premorbid from newly acquired impairments, but she also had to select management strategies that did not rely heavily on intact executive function. Mrs. Kelsey's family struggled with the new setback in her status and expressed pessimism that intervention, in any form, could benefit the patient.

Fortunately, Mrs. Kelsey experienced a degree of spontaneous recovery and was able to express a desire to receive a course of speech-language therapy to maximize her communicative potential. Somewhat ironically, the new stroke ended up being to Mrs. Kelsey's advantage, as she had exhausted her insurance's allotment for therapy given the diagnosis of frontotemporal dementia. The new diagnosis of stroke and aphasia triggered a new allotment of sessions, and the clinician was able to address not only the difficulties associated with the new aphasia but also the declines in cognitive function that had occurred since therapy had been discontinued. Mrs. Kelsey's family members, who participated in the therapeutic process, ultimately expressed satisfaction with her therapy, with respect to both Mrs. Kelsey's language abilities and their own success in implementing communicative and cognitive strategies.

Traumatic Brain Injury

Traumatic brain injury (TBI) results when external forces (e.g., sudden impact of striking one's head on a car dashboard in a car accident, or on the ground because of a fall) cause brain damage that leads to loss or alteration of consciousness, and/or temporary or permanent physical, cognitive, emotional, and behavioral impairments (Cornis-Pop et al., 2012; National Head Injury Foundation Task Force on Special Education, 1989). Similar to RHD, communication problems following TBI are typically referred to as "cognitive-communicative disorders" to capture that for most TBI patients, there is a stronger cognitive, rather than linguistic, basis to their communicative limitations. Typically, the type and severity of cognitive-communicative disorders displayed by a given patient with TBI will depend on the patient's stage of TBI recovery and the location and extent of his or her brain damage. Whereas Chapter 3 provides further description of the mechanisms of TBI, a summary of cognitive and communicative symptoms associated with TBI is presented in this chapter.

Stages of Recovery

As patients recover from a TBI, they may progress through one or more of the following stages: (1) a period of impaired consciousness, (2) post-traumatic amnesia or a phase of severe confusion and disorientation, (3) a rapid recovery phase of about three to six months in which they experience significant progress, and (4) a long-term-plateau recovery phase in which they experience more gradual progress. Understanding these recovery phases is germane to providing families with appropriate education and counseling, particularly during the acute stages, in which patients may have impaired consciousness or profound confusion. Accordingly, a more detailed description of disorders of consciousness and post-traumatic amnesia is provided below.

Disorders of Consciousness

Coma. Patients who are in a **coma** exhibit no or minimal organized or purposeful response to external stimuli within their environment, including intrinsic stimulation or need (e.g., hunger) (Giacino & Whyte, 2005; R. S. Howard, 2008). That is, even following exposure to painful, tactile, auditory, olfactory, kinesthetic, or visual stimuli, these patients display no overt behavioral responses. Coma is more likely if the TBI was associated with rotational external forces; if there is diffuse, bilateral cortical and subcortical brain damage; and if the areas of the brain associated with arousal and awareness are compromised (e.g., brain stem regions such as the reticular formation) (R. S. Howard, 2008; Zeman, 1997).

In the acute stages, coma duration and depth are quantified and qualified because these variables can help guide predictions about survival and head injury severity (Formisano et al., 2004; R. S. Howard, 2008; Lieberman et al., 2003). For example, when diagnosing TBI severity, one of the criteria relates to coma duration (Yeates, 2010): (a) In mild TBI, if there is loss of consciousness, it must be for less than 30 minutes; (b) in moderate TBI, coma persists longer than 30 minutes but less than 24 hours; and (c) in severe TBI, coma may persist for 24 hours or longer (see also Table 2-7). To document coma depth, the Glasgow Coma Scale (GCS) (G. Teasdale & Jennett, 1976) is most frequently used. For this scale, clinicians determine the patient's level of eye opening (e.g., never opens eyes vs. will open eyes if asked to do so), best verbal response (e.g., produces only sounds and unintelligible word approximations vs. produces words but these words do not make sense), and best motor response (e.g., displays abnormal extension posture vs. can complete simple motor tasks). GCS scores vary from a minimum of 3, indicating no response to external stimulation, to 15, indicating good orientation and alertness. When patients' scores rise above 8, they are no longer considered to be in a comatose state.

Vegetative State. Whereas most patients with TBI will progress from coma to a phase of post-traumatic amnesia, a small percentage will appear to awaken from coma (i.e., open their eyes) but will continue to demonstrate no willful, sustained, or reproducible

TABLE 2-7
Criteria for Severity Levels of Traumatic Brain Injury

SEVERITY LEVEL	TIME IN COMA	TIME IN POST-TRAUMATIC AMNESIA	GLASGOW COMA SCALE SCORE	OTHER
Mild	<30 minutes	<24 hours	13-15	Transient neurological abnormalities (e.g., seizure)
Moderate	≥30 minutes but <24 hours	≥24 hours but <1 week	9-12	
Severe	≥24 hours	≥1 week	3-8	

interaction with their external or internal environment and no communication ability (Giacino & Malone, 2008; R. S. Howard, 2008; Zeman, 1997). The term **vegetative state** may be used to describe patients with this type of consciousness disorder. If the vegetative state persists for longer than one month, the term "persistent vegetative state" may be applied, and if it persists for longer than a year after a TBI, it may be referred to as "permanent vegetative state." Although "vegetative" may be construed to have negative connotations, it is used to indicate that essential (i.e., "vegetative") life-sustaining abilities—such as breathing, digestion, and sleep-wake cycles—have recovered. In addition to eye opening, patients in this state also may display abnormal or spontaneous motor responses, such as primitive reflexes (e.g., grasp reflex), teeth grinding, chewing, and even smiling or grunting. Vegetative state is most frequently seen in patients with TBI who suffer profound cortical damage but have relatively intact brain stem functioning (Beuthien-Baumann et al., 2003). The longer the duration of vegetative state, the less likely it is that patients, regardless of age, will show improvements, and after one year in this state, it is unlikely that patients will recover even a rudimentary awareness of their environment (R. S. Howard, 2008; Zeman, 1997).

> **Persistent Vegetative State: Hot Topic in the News**
>
> Worldwide, management of persistent vegetative state (PVS) remains a hot topic, given some of the cases that have received widespread coverage in the popular media. For example, in the 1980s, there was a case involving Nancy Cruzan, a young woman who, subsequent to a severe TBI, entered into PVS. After three years of being in PVS, the woman's parents asked for the "right to die" for their daughter, given that she would not have wanted to live in such a state. Because the young woman had completed a living will, however, the State of Missouri would not approve the parents' request, a decision with which the U.S. Supreme Court later upheld. Ultimately, further evidence was obtained to document that it was indeed the woman's wish not to be treated in the case of such medical circumstance. The courts approved the withdrawal of artificial nutrition and hydration, leading to the woman's passing. For further description of this case, as well as other publicized cases pertaining to vegetative state, see R. S. Howard (2008).

Minimally Conscious State. Subsequent to coma or vegetative state, some patients may progress into a **minimally conscious state**, in which there are minimal but distinct intermittent periods of self- and environmental awareness (Costa & deMarco, 2011; Giacino & Malone, 2008; R. S. Howard, 2008). To receive this diagnosis, a patient must demonstrate at least one of the following: (a) attempts to follow simple commands; (b) can produce a yes/no response, regardless of accuracy or modality; (c) can produce intelligible verbal output; and/or (d) produces nonstereotypical movements or behaviors either spontaneously (but not reflexively) or in response to stimulation (e.g., visually tracks someone as he or she walks across the room). According to Giacino and Whyte (2005), a patient progresses out of the minimally conscious state once he or she can either (a) respond, in any modality, to six yes/no questions across two consecutive evaluations and thus demonstrate reliable and consistent communication, or (b) distinguish and use at least two common objects across two consecutive evaluations and thus demonstrate functional object use.

Post-Traumatic Amnesia. Fortunately, the majority of patients who emerge from coma will progress into a phase of **post-traumatic amnesia (PTA)** rather than a vegetative state. PTA refers to an acute and commonly temporary recovery phase in which patients are extremely confused and disoriented. More specifically, patients in PTA are disoriented to person (e.g., their name, marital status, address, birthday), time, and place; have incoherent language output and impaired language comprehension; and experience emotional and behavioral disturbances, such as marked agitation, **lability** (i.e., difficulty controlling one's emotions), impulsivity, and possible physical or verbal aggression. These symptoms are related to severe memory, attention, and executive function deficits that include problems remembering daily events and circumstances that transpired prior to and since their TBI; impaired sustained and focused attention (i.e., poor concentration); decreased processing speed; and impaired awareness of their cognitive, physical, and behavioral difficulties. Because of these widespread cognitive problems, the term "post-traumatic confusion" may be used instead of PTA to denote that these patients' problems extend well beyond amnesia.

Given their substantial attention, memory, and executive function impairments, patients do not typically remember their time in PTA. In fact, the criterion for emerging from PTA is the return of continuous, accurate, and reliable memory. Like coma duration, length of PTA can provide information pertaining to TBI severity, in that the longer patients remain in PTA, the more likely it is that they will have persistent symptoms and poorer functional recovery (Formisano et al., 2004; Yeates, 2010). Table 2-7 lists the lengths of PTA associated with the different severities of TBI, along with other TBI severity criteria. Because of the significant confusion and agitation associated with this phase of recovery, formal assessment and active rehabilitation services do not begin until patients with TBI have emerged from PTA.

Cognitive Symptoms

Regardless of head injury severity, deficits of perception, attention, memory, and executive functioning are a frequent if not an invariable consequence of TBI and, in many cases, are stronger predictors of functional outcome than physical status (Bush et al., 2003; Cornis-Pop et al., 2012; Hoofien, Gilboa, Vakil, & Barak, 2004) (see included DVD: Patient 2). The exact type and severity of these cognitive disorders will be dependent, at least in part, on the location and extent of neural structures and pathways that were compromised by the head injury. For instance, if a given patient with TBI suffered brain damage that was more prominent in the right hemisphere, that patient's perception, attention, memory, and executive functioning deficits would most likely be similar to those previously described for patients with RHD. As will be reviewed in Chapter 3, however, certain brain regions are especially vulnerable in head trauma (e.g., frontal lobes, anterior portions of the temporal lobes), and thus certain cognitive symptoms are particularly common following TBI. Accordingly, what follows is a description of attention, memory, and executive functioning problems associated with TBI, with a special emphasis on those that occur most frequently. Perceptual problems are not reviewed here, as when they occur, they will include one or more of the auditory and/or visual perceptual deficits described in the preceding section on RHD symptoms.

Attention Problems

Attention impairments are widespread among patients with TBI, regardless of their head injury severity (Azouvi, Couillet, Leclereq, Martin, Asloun, & Rousseaux, 2004; Azouvi, Vallat-Azouvi, & Belmont, 2009; Galbiati et al., 2009; King & Kirwilliam, 2011; Ziino & Ponsford, 2006), and are important to quantify and qualify because they can contribute to other cognitive deficits (e.g., memory and executive functioning), communication problems (e.g., difficulty with topic maintenance or switching due to sustained or alternating attention limitations, respectively), and, consequently, poor rehabilitation and functional outcomes (Ginstfeldt & Emanuelson, 2010; Knight et al., 2006; Slovarp, Azuma, & LaPointe, 2012). Attention problems are typically most apparent acutely, particularly when patients are still in PTA. In the earlier stages of recovery, it is not uncommon for most, if not all, attention functions (i.e., sustained, selective, alternating, and divided attention) to be severely compromised. Because of these often profound attention impairments, most patients are inappropriate candidates for formal assessment or direct treatment at this point in their recovery because they lack the fundamental attention skills necessary to attend to the clinician, process task stimuli, and plan and carry out task responses.

As patients emerge from PTA, deficits of more basic attention functions (i.e., attention orienting) tend to resolve rapidly while impairment of more complex attention skills persist (Ginstfeldt & Emanuelson, 2010; King & Kirwilliam, 2011; Ryan & Warden, 2003). Several case reports indicate that left or right neglect syndrome may be another long-term attention problem following TBI (e.g., Cocchini, Beschin, & Della Sala, 2002; Grossi, Lepore, Napolitano, & Trojano, 2001). More frequently, however, patients with TBI in the chronic stages of recovery, particularly those who have suffered mild injuries, will demonstrate relatively intact attention functioning during simple or more routine daily activities, but will continue to report or display enduring attention problems when completing cognitively demanding tasks or when exposed to highly distracting or stressful environments (Azouvi et al., 2004, 2009; Cornis-Pop et al., 2012; King & Kirwilliam, 2011). Even when they may be performing attention tasks well, such performance may come at a greater cost: Compared to their non–brain-damaged peers, TBI patients report higher fatigue when completing attention tasks and also show physiological signs (e.g., overactivation in neural regions supporting attention; greater increases in blood pressure) that they are putting forth great effort to complete such tasks (M. Kramer et al., 2008; Ziino & Ponsford, 2006).

Memory Problems

A variety of memory abilities are compromised by TBI and can lead to problems completing many everyday activities, poor vocational and educational outcomes, and, relatedly, high levels of caregiver burden (Azouvi et al., 2009; Schmitter-Edgecombe & Wright, 2004; Vakil, 2005) (see included DVD: Patients 2, 4). Even in cases of mild TBI, working memory appears to be particularly vulnerable following TBI (Azouvi et al., 2009; King & Kirwilliam, 2011; Slovarp et al., 2012): Impairments of the executive component of working memory are reported more frequently than the buffer components, which appear to remain relatively preserved subsequent to TBI. Furthermore, working memory deficits appear to be strongly associated with a number of TBI language impairments, including poor auditory comprehension and discourse production problems, such as inadequate use of pronoun antecedents (Bittner & Crowe, 2006; Moran & Gillon, 2004; Turkstra & Holland, 1998). Problems with memory encoding and strategic learning (i.e., the ability to focus on learning the most important or relevant information while disregarding less important or relevant information) are also common subsequent to TBI (Cook, DePompei, & Chapman, 2011; Gamino, Chapman, & Cook, 2009; Geary, Kraus, Rubin, Pliskin, & Little, 2010), including lack or ineffective use of encoding strategies (e.g., semantic clustering, chunking, rehearsal). Whereas all aspects of long-term memory may be negatively affected by TBI, most frequently problems with episodic memory are reported, including difficulties with recency discrimination (i.e., how long ago in one's past an event or episode occurred) and prospective memory (Knight et al., 2006; Manning, Gordon, Pearlson, & Schretlen, 2007; Vakil, 2005).

Often episodic and other long-term memory deficits are part of **retrograde amnesia** in patients with TBI, which may be continuous or interrupted (i.e., intermittent "islands" of memories stored prior to the TBI are inaccessible) (Azouvi et al., 2009; Piolino et al., 2007; Vakil, 2005). Over time, most patients experience a shrinkage in their amnesia (i.e., a reduction in the amount of their past declarative and/or nondeclarative memories that they cannot recall); however, they typically are never able to recall the circumstances of their accident, most likely because the sudden onset of their brain damage interfered with encoding the events that occurred immediately prior to and during their accident.

Anterograde amnesia is another common memory problem following TBI that relates to difficulties storing and retrieving new long-term memories or, more generally, new information, regardless of modality (Azouvi et al., 2009; Mathias, Beall, & Bigler, 2004; Vakil, 2005). Anterograde amnesia will directly affect TBI patients' orientation; that is, in the presence of anterograde amnesia, maintaining orientation to the date and one's location and circumstance (e.g., nature of one's injuries) is difficult. In many cases, inadequate use of deliberate encoding (e.g., chunking, semantic associations) and retrieval strategies, as mentioned above, underlies anterograde memory problems.

For instance, researchers have shown that the word-list recall of patients with TBI can be significantly improved if they are given training in the use of encoding strategies (Azouvi et al., 2009; Richardson & Barry, 1985).

Even though many aspects of memory are susceptible to TBI, others are commonly spared or relatively intact, and it is these memory skills that are often exploited in cognitive rehabilitation programs (see Chapter 9). More specifically, procedural and other types of nondeclarative memory are often areas of relative strength for many patients with TBI, even those who have suffered severe injuries (Azouvi et al., 2009; Vakil, 2005; Ward, Shum, Dick, McKinlay, & Baker-Tweney, 2004). Indeed, recent investigations have identified positive outcomes when treatment involved the use of the patients' procedural memory skills to learn verbal, visual, and other forms of new information (Cohen et al., 2010; Lloyd, Riley, & Powell, 2009; Turkstra, 2001).

Executive Functioning Problems

Given that the neural regions proposed to support executive functioning (e.g., frontal lobes) are frequently damaged in TBI, it is not surprising that executive function deficits—including disinhibition, anosognosia, concrete and/or inflexible problem solving and reasoning, lack of initiation, and poor planning—are pervasive among patients representing the spectrum of TBI severity levels (Azouvi et al., 2009; Godefroy et al., 2010; Miotto et al., 2010; Morton & Barker, 2010) (see included DVD: Patients 2, 4, 7). These high-level cognitive problems may be due to impairments of the executive functions themselves or to deficits in one or more of the other cognitive domains (e.g., attention) that support executive functioning (O'Keeffe, Dockree, Moloney, Carton, & Robertson, 2007; Rath et al., 2004; Rios, Perianez, & Munoz-Cespedes, 2004). Further, given the complexity of executive functions, an impairment of a given executive function may reflect a deficit in one or more subcomponent abilities. For example, a problem-solving deficit might reflect a deficiency in one or more of the following abilities: (a) identification of the problem, (b) generation of possible solutions, (c) selection of the most appropriate solution, (d) execution of that solution, or (e) determination of whether the problem was resolved (W. Gordon, Cantor, Ashman, & Brown, 2006). Relatedly, different types of **anosognosia**, or awareness deficits, have been identified (O'Keeffe et al., 2007; Sohlberg & Mateer, 2001). In an intellectual awareness deficit, patients fail to understand that a certain ability (or several abilities) is impaired, whereas in an emergent awareness deficit, patients might be able to acknowledge they have a deficit but remain unable to recognize when that deficit is negatively affecting their performance or well-being. Finally, in an anticipatory awareness deficit, patients have difficulty identifying when a problem might occur in the future.

Importantly, research suggests that executive function deficits underlie certain pragmatic and discourse-level communication symptoms in patients with TBI (McDonald & Flanagan, 2004; Turkstra & Flora, 2002). Executive function deficits that appear to be particularly influential negative outcome predictors and sources of caregiver distress include unawareness of deficits and cognitive inflexibility (Hart et al., 2003; Hoofien et al., 2004; Morton & Barker, 2010). Thus, the detection and treatment of executive function impairments will be vital to success of TBI patients in rehabilitation and in their eventual social, educational, and vocational reintegration.

Communication Symptoms

Variable language profiles may result following TBI. For example, if patients suffer more discrete dominant hemisphere lesions subsequent to their TBI, they may present with language symptoms consistent with an aphasia diagnosis (Demir et al., 2006; Vukovic et al., 2008) (see included DVD: Patients 4, 7). More frequently, however, TBI is associated with more diffuse brain damage, and in these cases, pragmatic and discourse deficits beyond the lexical-semantic or morphosyntactic levels are most prominent (Coelho, 2007; Dardier et al., 2011; J. Douglas, 2010; McDonald & Flanagan, 2004) (see included DVD: Patient 2). Like cognitive-communicative disorders associated with RHD, pragmatic and discourse production and comprehension problems are proposed to be primarily a product of other cognitive deficits (e.g., Theory of Mind and social cognition issues, impaired focus attention, working memory limitations) rather than solely a disordered linguistic system, and accordingly are also referred to as "cognitive-communicative disorders." Regardless of lesion location, anomia is fairly common subsequent to TBI, in which the speed (rather than the accuracy) of lexical-retrieval processing appears particularly vulnerable (Bittner & Crowe, 2006; Douglas, 2010; Miotto et al., 2010).

Overall, there is much overlap in the types of cognitive-communicative symptoms associated with TBI and those associated with RHD, which were already described in this chapter. For example, frequently reported pragmatic and discourse deficits following TBI, regardless of severity, include poor topic management skills (e.g., excessive or infrequent topic initiation, inappropriate or egocentric topic choices [see included DVD: Patient 2b]), turn-taking issues (e.g., monopolizing or failing to contribute to the conversation), inadequate discourse cohesion (e.g., nonspecific use of pronouns), decreased discourse informativeness (e.g., inclusion of irrelevant details, confabulation, perseveration) (see included DVD: Patient 7), impaired macrostructure (e.g., failure to include or correctly sequence essential story episodes), and difficulties processing implied information or figurative language (e.g., problems identifying the moral of a story, concrete interpretation of indirect speech acts) (Angeleri et al., 2008; Carlomagno, Giannotti, Vorano, & Marini, 2011; Coelho, 2007; Dardier et al., 2011; Douglas, 2010; M. Wong, Murdoch, & Whelan, 2010). Like patients with RHD, TBI survivors are more likely to demonstrate pragmatic and discourse difficulties when the social setting or communicative activity is more demanding or unfamiliar (e.g., responding to hints such as "It's noisy in here" would be more difficult than responding to conventional indirect requests such as "Could you turn down the television?").

Again, the types of cognitive-communicative problems exhibited by a given patient with TBI will be dependent on, at least in part, the location of that patient's brain damage and the other cognitive abilities that have been compromised. For instance, patients with TBI who suffer damage to orbitofrontal regions are often highly disinhibited; thus, their language output and input abilities reflect this disinhibition (e.g., excessive topic switching, inappropriate vocabulary or topic choices). In contrast, patients with TBI with damage to the dorsolateral frontal cortex are frequently apathetic (i.e., impaired initiation) and, accordingly, are more likely to have more passive or impoverished language profiles (e.g., infrequent conversational initiation or turns, incomplete responses). Because of the direct relationship between pragmatics and successful social interactions, appropriate management of pragmatic and discourse problems is essential to facilitating resumption of participation in previous or new social activities for patients with TBI.

Dementia

Dementia refers to a set of cognitive, communicative, and behavioral symptoms that are caused by a variety of progressive medical or neurological conditions (see included DVD: Patients 8, 9). More specifically, a diagnosis of dementia will be considered if patients demonstrate, in addition to memory problems, unremitting deterioration in one or more of the following areas: perception, language, executive functioning, or praxis (Alzheimer's Association, 2012; American Psychiatric Association, 1994); additionally, these symptoms must be sufficiently significant so that they negatively affect daily social and occupational functioning. This latter criterion is particularly important when distinguishing dementia from another possible diagnosis, **mild cognitive impairment (MCI)**. Mild cognitive impairment is identified when an individual demonstrates a cognitive decline that is greater than that expected, given that individual's age and level of education (Alzheimer's Association, 2012; Libon et al., 2010); however, the cognitive decline in MCI should not be interfering with the individual's social and vocational functioning. Cognitive decline in MCI may be circumscribed, affecting just one cognitive domain (e.g., amnestic MCI, in which only memory is problematic), or multidomain (e.g., memory and word retrieval difficulties). Although MCI does not interfere with daily activities, it is of concern given that compared to healthy aging adults, individuals with MCI are at greater risk for developing dementia.

The types, severity, and breadth of cognitive and communicative symptoms with which a patient with dementia presents will be dependent on (a) what disease (e.g., Alzheimer's vs. Parkinson's vs. Lewy body disease) is causing the dementia, as different diseases will affect different brain regions and different neurotransmitter systems (see Chapter 3 for a description of some of the more common reversible and irreversible causes of dementia), and (b) the disease stage in which the patient currently is (e.g., subtle vs. profound changes during early vs. late stages, respectively). Accordingly, dementia is characterized by a diverse set of communicative and cognitive impairments, most of which have already been described in the preceding aphasia, RHD, and TBI sections of this chapter. Because many of these specific symptoms have been previously reviewed, a more general summary of cognitive and communication problems associated with dementia is provided below.

Dementia Types Based on Lesion Location

Dementia sometimes has been classified on the basis of what part of the brain is involved in the dementing disease or condition. For example, the dementia associated with Alzheimer's disease and Pick's disease is sometimes referred to as "cortical dementia" because the pathological changes associated with each of these diseases primarily affects cortical areas. In contrast, Parkinson's disease, Huntington's disease, progressive supranuclear palsy, Wilson's disease, and multiple sclerosis are associated with subcortical dementia because each of these diseases produces alterations in primarily subcortical structures. This classification system also was designed to demarcate differences in the cognitive and behavioral profiles of patients with cortical versus subcortical dementia. For example, in subcortical dementia, initial symptoms are typically motoric in nature (e.g., dysarthria, gait disturbances), while language abilities remain intact. In contrast, in cortical dementia, initial symptoms are typically cognitive or behavioral in nature, and language is compromised.

Over the past two decades, however, research has accumulated to indicate that patients with subcortical dementia may present with both language comprehension and production difficulties (L. Murray, 2000b, 2008b; L. Murray & Stout, 1999), and, in at least some cases, their initial symptoms may consist of cognitive or behavioral problems (NINDS, 2010, 2011a; Troster, 2011). In fact, there is overlap not only in terms of cognitive profiles but also in terms of which areas of the brain are damaged in cortical and subcortical dementia (Alzheimer's Association, 2012; Julian, 2011; Ritchie & Lovestone, 2002). Consequently, clinicians would be well advised to avoid the terms "cortical dementia" and "subcortical dementia" when describing their patients with dementia.

Perceptual Problems

Because auditory and visual perceptual problems are often a product of either right hemisphere damage or bilateral brain damage, and because many dementing diseases cause not only right hemisphere but also bilateral brain damage, perceptual disorders are common among patients with dementia (Alzheimer's Association, 2012; Barton, 2011; Chu & Selwyn, 2011; Lewis et al., 2006; Troster, 2011; Uc et al., 2006) (see Table 2-6). For example, because Alzheimer's disease affects predominantly posterior regions of both hemispheres, patients with this disease often display problems with both basic and complex visuospatial discrimination, prosopagnosia (i.e., facial recognition deficits), achromatopsia (i.e., problems perceiving colors), or propopagnosia (i.e., a disorder in which patients do not recognize their own image in a mirror) (Barton, 2011; Fukui & Lee, 2009; Oda, Ohkawa, & Maeda, 2008). In contrast, patients with frontotemporal dementia, which, as the name implies, affects predominately anterior brain regions, may be more likely to present with auditory perceptual deficits, including auditory agnosia and complex nonverbal sound perception difficulties (Goll et al., 2010; Kaga, Nakamura, Takayama, & Momose, 2004). Importantly, perceptual problems can have negative effects on the language and other cognitive abilities of patients with dementia and, consequently, on their completion of a variety of daily activities (Fukui & Lee, 2009; Glosser et al., 2002; Rankin et al., 2009; Uc et al., 2006).

Attention Problems

All attention functions and modalities may be compromised in dementia, with attention problems one of the earliest symptoms in many types of dementia (C. G. Ballard, 2004; Chiu et al., 2004; Chu & Selwyn, 2011; Sieroff, Piquard, Avclair, Lacomblez, Derovesne, & Laberge, 2004; Troster, 2011). Whereas in the early stages of most dementing diseases, only more complex aspects of attention (e.g., attention switching, divided attention) are deficient, as these diseases progress, more basic attention functions (e.g., sustained attention) will also deteriorate. As with the other cognitive domains, there is heterogeneity in the types and severity of attention problems observed across dementing diseases. For example, attention problems are prominent in the early and middle stages of dementia with Lewy bodies, more so than in Alzheimer's or Parkinson's disease (Mahendra, Scullion, & Hamerschlag, 2011; K. W. Park et al., 2011).

It should also be noted that neglect syndrome may occur in some forms of dementia (Ishiai et al., 2000; Liu, McDowd, & Lin, 2004; Oda et al., 2008). Although neglect does not appear to be a frequent problem, Foldi, LoBosco, and Schaefer (2002) have suggested that (a) other cognitive problems mask neglect symptoms, (b) only a subset of patients with predominantly right hemisphere involvement develop neglect, and/or (c) bilateral neural deterioration nullifies attentional bias effects and, thus, patients have problems attending to both sides.

Memory Problems

Strikingly different memory profiles can be observed among patients with dementia, depending on the etiology of their dementia. For example, in **Alzheimer's disease (AD)**, persistent memory decline is a hallmark symptom, even in the earliest stages of the disease (Mahendra et al., 2011; Park et al., 2011; Xie et al., 2010) (see included DVD: Patient 8). Over time, patients with AD will deteriorate from initially mild working and episodic memory problems (e.g., disoriented to place, misplacing personal items) to profound anterograde and retrograde amnesia and thus impairment of most memory stores and functions (e.g., working memory, episodic memory, semantic memory, encoding and retrieval strategies). Interestingly, however, procedural memory remains an area of relative strength well into the disease process, a finding that has been capitalized on in many dementia treatment programs (see Chapter 10).

In contrast to the pattern of memory decline associated with AD, less prominent memory problems are observed in the early stages of other forms of dementia, including the progressive nonfluent aphasia and behavioral variants of frontotemporal dementia (J. Reilly, Rodriguez, Lamy, & Neils-Strunjas, 2010; Xie et al., 2010). In other dementias, circumscribed rather than broad memory deficits are observed. For example, in dementias associated with primarily subcortical degeneration (e.g., Parkinson's disease), procedural memory appears most vulnerable (Park et al., 2011; Zgaljardic, Borod, Foldi, & Mattis, 2003). As the name implies, the semantic dementia variant of frontotemporal dementia is characterized by semantic memory deficits with relative preservation of other declarative and nondeclarative memory abilities (Kertesz, 2010; Rosen & Viskontas, 2008). Despite these different patterns of memory decline, the vast majority of patients in the final stages of dementia will experience significant impairment of most (if not all) aspects of memory.

Executive Functioning Problems

Patients with dementia, regardless of the etiology of their dementia, invariably present with some form of executive dysfunctioning (Godefroy et al., 2010; Kertesz, 2010; Troster, 2011). As just discussed with respect to memory problems, however, the type and severity of executive dysfunctioning can vary dramatically across the many dementing diseases. For instance, in the behavioral variant of frontotemporal dementia, the most striking initial symptoms are typically executive function deficits, such as cognitive and social disinhibition, anosognosia, perseveration, and cognitive inflexibility (Eslinger et al., 2011; Kertesz, 2010). In contrast, in AD, executive function problems such as impaired reasoning and planning are less prominent compared to memory and language impairments, and, according to some research, are possibly a product of other cognitive deficits (Godefroy et al., 2010; Park et al., 2011; Slachevsky et al., 2004). In **Parkinson's disease** (see included DVD: Patient 9), early deterioration of executive functioning is also common, but at least some of these executive function deficits, such as initiation and planning problems, are infrequently observed in early frontotemporal dementia (Godefroy et al., 2010; Pagni et al., 2011; Troster, 2011). Regardless of these differences, by the middle and late stages of most dementing diseases, executive function deficits are significant and typically result in complete patient dependence and, consequently, significant caregiver burden (S. T. Chen, Sultzer, Hinkin, Mahler, & Cummings, 1998; Godefroy et al., 2010; Torti, Gwyther, Reed, Friedman, & Schulman, 2004).

Communication Symptoms

Communication problems are common in dementia, regardless of etiology (Kempler & Goral, 2008; Reilly et al., 2010; Rousseaux, Seve, et al., 2010; Zgaljardic et al., 2003), but the profile of language symptoms varies across dementia types. In the early stages of AD and many cases of vascular dementia, language problems such as anomia (particularly for nouns) (see included DVD: Patient 9b), writing difficulties (see included DVD: Patient 8n), and impaired comprehension of complex or figurative linguistic material are prominent symptoms (Kempler & Goral, 2008; Mahendra et al., 2011; L. Murray, 2010;

Neils-Strunjas, Groves-Wright, Mashima, & Harnish, 2006) (see included DVD: Patient 8i). In contrast, in the nonfluent progressive aphasia variant of frontotemporal dementia, morphosyntactic deficits and nonfluent output (see included DVD: Patient 10g) are often noted prior to or in addition to lexical-semantic difficulties (particularly for verbs), whereas the behavioral variant of frontotemporal dementia is characterized by relative preservation of speech and basic language abilities (Eslinger et al., 2011; Reilly et al., 2010). Furthermore, in other forms of dementia, such as that associated with Parkinson's disease, only more subtle, high-level language abilities (e.g., processing of complex, infrequent syntactic forms) appear compromised (L. Murray, 2008a; L. Murray & Stout, 1999; Rousseaux, Seve, et al., 2010).

By the middle stages of AD and some other dementing diseases (e.g., Huntington's disease, vascular dementia), language problems are more diverse and severe in that patients' spoken, written, and nonverbal output becomes vague, perseverative, and difficult to follow; their discourse skills begin to decline (e.g., impaired topic maintenance and shifting); and comprehension of both concrete and figurative spoken and written language becomes difficult (Groves-Wright, Neils-Strunjas, Burnett, & O'Neill, 2004; Kempler & Goral, 2008; Reilly et al., 2010; Rousseaux, Seve, et al., 2010). By the final stages of many forms of dementia, patients are often able to produce little meaningful output and often become completely mute. Their language comprehension abilities are similarly ravaged by whatever disease is causing their dementia.

The underlying source of communication disorders in patients with dementia will vary according to not only the etiology of their dementia, but also the stage or severity of their dementing illness. For instance, the word retrieval and comprehension deficits of patients with the semantic dementia variant of frontotemporal dementia are a product of their semantic memory impairments (Gorno-Tempini et al., 2011; Reilly et al., 2010), whereas the syntactic processing difficulties of patients with Parkinson's disease have been associated with cognitive deficits such as attention and working memory limitations (Hochstadt, Nakano, Lieberman, & Friedman, 2006; L. Murray, 2008a). In Alzheimer's disease, word retrieval difficulties may initially reflect problems with lexical access, but over time, spoken and written word retrieval will be additionally compromised by semantic memory and other cognitive impairments (e.g., perseveration, selective attention deficits) (Kempler & Goral, 2008; Neils-Strunjas et al., 2006).

Because communication abilities are necessary not only for the completion of daily activities (e.g., reading directions on medications) but also to maintain social interactions, research indicates that the communication breakdown associated with dementia can lead to problem behaviors (e.g., patients may act out because they are no longer able to communicate their needs), significant caregiver burden, and social isolation and depression in both the patient and the caregiver (J. A. Small, Geldart, & Gutman, 2000; J. A. Small, Geldart, Gutman, & Clarke Scott, 1998; Savundranayagam & Orange, 2011). Importantly, as will be reviewed in subsequent treatment chapters (Chapters 9 through 12), researchers are continuing to develop new approaches to helping patients with dementia maintain their communicative and cognitive abilities, despite the progressive nature of this adult neurogenic language and cognitive disorder.

Summary

The number, variety, and complexity of underlying linguistic and cognitive impairments characterizing neurogenic language and cognitive disorders can seem overwhelming. By considering the impairments within the framework of the process model depicted in Figure 1-3, however, readers may gain a clearer understanding of the relationships among impairments associated with the various neurogenic language disorders. The review of etiologies commonly associated with neurogenic language disorders provided in Chapter 3 will reveal additional relationships among impairments in body structure and body function and resulting communication limitations.

Discussion Questions

1. Which aphasia symptoms might be exhibited by non-aphasic individuals (i.e., people without cognitive or language impairment)? Discuss how these normal "slips" are like and unlike true aphasia.
2. Discuss the similarities and differences between the communication difficulties experienced by individuals with aphasia and those with right hemisphere disorders.
3. How are depictions of amnesia in popular media (movies, television, books) consistent with the descriptions presented in this text?
4. How are the memory impairments experienced by individuals with traumatic brain injury similar to and different from those experienced by individuals with dementia?

Neuropathology of Neurogenic Language and Cognitive Disorders

chapter 3

Learning Objectives

After reading this chapter, you should be able to:

- List the major arteries that provide blood flow to the brain
- Describe the two major types of stroke
- Identify different types of benign and malignant tumors
- Describe two infections that may cause neurogenic language disorders
- Contrast open head, closed head, and blast injury
- Differentiate primary and secondary forms of structural and physiological damage associated with traumatic head injury
- Distinguish between reversible and irreversible causes of dementia
- Describe at least two etiologies of irreversible dementia

Key Terms

- Alzheimer's disease (AD)
- aneurysm
- arteriovenous malformation (AVM)
- blast injury
- carotid arterial system
- closed head injury
- contrecoup effect
- diffuse axonal shearing
- embolus
- frontotemporal lobar degeneration (FTLD)
- hemorrhagic stroke
- hypoxic-ischemic brain injury
- irreversible dementia
- ischemic stroke
- open head injury
- paraneoplastic syndromes
- reversible dementia
- stroke/brain attack
- thrombosis
- transient ischemic attack (TIA)
- traumatic brain injury (TBI)
- tumor/neoplasm
- vascular dementia
- vertebrobasilar arterial system

Introduction

Neurogenic language and cognitive disorders are caused by a variety of pathologies that affect the structure and function of the central nervous system. The severity, type, and eventual outcome of our patients' neurogenic language and cognitive disorders will depend, at least in part, on the site and extent of their brain damage. Therefore, it is important that we, as clinicians, understand at least basic information about the nature, course, and medical treatment of these pathologies. This chapter provides a description of the major types of pathology that most frequently underlie acquired neurogenic linguistic and cognitive deficits.

Familiarity with these pathologies will not only enhance our competency in managing the neurogenic language and cognitive disorders experienced by our patients but also improve our skill in communicating more effectively with the variety of other professionals with whom we may interact in educational or health-care settings.

Stroke

A **stroke** refers to any disruption in blood flow to the brain. Sometimes referred to as "cerebrovascular accident" or, more recently, **brain attack**, stroke is the third leading cause of death following heart disease and cancer, and accounts for approximately 1 out of every 18 deaths in the United States (Roger et al., 2011). Stroke is also the leading cause of adult disability in the United States. Unfortunately, the number of new and recurrent stroke cases reported each year remains high, with an estimated 795,000 cases each year in the United States (Roger et al., 2011). Stroke also is the most common cause of aphasia (Code & Petheram, 2011; Sinanovic et al., 2011) and right hemisphere cognitive-communicative disorders (Lehman Blake et al., 2002; Tompkins, 1995), and it's the second-most-frequent cause of dementia (Fratiglioni & Rocca, 2001; Wharton et al., 2011). Despite these sobering statistics, several studies have documented inadequate public knowledge about stroke, including risk factors and symptoms (Fisher, 2003; Roger et al., 2011). For example, in 2007, Zerwic, Hwang, and Tucco reported that among patients who had already suffered a stroke, only about 60% could accurately identify one stroke risk factor and only about 55% could identify one stroke symptom.

As clinicians, it is our job to treat the variety of communication and cognitive deficits that may result from stroke. Because an important aspect of treatment involves educating our patients and their caregivers about stroke, as well as about their communication and cognitive problems, clinicians must be cognizant of the mechanisms, outcomes, and medical management of stroke. To better understand the causes and consequences of stroke, it is helpful first to review the normal pattern of blood supply to the brain.

Blood Supply

Although the brain typically accounts for only 2% of our body weight, it requires about 17% of our cardiac output and expends about 20% of the oxygen used by our entire body. Because the brain is unable to store oxygen, glucose, or other nutritional substances, even a brief interruption of blood flow can affect its functioning. For example, obstruction of blood flow for about 10 seconds will result in unconsciousness, and as little as two to three minutes of blood flow cessation may cause permanent brain damage. The body is able to meet the blood supply demands of the brain via two major arterial systems: the carotid and the vertebrobasilar systems. As depicted in Figure 3-1, both of these arterial systems arise from the aorta, the major artery from the heart. The brachiocephalic (innominate) artery comes directly off the right side of the aortic arch.

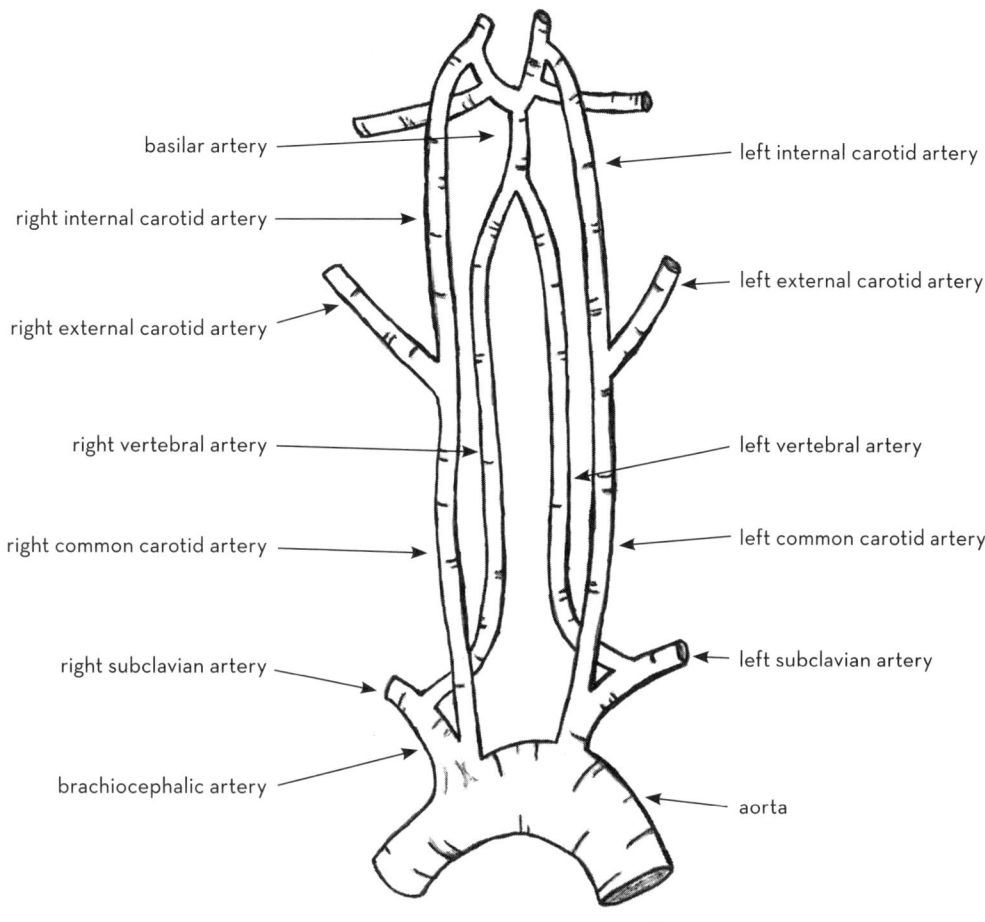

Figure 3-1. Carotid and vertebral basilar systems as they arise from the aorta. These two arterial systems are the basis of the cerebral vascular system.

This artery then subdivides into the right common carotid and right subclavian arteries. On the left side, the left common carotid comes off of the apex of the aortic arch, and then, in turn, sends off a branch, which is called the left subclavian artery.

The **carotid arterial system** begins at the left and right common carotid arteries. These two arteries ascend laterally to the trachea; at about the level of the larynx, each divides into external and internal carotid arteries. The internal carotid arteries are of particular importance because they enter the skull to provide the brain's anterior blood supply. Specifically, each internal carotid artery subdivides into an anterior and a middle cerebral artery. The anterior cerebral arteries supply the medial surfaces of the two cerebral hemispheres, as well as the superior borders of the frontal and parietal lobes (see Figures 3-2A and 3-2B). The middle cerebral arteries travel along the lateral fissure to supply most of the lateral surface of the cerebral hemispheres, including superior and lateral portions of the temporal lobes and the lateral surfaces of the frontal lobes (see Figure 3-2A). Consequently, the middle cerebral artery is of particular importance because it provides blood flow to the major speech and language brain areas

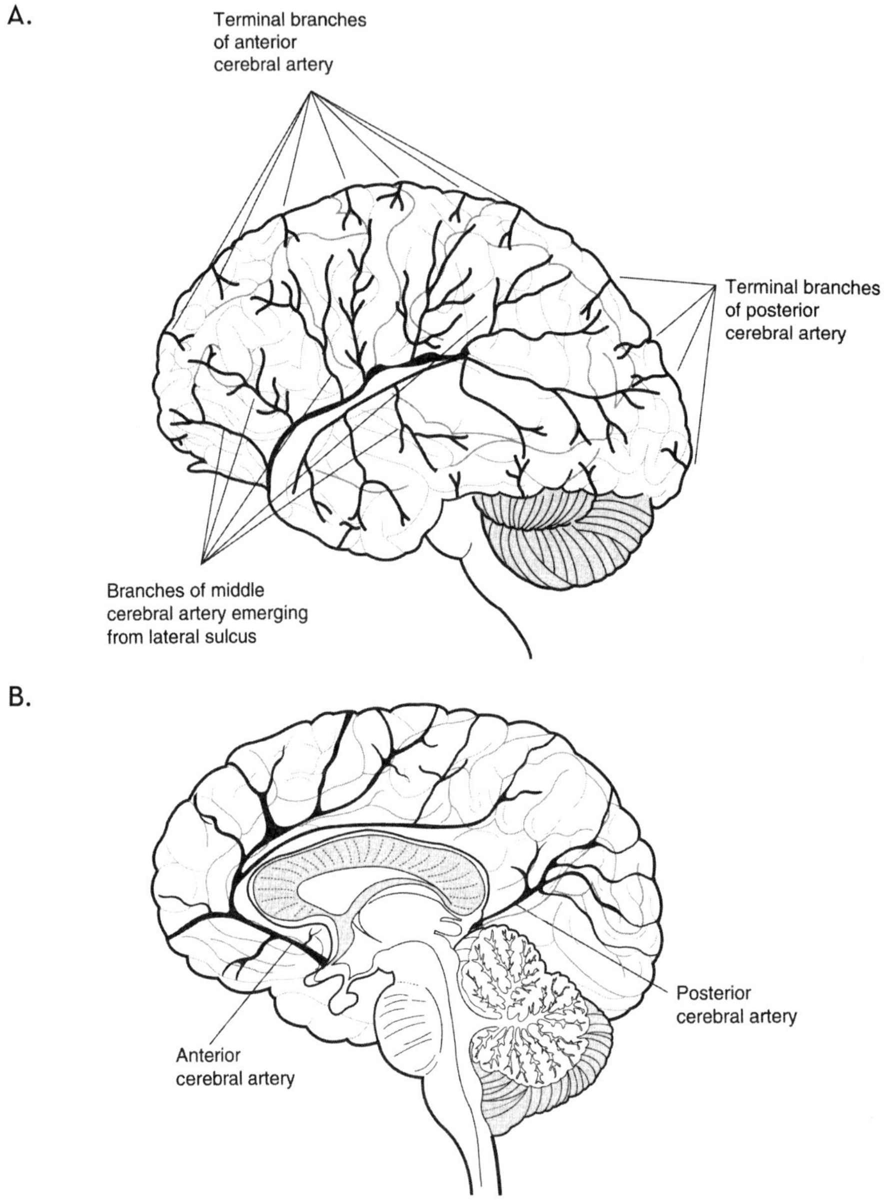

Figure 3-2. Cerebral vascular system. (**A**) Lateral view of the left side of the brain and the left middle cerebral artery that supplies most of the lateral aspects of the left hemisphere. Also shown are the terminal branches of the left anterior cerebral artery supplying superior aspects of the frontal and parietal lobes, and the terminal branches of the left posterior cerebral artery supplying inferior aspects of the temporal lobe and lateral aspects of the occipital lobe.
(**B**) Medial view of the right side of the brain and the right anterior cerebral artery supplying medial aspects of the frontal and parietal lobes, and the right posterior cerebral artery supplying medial aspects of the occipital lobe.

(i.e., perisylvian language zone), including Broca's and Wernicke's areas. The middle cerebral artery also sends off smaller branches called the "lenticulostriate arteries" to supply deep structures such as the basal ganglia and internal capsule.

The **vertebrobasilar arterial system** arises from the left and right subclavian arteries. Each of the subclavian arteries branches into a vertebral artery. These vertebral arteries ascend toward the brain via small holes in the upper vertebrae of the spine. They enter the skull through the foramen magna, and at the level of the pons, they unite to form one basilar artery (see Figure 3-3). The basilar artery then subdivides into the right and left posterior cerebral arteries. The posterior cerebral arteries provide blood to the occipital lobes as well as medial and inferior portions of temporal lobes (see Figures 3-2A and 3-2B). The posterior cerebral arteries also send arterial branches deep into the cerebral hemispheres to supply blood to important subcortical structures, such as the thalamus.

The carotid and vertebrobasilar artery systems are connected with each other through a ring of arteries referred to as the **Circle of Willis** (see caption of Figure 3-3). Located at the base of the brain, the Circle of Willis provides a collateral circulation system that can help compensate for a blockage in one of the major cerebral arteries. For

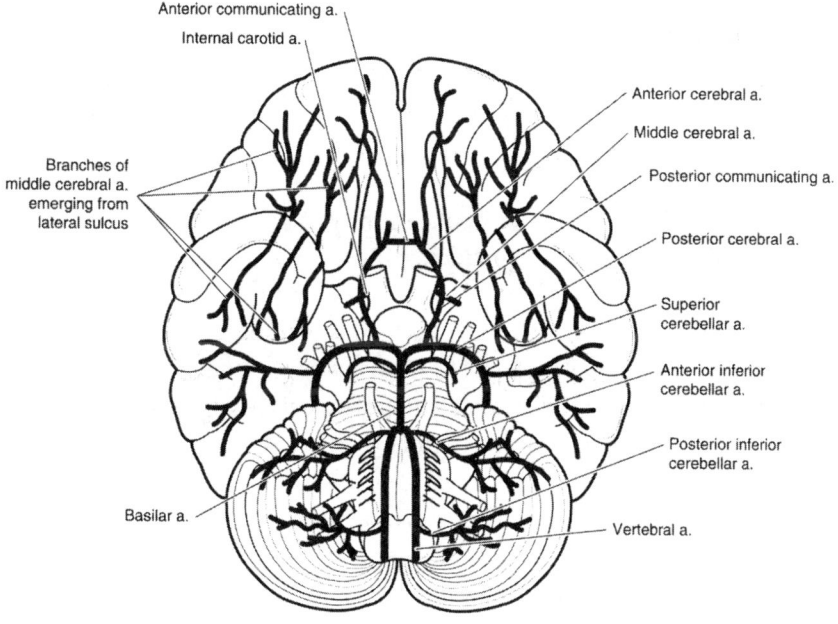

Figure 3-3. Inferior view of the brain and the cerebral vascular system. The posterior cerebral arteries are shown arising from the vertebral basilar system. Also depicted is the Circle of Willis—the ring of arteries that connects the carotid and vertebral basilar arterial systems and provides collateral cerebral circulation. The following arteries make up the Circle of Willis: posterior cerebral arteries, posterior communicating arteries, middle cerebral arteries, anterior cerebral arteries, internal carotid arteries, and anterior communicating artery.

example, if there is occlusion of the left internal carotid artery that in turn is reducing blood flow through the left middle and anterior cerebral arteries, the right carotid artery and the basilar artery can provide alternate sources of blood flow via the anterior communicating artery and the left posterior communicating artery, respectively. Unfortunately, with age, these communicating arteries often become less viable alternative blood flow routes due to narrowing associated with vascular disease.

Certain lateral areas of the hemispheres have some backup protection from blood flow occlusions because they are located where the distributions of major cerebral arteries overlap (Figure 3-2A). These areas are referred to as "watershed areas" or "watershed zones." The anterior watershed zone is found on the lateral surface of frontal and parietal lobes where the anterior and middle cerebral arteries meet, whereas the posterior watershed zone is found on the lateral surface of the occipital and temporal lobes where the middle and posterior cerebral arteries meet. Therefore, if blockage occurs in the posterior cerebral artery, there might be little damage to brain tissue within the posterior watershed area because this tissue is still receiving blood supply from the neighboring branches of the middle cerebral artery.

Stroke Risk Factors

Despite some built-in protective mechanisms within the cerebral circulatory system, every 40 seconds in the United States an individual suffers a stroke (Roger et al., 2011). Risk factors that increase an individual's likelihood of having a stroke include the following (L. B. Goldstein et al., 2010; Roger et al., 2011):

- *Age* (whereas the incidence of stroke in the general population is approximately 2 per 1,000 individuals, this incidence increases to 1 per 100 individuals for adults over 70 years of age)
- *Hypertension or high blood pressure*, which is defined as having a systolic pressure of equal to or greater than 140 mmHg and/or a diastolic pressure of equal to or greater than 90 mmHg, using an antihypertensive medication, or being told by a health-care professional more than once that you have high blood pressure
- *Heart disease*, including heart attacks or cardiac arrhythmias
- *Diabetes*, which speeds up the process of atherosclerosis (i.e., hardening of the arteries) and currently affects more than 18 million American adults
- *Smoking*, which narrows blood vessels throughout the body and doubles one's risk of ischemic stroke (see below for description)
- *Obesity*, with 68% of American adults and 32% of American children overweight or obese (i.e., body mass index > 30 kg/m^2), and abdominal fat being particularly dangerous
- *Substance abuse* (e.g., alcohol), which can lead to restriction of arteries, increased blood pressure, or both

- *High cholesterol* (> 200 mg/dL), which affects close to 100 million American adults
- *Transient ischemic attacks* (see below for description)
- *Depression*, particularly in individuals who are younger than 65 years of age
- *Physical inactivity*

In terms of sex differences, 30% more men suffer strokes than women (L. B. Goldstein et al., 2010; Roger et al., 2011). This does not, however, translate into all good news for women. For example, each year in the United States, more women than men die from stroke, and more than twice as many women die from stroke than from breast cancer. Women also experience greater disability than men do subsequent to stroke. Additionally, women over 30 years of age who take high-estrogen oral contraceptives and who smoke have a stroke risk rate that is 22 times higher than that of the average individual; use of postmenopausal hormones can also increase a woman's stroke risk. There are also racial differences in terms of stroke occurrence: Whereas strokes are more common among African Americans and American Indians than among Caucasians, they are less common among other minority populations, such as Asians.

Individuals who live in the southeast part of the United States also seem to be at a higher risk for suffering a stroke. States such as North Carolina, South Carolina, Georgia, Tennessee, Mississippi, Florida, Alabama, Arkansas, and Louisiana are often referred to as the "stroke belt" because of their high stroke incidence and mortality rates (Roger et al., 2011). For example, stroke mortality is 20% higher in the stroke belt than in the United States as a whole. Factors that may contribute to these rates include a higher-than-average population of African Americans and elderly individuals, as well as the traditional diet associated with these geographic areas. Unfortunately, the "stroke belt" is stretching, as recent survey data have indicated that Oklahoma and Alabama now have the highest stroke prevalence rates. In contrast, Colorado has the lowest stroke rate in the United States.

It is also important to be cognizant that stroke may affect children (Roach et al., 2008; Roger et al., 2011). Stroke in children most frequently occurs within the first 30 days following their birth. As with adults, stroke is more common among African American children than other ethnicities, and boys are at greater risk than girls are. Unlike with adults, however, hemorrhagic strokes are more common than ischemic strokes (see next section for a description of these types of strokes). Unfortunately, approximately 40% of children who suffer a stroke will acquire moderate to severe disabilities, such as cognitive and sensory impairments, cerebral palsy, and epilepsy.

Types of Stroke

Although a number of diseases and complications of diseases or trauma cause strokes (e.g., lupus, blast injuries), there are only two major types of stroke: ischemic and hemorrhagic (see Figure 3-4).

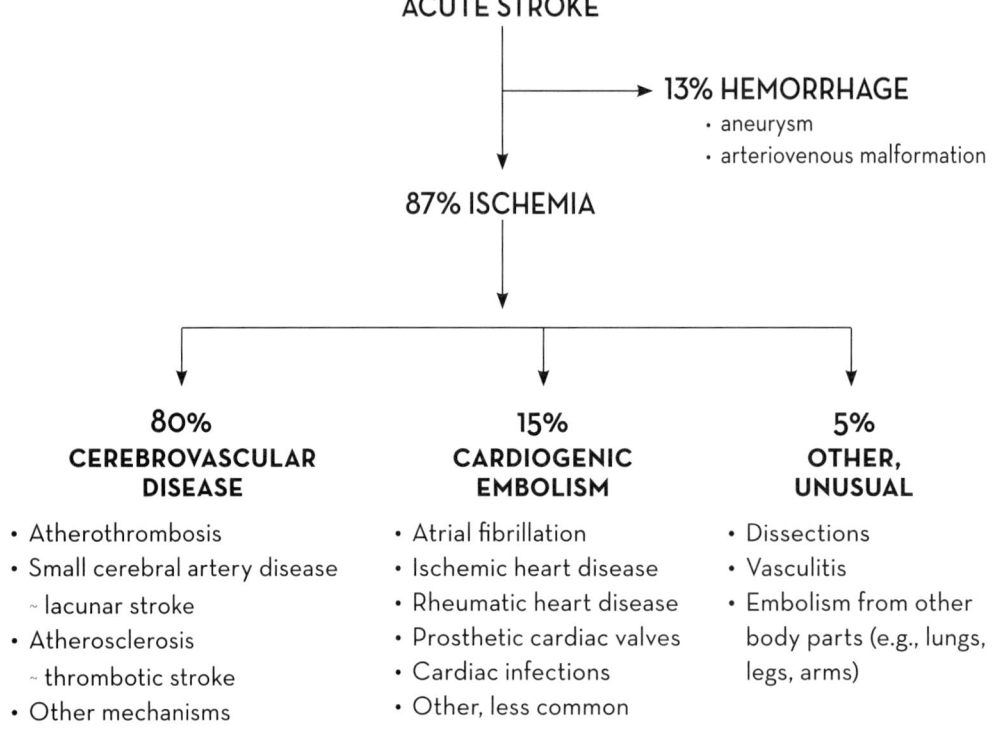

Figure 3-4. The two major types of stroke and their respective causes.

Ischemic Stroke

Ischemic strokes are the more common and account for about 87% of all strokes (Roger et al., 2011). In an **ischemic stroke**, there is a deficiency in blood flow to the brain due to blockage of an artery (Suarez, 2000). If the patient suffers a very small ischemic stroke, it may be called a "lacunar stroke." Lacunar strokes typically involve small penetrating arteries that supply blood to structures deep within the brain (e.g., basal ganglia, internal capsule, thalamus) and result in a very small area of brain damage (i.e., 2 to 15 mm^2).

The term "**infarct**" is used to describe the area of dead brain tissue that results from ischemia or blood flow deprivation. Two types of blockages may cause an ischemic stroke. One type is referred to as a **thrombosis**. In a thrombotic stroke, there is a buildup of atherosclerotic or fatty plaque on an artery that provides blood flow to the brain (Reinmuth, 1997). The process of forming the thrombosis or occlusion may take minutes or weeks, in part reflecting the size or number of affected arteries. The other type of ischemic stroke is due to an **embolus**. In an embolic stroke, a clot forms or a piece of fatty plaque breaks off from elsewhere in the circulatory system and then travels to block off a smaller artery that supplies blood to the brain. The most common source of emboli is the heart, although clots may arise from disease or trauma to other parts of the body as well (e.g., lungs, legs, arms). In comparison to a thrombotic stroke, the clinical onset of an embolic stroke is typically faster, with maximal neurological symptoms manifesting themselves within seconds or minutes. For many patients, the exact mechanism of an ischemic stroke is never determined, so the medical charts of many patients indicate that they had a "thromboembolic" stroke.

Transient Ischemic Attack. A frequent precursor to an ischemic stroke is a **transient ischemic attack (TIA)**, which is a small and temporary disruption of blood flow to the brain, usually caused by small emboli that briefly become lodged in the cerebral vasculature prior to being broken up (Easton et al., 2009; Hadjiev & Mineva, 2007). It is estimated that about 5 million people in the United States have had a TIA (Roger et al., 2011), although this number is likely much higher, as many individuals who suffer a TIA do not report it to their health-care provider. During a TIA, an individual experiences the abrupt onset of stroke symptoms—such as blurring or double vision, weakness or numbness of a limb or one side of the body, speech problems, aphasia, or dizziness (i.e., vertigo). Whereas in older definitions and descriptions of TIA, symptoms were allowed to persist up to 24 hours, most TIAs resolve within an hour (Hadjiev & Mineva, 2007; Johnston, 2007). Accordingly, more recent views prescribe that symptoms should not last longer than 1 hour (Easton et al., 2009). When people who suffer a TIA are examined acutely, no infarction should be observed, though permanent brain damage is frequently later identified. Furthermore, there is about a 3 to 10% chance of suffering a stroke within 2 days of experiencing a TIA, a 10 to 20% chance during the first year, and a 30 to 60% chance within five years (Johnston, 2007; Roger et al., 2011). TIAs are also associated with greater risk of cardiac events (e.g., heart attack) (Easton et al., 2009). Accordingly, it is vital that TIAs be taken seriously. Unfortunately, it is estimated that around 50% of people who experience a TIA do not report it to their health-care practitioner (Roger et al., 2011).

Medical treatment for a TIA focuses on either reducing the development of thrombi or the release of emboli (R. Adams et al., 2008; Easton et al., 2009; Johnston, 2007). In the case of thrombosis, plaque buildup within the carotid artery (i.e., when the artery is more than 50% blocked) may be removed by a surgical procedure called **endarterectomy**. Although endarterectomies may successfully reduce a patient's chance of suffering a stroke, in a small proportion of patients they may induce an embolic stroke if a piece of plaque is dislodged during the arteriogram (i.e., the radiological procedure used to visualize the arteries; see also Chapter 4) or the surgical procedure itself (Hartmann et al., 1999). Another treatment option is to prescribe anticoagulants such as heparin or warfarin (e.g., Coumadin) to prevent thrombus formation and, consequently, the release of emboli (Adams et al., 2008; Johnston, 2007). Antiplatelet medications such as aspirin, clopidogrel, or extended-release dipyridamole also may be used, as they help reduce the buildup of plaque on existing thrombotic areas. Taking one aspirin or fewer a day has been shown to reduce the risk of further TIAs, strokes, and even death—particularly in men (Albers & Tijssen, 1999). Finally, medications to reduce cholesterol or blood pressure levels may also be prescribed following a TIA (Adams et al., 2008; Johnston, 2007).

Hemorrhagic Stroke

The other major type of stroke, **hemorrhagic stroke**, occurs when an artery bursts and causes blood to escape and flood surrounding brain tissue. The buildup of blood is called a **hematoma**, and this pool of blood is dangerous because it can displace and compress adjacent brain tissue, arteries, or cranial nerves. Hemorrhagic strokes are most frequently associated with aneurysms, arteriovenous malformations, or a long medical history of hypertension. An **aneurysm** is a weak or thin spot on a blood vessel that causes the vessel to dilate or balloon (see Figure 3-5). Aneurysms are often present from birth and remain asymptomatic until they grow so large that they exert pressure and consequently affect the functioning of adjacent brain structures, or until they burst. If identified prior to a stroke, aneurysms may be treated by clipping the neck of the dilation or by spraying the dilation and adjacent vessels with plastics. An **arteriovenous malformation (AVM)** is a defect in the communication links between arteries and veins (i.e., regions in which oxygenated blood from arteries mixes with deoxygenated

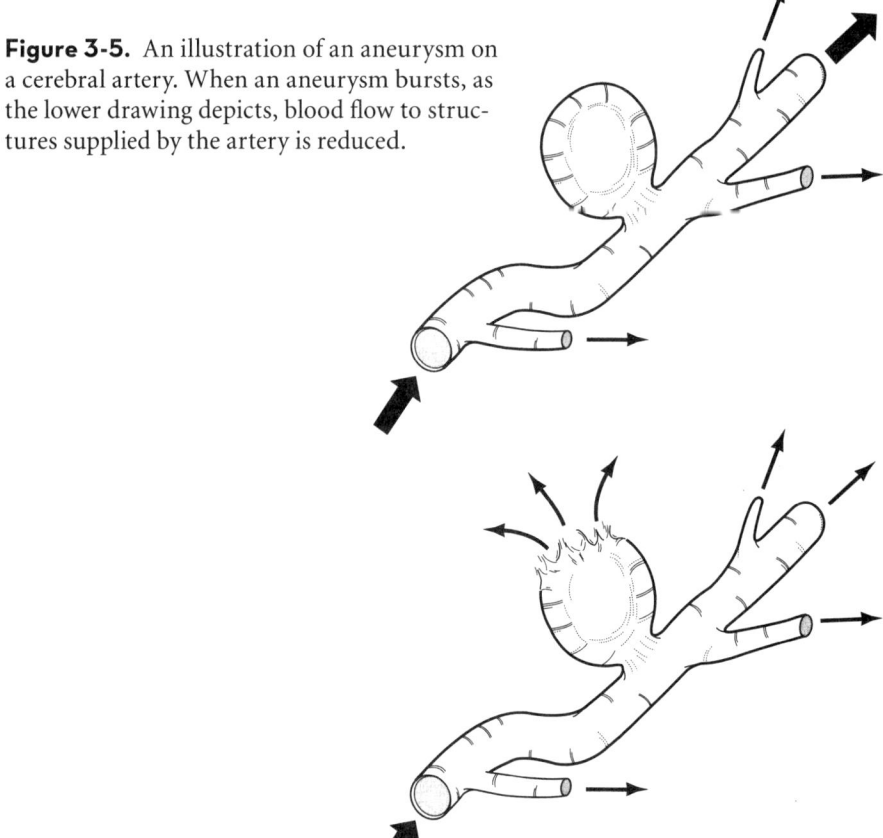

Figure 3-5. An illustration of an aneurysm on a cerebral artery. When an aneurysm bursts, as the lower drawing depicts, blood flow to structures supplied by the artery is reduced.

blood from veins) and consequently results in weakened arterial walls. Like aneurysms, AVMs are present from birth and usually remain asymptomatic until early adulthood, when they can cause seizures or hemorrhages. When identified, AVMs may be removed with surgery or radiation, or embolized (filled with a material to prevent blood flow into the AVM) to prevent stroke.

Hemorrhagic strokes are often classified according to where they occur. For example, an intracerebral hemorrhage, which accounts for about 10% of all strokes (Roger et al., 2011), is one in which blood invades tissue within the brain. A severe headache is the most prominent early clinical symptom of an intracerebral hemorrhage, but patients may also experience nausea, vomiting, and loss of consciousness. In a subarachnoid hemorrhage, which accounts for about 3% of all strokes, blood spills into the pia-arachnoid space surrounding the brain. This type of hemorrhage is frequently caused by a ruptured aneurysm in the area of the Circle of Willis, or by a hemorrhaging AVM.

Stroke Survival

Patients who suffer an ischemic stroke have the best chance of surviving, whereas those who suffer an intracerebral hemorrhagic stroke have the least chance of surviving. Although hemorrhagic strokes are associated with higher morbidity rates, patients who survive a hemorrhage often have a better recovery than survivors of ischemic stroke do. That is because, following successful acute medical treatment, hemorrhagic strokes tend to produce less permanent brain damage compared with ischemic strokes (Reinmuth, 1997).

Stroke Treatment

Although strokes were previously referred to as "cerebrovascular accidents," they have been more recently called **brain attacks**. This change in terminology has been instigated to emphasize that, like heart attacks, strokes should be treated as a medical emergency. That is, whereas in the past there was little that could be done to help a patient who was experiencing stroke symptoms, there are now medical treatments available that can be administered acutely to help prevent or reduce permanent brain damage and, consequently, the disability caused by strokes.

The first step to treating stroke is to recognize the symptoms (e.g., dizziness, confusion, severe headache, one-sided numbness or weakness, slurred speech) so that the patient can get immediate medical attention. Once at the hospital, the physicians will try to determine whether the patient is presenting with an ischemic or hemorrhagic stroke. If it is an ischemic stroke, the patient may be a candidate to receive drug treatments designed to reverse or minimize permanent brain damage. For example, intravenous thrombolytic therapy involving drugs such as rtPA (recombinant tissue plasminigen activator) can be given within the first three hours of stroke onset to break up blood clots by speeding up the body's natural clot-dissolving process (Falluji, Abou-Chebl, Rodriguez Castro, & Mukherjee, 2011; Suarez, 2000); recent research suggests that this time window can be extended to 4.5 hours, albeit with more moderate positive outcomes (Molina, 2011). Unfortunately, the vast majority of stroke patients do not receive rtPA because of one or more of the following (Katzan et al., 2000; Molina, 2011; Roger et al., 2011): (a) Patients wait too long to seek medical treatment and thus miss the critical three-hour window in which rtPA has been shown to be effective; (b) some patients who arrive at the hospital in time may have characteristics (e.g., traumatic brain injury within the previous three months, major surgery within the previous two weeks, evidence of bleeding or skull fracture) that contraindicate the use of rtPA (i.e., they have an increased risk of hemorrhaging if the drug were to be used); and (c) many hospitals lack the resources or personnel required for effective provision of rtPA (e.g., between 2004 and 2007, 64% of American hospitals did not give rtPA; Kleindorfer, Xu, & Moomaw, 2009).

There are other treatment strategies for acute ischemic stroke. For example, there are surgeries aimed at mechanically disrupting and removing the clot (Falluji et al., 2011; Molina, 2011); such surgeries may or may not be used in concert with thrombolytic drugs. Like rtPA, there are strict guidelines pertaining to which patients may qualify for surgical intervention.

Another acute treatment option currently under development is the use of neuroprotective agents (Fisher, 2011; Ginsberg, 2008). Agents such as nimodipine (a calcium channel blocker), citicoline (contributor to several neurophysiological functions, including increasing levels of dopamine and noreinephrine), and magnesium (an inhibitor of excitatory neurotransmitters and a calcium channel blocker) can protect brain tissue directly adjacent to the infarct (i.e., penumbra) from the biochemical and molecular changes that occur when its blood flow is reduced and that, if left unchecked, cause irreversible damage. Unfortunately, to date, clinical trials have been disappointing for most neuroprotective drugs despite positive outcomes in animal studies. Most recently, another neuroprotective therapy—therapeutic hypothermia, or cooling therapy—has been evaluated and has produced some positive but still preliminary outcomes (Klassman, 2011). Hypothermia serves as a neuroprotective agent because it reduces the brain's metabolic rate and oxygen consumption, which in turn, slows down the cascade of negative effects associated with ischemia. Despite the lack of compelling evidence thus far, neuroprotection research continues because neuroprotective agents have the potential to salvage brain tissue and have advantages over rtPA administration (e.g., increasing the three-hour treatment window of thrombolytic drugs to twenty-four hours and being simpler to administer) (Fisher, 2011; Ginsberg, 2008; Klassman, 2011). Consequently, neuroprotective agents could improve ischemic stroke management in both developed as well as developing countries around the world.

Tumor

Although not as common as strokes, brain **tumors**, or **neoplasms**, also may cause neurogenic language and cognitive disorders. It is estimated that each year, approximately 66,300 individuals in the United States will be diagnosed with a brain tumor (American Brain Tumor Association [ABTA], 2012). It is further estimated that for every 100,000 people in the United States, just over 200 have a brain tumor diagnosis (Porter, McCarthy, Freels, Kim, & Davis, 2010). In children, brain tumors are the second-most-common type of malignancy, with leukemia being the most common. Tumors are tissue masses that arise from an abnormally fast rate of cell reproduction. As the tumor grows, it progressively takes up more and more intracranial space, and consequently causes more and more compression or destruction of surrounding brain tissue, cranial nerves, and blood vessels. Onset of tumor symptoms reflects this progressive growth and is characterized by the gradual appearance of problems with communication, cognition, or both; as the tumor continues to grow, communication and cognitive abilities continue to deteriorate. The specific symptoms that a patient may experience will depend on the location of the tumor.

Brain tumors may be benign or malignant (ABTA, 2012). Benign brain tumors are noncancerous; do not spread or metastasize to other parts of the body; and occur more frequently, accounting for about two thirds of new brain tumor cases each year (Porter et al., 2010). Malignant brain tumors are cancerous and often recur despite treatment efforts; they may invade other parts of the body, or themselves be the product of cancer elsewhere in the body that has infiltrated the brain. Fortunately, in recent years, survival rates for malignant brain tumors have been increasing (ABTA, 2012). Brain tumors may also be classified as primary or metastatic. *Primary brain tumors* arise from pathology within the brain. In contrast, *metastatic brain tumors*, which are more common, arise from cancer that began elsewhere in the body (ABTA, 2012; Fox, Cheung, Patel, Suki, & Rao, 2011). Most frequently, metastatic brain tumors are a product of lung and breast cancer.

There are many different types of intracranial tumors, each of which is named according to its tissue origin. A common tumor source within the brain is the supportive, or glial, cells (ABTA, 2012). For example, a common type of tumor in adults is a glioblastoma multiforme, also known as a "high-grade astrocytoma" (Wen et al., 1995). Glioblastomas are malignant, and treatment may include chemotherapy, radiation, or surgical removal (i.e., resection). Life expectancy following treatment for a glioblastoma varies from less than one year to about six years, depending on the size of the tumor and how fast the tumor is growing. Meningiomas arise from the arachnoid tissue that sheaths the brain and are the most common type of primary brain tumor (ABTA, 2012). Meningiomas are benign, typically occur during adulthood, and are more common in women than in men. These tumors grow quite slowly, giving the brain time to accommodate, and thus they cause few symptoms for a long time period. Prognosis is often favorable, as these tumors do not invade cortical tissue, tumor recurrence rates are low, and surgery is typically successful in removing the entire tumor.

How Big Tumors Can Cause "Little" Symptoms

Because some tumors have a very slow growth rate, patients may show minimal symptoms for some time. This phenomenon is sometimes referred to as the "serial lesion effect" and indicates that because of the slow, progressive nature of some tumors, the brain tissue and the neural circuits they support are able to adapt over time to the presence of the invading tumor. For example, I recently received a referral to assess a patient as part of a research study investigating attention and language abilities following right hemisphere brain damage. The patient's medical records indicated that she had recently undergone surgery to remove a large right frontal lobe meningioma. According to the patient's husband, the tumor had been the size of a golf ball. Based on this information about tumor size and location (note that the patient had not received any previous speech-language pathology or neuropsychology services), I was predicting that the patient would demonstrate significant difficulty on a number of the pragmatic and cognitive tests I had planned. During the assessment, however, I soon discovered that my expectations were wrong, as the patient scored within and even above the normal range on most measures. I attributed the preservation of her linguistic and cognitive abilities not only to successful medical treatment of her tumor but also to the serial lesion effect.

Related to malignant tumors either in the brain or elsewhere in the body is another potential etiology of acquired communication and cognitive disorders, **paraneoplastic syndromes**. Paraneoplastic syndromes encompass a group of relatively rare disorders that result when one's immune system reacts abnormally to a cancerous tumor in the body or when the tumor secretes certain chemicals (NINDS, 2009; Pelosof & Gerber, 2010). For example in the case of an abnormal immune system response, cancer-fighting T cells (white blood cells) erroneously attack healthy nervous system cells, resulting in progressive neurological deterioration and numerous possible symptoms, including motor disturbance (e.g., dysarthria), perceptual disturbance (e.g., vision problems), and cognitive disturbance (e.g., dementia). Paraneoplastic syndromes are more common in middle- or older-age adults and in certain cancers (lung, ovarian, lymphatic, and breast cancer), with about 8% of all cancer patients being affected by these syndromes (Pelosof & Gerber, 2010). Typically, tumors that are more advanced will be associated with more progressive and involved neurological damage.

Infection

Certain bacterial and viral infections may invade the central nervous system to produce any number of neurogenic communication and cognitive problems. In terms of bacterial infections, bacterial meningitis and brain abscesses are the most common. Bacterial meningitis is associated with inflammation of the pia and arachnoid tissues that cover the brain. Symptoms include fever, fatigue, headache, a stiff neck, and, if severe, coma. Because this type of infection spreads rapidly, prompt medical treatment in the form of antibiotics is essential. In brain or intracerebral abscess, bacteria from another infection in the body attack a focal brain site. The inflammation caused by this infection leads to destruction of brain tissue, and may also exert pressure on adjacent brain structures and blood vessels. Brain abscesses are treated with both antibiotics and surgery to drain the abscess. Localized symptoms such as sensory loss or aphasia may occur prior to treatment, as well as persist following treatment if the abscess or its removal results in permanent brain damage.

The central nervous system also is vulnerable to viral infections, such as herpes simplex encephalitis, viral meningitis, West Nile Virus, and syphilis. In acquired immune deficiency syndrome (AIDS), the human immunodeficiency virus (HIV) may invade the brain and cause widespread damage (particularly to white matter and subcortical brain structures) and, consequently, dementia (sometimes referred to as "HIV encephalopathy") (Chu & Selwyn, 2011; Schouten, Cinque, Gisslen, Reiss, & Portegies, 2011). Initial research indicated that approximately 15 to 30% of AIDS patients would develop dementia, usually in the later stages of this infection (Clifford, 2000; Heaton et al., 2001). The development of antiretroviral drugs, the pharmacotherapy used to treat HIV, led to a significantly reduced prevalence of dementia among AIDS patients, with current estimates of less than 10% (Heaton et al., 2011; Schouten et al., 2011). Recently, however, clinicians and investigators have found that long-term patients (i.e., infected for many years and using the antiretroviral therapy for many years) are presenting with impairments that affect a number of cognitive domains, and an estimated 30 to 70% of HIV patients score within the impaired range on neuropsychological tests. Most commonly, these cognitive impairments do not appear severe enough for a dementia classification and are instead referred to as "HIV-associated neurocognitive disorders," or HAND. Importantly, presence of HAND is associated with an increased risk for early mortality and is one of the most distressing symptoms for HIV patients. A recent meta-analysis by Al-Khindi, Zakzanis, and van Gorp (2011) revealed few differences in neuropsychological status between HIV patients who were taking antiretroviral drugs and those who were not, indicating the need to develop treatments that address the cognitive-linguistic symptoms caused by HIV infection.

For other viral infections, some antiviral medications are available; however, treatment for many of these infections is palliative. That is, care focuses on making the patient as medically stable and comfortable as possible while waiting to see if the patient's own immune system can successfully eliminate the infection.

Scary Mosquitoes?

Over the past decade, there has been increased public awareness concerning West Nile Virus, as each spring or summer news reporters often do a story or two on how rampant the virus is in their state. Mosquitoes acquire the virus from birds and then pass it on to humans when they bite us. This virus may become a concern, as it can invade the brain and cause meningitis, encephalitis, or both, which in turn can cause permanent brain damage and disability. However, despite fears that the media might stir up regarding West Nile Virus, it is important to keep in mind that only around 1% of people who acquire the virus actually develop neurological symptoms (S. Brady, Miserendino, & Rao, 2004), and most people won't even know if they've been bitten by a "scary" mosquito.

Traumatic Brain Injury

The National Head Injury Foundation (1989) defined **traumatic brain injury (TBI)** as an insult to the brain produced by external forces that may cause a variety of temporary or permanent physical, cognitive, emotional, and behavioral impairments. It is the leading cause of death and disability in the world for the general population (Bruns & Hauer, 2003). Currently in the United States, it is estimated that each year 1.7 million people suffer a TBI, with TBI contributing to approximately one third of all injury-related deaths (Faul et al., 2010). The Centers for Disease Control and Prevention (CDC, 2012) have estimated that approximately 5.3 million, or 2%, of all Americans are presently living with disabilities caused by TBI. Additionally, TBI is the most common cause of death and disability among children in the United States, resulting in an estimated 500,000 emergency room admissions and more than 7,000 deaths each year (Faul et al., 2010; Langlois, Ruthland-Brown, & Tomas, 2004). Also contributing to the prevalence of TBI in the United States is the number of soldiers deployed to conflicts in Iraq and Afghanistan; approximately 20% of these troops are estimated to have experienced a TBI (H. Golding, Bass, Percy, & Goldberg, 2009). Unfortunately, these statistics may represent an underestimation of the true occurrence rate of TBI, given that many individuals may not seek medical assistance for a head injury and individuals who are not hospitalized for their TBI are frequently not included in incidence or prevalence studies.

"Show Me the Money!"

As just reviewed, TBI is quite prevalent in the United States, affecting individuals across all age groups and frequently resulting in permanent brain damage and thus disability. Despite this prevalence, however, funding for TBI research, whether basic (e.g., identifying mechanisms of cell death in TBI) or applied (e.g., developing and evaluating new cognitive prostheses), is lacking. A National Institutes of Health (NIH) report recently noted that even though the number of people suffering a TBI each year outnumbers those diagnosed with breast, lung, prostate, brain, and colon cancer combined, in 2009, research for these five cancers received approximately two billion dollars in funding, whereas TBI research received only about 4% of that, eighty-six million dollars (NIH, 2011).

TBI Risk Factors and Causes

There are a number of populations who are at greater risk than others for suffering a TBI. In terms of age, children between the ages of 0 and 4 years, older adolescents between the ages of 15 and 19, and the elderly (i.e., 65 years and older) are more apt to sustain a TBI than other age groups, with individuals between 15 and 24 years of age having the highest TBI rates (Bruns & Hauer, 2003; Faul et al., 2010; McKinlay et al., 2008). Not only is TBI more common among the elderly than in the general population, but prognosis for recovery from TBI is poorer for elderly patients. For example, elderly patients with TBI have longer hospital stays and are more likely to die from their injuries compared to younger patients with TBI (Bruns & Hauer, 2003; Sendroy-Terrill, Whiteneck, & Brooks, 2010). Regardless of age, males have higher rates of TBI compared to females (CDC, 2012; Faul et al., 2010; McKinlay et al., 2008). Other risk factors for TBI include the following: (a) low socioeconomic level (Kraus & McArthur, 1996; A. K. Wagner, Sasser, Hammond, Wiercisiewski, & Alexander, 2000), (b) pretraumatic psychiatric illness or family dysfunction (McGuire, Burright, Williams, & Donovick, 1998), (c) substance abuse (e.g., 56% of patients have a positive blood alcohol concentration upon diagnosis of TBI) (Bombardier & Thurber, 1998; NINDS, 2011b; Wagner et al., 2000), and (d) previous TBI (i.e., after suffering a TBI, a patient has a three times greater risk of suffering another TBI compared to the general population).

Although motor vehicle accidents (including when the victim is a vehicle occupant or a pedestrian/bicyclist) used to be the most frequent cause of TBI in the general population, they now only account for the most TBI-related deaths (CDC, 2012; Faul et al., 2010). Instead, falls are currently the leading source of TBI in the U.S., with the highest rates of fall-related TBI among the elderly and young children (Faul et al., 2010; McKinlay et al., 2008; Sendroy-Terrill et al., 2010). In fact, falls are responsible for more than 50% of all accidental deaths in adults aged 65 years or older. In addition to normal aging effects on postural stability, a number of medical factors may account for the high rates of falling among the elderly (Isaacson & Rubin, 1999; Luukinen, Viramo, Koski, Laippala, & Kivela, 1999; Sullivan et al., 2009); these include medical conditions such as stroke, postural dizziness, hip disease, Parkinsonism, and diabetic neuropathy, which may affect the elderly adult's balance, coordination, or both. Other common causes of TBI include assaults (e.g., gun wounds, physical abuse), suicide attempts, and sports and recreation accidents (Bruns & Hauer, 2003; CDC, 2012; Faul et al., 2010; Wagner et al., 2000).

Types of TBI

As previously mentioned, traumatic brain injury occurs when an external force is of sufficient strength to compromise brain structures or functioning. The external force may be created by projectiles striking the head (e.g., bullets, baseballs, clubs), by the head suddenly striking a stationary object (e.g., a car windshield, a floor, a bathtub), or by sudden changes in pressure (e.g., being near an explosion). When the skull is fractured or penetrated by an external force and the contents of the skull are exposed, the injury is referred to as an **open head injury**. In contrast, when the skull is not pierced by the external force and thus stays intact, the injury is referred to as a **closed head injury**. Individuals who have been shot or struck on the head by a sharp object typically suffer an open head injury, whereas individuals who have been involved in a car accident or who have fallen typically suffer a closed head injury. In open head injuries, brain damage is frequently focal or localized and the resulting functional impairments are likewise circumscribed. For example, if the focal brain damage affects the left hemisphere, the patient with TBI may present with aphasia. In closed head injuries, brain damage is typically more diffuse, affecting widespread areas of the brain, and consequently causes an array of cognitive and communicative deficits.

Blast Injuries

TBI can also result from **blast injuries**. Blast injuries are common among those serving in current Middle East conflicts, and it has been estimated that 60 to 90% of blast injury survivors may present with a TBI (Okie, 2005; Scott, Belanger, Vanderploeg, Massengale, & Scholten, 2006). Blast injuries occur when the brain and other body parts and organs suffer barotraumas (i.e., trauma due to pressure changes) (Kocsis & Tessler, 2009; Roth, 2007; Schneider, Haack, Owens, Herrington, & Zelek, 2009). Following a blast or explosion, there will be a shockwave of pressurized air followed by an incredibly forceful gust of wind, both of which can produce barotraumas via accelerating and decelerating tissues and organs of different densities, which can cause destructive stretching and shearing. The extent and degree of a blast injury will be dependent on such factors as the peak pressure to which the individual is exposed, the duration for which the individual is exposed to the excessive pressure, how close the individual is to the explosion, and the presence and types of barriers and protective gear.

Explosions or blasts can cause a variety of physical consequences, and these have been classified as the following (Kocsis & Tessler, 2009; Roth, 2007; Schneider et al., 2009):

(a) *Primary effects result from barotraumas*—Parts of the body that involve an air–fluid interface are particularly vulnerable to barotraumas (e.g., middle and inner ear, eyeballs, lungs). In addition to directly affecting tissue integrity, barotraumas can result in air or fat embolisms and consequently lead to stroke and can also cause cerebral contusions (i.e., closed head injuries).

(b) *Secondary effects result from flying debris*—These can result in injuries such as eyeball penetration and open head injuries. Infections may also occur if there are bacteria on the flying debris.

(c) *Tertiary effects are caused by body displacement*—This can include falling because the floor caved in due to structural damage or being actually thrown off one's feet by a blast. Both open and closed head injuries may occur subsequent to tertiary effects.

(d) *Quaternary effects include injuries related to burns and exposure to toxins such as gases, radiation, and excessive dust*—These injuries might include breathing disorders such as asthma, burns, and anoxic brain damage.

Therefore, blast injury survivors may present with a closed head injury, open head injury, or both, along with other bodily injuries. Consequently, they frequently experience a wide variety of symptoms, such as vision and hearing loss, fractures, respiratory disorders, spinal cord damage, amputations, sleep disorders, and emotional or psychiatric conditions (e.g., post-traumatic stress disorder) (Chen & Huang, 2011; Roth, 2007). Because blast injury survivors typically have so many overt, external injuries, their cognitive-communicative symptoms may go undiagnosed or untreated for some time (H. Belanger, Scott, Scholten, Curtiss, & Vanderploeg, 2005; Chen & Huang, 2011).

Pathophysiological Consequences of TBI

A number of pathophysiological changes take place within the brain subsequent to a TBI. These structural and physiological changes are often categorized according to whether they are the product of primary versus secondary damage (Graham, 1999). *Primary damage* refers to brain damage caused by the external or mechanical forces involved in the accident or trauma. In contrast, *secondary damage* refers to brain damage that is not mechanically generated and may develop hours to weeks following the head injury. Secondary damage is a product of complications arising from the primary damage or represents a pathophysiological process independent of the original, primary damage.

Types of Primary Damage

Type of primary damage depends, at least in part, on whether the patient suffered an open or closed head injury. In an open head injury, the primary damage is typically localized around the area of contact or the path of the penetrating object. Fragments of the skull, shattered pieces of the bullet, and debris from the penetrating object also may lacerate the brain. One type of primary damage associated with open head injuries is skull fractures, in which a bone or bones of the skull have been broken and consequently lacerate brain tissue. Contusions or bruises also form around the site of impact, as blood vessels also are typically lacerated by the injury. If the contusion is severe, resulting in an accumulation of blood that begins to displace brain mass, it may be diagnosed as a hematoma or blood clot (Table 3-1) (Graham, Adams, Nicoll, Maxwell, & Gennarelli, 1995; Mackay, Chapman, & Morgan, 1997). Hematomas may form within brain tissue (i.e., intracerebral hematomas) or between the skull and brain tissue (i.e., epidural hematomas, subarachnoid hematomas, or subdural hematomas).

Contusions are a common form of primary damage following closed head injuries, and typically are found on the crests of gyri on the surface of the cerebral hemispheres. **Contrecoup effect** or **contrecoup injury** is the term used when contusions occur both

TABLE 3-1
Types of Hematomas or Blood Clots

TYPE	DESCRIPTION
Intracerebral hematoma	• Blood accumulation within brain tissue • Commonly found within the frontal and temporal lobes following a closed or diffuse head injury
Epidural hematoma	• Blood accumulation between the skull and the dura • Usually the result of arterial bleeding and thus enlarge rapidly • Frequently associated with skull fractures
Subarachnoid hematoma	• Blood accumulation between the arachnoid and pia maters • May cause compression of cerebral arteries or obstruction of the flow of cerebrospinal fluid
Subdural hematoma	• Blood accumulation underneath the dural membrane and above the arachnoid mater

at the site of impact (i.e., "coup") and at the opposite side of the brain (i.e., "contre"). That is, the force of the impact causes inward skull impression directly below the site of contact, and then also causes negative pressure changes (i.e., cavitation) to produce damage on the diametrically opposite side of the brain (D. Pang, 1985) (Figure 3-6). Contrecoup effects are commonly seen in head injuries that result from car accidents that involve high-speed stops, and in shaken baby syndrome (NINDS, 2011b). In addition to contrecoup injury, certain brain regions are at great risk for contusions following a closed head injury. For example, contusions often form on inferior and lateral surfaces of the frontal and temporal lobes because brain tissue and blood vessels can hit sharp, bony prominences located in those anterior areas of the skull. Contusions also are frequently found near the corpus callosum, cerebral peduncles, and cerebellar peduncles because these structures are located next to strong tentorial membranes against which they may strike and bounce during a closed head injury. In non-impact, blast-induced TBI, contusions can be quite small and spread out, producing a "pepper-spray pattern" (Chen & Huang, 2011).

Diffuse axonal shearing or injury also occurs following closed head injuries and is caused by high-velocity rotation of the brain relative to the skull. As illustrated in Figure 3-7, this movement produces microscopic damage, such as shearing axons from their myelin sheath or tearing of the axons themselves (Chen & Huang, 2011; Maxwell, Watt, Graham, & Gennarelli, 1993; NINDS, 2011b). Diffuse axonal shearing frequently affects brain tissue at gray–white matter junctions, particularly in those cerebral areas already identified as vulnerable in terms of contusions (e.g., inferior frontal lobe, cerebellar peduncles). Diffuse axonal shearing has been identified as the major form of both focal and diffuse primary damage following closed head injury and is thought to be fundamental in causing impairments of consciousness.

Neuropathology of Neurogenic Language Disorders 99

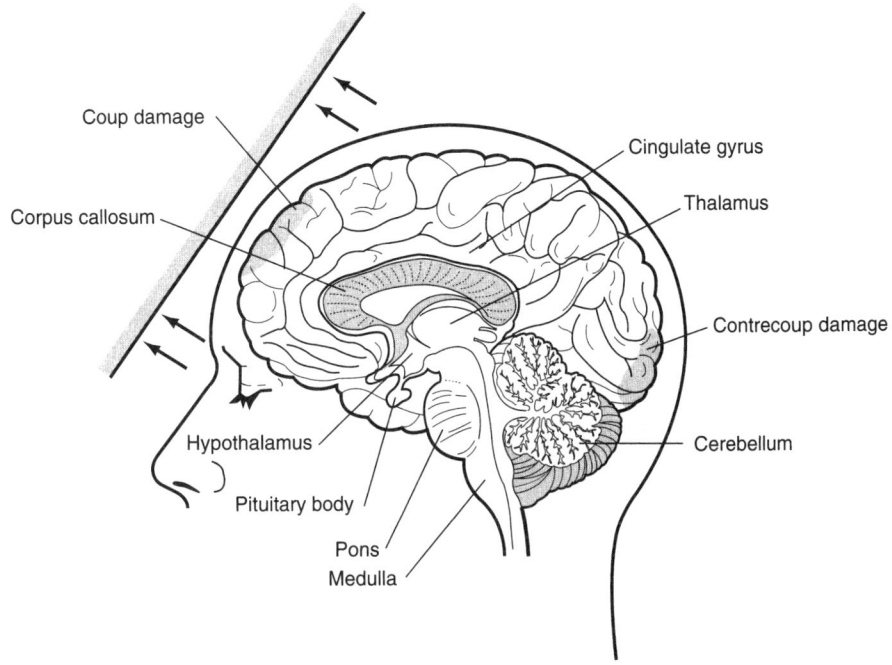

Figure 3-6. An illustration of coup (i.e., contusion and cavitation at the site of the external impact) and contrecoup (i.e., contusion and cavitation at the side of the brain opposite to the external impact) brain damage.

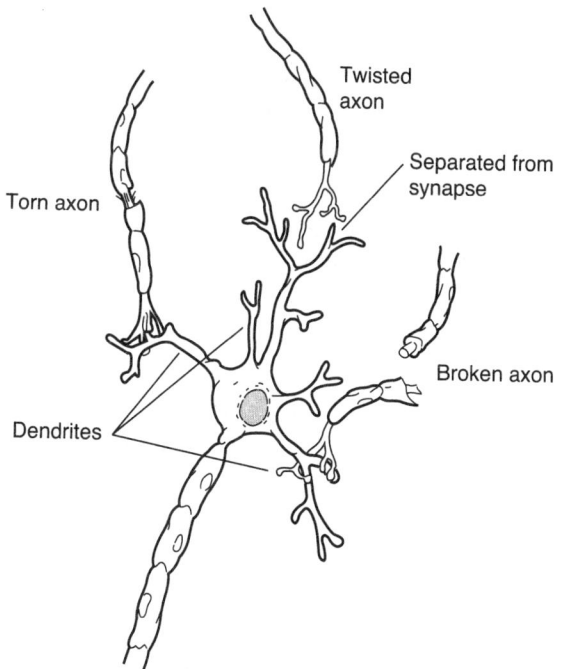

Figure 3-7. Examples of different forms of diffuse axonal shearing that may occur due to a traumatic brain injury.

Type of Secondary Damage

The thrust of medical management for both open and closed head injuries is to prevent or minimize secondary forms of brain damage (Chen & Huang, 2011; Dearden, 1998; Graham et al., 1995; Mackay et al., 1997). Of the various complications that may occur, edema or swelling is quite common, particularly if the blood–brain barrier (i.e., the protective layer of blood vessels and tissue that shelters the brain from toxic substances) is compromised. It is the product of increased intra- and extracellular fluid in brain tissues. Edema disrupts brain functioning because there is little room within the cranium for the brain to expand. Consequently, edema tends to co-occur with increased intracranial pressure, as brain tissue and blood vessels squeeze against the skull. Prolonged increased intracranial pressure (particularly when pressure exceeds 20 mmHg) is of concern because it can cause hypoxia (decreased oxygen in brain tissue), ischemic brain damage (cell death or infarction due to inadequate blood supply), or both. Hypoxia and ischemia also may be produced by decreased respiration (e.g., chest injuries that obstruct breathing) and low arterial blood pressure (e.g., excessive blood loss due to skeletal injuries).

Medical treatments for edema and high intracranial pressure include drugs to decrease metabolic activity (e.g., sedatives or antiseizure medications), fluid restriction to increase osmotic pressure to draw fluid off of the brain, and surgery to create a bone flap (i.e., cutting a hole in the skull to allow the brain more room to expand), to drain cerebrospinal fluid (i.e., ventriculostomy), or to insert a pressure transducer that allows continuous monitoring of intracranial pressure (Dearden, 1998; NINDS, 2011b; Pentland & Whittle, 1999). Hypoxia may be prevented or treated by ensuring that the patient has an adequate airway (e.g., inserting tracheostomy or endotracheal tubes) and by providing supplementary oxygen.

Another possible form of secondary damage is infection (Landesman & Cooper, 1982). Infections are particularly frequent among blast injury survivors (Dau, Oda, & Holodniy, 2009). Specific infections such as meningitis and cerebral abscesses are common following open head injuries and skull fractures, and are treated with antibiotics to prevent outcomes that range from increased intracranial pressure to mortality.

Patients with TBI in both acute and chronic care facilities also typically suffer from a variety of other medical complications (NINDS, 2011b; Pentland & Whittle, 1999). In some cases, these medical complications have direct effects on the patients' communication abilities. For example, prolonged intubation or use of endotracheal tubes may damage the vocal folds or nerves controlling phonation, leading to voice disorders. Other medical complications, such as contractures (i.e., decreases in joint range of motion due to shortening and other changes in muscles, tendons, and ligaments) and pressure sores can cause severe pain, which in turn can negatively affect a patient's ability and willingness to participate in speech-language assessment or treatment activities. Finally, any time the brain is injured, an individual is at risk for seizures. For patients with TBI, onset of seizures typically occurs within the first year or two post-trauma. It is estimated that approximately 5% of all patients with TBI will experience seizures, with more frequent incidence rates among pediatric patients and patients with open head injuries, regardless of age (Ludwig, 1993).

Hypoxic-Ischemic Brain Injury

Another etiology that may produce neurogenic language or cognitive disorders is **hypoxic-ischemic brain injury** (Anderson & Arciniegas, 2010; Sinanovic et al., 2011). A diagnosis of hypoxic-ischemic brain injury is given when damage to brain tissue or functioning is a consequence of drastically reduced levels of oxygen (i.e., hypoxia), decreased blood supply (i.e., ischemia), or both (Arciniegas, 2010; Busi & Greer, 2010). Common causes of hypoxic-ischemic brain injury include incomplete suffocation (e.g., near-drowning, near-hanging), cardiac arrest (i.e., heart attack), respiratory arrest, exposure to poisonous gas (e.g., carbon monoxide), sedative intoxication, and, in newborns, delivery complications that compromise the baby's respiration and/or circulation.

The presence and severity of permanent brain damage subsequent to hypoxic-ischemic brain injury will vary depending on the amount of time the brain was exposed to decreased oxygen levels, blood perfusion, or both, with longer exposure more likely to cause irreversible damage (Arciniegas, 2010). Importantly, this type of injury differs from ischemic stroke in that it puts the entire brain at risk of damage, whereas a stroke—because of blockage of one or a few cerebral blood vessels—typically puts a more focal area of the brain at risk. Further, certain brain areas are more vulnerable to hypoxic-ischemic brain injury, including the superior brainstem; cerebellum; white matter and subcortical structures that rely on small, penetrating blood vessels (e.g., basal ganglia, thalamus); cortical watershed areas; and parts of the hippocampus (Busi & Greer, 2010).

Progressive Neurological Diseases

Most, if not all, progressive neurological diseases initially or over time will produce neurogenic language and/or cognitive disorders. The types and severity of the neurogenic language and cognitive disorders will depend on the neuroanatomical and neurophysiological consequences of the progressive neurological disease. Similarly, the onset (e.g., sudden vs. gradual onset; initial language vs. memory deficit) and rate of progression (e.g., rapid vs. protracted) of language and cognitive symptoms will also vary depending on the type and severity of the progressive neurological disease. Although it is not the responsibility of clinicians to diagnose the type of progressive neurological disease with which their patients present, they must be cognizant of the numerous types of diseases so as to assess, treat, and counsel these patients appropriately. Examples of some of these diseases include:

- Alzheimer's disease (AD)
- Creutzfeld-Jakob disease
- Dementia with Lewy bodies
- Frontotemporal dementia or dementia of the frontal lobe type
- Human immunodeficiency virus encephalopathy

Huntington's disease (HD)
Korsakoff's disease
Multiple sclerosis
Paraneoplastic syndromes
Parkinson's disease (PD)
Pick's disease
Progressive supranuclear palsy
Repeated traumatic brain injury (e.g., dementia pugilistica)
Vascular (i.e., multiple strokes) dementia
Wilson's disease

A description of some of the above progressive neurological diseases capable of producing neurogenic language and cognitive disorders is provided below.

Alzheimer's Disease

The most common cause of dementia, particularly in North America, is **Alzheimer's disease (AD)** (Alzheimer's Association, 2012). It is estimated that approximately 60 to 80% of the dementia population has AD. In terms of the general population, 5.4 million Americans are estimated to have AD, 5.2 million of whom are ages 65 or older (Alzheimer's Association, 2012; Hebert, Scherr, Bienias, Bennett, & Evans, 2003; Plassman et al., 2007); among Americans aged 85 or older, 45% have AD. It is further estimated that in the United States, every 69 seconds someone develops AD and that for people 65 years or older, one out of every eight will have AD. Across all age groups, AD is the sixth-leading cause of death among Americans. It is important to keep in mind that with the elderly being the fastest growing segment of the U.S. population and with longer life expectancies, the projected number of Americans with AD may triple by the year 2050.

Although the exact cause of AD has yet to be specified (see below), a variety of risk and protective factors have been identified (see Table 3-2) that may increase or decrease, respectively, an individual's chance of developing this dementing illness (Alzheimer's Association, 2012; Fratiglioni & Rocca, 2001; O'Brien et al., 2003). For example, individuals who have inherited apolipoprotein E-ε4 (APOE-ε4), which is linked to a protein that carries cholesterol in our bloodstream, from one parent have an increased risk of developing AD. Those who inherit this form of the APOE from both parents will be at even greater risk of developing AD in their lifetime. Certain demographic groups also appear more vulnerable to AD. For example, as with stroke, certain ethnicities are at greater risk for developing AD; in the United States, these include older African American and Hispanic adults, who are 2 and 1.5 times, respectively, more likely than older Caucasian adults to have AD (Alzheimer's Association, 2012). Although more women than men have AD (about two thirds of Americans with AD are women), this is a reflection of the well-documented fact that women have a longer life span than men do (Plassman et al., 2007).

TABLE 3-2
Risk and Protective Factors Associated With Alzheimer's Disease

RISK FACTORS	PROTECTIVE FACTORS

• Old age
• Down syndrome or family history of Down syndrome
• History of leukemia
• Advanced age of mother at birth
• Family history of Alzheimer's disease
• Presence of APOE type 4 allele (APOE-ε4)
• History of traumatic brain injury, particularly if:
  ~ in presence of APOE-ε4
  ~ had a moderate or severe TBI
  ~ had repeated TBIs
• Mild cognitive impairment (MCI) diagnosis
• Cardiovascular disease risk factors
  ~ high blood pressure
  ~ high cholesterol
  ~ smoking
  ~ diabetes
  ~ physical inactivity
  ~ obesity
	• Rich social network
	• Early diagnosis and treatment of vascular disorders
	• Staying mentally active
	• Staying physically active
	• Possibly high education levels

Currently, the most accurate means of confirming a diagnosis of AD is the identification of neuropathological markers upon autopsy. For example, the pathologist will look for neurofibrillary tangles (i.e., unusual triangular and looped fibers in the cytoplasm of neurons made up of twisted strands of the protein tau), which are typically most pronounced in the inferior temporal lobe, posterior association regions, and Wernicke's area, and neuritic or senile plaques (i.e., aggregations of the protein fragment beta-amyloid), which are most pronounced in the medial temporal lobes (Alzheimer's Association, 2012; Wharton et al., 2011). The brains of patients with AD also show widespread cortical atrophy and ventricular dilation. Importantly, bilateral areas of the brain are affected, although involvement may not necessarily be symmetrical (Cummings, 2000).

Because confirmation of AD can only be made post mortem, the terms "probable AD dementia" or "possible AD dementia" have been recently adopted (McKhann et al., 2011). To help physicians and clinicians reliably make these probable and possible AD diagnoses in patients who are still living, a number of behavioral and medical criteria have been developed (see Table 3-3). In particular, these criteria are aimed to help rule out other possible causes of dementia, such as depression, stroke, alcoholism, malnutrition, or other neurological and medical disorders.

Finding the cause of AD is the major thrust of much research. It is known that in a very small percentage of AD cases, perhaps less than 1%, the cause is genetic (Alzheimer's Association, 2012) due to an autosomal dominant inheritance pattern (Lid-

TABLE 3-3
Clinical Criteria for Probable and Possible Alzheimer's Disease (AD)

PROBABLE AD	POSSIBLE AD
Dementia	Dementia
Gradual onset	Atypical course (e.g., sudden onset)
Observed or reported gradual worsening of cognitive symptoms	Insufficient evidence of progressive decline

Initial and most prominent cognitive symptom in one of the following:
a. Amnestic profile (i.e., memory)
b. Nonamnestic profile
   ~ Language/word retrieval
   ~ Visuospatial ability
   ~ Executive functioning
	Initial and most prominent cognitive symptom in one of the following:
	a. Amnestic profile (i.e., memory)
	b. Nonamnestic profile
	   ~ Language/word retrieval
	   ~ Visuospatial ability
	   ~ Executive functioning

Negative history of: a. Stroke b. Core symptoms of dementia with Lewy bodies c. Core symptoms of frontotemporal dementia d. Core symptoms of semantic or nonfluent primary progressive aphasia e. Another concurrent neurological disorder or non-neurological, medical disorder	Mixed etiology (e.g., concurrent cerebrovascular disease, taking medications that could compromise cognition)

dell, Lovestone, & Owen, 2001). These genetic cases tend to be associated with an early onset of AD (i.e., younger than 65 years of age). So far, researchers have identified at least four genes that, when abnormal, may produce AD:

- AD1—Located on chromosome 21 and has been associated with the high incidence of AD among individuals with Down syndrome
- AD2—Apolipoprotein E (apoE), which is found on chromosome 19 and is described as a risk-modifying gene (i.e., the presence of this abnormal gene is not sufficient to produce AD)
- AD3—Located on chromosome 14 and may be responsible for as many as 5% of AD cases
- AD4—Not as common as AD3 and is found on chromosome 1

Another possible cause of AD revolves around abnormalities in neurotransmitters and neuromodulators (Ritchie & Lovestone, 2002). For example, patients with AD have decreased levels of choline acetyltransferase, a chemical responsible for making acetylcholine, a neurotransmitter known to be important for learning and memory. The mechanism responsible for these neurotransmitter deficiencies, however, has yet to be determined. Other possible causes of AD, which have so far received little empirical support, include exposure to toxins such as aluminum or silicon, immunologic disorders, and nutritional deficiency. Some recent research also suggests that chronic exposure to high levels of pesticides may increase one's risk for AD (Parron, Requena, Hernandez, & Alarcon, 2011).

Pick's Disease and Other Types of Frontotemporal Lobar Degeneration

Pick's disease is another cause of irreversible dementia. This relatively rare disease typically occurs between the ages of 40 and 60 years and more frequently affects women than men (Rossor, 2001). Like AD, a diagnosis of Pick's disease can only be confirmed upon autopsy. At that time, the pathologist examines the brain for the presence of neuropathological markers such as Pick bodies and atrophy in the anterior frontal and temporal cortices (Kertesz, 2010; Yokota et al., 2009). Close to two thirds of Pick's disease cases that go to autopsy show asymmetrical atrophy, with greater left than right hemisphere atrophy being most common (Binetti, Locascio, Corkin, Vonsattel, & Growdon, 2000). Behaviorally, Pick's disease can be distinguished from AD because in Pick's, personality changes (e.g., socially inappropriate behavior, disinhibition) and reduced verbal output are prominent early in the disease, whereas memory and visuospatial skills may be spared until later stages of the disease (Binetti et al., 2000; Yokota et al., 2009); the reverse behavioral profile is more common in AD.

More recently, some researchers have proposed that Pick's disease may encompass or be a subtype of **frontotemporal lobar degeneration (FTLD)**, which produces similar behavioral and cognitive symptoms (Grossman et al., 2007; Kertesz, Hillis, & Munoz, 2003; Yokota et al., 2009). The term "FTLD" was coined when it was found that some patients with the behavioral symptoms of Pick's disease did not have the characteristic neuropathological markers of the disease (i.e., absence of Pick's bodies and AD pathology) (Kertesz, 2010). It is estimated that FTLD accounts for 5 to 20% of all dementia cases, and more frequently affects men than women (Bird et al., 2003; Grossman et al., 2007; Kertesz, 2010). FTLD tends to manifest after the age of 40 years, and, typically, patients with FTLD are younger than patients with AD. FTLD also differs from AD in that whereas disturbed levels of the neurotransmitter serotonin have been identified in FTLD, cholinergic levels are compromised in AD. FTLD is also associated with less hippocampal atrophy compared to AD (Xie et al., 2010).

Although the cause of FTLD remains unknown, progress has been made in identifying biomedical characteristics (Bird et al., 2003; Grossman et al., 2007; Yokota et al., 2009). For example, at least two pathology variants have been determined: (a) tau-positive inclusions or pathology, which is associated with frontal and parietal atrophy and progressive nonfluent aphasia as a prominent symptom, and (b) ubiquitin-positive, tau-negative inclusions or pathology, which is associated with frontal and temporal atrophy and semantic dementia as a prominent symptom. The latter type of FTLD is more common, occurring in about 40 to 60% of FTLD patients. A possible familial form of FTLD may also exist, which has been linked to mutations of the tau gene on chromosome 17 (Kertesz, 2010); the genetic variant appears to be quite rare, accounting for less than 5% of FTLD cases.

A Progressive Disorder With a Progressing Diagnosis

In many cases, the exact cause of patients' progressive communicative and cognitive deterioration is either only determined upon autopsy or, if an autopsy is not completed, never confirmed. For example, a couple of years ago, a patient was referred to our clinic to receive treatment services for what his neurologist had diagnosed as primary progressive aphasia (see Chapter 2 for a more detailed description of this neurogenic language disorder). Indeed, this patient did initially report and present with relatively isolated progressive language decline in the form of increasing difficulty with word finding and sentence formulation. However, over the first few months that this patient attended individual and group therapy in our clinic, he began to demonstrate significant behavioral symptoms (e.g., inappropriate spending with his credit card) and motor symptoms (e.g., periodic falling, gait disturbance, dysarthria). The onset of these symptoms negated a diagnosis of primary progressive aphasia, which is typically only given when patients demonstrate isolated declines in their language for at least two years; in contrast, this patient was still within the first year of the onset of his language decline. Given the striking behavioral problems that this patient was developing, we hypothesized that he might be presenting with a variant of frontotemporal dementia, which is associated with both language and behavioral symptoms. The breadth and severity of motor symptoms with which this patient was presenting, however, were not consistent with frontotemporal dementia. We were aware, though, that his sister had recently passed away from amyotrophic lateral sclerosis (ALS, or Lou Gehrig's disease), and consequently wondered if he might be presenting with more than one progressive disease.

We continued to provide this patient and his wife with support for his deteriorating communication abilities, which were soon confounded by the onset of additional cognitive impairments (e.g., memory and attention problems). For instance, although we quickly tried to identify an electronic augmentative communication system that would allow this patient to circumvent his rapidly escalating motor speech deficits, by the time his system arrived and we had begun training with the device, his cognitive and behavioral problems were interfering with successful device use (e.g., he could not remember how to access items not displayed on the main page of the device). Unfortunately, the patient's overall cognitive, communicative, behavioral, and motoric functioning deteriorated rapidly, and about 18 months after his initial referral to our clinic, his wife was no longer able to care for him within their home. The patient was admitted to a nursing home, but within a few weeks passed away.

The patient's wife did seek an autopsy to determine the cause of her husband's neurological disease and subsequent death. She was particularly interested in finding out whether there might be a genetic component to whatever disease caused his demise, given that they had children and grandchildren. The results of the autopsy indicated that he did display some pathological changes consistent with Pick's disease or frontotemporal dementia. Other changes, however, suggested more widespread, nonspecific neural degeneration. Therefore, although the patient's wife never received a specific diagnosis, the autopsy findings did allay her fears somewhat, as ALS was ruled out. She also received comfort in knowing that the results of her husband's autopsy would be used to further research the understanding of frontotemporal dementia and other, related progressive neurological diseases.

Parkinson's Disease

Parkinson's disease (PD) affects about 1.6% of Americans over the age of 65 (Wright Willis et al., 2010). It is more common in men than in women and among Caucasians versus other ethnicities. Like AD, the prevalence and incidence of PD increase with age, and thus is of concern, given the rapidly growing aging population (Boland & Stacy, 2012). PD is associated with deterioration of subcortical structures (e.g., the substantia nigra) and decreased levels of the neurotransmitter dopamine (Albin, Young, & Penny, 1995; Rinne et al., 2000); over time, disrupted functioning of other cortical areas (e.g., frontal lobe) and subcortical areas (e.g., putamen, globus pallidus) with which the substantia nigra connects and other neurotransmitter systems (e.g., cholinergic, serotonergic) will occur (Boland & Stacy, 2012; Schapira, 2009). It is not yet known what causes PD in the majority of patients, although in a small percentage of cases, there appears to be a genetic origin, and twin studies (Warner & Schapira, 2003) and epidemiological data (Parron et al., 2011; Wright Willis et al., 2010) indicate that environmental factors (e.g., herbicide and/or pesticide exposure; industrial pollution) may contribute to PD onset.

Hallmark motor symptoms of PD include dysarthria, bradykinesia (i.e., slowed movement), resting tremor, rigidity, gait and posture disturbances (and consequently, frequent falling), micrographia (i.e., a mechanical disruption of writing that results in extreme reductions in letter size; see Figure 3-8), and depression (Boland & Stacy, 2012; Heisters, 2011). Nonmotor symptoms also occur in PD, affecting psychiatric well-being (e.g., depression, psychosis), sensation (e.g., pain, degraded or loss of sense of smell), and language and cognition; these nonmotor symptoms may actually precede motor symptoms in many patients (Boland & Stacy, 2012). Whereas about 50 to 80% of PD patients will develop language and cognitive symptoms, in only around 20 to 30% will these symptoms be severe enough to be diagnosed as irreversible dementia (Heisters, 2011; Muslimovic, Post, Speelman, De Haan, & Schmand, 2009). Generally, patients with PD who develop dementia tend to be older, have had the disease for a shorter period of time, and display a faster rate of disease progression when compared with patients who have PD but do not develop dementia.

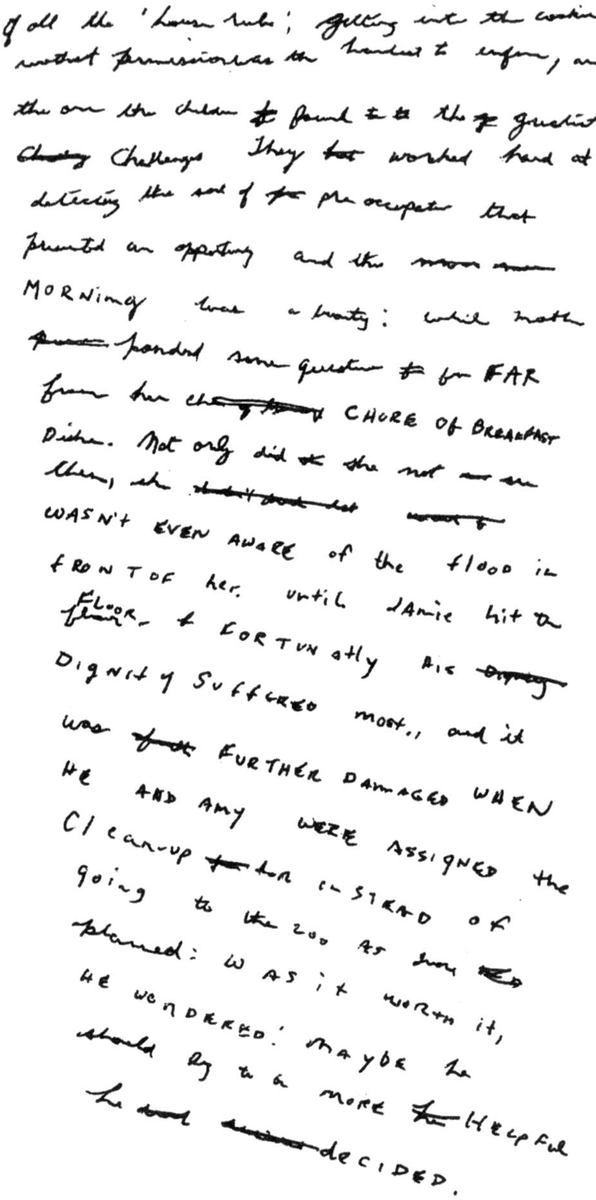

Figure 3-8. A sample of micrographia in the writing of a patient in the middle stages of Parkinson's disease. Note that the patient's strategy is to switch to printing when her writing becomes so small that even she can't read what she has written.

Huntington's Disease

Another subcortical disease that can produce neurogenic language and cognitive disorders is Huntington's disease (HD). More than 15,000 individuals in the United States suffer from HD, with an additional 150,000 having a 50% chance of inheriting the disease (NINDS, 2010). Age of symptom onset typically occurs somewhere between 35 and 50 years, with death following 15 to 20 years after symptom onset (C. A. Ross & Tabrizi, 2011; Sutton-Brown & Suchowersky, 2003). It is commonly observed that earlier symptom onset is associated with faster disease progression (NINDS, 2010). For example, in the early-onset or juvenile variant of HD, in which symptom onset occurs before age 20, death often occurs within 10 years following the appearance of symptoms.

In HD, the caudate nucleus and putamen undergo gradual deterioration, which are eventually followed by atrophy of subcortical white matter, the cerebral cortex, certain parts of the hypothalamus, and other brain regions (NINDS, 2010; C. A. Ross & Tabrizi, 2011; Weir, Sturrack, & Leavitt, 2011). HD is an autosomal dominant disease caused by a mutation of the huntingtin gene on chromosome 4. "Autosomal dominant" means that the mutated gene is located on a chromosome other than the sex-linked twenty-third chromosome, and that even if only one parent is carrying one copy of this mutated gene, that parent will develop the disease, and there is a 50% chance of passing the disease on to all children born to that parent. In rare cases, chronic drug abuse may also lead to HD.

Common symptoms of HD include chorea that affects speech (i.e., dysarthria), walking, swallowing (i.e., dysphagia), and other motor skills; bradykinesia; rigidity; and psychiatric problems such as depression and anxiety (Ross & Tabrizi, 2011; Sutton-Brown & Suchowersky, 2003; Weir et al., 2011). Unlike PD, HD always is associated with an **irreversible dementia**, which in some patients may actually precede motoric symptoms (Ross & Tabrizi, 2011; Weir et al., 2011).

Multiple Sclerosis

Multiple sclerosis (MS) is the most common, nontraumatic, disabling neurological disease among young and middle-aged adults. It is estimated that between 250,000 and 400,000 Americans are living with MS, with about 200 people being diagnosed with MS each week (Lewis et al., 2006; NINDS, 2011a). Although symptom onset is most common between the ages of 20 and 40, a small number of individuals, 2 to 5% of those with MS, will develop the disease in childhood (Julian, 2011). Generally, a diagnosis of MS often doesn't occur until later because symptoms can be transitory (i.e., a relapsing-remitting progression pattern). Certain individuals are at greater risk of developing MS (NINDS, 2011a). These include Caucasians, women, and people living in temperate climate zones (e.g., northern U.S., Canada, England). Although this latter risk factor suggests an environmental contribution to MS (Parron et al., 2011), as with the majority of progressive neurological diseases, the cause of MS remains unknown, with researchers continuing to explore both genetic and environmental factors (Lewis et al., 2006; NINDS, 2011a).

It is known, however, that MS causes patches of inflammation in white matter (called "plaques"), which in turn lead to demyelinating lesions and axonal damage within the white matter of the cerebrum, brain stem, cerebellum, and spinal cord; over time, diffuse cerebral atrophy may also occur (Julian, 2011; Lewis et al., 2006; NINDS, 2011a). In addition to motor symptoms (e.g., weakness, dysarthria, dysphagia, ataxia), psychiatric symptoms (e.g., depression, paranoia), and sensory symptoms (e.g., auditory processing difficulties, numbness, visual problems such as double vision and/or visual field cuts), somewhere between 40 and 70% of MS patients will experience cognitive and linguistic symptoms, which may over time progress into dementia. Notably, cognitive problems may be present when other MS symptoms are not, and have been found to negatively influence quality of life, functional status, and the integrity of motor skills (Benedict et al., 2011).

Korsakoff's Disease

Chronic alcohol abuse can lead to a condition called "Korsakoff's disease" that is characterized by an irreversible dementia (Kopelman, Thomson, Guerrini, & Marshall, 2009; NINDS, 2007). Like Wernicke-Korsakoff syndrome, which may result from dietary deficiencies and eating disorders (e.g., anorexia, effects of chemotherapy), Korsakoff's disease, which is sometimes also referred to as "Korsakoff's amnesic syndrome," results from, at least in part, a lack of thiamine (vitamin B1). In addition to this nutritional deficiency, chronic alcohol use can have other direct toxic effects on the brain (e.g., exposure to metabolic toxins), as well as indirect effects such as TBI. Neuropathological changes associated with Korsakoff's disease include unilateral or bilateral damage to the thalamus, mammillary bodies, cerebellum, and diencephalic structures (e.g., hypothalamus, mammillary bodies); widespread cortical atrophy, often most marked in the frontal lobes, may also occur. These neural changes are associated with the hallmark symptoms of memory and learning deficits (i.e., problems acquiring new memories and retrieving existing memories) and confabulation. Chronic abuse of other drugs, such as cocaine, also may cause permanent cognitive impairments that can progress in severity over time (Ardila, Rosselli, & Strumwasser, 1991).

Multiple Strokes, or Vascular Dementia

There are a number of medical conditions and diseases that can cause an individual to suffer multiple strokes or experience progressive damage to the cerebral blood vessels (e.g., hypertension, small vessel disease, diabetes, lupus erythematosus). Whereas the initial one or two strokes might cause deficits associated with focal lesions (e.g., aphasia), further strokes can lead to progressive decline of a broad range of language and cognitive abilities referred to as "vascular dementia." In fact, the second most frequent cause of irreversible dementia in the elderly, accounting for about 20 to 30% of all dementia cases, is **vascular dementia** (Alzheimer's Association, 2012; Fratiglioni & Rocca, 2001; O'Brien et al., 2003). In fact, vascular lesions are extremely common in individuals who have been diagnosed with AD, with one autopsy study finding that among their cases who fulfilled the diagnostic criteria for a pathological diagnosis of AD (e.g., had sufficient levels of some of the pathological markers described above when reviewing AD), only 21% had pure AD (Fernando & Ince, 2004); the rest of the cases had a mix of AD pathology and vascular lesions.

The same factors that put individuals at risk for suffering one stroke also put them at risk for suffering multiple strokes (e.g., hypertension, cigarette smoking). It has also been suggested that one's risk for developing vascular dementia may be increased if one has a history of high alcohol consumption, psychological stress in early life, and a lower level of formal education (Mahendra & Engineer, 2009). Recent research efforts have also been exploring a genetic component to vascular dementia (del Rio-Espinola et al., 2009; Leblanc, Meschia, Stuss, & Hachinski, 2006). For example, a few genes have been identified that can make the brain more susceptible to stroke: (a) cerebral autosomal dominant arteriopathy with subcortical infarcts and leucoencephalopathy, or CADASIL, which has been linked to a mutation on chromosome 19 and causes small vessel disease in the brain and other organs and, consequently, lacunar strokes in middle age (i.e., symptom onset around 46 years of age), and, (b) hereditary cerebral hemorrhage with amyloidosis-Dutch type, or HCHWA-D, which can cause multiple hemorrhagic strokes.

In contrast to the progressive neurological diseases described above, in which symptom onset is gradual and progressive, vascular dementia is associated with symptoms that have an abrupt onset (co-occurring with stroke onset) and that over time tend to show a stepwise deterioration. Furthermore, unlike patients with one of the previously mentioned progressive diseases, patients with vascular dementia can have focal neurological symptoms and signs and may show an interim recovery of lost function (i.e., spontaneous recovery) following each of their strokes.

Despite these differences, one form of vascular dementia, angular gyrus syndrome, is often confused with AD and pseudodementia (Benson, Cummings, & Tsai, 1982; Nagaratnam, Phan, Barnett, & Ibrahim, 2002; Vallar, 2007). Angular gyrus syndrome is caused by multiple lesions to posterior and inferior parietal regions of the left hemisphere. It is difficult to discern this syndrome from AD and pseudodementia (i.e., cognitive symptoms due to depression) because symptoms such as disorientation, anomia, and depression are characteristic of all three disorders, and because the lesions that produce angular gyrus syndrome are often so small they are not detected by CT scans.

Reversible Causes of Language and Cognitive Disorders

It is important to keep in mind that language and cognitive disorders may also appear in a number of conditions that when treated promptly and appropriately, will lead to partial or complete eradication of the language and cognitive symptoms. For example, an estimated 10 to 30% of dementia cases are **reversible** in that they can improve with appropriate medical treatment. Some reversible causes of neurogenic language and cognitive disorders are described below:

Depression (pseudodementia)
Medications (e.g., side effects from certain anticholinergic or antihypertensive drugs)
Infection (e.g., meningitis, encephalitis, urinary tract infection, West Nile Virus)

Hearing loss
Electrolyte imbalance
Tumors
Normal pressure hydrocephalus
Mental and/or sensory deprivation
Renal failure (dialysis dementia)
Thyroid disease and other metabolic disorders
Toxin exposure (e.g., lead poisoning)
Vitamin deficiency (e.g., pellagra, Wernicke-Korsakoff syndrome)

Depression may cause dementia and accounts for nearly 15% of all dementia cases (Rabins, 1983). Although depression does not always produce language and cognitive symptoms severe enough to qualify as dementia, approximately 10 to 20% of the depressed elderly will develop overt cognitive problems, sometimes referred to as **pseudodementia** (Beats, Sahakian, & Levy, 1996; Nussbaum, 1994). With respect to elderly patients, neither neuropsychological assessment nor biomedical methods (e.g., neuroimaging, neuroendocrine sampling) have proven sensitive or specific enough to permit timely, affordable, and confident diagnostic discrimination between pseudodementia and early or mild forms of irreversible dementia etiologies such as Alzheimer's disease (Dobie, 2002; Maynard, 2003; Saez-Fonseca et al., 2007). Differential diagnosis is difficult because (a) pseudodementia has widespread cognitive symptoms (e.g., impaired memory and reasoning, visuospatial deficits) and behavioral issues (e.g., social withdrawal, apathy) that are indistinguishable from those of early Alzheimer's disease (Dobie, 2002; Wright & Persad, 2007); (b) presentation of depression in the elderly often is atypical in that their affective symptoms (e.g., depressed mood, feelings of worthlessness) may appear to be absent or secondary to their cognitive symptoms (Gallo, Rabins, & Anthony, 1999); and (c) definitive diagnosis of Alzheimer's disease is possible only via autopsy to confirm Alzheimer-type neuropathology. Consequently, approximately 40% of dementia cases referred for psychiatric services will later receive a diagnosis of depression with reversible cognitive changes (Maynard, 2003; Rabins, 1983), and 5 to 20% of thoroughly evaluated patients who receive an initial diagnosis of irreversible dementia are rediagnosed with depression at a later date (Feinberg & Goodman, 1984).

Numerous medications and toxic substances may also produce reversible dementia. For example, dementia is a well-documented side effect of many anticholinergic drugs, including sedatives, antidepressants, anti-arrhythmics, and some antihypertensive medications (R. A. Stein & Strickland, 1998; Vogel, Carter, & Carter, 2000). As another example, one recent study identified greater attention deficits and fatigue levels in patients with multiple sclerosis who were taking medications with central nervous system effects versus those who were not (Oken et al., 2006). Exposure to toxins such as lead, mercury, or certain insecticides may also cause cognitive problems (Parron et al., 2011). Notably, prolonged exposure to these toxins, particularly in children, may lead to irreversible dementia.

A number of medical conditions, when left untreated, may also produce language and cognitive symptoms. These include metabolic disorders (e.g., thyroid or liver disease), hydrocephalus, vitamin deficiency (e.g., pellagra or B3 deficiency; Wernicke-Korsakoff syndrome or thiamine deficiency), renal failure (sometimes referred to as "dialysis dementia"), infection (e.g., meningitis, syphilis, encephalitis), and tumors (Alzheimer's Association, 2012; Harciarek, Beidunkiewica, Lichodziejewska-Niemierko, Debska-Slizien, & Rutkowski, 2009; Pantiga, Rodrigo, Cuesta, Lopez, & Arias, 2003; Sahin, Gurvit, Bilgic, Hanagasi, & Emre, 2002). Although some of these medical disorders may eventually lead to permanent dementia, there is the potential to reverse the language and cognitive symptoms if the etiology is identified and treated early in the course of the disorder.

Summary

This chapter reviewed several diseases, medical conditions, and drugs that may produce neurogenic language and cognitive disorders. Further information pertaining to many of these diseases and medical conditions is provided in the remaining chapters of this book; for example, in Chapter 12, a list of online information resources, some of which pertain to these diseases and conditions, that are appropriate for clinicians as well as patients and their caregivers is provided (see Table 12-4). It is important to be aware that suffering from one of these diseases or conditions does not negate the possibility of acquiring another of these etiologies. Thus, in many patients there are numerous reasons for their neurogenic language or cognitive disorder (e.g., a patient with dementia who has a history of stroke and Parkinson's disease; a patient with Huntington's disease who suffers a fall and, consequently, a TBI). Accordingly, a comprehensive assessment, as will be reviewed in several subsequent chapters, is essential to identifying behaviors that can lead to the most accurate determination of the etiology or etiologies of each patient's neurogenic language or cognitive disorder.

Discussion Questions

1. Have you ever experienced any of the symptoms associated with stroke? Discuss why individuals experiencing stroke symptoms might delay medical evaluation.
2. Consider the following age groups: 1-5 years old, 10-25 years old, 30-50 years old, and 60-90 years old. Which potential causes of neurogenic cognitive or language disorders are each of these age groups at greatest risk for experiencing?
3. Why is it important for speech-language pathologists to understand the nature of the conditions leading to neurogenic language or cognitive disorders?

A General Model of Assessment

chapter 4

Learning Objectives

After reading this chapter, you should be able to:

- List four general goals of assessment
- Describe factors that influence the determination of specific assessment goals
- Describe the primary job responsibilities of the variety of health-care professionals with whom speech-language pathologists may interact
- Identify pertinent information to collect for a case history
- Define the psychometric properties of reliability, validity, and standardization
- Differentiate the strengths and weaknesses of test batteries versus tests of specific linguistic and cognitive functions
- Describe the difference between qualitative and quantitative assessment information
- Identify why a caregiver assessment might be needed
- List important information that should be included in diagnostic reports

Key Terms

- neuropsychologists
- occupational therapists
- premorbid abilities
- qualitative information
- reliability
- sensitivity
- specificity
- standardization
- team approach
- validity

Introduction

Clinicians who assess and treat adults with neurogenic language or cognitive disorders may work in a variety of employment settings (e.g., acute care hospital, skilled nursing facility, home health) and with a variety of patient populations (e.g., varying in age, neurological disorder, time postonset of the language disorder). Despite this variability, there are some generalities among the procedures used to quantify and qualify the acquired linguistic and cognitive impairments and activity and participation restrictions of their patients. Accordingly, the purpose of this chapter is to describe general assessment guidelines and procedures germane to planning an evaluation of a neurogenic language or cognitive disorder, regardless of whether the patient presents with aphasia, right hemisphere brain damage (RHD), traumatic brain injury (TBI), and/or dementia. Specifically, this chapter defines what an assessment is and reviews both general and specific assessment goals. Next, general assessment procedures are described, followed by a brief review of assessment report writing.

Assessment: Definition and Goals

An assessment represents an organized evaluation of the multiple factors (e.g., amount of environmental support) and abilities (e.g., morphosyntactic ability, problem-solving skills) that may influence a patient's language and cognitive functioning. The general purposes of an assessment include (Murray & Chapey, 2001; Murray & Coppens, 2011) the following: (a) quantifying and qualifying communication and cognition strengths as well as weaknesses, (b) identifying the presence and possible influence of concomitant disorders, (c) establishing treatment goals, and (d) providing an informational basis from which to make predictions regarding recovery and treatment outcomes.

To satisfy these assessment goals, a clinician should ideally be completing an in-depth evaluation. Currently, however, there is a growing tendency for health-care/insurance agencies to prescribe quick and cheap—versus comprehensive and, consequently, more costly—language and cognition evaluations. Nevertheless, clinicians should, at the very least, attempt to obtain adequate time and financial support to complete the type of methodical assessment that is necessary to depict accurately their patients' linguistic and cognitive abilities, and thus plan individualized and appropriate treatment goals and procedures. Clinicians must be proactive and educate health-care/insurance agencies about the subsequent time and financial savings associated with a thorough assessment. As Brookshire (1997) advised, it is clinicians' ethical responsibility "to ensure that gains in economy and efficiency do not come at the expense of their understanding of their patients' impairments and do not compromise their ability to provide the most efficacious treatment for those impairments" (p. 206).

The Quest for Diagnostic Time!

Clinicians across health-care disciplines are constantly being challenged by reimbursing agencies to streamline and thus reduce costs associated with diagnostic services. However, there are discrepancies in terms of how much time each of these disciplines is customarily allotted for evaluations. For instance, the mean neuropsychology evaluation time cited by Sweet, Nelson, and Moberg (2006), when they were raising concerns about shrinking assessment times, was approximately four hours. Based on our clinical experiences, this average time amount well exceeds that of most speech-language pathology assessments, regardless of work setting. Accordingly, speech-language pathologists might point out this incongruity when advocating for longer assessment times for their patients.

Specific Assessment Goals

Specific assessment goals define the nature and focus of the assessment (for examples, see Table 4-1). These goals are dictated by a variety of work-setting and patient-related factors. For example, the assessment provided to patients in temporary acute care units will differ from that provided to patients in rehabilitation units or facilities or in skilled nursing facilities, or those receiving home health services (J. Duffy, Fossett, & Thomas, 2011). Acute care assessment goals tend to focus on (a) immediate physical survival (e.g., presence and severity of dysphagia), (b) basic communication needs (e.g., determining the reliability of yes/no responses, presence of motor speech vs. language disorder), and (c) the need for caregiver (family and medical staff) education and counseling. In contrast, subacute, rehabilitation, outpatient, and long-term care assessment goals are more comprehensive and should include a detailed examination of specific linguistic and cognitive abilities (see Chapter 13 for more information about health-care settings).

TABLE 4-1
Examples of Specific Assessment Goals

INFLUENTIAL FACTOR		EXAMPLE GOAL
Work setting	Acute care	• Determine caregivers' understanding of patient's current deficits.
		• Determine presence or absence of dysphagia.
		• Identify presence/absence of common right hemisphere cognitive-communicative deficits.
	Long-term care	• Describe nature and severity of patient's neglect.
		• Examine patient's productive discourse abilities in terms of macrolinguistic variables.
ICF model	Structure and function level	• Describe nature and severity of patient's neglect.
		• Examine patient's ability to understand spoken and written figurative language.
	Participation level	• Determine patient's current perception of his or her ability to participate in social gatherings.
		• Determine caregivers' current perception of the patient's ability to participate in social gatherings.
Lesion location	Right hemisphere	• Examine patient's productive discourse abilities in terms of macrolinguistic variables.
		• Examine patient's ability to understand spoken and written figurative language.
	Left hemisphere	• Determine type and severity of aphasia.
		• Examine patient's productive discourse abilities in terms of microlinguistic variables.

Note. ICF = International Classification of Functioning, Disability, and Health (World Health Organization, 2001).

Clinicians also should take into consideration the World Health Organization's (WHO, 2001) International Classification of Functioning, Disability, and Health (ICF) when deciding on specific assessment goals and procedures. Traditionally, the goal of assessment has been to evaluate the type and degree of language and/or cognitive impairment (i.e., ICF level of body structure and function). Consequently, the vast majority of standardized tests that are currently available assess linguistic (e.g., *Western Aphasia Battery* [Kertesz, 1982], *Boston Naming Test* [Kaplan, Goodglass, & Weintraub, 2001]) and/or cognitive (e.g., *Delis-Kaplan Executive Function System* [Delis, Kaplan, & Kramer, 2001]; *Wechsler Memory Scales-IV* [Wechsler, 2009]) impairments (see Chapters 6 and 7, respectively). More recently, however, there has been a trend in health care to determine how these impairments impact patients' daily activities and communication interactions (i.e., ICF level of limitations of personal activities), as well as their ability to resume their premorbid social and vocational roles and activities (i.e., ICF level of restrictions to participation in society). Accordingly, there is now a need to develop new, or utilize existing, tests (e.g., *ASHA Functional Assessment of Communication Skills for Adults* [Frattali, Thompson, Holland, Wohl, & Ferketic, 1995]) that assess the extent to which patients' well-being and social and vocational lifestyle have been compromised by their neurogenic language or cognitive disorder (Simmons-Mackie, Threats, & Kagan, 2005; Turkstra et al., 2005) (see Chapter 8). It is particularly essential that test developers begin to design measures appropriate for patients with language deficits such as aphasia, as most existing tests for assessing problems at the ICF activity and society participation levels were created for patients with primarily physical deficits and, more recently, for patients with nonlinguistic cognitive disorders. Therefore, when using these tests with aphasic patients, clinicians must make guarded interpretations of the reliability and validity of their findings.

When setting specific assessment goals, particularly in rehabilitation, outpatient, home health, and long-term care settings, clinicians should ensure that their assessment protocols address each of the ICF levels (WHO, 2001) (i.e., body function and structure, activities participation, and contextual factors). It is important to incorporate assessment procedures specific to each of these levels, because research indicates there is no one-to-one correspondence among these levels (Chaytor & Schmitter-Edgecombe, 2003; Irwin, Wertz, & Avent, 2002; Samsa & Matchar, 2004; Silverberg & Millis, 2009). That is, although clinicians might assume that patients who display severe impairments would also suffer severe activity and participation limitations, this is not necessarily the case. Likewise, it is not possible to identify influential contextual factors (e.g., communication barriers and facilitators) via impairment-based tests, and failure to identify these factors can lead to under- or overestimating how well patients will function when they return to their typical daily environments (K. Brown et al., 2006; Constantinidou et al., 2012; Schmitter-Edgecombe, Parsey, & Cook, 2011).

Deficit Severity Is in the Eye of the Beholder

Clinicians should never make assumptions about the impact of linguistic or cognitive impairments on their patients' participation in daily activities and social interactions. Take, for example, the following two patients who were receiving aphasia therapy in an outpatient rehabilitation clinic. Mr. McKibbin presented with a severe writing impairment following his stroke two months ago, and Ms. Ross presented with a mild reading deficit following her stroke four months ago. Whereas we might presume that Mr. McKibbin would also report greater daily activity and society participation setbacks compared to Ms. Ross, he does not: Writing is not (and was not even prior to his stroke) an essential communication skill for Mr. McKibbin, a retired bricklayer who currently spends most of his days golfing with his wife (who records their golf scores). In contrast, Ms. Ross is currently completing a doctorate degree in education and, consequently, in addition to a mild reading impairment, presents with significant daily activity limitations and society participation restrictions. She is unable to complete reading assignments with the accuracy and speed with which she could prior to her stroke, and her success as a doctoral student and, subsequently, a professor is now being jeopardized.

In addition to the ICF levels of disease/disorder, clinicians should consider other patient-related factors (e.g., lesion location, progressive vs. static brain damage, caregiver support) when developing specific assessment goals. For example, a request to evaluate a patient who has suffered a right hemisphere stroke would definitely suggest different specific assessment goals (e.g., analysis of visuospatial skills, analysis of high-level language comprehension abilities) than a request to evaluate a patient who has suffered a left hemisphere stroke (e.g., analysis of productive grammar skills, analysis of basic auditory comprehension abilities). Likewise, a review of the patient's **premorbid abilities** (e.g., literacy skills, number and types of languages most frequently used, pragmatic profile) also is useful when setting specific assessment goals.

Assessment Approach Considerations

It is very important that when planning assessments, clinicians take into consideration their role on the health-care team. Throughout most countries in the world, the **team approach** to health-care delivery is viewed as the optimal method for providing medical and rehabilitative services (Cornis-Pop et al., 2012; Langhorne & Duncan, 2001; E. Miller et al., 2010; Turkstra et al., 2005). Team organizational designs require establishing and maintaining collaboration among professionals from a variety of disciplines (Table 4-2). Because the precise composition of these health-care teams may vary from work setting to work setting (e.g., rehabilitation ward vs. skilled nursing facility) and from patient to patient (e.g., comatose vs. mildly impaired traumatic brain injury patient), it is essential that speech-language pathologists first determine what professions are represented on the health-care team to which they have been assigned. This is an important first step, as a number of team members may be capable of and interested in assessing the communication and cognition abilities of adults with neurogenic language

TABLE 4-2
Professions Frequently Found on Health-Care Teams Serving Adults With Neurogenic Language or Cognitive Disorders

PROFESSION	RESPONSIBILITIES
Audiology	Assess hearing abilities and balance/dizziness problems. Provide appropriate hearing devices and education/counseling.
Behavioral psychology	Assess behavioral problems and develop and monitor implementation of behavioral modification programs.
Clinical/rehabilitation psychology	Assess psychosocial status (e.g., depression, grief, anxiety) and needs of patient and family. Provide counseling or make recommendations for and monitor outcomes of other treatments (e.g., pharmacological treatment).
Neuropsychology	Assess cognitive abilities, including perception, attention, memory, executive functions, and language. Seldom directly involved in developing or providing communicative-cognitive treatment programs.
Nursing	Apply and monitor daily medical care, as well as educate, counsel, and train patient and family regarding ways to manage their own daily care. Essential to implementing behavioral treatments developed by other team members (e.g., encouraging patient use of a communication board; using appropriate behavioral modification techniques). Can be certified to specialize in rehabilitation nursing.
Nutrition	Assess nutritional (e.g., daily caloric intake) and hydration status and needs and develop dietary plans.
Occupational therapy	Assess fine motor and sensorimotor abilities, skills involved in completing activities of daily living (e.g., grooming, cooking), and, in some settings, cognitive abilities (e.g., perception, attention, problem solving) as they pertain to activities of daily living. Develop and provide treatment programs for deficits in those areas that they assess, including provision of and training with adaptive devices (e.g., switches, special eating utensils).
Physiatry	Determine the type of medical (e.g., laboratory tests) and rehabilitation (e.g., speech-language pathology, rehabilitation psychology) services needed and make requisitions for these services.
Physical therapy	Assess gross motor, balance, and postural abilities, such as those involved in walking and transferring (e.g., moving from a wheelchair to a bed). Develop and provide treatment programs for deficits in assessed areas, including provision of and training with adaptive devices (e.g., wheelchair, quad cane).
Speech-language pathology	Assess and provide treatment programs for motor speech, voice, language, cognitive, and swallowing disorders. Treatment includes not only individual services to patients but also group therapy for patients, and education and counseling of patients and their caregivers.
Social work	Assess social support status and needs, and make recommendations for and assist in implementing patient discharges (e.g., arranging home health services, identifying financial concerns and possible funding sources). Sometimes provide patient and family counseling.

TABLE 4-2 (*continued*)

PROFESSION	RESPONSIBILITIES
Therapeutic recreation	Assess social interaction and leisure needs. Plan and implement recreational and, when possible, community-based activities to improve physical, social, emotional, behavioral, and communicative-cognitive functioning.
Vocational rehabilitation	Determine appropriate vocational goals by identifying current work tolerance, past work history (to pinpoint transferable skills that are compatible with the patient's current physical, cognitive, and behavioral limitations); evaluating potential work environments and government or disability compensation funding.

or cognitive disorders. Furthermore, depending on geographic location in the United States or Canada, by administering certain cognitive tests, a speech-language pathologist may actually violate professional guidelines of that state or province. For example, frequently, only psychologists are licensed to purchase, administer, and/or interpret the results of certain tests of executive functioning (e.g., *Wisconsin Card Sorting Task* [Grant & Berg, 1993]), as well as many cognitive test batteries (e.g., *Wechsler Adult Intelligence Scale-IV* [Wechsler, 2008]; *Wechsler Memory Scale-IV* [Wechsler, 2009]). Therefore, the health-care team needs to determine who is responsible for assessing which communicative and cognitive abilities so as to avoid redundant testing procedures and, perhaps, breaching professional restrictions.

Same Testing for Different Purposes

Several assessment procedures utilized by speech-language pathologists within the context of communication assessment are also utilized by other disciplines for different purposes. A good example is the use of the *Boston Naming Test* (BNT; Kaplan, Goodglass, & Weintraub, 2001; see Chapter 6) by neuropsychologists. It is not unusual for the quantitative information provided by the BNT to be considered in a broader assessment of verbal recall abilities—for example, in contrast to nonverbal recall. The BNT also incorporates cueing strategies that are not taken into account in the quantitative results, and are therefore often not of great interest in the final interpretation by neuropsychology. In contrast, qualitative information about how the patient responds to semantic and phonemic cues is highly valuable to the speech-language pathologist in developing treatment recommendations. Therefore, this is a situation where the speech pathologist may opt to re-administer a test that has been previously administered for a different purpose.

Preferably, *all* team members should directly or indirectly contribute to the assessment of the communicative and cognitive abilities of patients with neurogenic disorders. Team members who are typically best qualified for, and most frequently responsible for, the direct examination of abilities that speech-language pathologists commonly evaluate include **neuropsychologists** (or rehabilitation psychologists, clinical psychologists, etc.) and **occupational therapists**. Importantly, even when these other team members are in charge of directly assessing the linguistic and cognitive abilities of patients with neurogenic language or cognitive disorders, speech-language pathologists must maintain as much active involvement as possible because of our unique expertise in examining and interacting with this patient population. Although these other team members often have had more training and experience in administering cognitive tests (i.e., attention, memory, and executive function assessment tools), speech-language pathologists typically are more educated about and proficient in accommodating test procedures for and interpreting the test results of patients with speech and language impairments. Likewise, when speech-language pathologists are responsible for the direct assessment of communication and cognition, it is very informative to interview other team members regarding their observations of a given patient's abilities. Their input will supplement direct assessment results by providing clinicians with a more comprehensive description of the patient's linguistic and cognitive abilities under varying communicative and cognitive circumstances (i.e., different communicative partners, activities, and settings), as well as assist with identifying contextual factors (i.e., a component of the ICF model) that may negatively or positively affect the patient's communicative and cognitive abilities.

Lastly, clinicians must not overlook that the patients themselves, as well as their family or significant others, are also integral members of the health-care team (Cornis-Pop et al., 2012; E. Miller et al., 2010; H. Murray et al., 2006). It is imperative that an assessment be driven by the needs voiced by patients (at least in those cases in which they are adequately cognizant of the type and extent of their impairments) and their families. Given the trend to incorporate ICF levels into current health-care practice, inclusion of patients and their families in the assessment process is essential to quantifying and qualifying problems at the body function and structure level, and in particular at the personal activities and participation in society levels; additionally, identifying influential contextual factors—both environmental and personal—requires patient and caregiver feedback. Auditing bodies, including the Joint Commission of Accreditation of Healthcare Organizations (JCAHO) and the Commission on Accreditation of Rehabilitation Facilities (CARF), also require documented patient input. Finally, obtaining patient and family input is necessary because discrepancies among the perceptions of patients, families, and health-care professionals regarding the nature of the problem and the types of medical and rehabilitation services required have been found (Code, Muller, & Herrmann, 1999; H. Murray et al., 2006; Schmitter-Edgecombe et al., 2011). Consequently, a team approach to assessment should include procedures for identifying perceptual discrepancies among team members, and then ensure that subsequent services resolve these discrepancies.

> **Community-Based Teams**
>
> All members of the health-care team are not necessarily employees of the same facility. A small acute-care hospital in rural Iowa employed only one speech-language pathologist, three physical therapists, and no occupational therapists. Therefore, some patients' health-care teams included occupational therapists as well as physician specialists (e.g., radiation oncologists) employed at the neighboring hospital. When a patient's care team extends beyond typical boundaries, special care must be taken to ensure that communication among team members is accurate and efficient. Furthermore, having team members in different geographic locations is likely to be a more common occurrence in the future as telemedicine and telerehabilitation become more widespread.

Getting Referrals

One might expect that the presence of a neurogenic language or cognitive disorder will be apparent to the patient, the patient's family, and the many health-care professionals the patient encounters during a hospital stay. There are a variety of neurogenic communication and cognitive disorders, however, that can go undetected while the patient is staying in structured health-care settings. For example, patients with cognitive-communication disorders subsequent to RHD or with mild aphasia frequently demonstrate little difficulty in participating in the somewhat superficial and concrete conversations that occur throughout the day as their medical and physical problems are being addressed. Likewise, patients with executive function deficits are often able to act or function appropriately when staying in a health-care facility because of the predictable and organized schedules of these institutions. That is, inherent to these facilities is the type of external structure and support that these patients need to compensate for their executive function problems (Constantinidou et al., 2012; Miyake et al., 2000; Schmitter-Edgecombe et al., 2011). Often it is only when these patients return to their homes, which tend to have less structured and controlled environments and routines, that they and/or their loved ones begin to observe the patients' higher-level or more subtle linguistic and cognitive deficits.

Another factor that may negatively affect referrals, particularly the assessment of patients with progressive disorders, is therapeutic nihilism (Cahill et al., 2008; Iliffe, Wilcock, & Haworth, 2006). That is, among some health-care providers and citizens in the general public, there remains the belief that referrals for evaluation and treatment of progressive conditions are futile or wasteful, given that the advancement of the condition cannot be stopped. For example, in 2003, Cleary, Donnelly, Elgar, and Hopper reported that over 75% of Canadian speech-language pathologist survey respondents indicated that they did not routinely receive referrals to either assess or treat dementia patients.

Consequently, in many medical settings, the clinician must educate other health-care professionals and team members regarding possible high-level linguistic and cognitive problems associated with neurogenic disorders such as mild aphasia, mild TBI, and RHD, as well as evidence supporting the provision of speech-language pathology services to individuals with progressive disorders. Information concerning general characteristics of the various neurogenic communication or cognitive problems, strategies to compensate for these problems, and treatment options for progressive disorders can be provided via in-service training, informal discussion, the provision of reading materials (e.g., handouts, pamphlets), or case presentations at clinical rounds. Such educational efforts will hopefully result in increases in the number of these at-risk patients who are referred for speech-language pathology services.

Assessment Procedures

A variety of information-obtaining procedures should be used when completing an assessment (see Figure 4-1). Typically, the initial assessment procedures, such as obtaining a case history and completing informal observations, serve as a broad screen to identify the areas that will require more detailed and formal or structured assessment. The next step of the assessment process following collection of case history, observational, and formal test data is to integrate and interpret these findings to make decisions regarding the presence of a neurogenic language or cognitive disorder, amount and type of treatment, and prognosis. Lastly, clinicians must keep in mind that assessment is an ongoing process: Following an initial evaluation, clinicians must continue to assess the accuracy and adequacy of their diagnostic and treatment decisions to ensure optimal provision of services to their patients.

Case History

Case history information is essential to determining the patient's premorbid abilities, and consequently to identifying the presence of a neurogenic language or cognitive disorder. This information is useful when planning subsequent assessment and treatment procedures as well. For example, information pertaining to the patient's interests and hobbies can be used to develop motivating treatment stimuli and activities. To gather case history information, clinicians should not only review their patients' relevant medical records but also interview the patients and their caregivers, including family and friends as well as other professionals on the health team.

Review of Previous and Current Medical Records
Medical charts and records contain the reports of all health-care team members who have already assessed or treated the patient and consequently provide a wealth of information about the patient's past and current levels of functioning. With respect to developing assessment and treatment plans, identifying the following information will be of particular interest to speech-language clinicians:

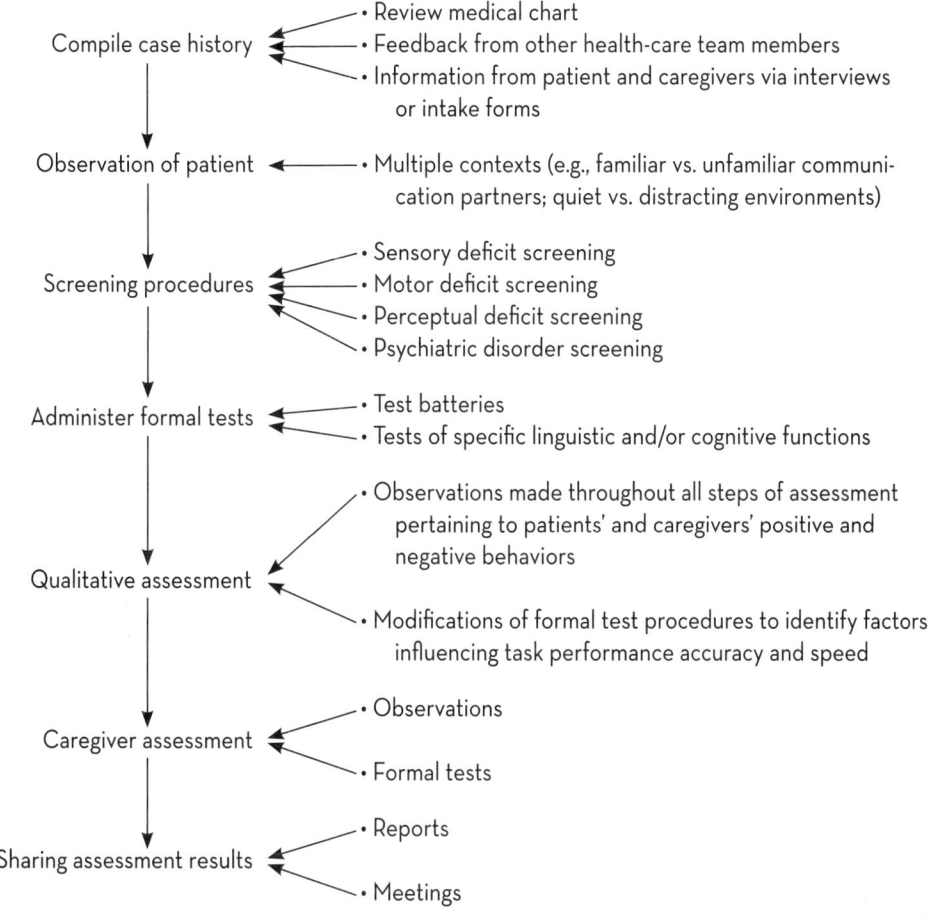

Figure 4-1. General steps to completing an in-depth neurogenic language or cognitive disorder evaluation.

1. Personal information, such as the patient's address, date and place of birth, educational background, past and current vocational status, ethnicity, and cultural background
2. Family and social history, including marital status, number of children, living situation (e.g., independent vs. assisted living), preferred social activities, and current level of family/social support
3. Past and present interests and hobbies
4. Premorbid speech and language abilities, including the languages that the patient uses, how frequently these languages are used, and competence and daily needs with respect to the various language modalities (e.g., pre-existing speech or language problems, such as developmental stuttering or dyslexia; prior to his stroke, although the spoken language skills of a given bilingual patient were comparable, his written Spanish skills were stronger than his written English skills)

5. Premorbid and present handedness
6. Past and present medical, neurological, and psychiatric status, including current medications, description of physical, cognitive, and behavioral symptoms, symptom onset and duration, and type (e.g., focal vs. diffuse damage) and location of brain damage

On the basis of this information, clinicians can begin to identify and implement appropriate assessment and treatment procedures. For example, information concerning the patient's age, education, and ethnocultural background can be used to identify formal tests with normative standards that are appropriate for that patient. Additionally, many formal linguistic and cognitive tests include questions pertaining to the above information; consequently, clinicians must know if their patients' responses to these test items are accurate.

With respect to reviewing patients' medical charts, speech-language clinicians also need to educate themselves regarding the assessment procedures, terminology, and abbreviations used by not only speech-language pathologists but also other health-care team members. This may be of particular importance when trying to interpret the assessment findings of neurologists and radiologists. Examples of some terms and abbreviations that clinicians will likely see in medical charts and reports are listed in Table 4-3 (for a more comprehensive list, see Ehrlich & Schroeder, 2009). Table 4-4 describes some of the more frequently used procedures that clinicians may encounter in neurology reports, and Table 4-5 reviews the different structural and metabolic assessment techniques used to quantify and qualify brain damage in patients with neurogenic language disorders (Baylor, 2003; Holdsworth & Bammer, 2008; Tartaglia, Rosen, & Miller, 2011).

Patient and Caregiver Interviews

Information concerning patients' premorbid and current levels of functioning as well as their assessment and intervention needs can also be obtained by interviewing patients and their caregivers (e.g., family members, friends, health-care providers, professional caregivers, community members). Conducting an initial interview with patients and caregivers not only provides clinicians with much-needed background information about their patients, but also gives clinicians an opportunity to establish rapport and mutual respect with patients and caregivers, qualities important to a therapeutic relationship. When an initial interview is not possible (usually due to time constraints), clinicians can obtain at least some of the same information by having patients and caregivers complete questionnaires.

One important question to ask during interviews pertains to what patients perceive to be their major problem or, perhaps more specifically, what they view to be their current communicative and cognitive weaknesses and strengths. Patients' responses to this line of questioning not only can identify the patients' treatment priorities and expectations, which sometimes differ from those of the clinician (e.g., a patient might be much more concerned about an apparently mild auditory comprehension problem than his obviously severe reading deficit) but also can provide data to assist in determining if

TABLE 4-3
Examples of Terms and Abbreviations Frequently Encountered in Medical Speech-Language Pathology

TERM OR ABBREVIATION	DEFINITION OR DESCRIPTION
ACVD	acute cardiovascular disease
ADL	activities of daily living (e.g., bathing, brushing teeth, dressing)
ADR	adverse drug reaction
A & O	alert and oriented
amb	ambulatory
aq	water
ASHD	arteriosclerotic heart disease
Ba	barium, barium sulfate
bid	twice daily
bil	bilateral
bp	blood pressure
bx	biopsy
c/o	complains of
CBR	complete bed rest
ck	check
CHF	congestive heart failure
COPD	chronic obstructive pulmonary disease
DAT	diet as tolerated
DG	diagnosis
DNR	do not resuscitate
DVT	deep vein thrombosis (i.e., blood clot that is often located in the leg)
DX, Dx	diagnosis
emb	embolism
ETOH	alcohol
FH	family history
F/U	follow-up
GERD	gastroesophagial reflux disease
HBP	high blood pressure
Hx	history of
HPN, HTN	hypertension (i.e., high blood pressure)
ICP	intracranial pressure
LOC	loss or level of consciousness
LOS	length of stay
MVA	motor vehicle accident
N/C	no complaints

(continues)

TABLE 4-3 (*continued*)

TERM OR ABBREVIATION	DEFINITION OR DESCRIPTION
NPO	nothing by mouth
OP, OPT	outpatient
PI	present illness
PNA, PN	pneumonia
p.r.n.	as needed
p.o.	by mouth
Px	prognosis
q.d.	every day
RO	reality orientation (a form of cognitive stimulation often provided to patients with dementia or in post-traumatic amnesia following traumatic brain injury)
ROM	range of motion
Rx	prescription; treatment
SNF	skilled nursing facility
STG	short-term goal
Sx	symptoms
UE	upper extremity
WNL	within normal limits

patients are unaware of (i.e., anosognostic) or in denial of their deficits. Patient interviews can also provide insight into patients' level of orientation (e.g., ability to correctly answer questions concerning personal background information), self-monitoring and correction skills (i.e., ability to determine whether they have made a mistake and, if so, to correct their error), and their pragmatic language abilities (e.g., ability to stay on topic or provide relevant vs. irrelevant information).

Clinicians must, however, keep in mind that a number of factors may limit the amount of information that neurogenic patients can supply. For example:

- Patients with aphasia may be unable to express information or comprehend interview questions due to their language problems.
- Patients with RHD or TBI may have little insight into the presence or severity of their deficits, due to cognitive impairments such as anosognosia.
- Patients with dementia or TBI may have memory limitations that reduce the amount or accuracy of the background information they share.
- Dysarthria or apraxia of speech, which limit speech production abilities, may further limit a patient's ability to respond to interview questions.
- Acute care patients may be too sick or medicated to participate in an interview (Duffy et al., 2011).

TABLE 4-4
Procedures Frequently Completed During a Neurological Examination to Identify the Presence and Possible Location of Nervous System Dysfunction

PROCEDURE	PURPOSE AND DESCRIPTION
Neck flexion	Checking for neck rigidity or stiffness, as these are indicative of a hemorrhage.
Auscultation	Applying a stethoscope over the carotid bifurcation (within the neck) to listen for evidence of bruits or abnormal pulsating sounds that indicate turbulent blood flow through an artery. Bruits are associated with artery stenosis or narrowing.
Palpation	Palpating the carotid arteries within the neck to feel for altered or unilateral pulsation that is indicative of arterial obstruction or occlusion.
Neuro-ophthalmologic exam	Inspecting the optic fundus or the vascular system at back of eye. Atherosclerosis, hypertension, diabetes, and other disorders produce recognizable retinal and vascular changes.
Motor function exam	Visually and manually inspecting muscular tone (e.g., spasticity vs. rigidity vs. flaccidity), bulk (e.g., wasting or hypertrophy), strength (e.g., hemiplegia or hemiparesis), and coordination, as well as inspecting for the presence of involuntary movements.
Sensory function exam	Assessing responses to primary sensory modalities (i.e., touch, pain, temperature, vibration, and position) and cortical sensations (e.g., two-point discrimination, stereognosis, graphesthesia).
Cranial nerve function exam	Examining for symptoms indicative of cranial nerve damage (e.g., lack of pupillary light reflex, impaired vertical and horizontal eye movements, presence of facial droop or asymmetry, asymmetrical soft palate movement, tongue deviation upon protrusion).
Reflex elicitation	Checking for the presence or absence of deep tendon reflexes (i.e., absence indicative of peripheral nerve damage, hyporeflexia indicative of lower motor neuron damage, and hyperreflexia indicative of upper motor neuron) and pathological or release reflexes (i.e., reflexes that are normal in infants but that disappear over first to second year of life) such as the Babinski sign (i.e., when the lateral aspect of the sole of the foot is stroked, the toes extend rather than flex), the snout reflex (i.e., tapping the upper lip causes an abnormal puckering response), the rooting reflex (i.e., when a cheek is tapped or stroked, there is an abnormal movement of the angle of the mouth toward the tap), or the grasp reflex (i.e., stroking the web between the thumb and first finger produces an abnormal involuntary grasp of the stroking fingers).
Exam of higher cognitive functions	Completing a brief screening of cognitive ability (e.g., orientation to person, place, and time) and emotional-behavioral functioning (e.g., lability).

Rather than avoiding interviewing patients who have one or more of the above confounding communication or cognitive issues, clinicians can utilize strategies to adjust the communication or cognitive demands of the interview process (Dalemans, Wade, van den Heuvel, & de Witte, 2009; Hellstrom, Nolan, Nordenfelt, & Lundh, 2007). As

TABLE 4-5
Procedures for Assessing Structural and Metabolic Changes Within the Brain

PROCEDURE	PURPOSE AND DESCRIPTION
Angiography	Injection of radiopaque material into an extracranial artery to obtain high-resolution x-ray images of the cerebral vascular system (i.e., arterial supply and venous drainage). Used to identify structural abnormalities of intracranial blood vessels (e.g., arterial stenosis or occlusion, aneurysms, arteriovenous malformations, vasculitis) or alterations in the positions of these vessels (e.g., displacement may be indicative of a cerebral tumor). May also be used to confirm brain death. This technique is considered invasive, with associated risks, such as dislodging arterial plaque, producing emboli, and negative reaction to the contrast medium.
Ultrasonography	Noninvasive imaging of the carotid bifurcation or intracranial blood vessels using Doppler technology. Ultrasound exams are less sensitive than other vascular imaging techniques but can be conducted at bedside.
Computer assisted tomography (CT)	X-ray cross-sectional images of the brain taken from various angles to identify the presence and location (within a few millimeters) of lesions. CT is also used to rule out reversible causes of dementia. This technique is considered invasive because of x-ray/radiation exposure. Another risk is a negative reaction to the contrast medium. Although this is an affordable, rapid, and widely available assessment procedure, it does not allow immediate (e.g., within 24 hours) visualization of thrombotic or embolic infarctions and may fail to identify lacunae or tiny lesions.
Magnetic resonance imaging (MRI)	Noninvasive images obtained by exposing the brain to a large magnetic field. Compared to CT scans, MRIs provide better visualization of gray versus white brain matter and small lesions, and quicker identification of infarction and edema (i.e., within 90 minutes). MRI also is useful for visualizing damage related to demyelinating diseases, tumors, infections, and degenerative diseases. Limitations of MRI include that it cannot be used with patients who have pacemakers or other metallic implants or prostheses because of the strong magnetic forces. Additionally, patients with movement disorders or who are uncooperative will require sedation to avoid movement during the long scanning time.
Magnetic resonance angiography (MRA)	Noninvasive imaging of extra- and intracranial blood vessels (e.g., identification of occlusions, aneurysms, arteriovenous malformations) based on MRI technology. MRA has fewer risks than angiography, but only allows imaging of the arterial or venous system during one examination unless scanning time is dramatically increased. Other limitations are similar to those mentioned for MRI.
Functional MRI (fMRI)	Collection of a series of MRI scans while the patient completes specific tasks to identify areas of brain activation. Associated with spatial resolution within a few millimeters and temporal resolution within a few seconds, although this resolution can be perturbed by neuropathology. fMRI is used not only in research to examine brain-behavior relations but also clinically to localize responses prior to neurosurgery and to examine brain activity in static and progressive forms of brain damage. Other strengths and limitations of fMRI are similar to those mentioned for MRI.

TABLE 4-5 (continued)

PROCEDURE	PURPOSE AND DESCRIPTION
Diffusion-weighted Imaging (DWI)	An MRI technique that measures the average distance that water molecules move by diffusion in a fixed time. DWI can identify acute infarction within minutes of stroke onset as well as subtle white matter changes. These images can also distinguish cysts from abscesses, and high-grade from low-grade tumors. DWI is particularly sensitive to even subtle motion, although techniques to address this concern are being developed. Across most neurodegenerative diseases, images generated by this MR technique are normal. Other strengths and limitations of DWI are similar to those mentioned for MRI.
Diffusion tensor imaging (DTI)	An MRI technique that, like DWI, measures water diffusion, but unlike DWI, measures diffusion in three directions. Thus, DTI allows examining the integrity of white matter tracts and, accordingly, is useful in identifying white matter pathology associated with traumatic brain injury, mild cognitive impairment, and several neurodegenerative diseases. Strengths and limitations of DTI are similar to those mentioned for DWI and MRI.
Perfusion-weighted imaging (PWI)	An MRI technique that involves injection of a contrast agent to provide information about blood flow, or hemodynamics, that allows visualization of not only the infarction but also brain tissue at risk for infarction (i.e., the penumbra). PWI can also be used in concert with MRA or DWI to evaluate the status of blood vessels (particularly small vessels) or identify the extent of ischemic brain injuries, respectively. Mismatch between the lesions identified via PWI versus DWI is used to make acute stroke management decisions (e.g., a large PWI lesion in concert with a small DWI lesion suggests a large penumbra and a good potential candidate for reperfusion therapy). Strengths and limitations are similar to those mentioned for other MRI techniques.
Positron emission tomography (PET)	Injection (or sometimes inhalation) of radioisotopes into an extracranial artery to visualize changes in regional cerebral blood flow (i.e., rCBF), cerebral glucose metabolism, or neurotransmitter levels. PET is particularly sensitive to early metabolic changes in mild cognitive impairment and several dementing diseases. This technique is invasive because of the exposure to radioactive material, and is expensive and not widely available because the radioactive material must be generated in an on-site cyclotron.
Single photon emission-computed tomography (SPECT)	Similar to PET, except the radioisotopes do not need to be generated by an on-site cyclotron. Although SPECT allows visualization of changes in cerebral blood flow (CBF), it is less precise than PET in terms of spatial resolution and identifying the etiology of CBF changes (e.g., tumor vs. stroke). Like PET, SPECT can also be used to examine neurotransmitter levels.

an example, Dalemans and colleagues (2009) provided a description of a variety of communication strategies and an interview format adaptation that proved effective when interviewing individuals with severe aphasia; these strategies and accommodations ranged from posing interview questions in both spoken and written modalities (including pictograms and drawings in the written version), limiting the length and complexity of questions, and allowing plenty of time for the individuals with aphasia to process the question and provide their response.

In addition to patients, it is equally important to interview family members, as well as health-care team members who have already assessed or treated the patient. The same questions should be posed to the patient's family and caregivers to identify any discrepancies in terms of perceptions of the patient's previous and current levels of functioning. Caregivers also should be asked to describe the communicative and cognitive style of the patient prior to the onset of neurological damage or disease. That is, the presence or severity of many communication and cognitive disorders can only be determined with respect to the patient's premorbid abilities. For example, it would be inappropriate to diagnose a patient who has RHD with aprosodia if the family reported that the patient had always sounded monotone.

There are a number of tools available, both commercially and in the research literature, to help clinicians structure interviews with or collect information and observations from caregivers or patients. For example, clinicians working with aphasic patients might have caregivers (or perhaps the patients themselves) complete the *Communicative Effectiveness Index* (CETI; Lomas et al., 1989). On the CETI, individuals rate the current communicative performance of patients with aphasia from *not at all able* to *as able as before the stroke* for a variety of daily communicative situations. Another example would be the *Clinician Interview-Based Impression of Change—Plus Caregiver Information* (CIBIC+; L. S. Schneider et al., 1997), which involves interviewing individuals with suspected dementia and their caregivers. The CIBIC+ interview focuses on 15 areas within the domains of general, cognitive, and behavioral functioning, as well as completion of activities of daily living. This interview tool was designed to be given at least twice: once at baseline prior to starting a treatment and then later during or after treatment to evaluate change since baseline. Upon completion of the follow-up interview, the clinician uses a 7-point scale (varying from 1, indicating marked improvement, to 7, indicating marked worsening) to rate the amount of change observed since the initial interview.

If clinicians opt to develop their own interview protocol or format, there are some format issues that should be taken into consideration. For instance, interviewing the patient and caregiver separately can often yield more information because caregivers may feel more comfortable discussing their concerns when the patient is not present. Additionally, comparing the responses of the caregiver and patient can assist the clinician in identifying awareness issues. Another issue pertains to the format of the interview questions. Nolin, Villemure, and Heroux (2006) found that when interviewed in the more typical open-question format (e.g., "Tell me what problems you're having since your head injury"), study participants with mild TBI reported fewer, and a narrower range of, symptoms compared to a "suggested response" interview (i.e., they were shown lists of possible TBI symptoms and asked to indicate which they were experiencing). In particular, out of 108 participants, none reported any social symptoms during the typical format interview, even though many of them reported problems such as difficulty participating in usual social activities, enjoying leisure activities, and maintaining friendships in the alternate format. Accordingly, developing a more structured interview format, perhaps geared toward the suspected neurogenic language or cognitive disorder (e.g., being sure to ask questions regarding neglect symptoms when interviewing a patient with RHD, being sure to ask questions regarding retrograde amnesia when interviewing a patient with TBI), may foster more feedback when interviewing patients, caregivers, or both.

Regardless of what type of interview or questionnaire format is used to collect information from patients and their caregivers, it is important to keep in mind that the data from such measures are at risk for reporter bias and thus need to be supplemented by data from other assessment methods (Dassel & Schmitt, 2008). Finally, in many assessment situations, it also is important to acknowledge that the interview will be the primary, or only, means of evaluating the ICF level of participation, as well as quality-of-life issues. Chapter 8 discusses several ways to include formal and informal measures of participation and quality of life as part of the interview portion of the evaluation.

Observations

Much information can be gleaned from a casual visit with patients and their family or caregivers. The main advantage of direct, informal observation is that it allows clinicians to examine the interaction between patients' behaviors and their daily environments, and thus may lead to identification of ICF contextual factors (e.g., communication partners, ambient noise levels) that positively or negatively affect patients' communicative and cognitive abilities. Observational sessions also allow clinicians to identify positive strategies (e.g., a spouse who always addresses his wife with left neglect on her right side, a patient with aphasia who uses gestures to augment her spoken output) and negative strategies (e.g., a caregiver who uses indirect requests with patients with RHD, a patient with dementia who avoids social situations) that enhance or hinder, respectively, the communication interactions of patients and caregivers (A. L. Holland, 1991).

Ideally, multiple informal observational samples should be completed to account for the variable behavior that is pervasive in adults with acquired neurogenic language or cognitive disorders. For example, the language abilities of patients with aphasia have been found to vary not only across different communication contexts, topics, and activities (e.g., D. Johnson & Cannizzaro, 2009; Mayer & Murray, 2003) but also within identical communication situations (e.g., Cameron, Wambaugh, & Mausycki, 2010; Freed, Marshall, & Chuhlantseff, 1996). Realistically, however, due to time and context limitations and, unfortunately, funding issues, most clinicians are able to complete only minimal amounts of observation and thus must acknowledge that they have a limited view of their patients' communicative behaviors in more naturalistic settings or circumstances. For instance, a clinician working in an outpatient clinic may be able to observe patients and caregivers/spouses interacting in the waiting room or during an occupational or physical therapy session, but have no opportunity to observe those patients' communication interactions in other, more frequently occurring settings, such as their place of work, their home, or even their daily trip to the grocery store.

In addition to providing preliminary insight into patients' communicative and cognitive abilities, initial observations and screening procedures are useful for identifying complicating conditions that interfere with patients' current levels of functioning or future recovery. Failure to identify these complicating conditions prior to formal assessment of communicative and cognitive abilities can result in inaccurate diagnostic and prognostic conclusions. Complicating conditions with which patients with neurogenic language or cognitive disorders frequently present and, consequently, of which clinicians must be cognizant include sensory deficits, motoric impairments, perceptual problems, and psychiatric disorders (for a further review of complicating conditions, see Chapter 5).

Initial Screening Procedures

Prior to direct evaluation of communication and cognitive abilities, it is important to document the presence or absence of conditions that may confound patients' performance on formal or informal measures of communication or cognition. Accordingly, screening for sensory, motor, perceptual, and psychiatric problems should be the next step when assessing patients with neurogenic language or cognitive disorders. Complicating conditions that commonly co-occur with neurogenic language and cognitive disorders, as well procedures for screening these confounding conditions, are described in Chapter 5.

Formal Test Procedures

Formal or structured tests allow clinicians to compare their patients' communicative and cognitive performances to normative standards. Generally, formal tests have the advantages of offering objective, quantifiable, and consistent administration procedures and, thus, assessment findings. Like any assessment method, however, formal tests have their disadvantages; in particular, they do not allow identifying or considering environmental factors (e.g., unstructured environments or tasks) or personal factors (e.g., motivation or anxiety level) that may be negatively or positively influencing a given patient's communicative or cognitive status (Constantinidou et al., 2012; Schmitter-Edgecombe et al., 2011; Turkstra et al., 2005).

Currently, a plethora of formal tests are available to assess the linguistic and cognitive status and functional outcome of adults with neurogenic language or cognitive disorders (see Chapters 6 through 8). These tests differ on a variety of levels, including (a) length (e.g., a bedside aphasia screening vs. a detailed aphasia battery), (b) scope (e.g., a test of verbal working memory vs. a memory test battery that assesses verbal and nonverbal short-, working-, and long-term memory), (c) test format (e.g., patient self-ratings vs. stimulus-response test), (d) target population (e.g., elderly populations vs. young adults, English- vs. Spanish-speaking, dementing disease vs. TBI), and (e) which ICF dimensions are assessed (e.g., body structure and function vs. activity and participation) (L. Murray, 2012a; L. Murray & Coppens, 2011). Each test format has certain advantages and disadvantages associated with its use. Consequently, there is no ideal test or battery for a given patient population or neurogenic disorder, and clinicians must be well informed regarding which test or tests would be most appropriate given the general and specific goals they have generated for a specific patient. Likewise, it is important for clinicians to keep abreast of new test developments, such as the release of new tests or new versions of existing tests by manufacturing companies, and the publishing of new normative data in the research literature for existing tests. Often clinicians may grow comfortable with administering a certain test or battery of tests, but these measures can quickly become outdated in terms of the test's theoretical framework, normative data, and even tasks and stimulus items.

For the vast majority of neurogenic patients, with the exception of those whose deficits are related to progressive brain damage, administration of formal test procedures, or, at the very least, outcome predictions based on formal test data should be postponed until they emerge from the acute stages of illness. For example, it is inappropriate to submit patients with TBI to an in-depth, formal cognitive-communicative examination while in the post-traumatic amnesia phase of recovery because of the widespread effects of this typically temporary confusional state. Likewise, many patients who have had strokes, particularly those with medical complications or those receiving numerous medications, are extremely confused and fatigued immediately following their brain attack. Consequently, formal test data from acute assessment sessions are typically confounded by the patients' current medical problems and thus are inaccurate reflections of the nature and severity of the linguistic and cognitive consequences of their brain damage (J. Duffy et al., 2011; A. Johnson, Valachovic, & George, 2006; R. Marshall, 1997).

Psychometric Properties and Considerations

Prior to administering any formal measure, clinicians should review the psychometric properties of the test to understand how best to utilize the test (e.g., Can repeated administrations of the test be used to document treatment effects? For which patients, if any, would the test be appropriate?) and interpret test data (Mitrushina, Boone, Razani, & D'Elia, 2005; Tate, 2010). Such an evaluation of a test's psychometric strengths and weakness is also consistent with evidence-based practice (ASHA, 2004a). Basic psychometric properties with which clinicians should be familiar include test reliability, validity, and standardization.

Reliability. **Reliability** refers to how similar test results are across repeated administrations of the test under comparable testing conditions (Mitrushina et al., 2005; Tate, 2010). The more consistent the data are from the repeated measurements, the more reliable the test is. To optimize reliability, tests should provide a thorough description of administration and scoring procedures to help clinicians prevent intra-examiner (i.e., repeated test administrations by the same examiner) and inter-examiner (i.e., repeated test administrations by different examiners) measurement error from negatively affecting test reliability.

Generally, clinicians should look for tests that report reliability coefficients that equal or exceed .80, as most researchers consider this to be an acceptable level of reliability (see Table 4-6 for a list of types of reliability and criteria). Clinicians should also be sure to check the reliability of not only the overall test but also individual subtests. This is particularly important when clinicians opt to administer only certain portions of comprehensive test batteries (e.g., *Wechsler Memory Scales–IV*). The test–retest reliability of a given measure should also be reviewed, particularly when the clinician wants to re-administer a test to monitor recovery. High test–retest reliability means that performance changes due to possible practice or artifactual improvements (or deterioration) are minimal. Lastly, as previously noted, the reliability of linguistic and cognitive tests is compromised when these tests are administered during the early, acute phases of recovery from sudden brain damage (e.g., stroke, TBI) because of the extensive physiologic changes that typically and rapidly occur during this time period.

Validity. When examining the psychometric adequacy of a test, clinicians need to review several types of **validity,** in particular, content, construct, criterion-related, and ecological validity (Mitrushina et al., 2005; Tate, 2010). **Content validity** refers to how-

TABLE 4-6
Types of Reliability and Validity and Criteria for Assessing Their Adequacy

TYPE	DESCRIPTION	ASSESSMENT CRITERIA[1]
Inter-rater reliability	Extent to which different raters agree on the score for the test	Correlation of $r \geq .80$ or Kappa $\geq .70$
Test–retest reliability	Extent to which scores from different administrations of a given test to a given individual agree	Correlation of $r \geq .80$
Split-half reliability/ internal consistency	Extent to which a test evaluates a single construct	Cronbach's alpha $\geq .80$
Content validity	Extent to which a test measures the behaviors it purports to measure	Test manual/article stipulates theoretical model on which test is based; test was developed by experts using extant empirical literature; test items and tasks appear to reflect behaviors of interest
Construct validity	Extent to which a test relates to other measures of the same behaviors, and thus measures a theoretical concept	Test manual/article stipulates significant relationships with other measures of the same behaviors and/or provides factor analysis results consistent with test's purpose
Predictive validity	Extent to which a test predicts whether an individual has adequate or inadequate performance or does or does not present with a disorder	Test manual/article stipulates that test predicts performance on other measures related to the concept or behaviors of interest

[1]Based in part on the criteria utilized by Turkstra et al. (2005) and advocated by Tate (2010).

well a test measures all of the behaviors that it purports to measure (Carmines & Zeller, 1979). For example, an aphasia test should assess all language behaviors that are viewed to be theoretically and functionally necessary for successful communication. **Construct validity** concerns how well a test relates to other measures of the same construct (e.g., working memory, syntax). For example, a naming test would be said to have good construct validity if patients' scores on that test correlated well with their scores on another naming test.

Criterion-related or **predictive validity** refers to how well a test predicts whether a patient has a deficit. For example, to have good criterion-related validity, a dementia test should distinguish patients with dementia from patients with mild cognitive impairment or other diagnoses as well as from adults without dementia and with no brain damage; similarly, a test of visual neglect that distinguishes patients with neglect from those without neglect would have good criterion-related validity. Recently, there has been increasing interest in a certain type of predictive validity—**ecological validity**. This type of validity refers to how well patients' test performances predict their behavior in daily, real-world settings. For example, to establish the ecological validity of a memory test, during test development it would need to be verified that the memory test scores corresponded well with the test sample's memory difficulties when they complete their typical, daily activities. See Table 4-6 for a list of types of validity and adequacy criteria.

Additional terms related to criterion-related validity that test users should understand are "sensitivity" and "specificity" (Pedraza & Mungas, 2008; Tate, 2010). **Sensitivity** refers to the proportion of individuals who have a given impairment and are identified by the test as having that impairment. For instance, a dementia test with only .60 sensitivity would be considered to have inadequate sensitivity, given that it only identifies 60% of individuals in a given sample who have dementia and, thus, misses identifying the other 40% of the sample that also have dementia. **Specificity** refers to the proportion of individuals who don't have a given impairment and are correctly identified by the test as not having that impairment. Overall, high sensitivity (i.e., > 90%) suggests that the test will allow confident exclusion of an impairment diagnosis, whereas high specificity (i.e., > 90%) suggests that the test will allow confident identification of an impairment.

Across most linguistic and cognitive tests, validity is usually the most problematic psychometric property (L. Murray & Ramage, 2000; Schmitter-Edgecombe et al., 2011). For example, the content validity of many tests of executive functioning has been questioned because these tests fail to include clear operational descriptions of which executive function or functions are being tested or which specific model of executive functioning the test was based on. Similarly, many linguistic and cognitive tests have unacceptable ecological validity because scores on these tests do not help clinicians reliably predict which clients are at risk for daily activity limitations, social participation restrictions, or both (Constantinidou et al., 2012; E. Miller et al., 2010; Schmitter-Edgecombe et al., 2011; Turkstra et al., 2005).

Standardization. To reduce measurement error and ensure a valid comparison of patients' performances to published normative data, test administration procedures should be standardized (Cronbach, 1990; Lezak, Howieson, & Loring, 2004). **Standardization** is achieved by giving the test to a large sample of individuals who represent the cross-section of the population with whom the test will be used in clinical practice. Over time, a test should be revised to improve or update its sampling and administration procedures and, consequently, expand its normative data to a greater variety of reference groups (e.g., greater minority representation or broader age range in the normative sample). Sometimes these standardization updates are published as commercially available, revised tests (e.g., *Wechsler Memory Scale–Fourth Edition* vs. *Wechsler Memory Scale–Third Edition* or *Wechsler Memory Scale–Revised*). Other times the updated normative data can only be found in the research literature. For example, numerous journal articles have been published to extend the normative sample for the *Boston Naming Test* to a wider population in terms of age, education, primary language, type of residence (i.e., community vs. institution), racial background, and socioeconomic status (e.g., Henderson, Frank, Pigatt, Abramson, & Houston, 1998; Rami et al., 2008) or to highlight limitations when used with populations not represented in published standardization samples (e.g., P. Roberts & Doucet, 2011). Further extension of the norms for many published linguistic and cognitive tests (e.g., *Western Aphasia Battery–Revised* [Kertesz, 2006]; *Arizona Battery for Communication Disorders of Dementia* [Bayles & Tomoeda, 1993]) remains an area of need, given that the demographic characteristics of the neurogenic patient population in North America continue to evolve slowly over time (Federal Interagency Forum on Aging-Related Statistics [FIFARS], 2010; Lorenzen & Murray, 2008b).

When selecting tests, clinicians must confirm that the characteristics of the standardization samples of the potential tests (e.g., age, primary language, education level) are consistent with those of their neurogenic patient (Marquez de la Plata et al., 2009; Molrine & Pierce, 2002). Failure to do so can lead to inaccurate interpretation of the patient's test performance, given that both test reliability and test validity may be compromised, resulting in test bias (Ardila, 2005; Marquez de la Plata et al., 2009; Pedraza & Mungas, 2008). That is, clinicians cannot assume that because a test has proven reliable and valid with a certain segment of the population, it will yield reliable and valid test scores with other segments of the population.

Ethnocultural Considerations

Related to the above discussion of the psychometric concept of standardization, clinicians must consider when selecting a formal test whether or not the test conforms to the ethnocultural background of the patient being assessed (Ardila, 2005; L. Murray, 2012a). Variables such as length of residency in the United States, English proficiency, education level, health beliefs and practices, the value that a given culture places on test stimuli and tasks, the process of formal testing, and different linguistic and cognitive skills have been found to influence patients' test performances, and thus must be considered when deciding on assessment priorities and procedures (Agranovich, Panter, Puente, & Touradji, 2011; Fyffe et al., 2011; Kennepohl, Shore, Nabors, & Hanks, 2004; K. Ross & Wertz, 2001). That is, clinicians must determine whether the stimuli and procedures involved in a given test are salient and appropriate for the cultural groups regularly represented on their caseload. To do so, clinicians should not only review standardization information for the given test as recommended above, but also familiarize themselves with the traditions and values of the ethnocultural population with whom they will be working and, if possible, conduct their own standardization and perhaps modification of the given test so that it does correspond with the ethnocultural backgrounds of their patient population. Failure to take these steps can lead to over- or underestimation of a given patient's current strengths and weaknesses and, accordingly, an inappropriate neurogenic language or cognitive disorder diagnosis and/or treatment recommendations.

Ethnocultural Variables

The issue of ethnocultural background may extend beyond typical conceptions, which are frequently limited to race or ethnicity (Ardila, 2005). Additional factors, such as age, education, religious affiliation, and vocational background, however, contribute to individuals' ethnoculture. For example, one of the first patients I evaluated as a clinical fellow was the former chief of staff of the hospital where I was employed. A well-educated, proud, and powerful man, he had strong feelings regarding what types of tasks were "worthy" of his time. Specifically, he refused to participate in any assessment tasks that included simple stimuli or responses. Instead, he would respond with a statement such as, "Well, everyone can do that."

In his case, most standardized tests failed to include *items salient to* his background and/or personality. Furthermore, few standardized tests include normative data from samples representative of individuals of his educational and professional history.

Test Batteries

A test is considered a test battery if it consists of several tasks or subtests, each designed to examine independently a different linguistic and/or cognitive ability. With respect to neurogenic language and cognitive disorders, there are test batteries available for each patient population (i.e., aphasia, RHD, TBI, and dementia). Aphasia test batteries (e.g., *Western Aphasia Battery–Revised* [Kertesz, 2006]) typically include subtests to evaluate basic skills in each language modality (i.e., listening, speaking, reading, and writing). Test batteries for RHD (e.g., *Mini Inventory of Right Brain Injury–Second Edition* [MIRBI-II; Pimental & Knight, 2000]), TBI (e.g., *Ross Information Processing Assessment–Second Edition* [Ross-Swain, 1996]), and dementia (e.g., *Arizona Battery for Communication Disorders of Dementia* [Bayles & Tomoeda, 1993]) include subtests to evaluate language as well as other cognitive abilities, such as memory, attention, and executive functioning, because of the diverse processes that may be compromised in these neurogenic disorders.

The main advantage to using test batteries is their efficiency and scope: They provide information concerning the integrity of a number of linguistic and/or cognitive functions in a relatively short period of time. Consequently, test batteries are often a good choice for an initial assessment to document general deficits and to identify areas that may require more in-depth testing. A disadvantage of test batteries is that they often lack a sufficient number of items to provide a precise and reliable characterization of a patient's abilities in each of the modalities or functions evaluated. Additionally, test batteries are often unsuitable for measuring change or recovery, because areas in which the patient improved or deteriorated may be underrepresented in the overall test score. Take, for example, the MIRBI-II, which contains only one item to assess reading comprehension. Because only one reading item is included, it becomes difficult for a clinician to determine whether the failure on this item of a patient with RHD should be attributed to a reading comprehension deficit or, perhaps, to visual neglect or one of the other cognitive deficits with which that patient presents. Likewise, during an initial evaluation, a patient might fail this item because of a severe reading deficit; following treatment, he might continue to fail this item because, even though his reading abilities improved, they did not improve to the level necessary to pass this item. Accordingly, use of test batteries is associated with a trade-off in that the benefits of their efficiency and scope are countered by their limitations of assessment depth and detail.

Tests of Specific Linguistic and Cognitive Functions

In the ideal clinical setting, which unfortunately has all but disappeared, the clinician should examine in detail all factors that may affect the communicative and cognitive performance of a patient with a neurogenic language or cognitive disorder. Therefore, clinicians often need to augment and in some cases substitute test batteries with tests of more specific linguistic or cognitive functions. For example, specific tests are essential when a patient bottoms out (i.e., fails all items) or reaches a ceiling (i.e., passes all items) on a test battery: These test performance patterns provide the clinician with little information concerning the patient's areas of relative strength or weakness and consequently must be supplemented with additional testing to allow for treatment planning. Compared to test batteries, tests of specific functions tend to provide a more precise quantification as well as qualification of the target linguistic or cognitive process, often by including more test items and, importantly, a more diverse range of item difficulty. As will be reviewed in Chapters 6 through 8, a plethora of tests for measuring specific linguistic and cognitive functions have been developed and are available both commercially and in the research literature. Whereas most of these tests discriminate problems at only the ICF body function level, there has been a recent thrust to develop tools for identifying activity and participation limitations as well.

When trying to choose which of these various tests might be most suitable for a given patient, clinicians should bear in mind some of the previously discussed patient characteristics and psychometric and ethnocultural factors. For example, a clinician trying to assess the memory abilities of a patient with aphasia will need to select a memory test that has relatively few linguistic demands so that the patient's score reflects that patient's memory, rather than memory *and* language abilities. Likewise, a clinician assessing an elderly patient must pay special attention to the test's normative data, as only a limited set of tests, particularly language tests that go beyond word retrieval assessment, provide norms for individuals over the age of 80 years, even though the most rapidly growing segment of the U.S. population is adults age 85 and older (FIFARS, 2010). As previously mentioned, in addition to checking test manuals for normative data, clinicians can search the research literature, where expanded normative data for many tests have been published. For instance, updated and/or more comprehensive norms for both language (e.g., *Controlled Oral Word Association Test*; A. Benton, Hamsher, & Sivan, 2001) and cognitive (e.g., the *Stroop Test*; Stroop, 1935) tests can be found in several recent research publications (e.g., Loonstra, Tarlow, & Sellars, 2001; M. Norman et al., 2011; Steinberg, Bileiauskas, Smith, & Ivnik, 2005).

When selecting tests, clinicians must also keep in mind that it is quite tricky to separate specific linguistic or cognitive functions (Constantinidou et al., 2012; L. Murray, 2012a; Stuss, 2011). This means that although a test may be marketed as assessing just one function, it may actually assess a number of functions. As an example, a reading comprehension test designed to examine reading accuracy and rate at the single-word through to the paragraph level will evaluate not only a number of linguistic functions (e.g., grapheme-phoneme conversion, lexical-semantic processing) but also several cognitive functions (e.g., visual attention and scanning when reading stimuli, verbal working memory when reading at the paragraph level). Thus, if a patient performs this reading comprehension test poorly, the clinician must have data pertaining to these various cognitive and linguistic functions to determine why the patient had difficulty on the reading test.

Qualitative Assessment Considerations

Most formal, standardized tests provide primarily quantitative information in that they compare a given patient's performance to normative data. Therefore, these tests are most useful for documenting the presence or absence of a neurogenic language or cognitive disorder (e.g., dementia) or symptom (e.g., verbal reasoning deficit). Clinicians must also keep in mind that in terms of treating neurogenic language or cognitive disorders, it is equally important to collect **qualitative information** about the patient's communication and cognitive skills (Constantinidou et al., 2012; L. Murray & Coppens, 2011). Qualitative information pertains to *how* a patient performs a given task (e.g., error types and patterns) and thus concerns the identification of influential task parameters and of patient strategies.

Qualitative information can be gleaned by (a) completing informal observations (as described earlier in this chapter), (b) taking notes about patients' behaviors during standardized testing (e.g., during a spoken naming test, the clinician notes that even though the patient with aphasia cannot verbally name many test items, he is able to write with his finger on the table the first letter of many of these items), (c) interviewing patients after they complete an assessment task (e.g., after completing an auditory comprehension test, the clinician asks the patient whether he had difficulty on the test because of one or more of the following: He did not understand the words or the grammar, he forgot the information as the test went on, or he had difficulty paying attention), or (d) implementing test modifications to determine how these modifications influence patients' performances (e.g., providing an initial letter during a spelling subtest). The terms "dynamic assessment" and "process assessment" are sometimes used to delineate the process of collecting qualitative information (i.e., the systematic identification of factors that facilitate or impede patients' communication or cognitive performance) (L. Murray & Coppens, 2011; Turkstra et al., 2005).

Common stimulus and administration modifications that might be considered when testing patients with neurogenic language or cognitive disorders include the following: (a) shifting the location of visual test stimuli to the unaffected hemispace or to a vertical versus horizontal display for patients with unilateral neglect or visual field deficits; (b) providing both written and oral instructions for patients with unaided hearing losses, visual problems (e.g., cataracts), or premorbid reading problems; (c) allowing for written or pointing responses for patients with motor speech deficits; (d) enlarging visual stimuli for patients with visual problems; and (e) using auditory trainers or other amplified headphones to help patients compensate for uncorrected hearing loss. Although some of these modifications may negate the use of test norms, the qualitative information gained by implementing these alterations is often more valuable in terms of making prognostic and treatment recommendations than basing prognosis and treatment recommendations on misinterpreted performance and inaccurate information.

Does Anyone Speak Urdu?

Given the growing ethnocultural diversity in the U.S. population, clinicians are likely to encounter patients with neurogenic language or cognitive disorders who do not use English or who use two or more languages, one of which may or may not be English. When asked to evaluate such a patient, clinicians must consider the following: (a) There is a much more restricted selection of language and cognitive tests developed for users of languages other than English, (b) translating English tests is not recommended because of the psychometric and cultural hazards that such translated versions can cause (L. Murray & Coppens, 2011; Roberts, 2008), and (c) each language a patient uses should be evaluated when quantifying and qualifying aphasia and cognitive-communicative disorders in bi- and multilingual patients (Lorenzen & Murray, 2008b; Paradis, 2004). Consequently, when evaluating a patient who doesn't use English or who uses English plus another language, clinicians will need to enlist the services of an interpreter if they are not proficient users themselves of these other languages. Ideally, the interpreter should not be a family member or social acquaintance, but should be familiar with the assessment process (and if not, should be trained by the clinician), health-care management issues (e.g., confidentiality), and neurogenic language or cognitive disorders (Langdon & Cheng, 2002; Roberts, 2008). When searching for interpreters, clinicians should determine if their health-care facility or company maintains a "language bank" of volunteers or might look for professional interpreters in their community. They just might find someone who does speak Urdu!

Caregiver Assessment

Given the increasing frequency and intensity with which caregivers are expected to participate in the rehabilitation process, it is important that clinicians collect some information about the caregivers of their patients with neurogenic disorders to see if they are willing and capable of participating. This information is very important, given that the caregiver's willingness and ability to provide help have been found to be a unique and, in some cases, more important predictor of functional outcome than brain damage factors such as lesion size or severity of cognitive deficits (A. Kramer & Coleman, 1999; Vangel, Vangel, Rapport, & Hanks, 2011). Likewise, there is a large literature indicating that caring for patients with neurogenic language or cognitive disorders can have negative effects on the physical and emotional well-being of not only the patient but also the patient's spouse, family, and other loved ones (Alzheimer's Association, 2012; Bakas, Kroenke, Plue, Perkins, & Williams, 2006b; E. Miller et al., 2010; H. Murray et al., 2006; Neugroschl & Wang, 2011; Vangel et al., 2011). Common negative consequences associated with caregiving include depression, guilt, anxiety, anger, and increased drug use, as well as the physical problems that can accompany these emotional problems (e.g., sleep and eating disturbances, increased vulnerability to getting colds and the flu). Consequently, Le Dorze and Brassard (1995) recommended that caregivers should "not merely be considered as partners in rehabilitation. They may in fact require specific attention for dealing with their problems. Failure to attend to their problems may also lead to further handicaps for both the aphasic person and his or her family and friends" (p. 252).

When a clinician is concerned about the emotional and/or physical health of a caregiver, a screening tool might be used to identify or substantiate quickly if there is reason for concern. An alternate or additional approach would be to refer the caregiver to a family physician, psychiatrist, psychologist, or social worker for an assessment. In terms of screening tools, clinicians could choose among the measures described in Chapter 5 or Chapter 8 if the caregiver's emotional well-being or quality of life, respectively, is of concern. Some tools specific to identifying caregiver needs, burden, or strain have also been developed (e.g., *Bakas Caregiving Outcomes Scale*; Bakas, Champion, Perkins, Farran, & Williams, 2006a), although other health-care professions (e.g., nursing, social work) more frequently administer these. In terms of making referrals, it is useful if the clinician can identify health-care professionals in the caregiver's community who are knowledgeable about the neurogenic language or cognitive disorder with which the caregiver's loved one presents. For instance, if the caregiver of a patient with aphasia is having problems with depression, it is often most helpful if the psychologist or counselor to whom the caregiver is referred has an understanding of the common social and emotional consequences of aphasia.

Caregiver assessment might also focus on the communicative and cognitive behaviors of the caregivers (Lock, Wilkinson, & Bryan, 2008; L. Murray & Coppens, 2011). Consistent with the ICF construct of contextual factors (WHO, 2001), it is important to document caregiver behaviors that may be exacerbating the communication or cognitive problems of the neurogenic patient. For instance, each day a caregiver might repeatedly question a patient in the early stages of dementia about what he did yesterday; although the caregiver's intent was to stimulate the patient's episodic memory abilities, such repetitive questioning might heighten the patient's awareness of his memory difficulties, leading to anxiety and, in turn, even greater memory difficulties. Formal and informal procedures that allow identifying caregiver behaviors that may be negatively affecting the communication or cognitive abilities of patients are described in Chapters 6 through 8.

It is important to keep in mind that just as patients' cognitive and communicative needs and abilities change over time, so too can the status of caregivers. That is, caregivers' needs, level of stress or burden, and communicative and cognitive behaviors should be viewed as dynamic. Accordingly, caregiver assessments ideally should occur throughout the recovery of patients with static brain damage or the evolution of patients with a progressive neurogenic disorder.

Sharing Assessment Results

A good assessment is achieved not only by selecting and completing the most appropriate and efficient assessment procedures, but also by organizing and condensing assessment results into a coherent and concise report. A well-written assessment report serves as the basis of intervention planning by specifying whether a patient requires treatment services and, if so, what treatment priorities and procedures may be most appropriate. Information in the following general areas should be included in a diagnostic report:

- *Background Information*—This includes a brief description of the patient's premorbid abilities and daily activities, current living and social situations, vocation, etiology and onset of the neurogenic language or cognitive disorder, previously identified concomitant symptoms, and previous speech-language pathology services.
- *Assessment Results*—This is a summary of current linguistic and cognitive strengths and weaknesses. This section should include the identification of factors that facilitate and hinder the patient's linguistic and cognitive abilities. Although typically it is not necessary to describe the observation and assessment procedures that were used, under some circumstances (e.g., a litigation case), this information may need to be included in the report.
- *Summary and Recommendations*—This is a synopsis of the assessment findings, including statements regarding the diagnosis—or, more specifically, the pres-

ence, type, and severity of the neurogenic language or cognitive disorder. Recommendations are included regarding whether or not treatment is needed, and if so, suggestions are provided regarding the treatment goals and therapy approach or procedures.

Importantly, these reports must be written so that team members outside the field of speech-language pathology, as well as caregivers and patients, can understand the contents, and thus the use of professional jargon, slang, and vague terminology must be avoided. Likewise, the length of diagnostic reports should be curtailed as much as possible. As Golper (1996) wrote, "Brief notes get read and long narratives do not" (p. 69). There is a rapidly growing literature documenting the importance of adjusting written documents to meet the health literacy of patients, caregivers, and other health-care providers outside of one's profession (e.g., Huff, 2011; Wynia & Osborn, 2010). This research should be consulted for strategies to ensure that reports and other written documentation shared with the health-care team are formatted at a level and in a manner that will maximize the reader's understanding.

When sharing assessment results with the patient, family, and significant others, clinicians should provide a verbal account at a family conference, as well as a written summary. Although medical or other professional terminology should be avoided, if it is introduced to the patient and caregivers (e.g., vocabulary related to the etiology or site of brain damage), the clinician might consider using visual illustrations to define and explain these terms. For example, when reviewing with a patient and his spouse what parts of his brain have been damaged by his TBI, the clinician might outline those areas on a diagram or model of the brain. Because patients and their caregivers can easily be overloaded with too much information at once (e.g., receiving reports from physical therapy, neuropsychology, physiatry, and occupational therapy all at the same time) and because patients and their caregivers are often overwhelmed and anxious because of the many issues they are currently facing (e.g., uncertain prognosis, financial concerns, the effects of the medical diagnosis on loved ones), clinicians should also consider reviewing assessment results and recommendations on more than one occasion to ensure that patients and caregivers understand the results and their implications and that they have had ample time to raise questions about these results (Luterman, 2008).

Summary

As Little and Doherty (1996) concluded, "There can be no 'ideal' measure or battery of measures which will provide the information required as economically and acceptably as possible in a psychometrically rigorous way" (p. 495). Therefore, for each patient, the clinician must begin by specifying the purpose of the assessment in terms of what information is needed and why. Only after the purpose of the assessment has been stipulated and complicating conditions (e.g., sensory or motoric problems) have been identified should a clinician begin to choose which formal linguistic and cognitive assessment procedures to use for a given patient. Likewise, clinicians must avoid relying solely on test scores, as "tests do not necessarily measure processes, and impairments in different processes can lead to similar test findings" (Stuss, 2011, p. 760). Only after taking into consideration the patient's motivation, attitude toward formal testing, coping style, environmental support, and other additional physical, behavioral, and social variables (e.g., fatigue, depression, side effects of medications), as well as information gleaned from informal assessment procedures (e.g., observations, task manipulations), should diagnostic and prognostic decisions be made. Finally, and perhaps most importantly, clinicians must acknowledge that assessment is an ongoing component of treatment and must occur at every phase of rehabilitation.

Discussion Questions

1. Generate cognitive, communicative, and emotional-behavioral characteristics that might negatively influence the amount and type of information gleaned from an unstructured interview with lots of broad questions (e.g., "What are your symptoms?").
2. Discuss how you could implement evidence-based practice (see Chapter 1) when selecting a formal test that will screen for the presence and type of dementia in a Spanish-English bilingual, elderly patient.
3. Explain why clinicians should not rely on just one type of assessment procedure (e.g., interviews, observation, test battery, informal assessment procedures) when assessing a patient with a neurogenic language or cognitive disorder who has been referred for both an evaluation and treatment.

Identifying Complicating Conditions

chapter 5

Learning Objectives

After reading this chapter, you should be able to:

- Describe sensory, motoric, perceptual, and psychiatric disorders that are important to identify prior to completing formal language or cognitive testing
- List formal and informal procedures used to identify sensory, motoric, perceptual, and psychiatric symptoms that commonly co-occur with neurogenic language and cognitive disorders

Key Terms

- agnosia
- apraxia
- ataxia
- bradykinesia
- chemosensory impairment
- depression
- dysarthria
- hemianesthesia
- hemianopia
- hemiparesis
- ideational apraxia
- ideomotor apraxia
- lability
- limb apraxia
- neurogenic stuttering
- presbycusis
- tinnitus

Introduction

Before administering formal or informal measures of language or communication, clinicians must determine whether their patients with neurogenic language or cognitive disorders present with any complicating conditions. That is, an important first step in the evaluation process is determining if patients have any pre-existing conditions or symptoms caused by the onset of brain damage or disease that may interfere with their performance of language or cognitive assessment tasks, may complicate their language or cognitive recovery, or both. Failure to identify these complicating conditions prior to assessing communicative and cognitive abilities can result in inaccurate diagnostic and prognostic conclusions.

Complicating conditions with which patients with neurogenic language or cognitive disorders frequently present and, consequently, of which clinicians must be cognizant include sensory deficits, motoric impairments, perceptual problems, and psychiatric disorders. Because these complicating conditions will confound assessment of a range of functions and activities, most health-care team members will be interested in determining the presence or absence of these conditions. Consequently, the screening of such conditions falls under the purview of several health-care professions (e.g., nursing, physiatry, speech-language pathology, physical therapy). Before administering any of the screening procedures reviewed in the following sections of this chapter, clinicians must determine which team members will be responsible for identifying which complicating conditions, and must additionally ensure that they have the appropriate qualifications and training to interpret the results of any screening tool they plan to administer (e.g., complicating visual conditions such as macular degeneration or diplopia should be confirmed by an optometrist or ophthalmologist).

Screening for Sensory Deficits

Auditory, visual, and even tactile sensitivity problems may negatively influence a patient's performance on tests of communicative or cognitive abilities. Patients with neurogenic language or cognitive disorders are at risk for hearing disorders because (a) many of these patients are older and thus commonly present with age-related hearing problems (i.e., **presbycusis**) (see included DVD: Patient 1) and (b) certain etiologies—such as traumatic brain injuries (TBI; particularly blast injuries, see Chapter 3) and infections (e.g., meningitis)—frequently cause not only neurogenic language and cognitive disorders but also hearing loss (Fausti, Wilmington, Gallun, Myers, & Henry, 2009; Federal Interagency Forum on Aging-Related Statistics, 2010) (see included DVD: Patient 4). For example, approximately 60% of patients with blast-related TBI will suffer a hearing loss as a direct result (e.g., physical trauma, noise exposure) and/or indirect product (e.g., infection, reaction to ototoxic drugs used to treat the infection) of the blast (Fausti et al., 2009). **Tinnitus** (a constant ringing in the ears) is also quite common following TBI, regardless of injury severity (Hoffer et al., 2010; Lew et al., 2006). Unfortunately, these hearing difficulties are often overlooked: Oleksiak, Smith, St. Andre, Caughlan, and Steiner (2012) reported that approximately 65% of their sample of veterans who had suffered a mild TBI and complained of at least moderate hearing difficulties did *not* receive an audiological referral.

Consequently, speech-language clinicians should ensure that each of their patients has recently had, at a minimum, a hearing screening and preferably a full audiological evaluation prior to administering any linguistic or cognitive tests. Determining the hearing acuity of patients with severe language impairments may be problematic if they have difficulty comprehending test instructions. With these patients, therefore, collaboration between the audiologist and speech-language clinician is imperative to ensure valid hearing assessment results. It also is important that for patients who require a hearing aid and/or other assistive listening devices, clinicians check that the devices are in proper working condition (e.g., hearing aid battery is charged, device is free of cerumen buildup) before administering linguistic or cognitive assessment or treatment procedures.

Vision also is frequently compromised in adults with neurogenic language or cognitive disorders (B. Greenwald, Kapoor, & Singh, 2012; Rosen & Viskontas, 2008; Rowe

& VIS Group UK, 2009; Rowe et al., 2011). Patients might present with (a) premorbid visual problems, such as myopia, presbyopia (i.e., age-related visual problems), cataracts, or macular degeneration (e.g., see included DVD: Patient 10); (b) visual deficits caused by their brain damage (e.g., Patient 1 on DVD) or neurological disease, such as visual field cuts (e.g., **left or right homonymous hemianopia**), nystagmus and other fixation deficits, diplopia (i.e., double vision), photosensitivity (i.e., intensified sensitivity to light), or optic neuritis (visual disorder found in multiple sclerosis and other medical conditions); or (c) both (Barton, 2011; Cockerham et al., 2009; Rowe et al., 2011). Visual problems are extremely common among patients with neurogenic disorders (B. Greenwald et al., 2012; Rowe & VIS Group UK, 2009), with one recent study identifying normal visual status in only 8% of their sample of stroke survivors (Rowe & VIS Group UK, 2009). Furthermore, Rowe et al. (2011) found that the vast majority of stroke patients (right, left, and bilateral stroke cases) who complained of reading difficulty had one or more visual impairments, rather than or in addition to a language disorder. In addition to affecting reading, such visual problems could compromise social communication abilities (e.g., poor eye contact related to an eye movement or fixation problem).

If an undiagnosed visual defect is suspected, clinicians should advocate for an ophthalmology or optometry referral. Likewise, clinicians should make sure that any visual assistive devices that their patients need are available and in suitable condition prior to completing their assessment. Clinicians also can help patients accommodate to visual field cuts by presenting visual stimuli in a vertical rather than horizontal display to reduce the possibility of inducing visual errors. Other possible accommodations include providing reading materials in enlarged text, ensuring adequate color contrast between the visual targets and their background (e.g., white text on black background vs. newsprint), and minimizing glare (see included DVD: Patient 10).

Many patients present with problems in sensing temperature, pain, touch, or movement (Rosen & Viskontas, 2008). In fact, it is estimated that 40 to 60% of stroke patients display some degree of somatosensory loss (Cary, 1995; Rathore, Hinn, Cooper, Tyroler, & Rosamond, 2002). If these problems affect only one side of the body, the patient may be diagnosed with **hemianesthesia**. Clinician awareness of tactile deficits is important in terms of providing tactile cues or feedback. For example, a clinician getting a patient's attention by touching his hand would want to touch this patient's right hand if the patient had suffered a right hemisphere stroke and presented with left hemianesthesia.

Other forms of sensory disturbances that patients with neurogenic language or cognitive disorders may experience include **chemosensory impairments**, that is, olfactory and gustatory problems (Reiter & Costanzo, 2010). Such sensory deficits are a common consequence of TBI, certain dementing diseases (e.g., Alzheimer's and Huntington's diseases), and even normal aging (Babizhayev, Deyev, & Yegorov, 2011; Reiter and Costanzo, 2010); for example, Reiter and Costanzo (2010) reported that around 20% of TBI survivors will experience olfactory dysfunction. Although smell and taste loss or distortions should not confound language and cognitive assessment procedures, they will be important to consider when examining neurogenic patients' perceptions of quality of life and, obviously, if swallowing or eating are areas of concern.

Screening for Perceptual Problems

Following brain damage, and in particular bilateral brain damage, patients may present with a variety of perceptual difficulties that must be identified so that these difficulties can be accounted for or accommodated during subsequent assessment procedures. These perceptual problems are due not to sensory loss (e.g., a hearing loss, presbyopia) but rather to a breakdown in interpreting and applying meaning to sensory information.

Auditory Perceptual Problems

When patients have difficulty recognizing auditory information despite accurate recognition of the same stimuli in other modalities, they are diagnosed with **auditory agnosia** (Rosen & Viskontas, 2008). Various types of auditory agnosia have been identified, including (a) pure word deafness, or impaired recognition of spoken language but relatively preserved recognition of other auditory stimuli; (b) auditory sound agnosia, or impaired recognition of nonverbal or environmental sounds (e.g., telephone ringing, frog croaking); and (c) amusia, or impaired recognition of musical rhythms or passages (Fausti et al., 2009; Slevc, Martin, Hamilton, & Joanisse, 2011; Vignolo, 2003). These auditory agnosias are typically rare, but when they do occur, they are more likely to be observed in patients with bilateral temporal lesions (Rosen & Viskontas, 2008). Additionally, problems perceiving pitch and loudness have been identified in patients with neurogenic language or cognitive disorders, most frequently those with RHD or TBI (Fausti et al., 2009; Tompkins, 1995). In contrast, unilateral left hemisphere damage is more likely to cause difficulties with auditory stimuli that require rapid temporal processing (Slevc et al., 2011). Research also suggests that patients with aphasia may experience difficulty processing nonverbal sounds (Saygin, Dick, Wilson, Dronkers, & Bates, 2003; Vignolo, 2003).

Currently, there are a limited number of tests available to identify auditory perceptual disorders, particularly for older patients (Table 5-1). For example, although the *SCAN-3 Tests for Auditory Processing Disorders in Adolescents and Adults* (Keith, 2009) offer evaluation of a number of auditory perceptual skills (e.g., perceiving speech that is degraded or in competition with another auditory signal), normative data for adults up to the age of only 51 are provided. Clinicians, therefore, must work closely with other team members, particularly the audiologist, when assessing for the presence of these types of perceptual problems. Regardless of which test or tests are used, it is important to rule out hearing loss, language comprehension and expression problems, and a lack of familiarity with test items prior to giving a diagnosis of auditory agnosia (this also applies to diagnosing agnosias in other sensory modalities).

TABLE 5-1
Tests of Auditory and Visual Perceptual Abilities

TEST	SOURCE	DESCRIPTION
Bender Visual Retention Test	Sivan (1991)	Assesses visual perception and memory, and visuoconstruction abilities utilizing a set of 10 visual designs
Hooper Visual Organization Test	Hooper (1983)	Assesses visual integration, or the ability to identify pictures of objects that have been cut up and rearranged; multiple-choice format also available (Schultheis et al., 2000)
Judgment of Line Orientation	Benton, Hamsher, Varney, & Spreen (1983)	Measures visuospatial judgment, or the ability to identify a target line orientation from an array of lines
Kent Visual Perceptual Test	Melamed (2000)	Assesses visual discrimination and visuomotor skills by requiring identification and copying, respectively, of various target visual stimuli
Letter or Star Cancellation	B. Wilson et al. (1987)	Measures visual search and scanning abilities by requiring the discrimination of target letters or stars, respectively, from an array of distracting visual stimuli
NAB Visual Discrimination Test	Stern & White (2009c)	Examines the ability to identify a target colorful design from an array of similar designs
Test of Visual Perceptual Skills–Third Edition	Martin (2006)	Measures a number of visual perceptual skills, including visual discrimination, visual closure, and figure-ground
Phoneme Discrimination	Benton, Hamsher, Varney, & Spreen (1983)	Assesses the auditory perceptual ability of discriminating pairs of nonsense syllables as being the same or different
SCAN-3 Tests for Auditory Processing Disorders in Adolescents and Adults	Keith (2009)	Includes auditory figure-ground, dichotic, temporal processing, and distorted signal listening tasks
Test of Auditory Perception	M. Williams (1990)	Measures the ability to discriminate and localize tone, word, and environmental sound stimuli
Test of Facial Recognition	Benton, Hamsher, Varney, & Spreen (1983)	Assesses the ability to match unfamiliar faces under different visual conditions (e.g., simple matching vs. matching target face with faces shown at different viewing angles)
Visual Object and Space Perception Battery	Warrington & James (1991)	Assesses the ability to identify images of objects, animals, or letters that have been degraded or are blackened silhouettes, and the ability to complete visual spatial tasks such as counting arrays of joined cubes

Visual Perceptual Problems

There are many visual perceptual problems with which adults with neurogenic language or cognitive disorders might present (for a comprehensive review, see Barton, 2011). Typically, these problems are more prevalent among patients with RHD or with bilateral brain damage (e.g., Alzheimer's disease, blast head injuries, Parkinson's disease) than those with unilateral left hemisphere damage (i.e., aphasia). First, many forms of **visual agnosia**, a disturbance in recognizing visual stimuli even though visual sensitivity is adequate to see the stimuli, have been identified, including (a) visual object agnosia, or impaired recognition of actual or pictured objects; (b) prosopagnosia, or impaired recognition of familiar faces; (c) autopagnosia, or impaired recognition of body parts; (d) environmental agnosia, or impaired recognition of familiar environments (e.g., one's own home); and (e) propopagnosia, or impaired recognition of pictures or a mirror image of oneself (Barton, 2011; Rosen & Viskontas, 2008; Rowe & VIS Group UK, 2009; Rowe et al., 2011; see also Table 2-6). Second, patients with neurogenic language or cognitive disorders may have complex visual discrimination and perception difficulties. For example, patients who can match pictures of objects viewed at the same angle may have difficulty matching or recognizing those objects when viewed from an unusual angle (e.g., identifying a cup viewed from the top vs. the side), when provided an incomplete or obstructed view (e.g., hatch marks cover part of the picture), or when presented with lots of competing background visual information (e.g., a figure–ground task). Problems with depth perception, visual scanning, movement perception (referred to as "akinetopsia"), and color perception (including achromotopsia, in which all colors are perceived to be dull or as shades of grey) are also possible. Most frequently, patients present with more than one visual sensory and perceptual problem (e.g., visual field cut *and* prosopagnosia *and* achromotopsia; Barton, 2011; Rowe et al., 2011).

Obviously, the presence of one or more of these visual perception deficits could not only negatively affect social communication skills (e.g., failure to perceive the facial expressions of one's communication partner) but also confound a patient's performance of many linguistic and cognitive test procedures, such as naming, describing, recalling, drawing, or copying objects, pictures, or geometric figures; such deficits also have implications regarding the selection of treatment activities and materials. Fortunately, there are a number of tests available to screen for the presence of visual perceptual difficulties (see Table 5-1). These tests are most frequently administered by neuropsychologists or occupational therapists. Many of these tests, however, must be adapted when administering them to adults with neurogenic language disorders who may have problems understanding test instructions or who may be unable to provide accurate verbal responses due to their linguistic deficits; thus, speech-language pathologists may be involved to assist with adapting visual perceptual test procedures or interpreting test findings. Importantly, researchers are beginning to acknowledge the need for these test adaptations: Modified versions of some tests can frequently be found in the research literature (e.g., Schultheis, Caplan, Ricker, & Woessner, 2000), and newly published tests have been developed to be suitable for a broad range of neurogenic patients (e.g., the *NAB Visual Discrimination Test*; Stern & White, 2009c).

Screening for Motoric Impairments

Adults with neurogenic language or cognitive disorders may present with a variety of motoric impairments that may not only directly or indirectly affect their expressive communication abilities (e.g., motor speech, writing, gesturing, facial expressions) but also affect their ability to fulfill the response requirements (e.g., speed and accuracy of a pointing response) of many frequently used linguistic and cognitive tests. Apraxia of speech and dysarthria are two common motoric problems that impact speech. Additionally, a number of motoric disorders may affect the limb and body movements of patients with neurogenic language or cognitive disorders.

Apraxia of Speech

The diagnosis of **apraxia of speech** refers to a motor programming deficit in which patients display difficulty with volitionally positioning their articulators, as well as planning and sequencing their movements, for the production of phonemes and phoneme sequences (Basso et al., 2011; Croot, 2002; Ziegler, 2002). Apraxia of speech is not a product of muscular weakness, slowness, or incoordination, particularly since patients are able to use the speech musculature without difficulty when completing reflexive or automatic motor acts. Frequently observed apraxia of speech symptoms include articulatory problems (e.g., consistent or inconsistent articulatory substitutions, distortions, omissions, repetitions, and additions) and prosodic disturbances (e.g., a decreased speech rate, abnormal stress patterns, excessive frequency or duration of pauses) (see included DVD: Patients 6a, 6b, 6d, 10). The variability of these symptoms appears to be influenced, at least in part, by speech context variables, such as the length and phonetic complexity of the word or utterance, word frequency, and type of speech activity (e.g., repetition task vs. reading aloud vs. spontaneous verbal output). Although apraxia of speech may occur following damage to many cortical and subcortical regions, it is most commonly associated with lesions to the premotor or parietal cortex, or insular regions of the left hemisphere, and consequently is frequently observed in patients with aphasia, TBI, and frontotemporal lobar degeneration (Dronkers, 1996; Kertesz, 2010; N. Miller, 2002). For example, it is estimated that around 25% of patients with aphasia will also present with apraxia of speech (Basso et al., 2011).

Because apraxia of speech and aphasia frequently co-occur, several aphasia batteries include subtests to assess for the co-existence of apraxia (e.g., *Boston Diagnostic Aphasia Examination–Third Edition* [BDAE-3; Goodglass et al., 2001]). There are also a number of tests designed to provide a more in-depth evaluation of the presence and severity of apraxia of speech, including the *Apraxia Battery for Adults–Second Edition* (Dabul, 2000) and the *Comprehensive Apraxia Test* (DiSimoni, 1989). Additionally, there are a few apraxia screening tools available, such as the *Quick Assessment for Apraxia of Speech* (Tanner & Culbertson, 1999c), that are designed to establish the presence or absence of apraxia of speech. Despite the availability of these tools, differentiating speech problems related to apraxia of speech from those related to certain types of aphasia (e.g., conduction aphasia, Broca's aphasia) remains difficult in many patients. Consequently, researchers continue to try to identify perceptual (see included DVD: Patient 10l, 10m, 10n), acoustic, and/or physiological measures that might in the future help clinicians reliably distinguish the apraxic versus aphasic verbal output problems of their patients (Croot, 2002; Ziegler, 2002).

Dysarthria

When a motor speech disorder is caused by impairments of speech musculature (e.g., weakness or excessive tone) and/or control (i.e., incoordination, imprecise movements), the diagnosis of **dysarthria** applies (F. A. Darley, Aronson, & Brown, 1975; Kent, Kent, Duffy, & Weismer, 1998; Urban et al., 2006). In dysarthria, one or many of the basic components of motor speech may be compromised, including respiration, phonation, resonance, articulation, and prosody. In contrast to apraxia of speech, many symptoms of dysarthria tend to be more predictable and more consistent across speaking contexts (see included DVD: Patient 9). The frequency and types of motor speech symptoms, however, can vary significantly among patients with dysarthria, depending on the location and etiology of their neurologic damage (see Table 5-2). Because most muscle groups involved in speech have bilateral upper motor neuron innervation (i.e., are controlled by both cerebral hemispheres), typically only patients who have suffered bilateral brain damage will present with persistent and severe dysarthria. Consequently, in terms of neurogenic language or cognitive disorder populations, patients with dementia or TBI are more apt to present with significant and enduring dysarthria than patients with aphasia or RHD, who often have suffered only unilateral brain damage and thus are more likely to present with a mild to moderate, mixed dysarthria if they have dysarthria (Kent et al., 1998; Urban et al., 2006).

To identify the presence, type, and severity of dysarthria, clinicians can use one of several commercially available tests, such as the *Assessment of Intelligibility of Dysarthric Speech* (Yorkston, Beukelman, & Traynor, 1984), the *Quick Assessment for Dysarthria* (Tanner & Culbertson, 1999d), the *Frenchay Dysarthria Assessment–Second Edition* (FDA-2; Enderby & Palmer, 2008), and the *Dysarthria Examination Battery* (Drummond, 1993), or one of the research protocols described in the research literature (e.g., J. Duffy, 2013; Kent, Weismer, Kent, & Rosenbek, 1989). These tools generally rely on auditory-perceptual judgments, along with an examination of the integrity of oral structures and musculature. For instance, with the FDA-2, clinicians rate their patients' reflexes (e.g., swallow reflex), respiration, lips, palate, larynx, tongue, speech intelligibility, and other variables (e.g., hearing, language, mood). Normative data for individuals ages 12 to 97 years are provided, including data both for individuals who have and for those who do not have dysarthria.

In addition to perceptual assessment (see included DVD: Patient 9c, 9d, 9f), clinicians should incorporate instrumental techniques (e.g., acoustic analyses, kinematic procedures) to provide further, and perhaps more reliable, quantification and qualifica-

TABLE 5-2
Types of Dysarthria

DYSARTHRIA TYPE	COMMON PERCEPTUAL FEATURES	ASSOCIATED NEUROLOGIC ETIOLOGIES (AND LOCATION)	POSSIBLE CO-EXISTING NEUROGENIC LANGUAGE OR COGNITIVE DISORDER
Spastic	Monopitch, monoloudness, reduced stress, slow speech rate, slow and regular alternate motion rates, harsh and strained voice, imprecise articulation	Stroke, TBI, tumor (bilateral upper motor neuron, motor cortex, internal capsule, corona radiata)	Aphasia, RHD, TBI
Flaccid	Hypernasality, breathy voice, short phrases, imprecise articulation*	Stroke, TBI, tumor (lower motor neuron, brainstem, spinal nerves, cranial nerves)	TBI
Hyperkinetic	Loudness variations, harsh and strained voice, irregular articulatory breakdowns, imprecise articulation, silent intervals	Stroke, TBI, tumor, Huntington's disease, dystonia (basal ganglia, putamen)	Dementia, TBI
Hypokinetic	Monopitch, mono- and reduced loudness, breathy and rough voice, short rushes of speech, imprecise articulation	Parkinson's disease, progressive supranuclear palsy (basal ganglia)	Dementia, TBI
Ataxic	Irregular articulatory breakdowns, irregular alternate motion rates, imprecise articulation, excess and equal stress, monopitch or variable pitch changes, slow rate	Stroke, TBI, tumor, Friedreich's ataxia, multiple sclerosis (cerebellum)	Dementia, TBI
Mixed	Varied and dependent on location of the multiple lesion sites	Stroke, TBI, multiple sclerosis, progressive supranuclear palsy, amyotrophic lateralsclerosis, olivo-pontine-cerebellar degeneration (diffuse brain damage/upper and lower motor neurons)	Dementia, TBI

Note. RHD = right hemisphere brain damage; TBI = traumatic brain injury. Table information synthesized from Kent et al. (1998), J. Duffy (2013), and Theodoros, Murdoch, and Goozee (2001).

*Variable depending on which cranial and/or spinal nerves were compromised by the brain damage.

tion of their dysarthric patients' motor speech problems (Kent et al., 1998; E. Miller et al., 2010).

> **Who Starts Stuttering in Adulthood?**
>
> Unfortunately, patients with neurogenic language or cognitive disorders are at risk for developing not only the motor speech problems described above but also other speech impairments, including **neurogenic stuttering**. Although less common than apraxia of speech or dysarthria, neurogenic stuttering has been reported following stroke, TBI, and onset of several progressive neurological diseases (e.g., Parkinson's disease) (Lundgren, Helm-Estabrooks, & Klein, 2010). As with any other condition associated with brain damage, the characteristics of neurogenic stuttering are variable, sometimes resembling developmental stuttering (e.g., stuttering on only certain sounds, word positions, or parts of speech; exhibiting secondary behaviors such as eye blinking or facial tics) and other times having unique features (e.g., stuttering in all word positions, lack of secondary behaviors) (Jokel, De Nil, & Sharpe, 2007). For a detailed description of neurogenic stuttering and the empirical literature aimed at characterizing this acquired speech disorder, see Lundgren et al. (2010).

Other Motoric Disorders

In addition to motor speech impairments, patients with neurogenic language or cognitive disorders often present with motoric disturbances of other muscular systems that in turn can have a negative effect on their communication abilities, their ability to complete linguistic and cognitive tests, or both. One of the most common of these motor disturbances is **hemiparesis**, a muscular weakness on one side of the body (Rathore et al., 2002); the term "**hemiplegia**" is applied when the disturbance is so severe that the one side of the body is paralyzed (see included DVD: Patient 5). In terms of cognitive-communication abilities, hemiparesis is most problematic when the patient's dominant side is affected, as commonly occurs in patients with aphasia (i.e., right hemiparesis). This weakness of the dominant hand and/or arm, or dependence on the nondominant hand and/or arm, can negatively affect the accuracy and speed of these patients' writing, typing, drawing, and gesturing.

Limb apraxia is a problem in executing skilled movements that is most frequently observed in patients with left hemisphere damage, particularly those with frontal or parietal lobe involvement, and that may or may not co-occur with other types of apraxia, such as oral apraxia or apraxia of speech (Rosen & Viskontas, 2008; Vanbellingen & Bohlhalter, 2011). Estimates regarding the prevalence of apraxia following onset of left hemisphere brain damage vary from 30 to 50%, with as many as 25% of these patients presenting with moderate to severe apraxia (Donkervoort, Dekker, van den Ende,

Stehmann-Saris, & Deelman, 2000; Vanbellingen & Bohlhalter, 2011; Vanbellingen et al., 2010). Limb apraxia can also appear following onset of right hemisphere brain damage, albeit of lesser frequency and severity than that associated with left hemisphere brain damage. Patients with progressive neurological disorders may also present with limb apraxia, including those with Alzheimer's, Parkinson's, or Huntington's disease. Importantly, limb apraxia is often persistent and considered a negative prognostic indicator, as it confounds recovery of activities of daily living, communicative gesture, gait, and transferring (e.g., moving from the bed to a wheelchair), and can reduce one's chance of returning to work (Vanbellingen & Bohlhalter, 2011).

Patients with limb apraxia have difficulty executing acquired and volitional movements of their fingers, wrists, elbows, and/or shoulders on both sides of their body (Rothi, Raymer, & Heilman, 1997; Vanbellingen & Bohlhalter, 2011). As in apraxia of speech, these execution problems are not a product of muscular, sensory, or cognitive impairments. Typically, movements involving distal versus proximal body parts, and movements or actions involving a tool or instrument (i.e., transitive) versus no tool, are more difficult for patients with limb apraxia. A diagnosis of **ideational apraxia** may be assigned if the patient displays difficulty completing or demonstrating the series of actions needed to complete tasks involving tools (e.g., preparing for and brushing one's teeth). A diagnosis of **ideomotor apraxia** may be given if the patient has difficulty pantomiming or imitating gestures (e.g., problems showing how to brush one's teeth, when asked to pretend to do so [without a toothbrush present]). Ideational and ideomotor apraxia may occur alone or concomitantly. Symptoms of limb apraxia can include content errors, in which the patient completes an incorrect movement or action (e.g., when asked to show how to blow a whistle, the patient gestures how to strike a match), and production errors, in which the correct movement or action is attempted but the spatial or temporal organization of the movement is in error (e.g., when gesturing how to brush his teeth, the patient performs the action with a flattened rather than gripped hand). Steps in more complex action sequences might also be omitted or performed in the wrong order (e.g., trying to put toothpaste on a toothbrush without taking the cap off of the toothpaste).

Because limb apraxia can result in problems performing commands that involve purposeful movements, and sometimes even in problems providing a reliable pointing or nodding response, clinicians should assess for limb apraxia before completing comprehension or other cognitive (e.g., memory, attention) testing to avoid misdiagnosing the problem. For a quick screen of possible limb apraxia, clinicians can administer the short apraxia subtests that many aphasia batteries include (e.g., BDAE-3; Goodglass et al., 2001). For a more in-depth and reliable evaluation (Butler, 2002; Vanbellingen & Bohlhalter, 2011), several protocols are described in the literature (e.g., *Test of Upper Limb Apraxia*; Vanbellingen et al., 2010), and there are a few commercially available tests, such as the *Test of Oral and Limb Apraxia* (Helm-Estabrooks, 1991), the *Apraxia Battery for Adults–Second Edition* (Dabul, 2000), and the *Naturalistic Action Test* (M. Schwartz, Buxbaum, Veramonti, Ferraro, & Segal, 2002). Because the strength of the relationship between formal apraxia test results and the integrity of performing activities of daily living has not yet been established, Vanbellingen and Bohlhalter (2011) recommended always pairing formal apraxia test results with observation of patients performing daily activities in their typical environments and feedback from patients and caregivers (e.g., self-report questionnaires).

There are a number of other motoric impairments that may compromise patients' ability to perform the types of movements and actions necessary to complete many linguistic and cognitive tests and daily activities, and that consequently should be identified early in the assessment process (Krauss & Jankovic, 2002; Lew et al., 2006). These other motoric impairments are more frequently observed in patients with TBI or in patients who have progressive neurological disease. For example, many patients with TBI or Parkinson's disease have **bradykinesia**, a motoric problem related to excessive muscle tone that causes decreases in the speed and range of these patients' movements and, in particular, negatively affects their ability to manipulate small objects such as a pen or pencil. Bradykinesia can also be reflected in reduced overall facial expression (see included DVD: Patient 9f), that could be easily mistaken for flat affect. Patients who have cerebellar involvement may present with **ataxia**, in which the accuracy, force, and timing of movements is disturbed. For example, when asked to point to a certain object on a comprehension test, the patient with ataxia might overshoot the target object and end up giving what appears to be an incorrect pointing response. Excessive and involuntary movement disorders such as chorea, hemiballismus, and tics may occur following TBI and are a defining characteristic of some progressive diseases (e.g., Huntington's disease). The abrupt and uncontrollable movements associated with these disorders may affect patients' ability to complete certain linguistic and cognitive test procedures, as well as their communicative skills (e.g., writing, facial expressions, speech).

Screening for Psychiatric Disorders

Psychiatric disturbances regularly co-occur with neurogenic language and cognitive disorders. For example, estimates of the prevalence of apathy in patients with Huntington's disease often exceed 70% (Krishnamoorthy & Craufurd, 2011), and depression is reported to occur in more than 60% of patients with TBI (King & Kirwilliam, 2011) and 80% of patients with Alzheimer's disease (Lopez, 2011). In some neurogenic disorders, such as the behavioral variant of frontotemporal lobar degeneration or dementia with Lewy bodies, psychiatric problems are the initial or hallmark symptom (Fatemi et al., 2011; Neugroschl & Wang, 2011). Regardless of etiology, patients with neurogenic language and cognitive disorders may present with one or more of the following emotional or psychiatric problems: delusions, hallucinations, agitation, anxiety (including agoraphobia), apathy, mania, disinhibition, irritability, euphoria, aggression, **lability** (i.e., difficulty controlling one's emotions that can manifest as excessive or inappropriate crying or laughing), sexual inappropriateness/dysfunction, low self-esteem, personality disorders (e.g., paranoid, schizoid, extravert), catastrophic reaction, and **depression**

(Fatemi et al., 2011; Jorge, Starkstein, & Robinson, 2010; King & Kirwilliam, 2011; Krishnamoorthy & Craufurd, 2011; Rhodes-Kropf, Cheng, Castillo, & Fulton, 2011; Woolley, Khan, Murthy, Miller, & Rankin, 2011; C. Yang, Huang, Lin, Tsai, & Hua, 2011).

Of these various psychiatric disturbances, depression is frequently reported to be the most prevalent among neurogenic patient populations (Byatt, Rothschild, Riskind, Ionete, & Hunt, 2011; Cobley, Thomas, Lincoln, & Walker, 2011; Fatemi et al., 2011; Neugroschl & Wang, 2011; Robinson & Spalletta, 2010; Sinanovic, 2010; Woolley et al., 2011). That is, although it is expected that patients who have suffered brain damage or have been diagnosed with a progressive neurological disease will experience some depression related to dealing with the negative effects of their brain damage or disease, many demonstrate significant and persistent depression (see included DVD: Patient 2), which in turn can compromise their ability to profit from rehabilitation and participate in daily activities and social interactions. Importantly, depression onset may occur at any time during recovery of a static lesion (e.g., TBI, stroke) or management of a progressive disease (e.g., Parkinson's disease, frontotemporal lobar degeneration) (E. Miller et al., 2010; Robinson & Spalletta, 2010; Sinanovic, 2010). Accordingly, clinicians working in the full gamut of health-care settings (e.g., acute care, long-term care) must remain vigilant to the onset of depression in their patients.

The psychiatric problems of patients with neurogenic language and cognitive disorders can originate from a number of factors, including premorbid psychiatric disorders, medication side effects, structural and physiological changes associated with brain damage, nutritional problems, and psychological reactions to dealing with acquired language or cognitive disorders along with other possible motor, sensory (particularly pain), and behavioral impairments (Byatt et al., 2011; E. Miller et al., 2010; Robinson & Spalletta, 2010; Woolley et al., 2011). Even genetics may play a role, as recent research has documented that siblings of Alzheimer's disease patients with psychotic symptoms have higher rates of psychosis compared with siblings of Alzheimer's disease patients who don't present with psychotic symptoms (Lopez, 2011). With respect to the ICF model (WHO, 2001), contextual factors may also instigate or contribute to psychiatric problems (Neugroschl & Wang, 2011; Rhodes-Kropf et al., 2011); for example, a lack of environmental and social stimulation, such as that encountered in some long-term care facilities, has been associated with agitation in patients with dementia.

Identifying and remediating psychiatric problems as quickly as possible is imperative. These problems have been shown to increase mortality rates; impact negatively patients' cognitive and communicative abilities, treatment outcomes, caregiver stress and burden levels, and quality of life; and, in patients with progressive diseases, increase the rate of disease progression, lead to early institutionalization, and even delay correct diagnosis of neurological disease (Byatt et al., 2011; Fucetola et al., 2006; Jorge et al., 2010; Krishnamoorthy & Craufurd, 2011; Lopez, 2011; Rhodes-Kropf et al., 2011; Robinson & Spalletta, 2010; Sinanovic, 2010; C. Yang et al., 2011).

Despite the prevalence of and negative consequences associated with psychiatric problems, there are few appropriate tools for diagnosing these problems in patients with neurogenic language or cognitive disorders (Cobley et al., 2011; E. Miller et al., 2010;

Robinson & Spalletta, 2010; C. Yang et al., 2011). Reliable assessment of psychiatric problems in patients with neurogenic language or cognitive disorders is difficult for several reasons:

1. Because most currently available assessment instruments were developed for psychiatric rather than neurological patient populations, many of them have linguistic, attention, memory, or executive function demands that exceed the capabilities of patients with neurogenic communication or cognitive disorders (see Table 5-3). For example, patients with aphasia may lack the linguistic skills necessary to comprehend or respond to interview-based or even checklist types of assessment tools, whereas patients with RHD, TBI, or dementia may have inadequate insight to complete self-rating scales accurately. It should be noted, however, that more recently developed measures of psychiatric well-being have been designed to minimize the reading proficiency level and length of time required to complete the measure; that is, many self-report measures are now written at a fifth-grade reading level or lower and take 10 minutes or less to complete (e.g., *Reynolds Depression Screening Inventory* [W. Reynolds & Kobak, 1998], *Clinical Assessment of Depression* [Bracken & Howell, 2004]). Therefore, patients with relatively mild reading impairments might be able to complete such measures.

2. A second confound to accurate assessment is that many of the signs used to diagnose psychiatric disorders may be obscured by the neurogenic language or cognitive problem or other concomitant neurological symptoms or medical complications. For instance, diminished prosody and flat facial expression are common among not only patients with RHD, TBI, or Parkinson's disease, but also those with depression. Likewise, many dementing illnesses cause sleep disturbances (e.g., Alzheimer's disease), another symptom used to diagnose depression. Consequently, depression and other psychiatric problems are often underdiagnosed in patients with neurogenic language or cognitive disorders because symptoms of the psychiatric problem are misattributed to the neurogenic disorder rather than to a possible co-existing psychiatric problem (Byatt et al., 2011; Krishnamoorthy & Craufurd, 2011; Woolley et al., 2011); the inverse may also occur, whereby patients are misdiagnosed with a psychiatric rather than or in addition to a neurogenic language or cognitive disorder.

3. Lastly, identifying psychiatric disorders in patients with neurogenic language and cognitive problems has proven difficult because of their variable presentation among this patient population. Whereas there have been primarily consistent findings with respect to the positive relationship between frontal lobe involvement and psychotic symptoms such as aggression and irritability (e.g., Lopez, 2011), variables such as lesion location and time postonset or severity of brain damage or disease have proven to be relatively unreliable predictors of whether patients will or will not present with psychiatric problems such as depression and anxiety (Jorge et al., 2010; King & Kirwilliam, 2011; E. Miller et al., 2010; Robinson & Spalletta, 2010).

Despite these obstacles to accurate identification of psychiatric problems, there are a few steps clinicians can follow to help ensure that the emotional stability of their patients is evaluated. First, as indicated in Table 5-3, there are some newer tests developed specifically for patients with acquired brain damage that clinicians might use.

TABLE 5-3
Measures of Psychiatric Well-Being

	SYMPTOMS ASSESSED					FORMAT		LINGUISTIC DEMANDS		
	Anxiety	Depression	Multi-dimensional	Irritability	Self-esteem	Observer-rated	Self-rated	Sentence-level	Word-level	N/A
Measures originally developed for psychiatric patients										
Beck Anxiety Inventory (Beck, 1993)	X						X	X		
Beck Depression Inventory–Second Edition (Beck, Steer, & Brown, 1996)		X					X	X		
Brief Symptom Inventory 18 (Derogatis, 2001)			X				X	X		
Centre for Epidemiological Studies Depression Scale (Radloff & Terri, 1986)		X					X	X		
Clinical Assessment of Depression (Bracken & Howell, 2004)		X					X	X		
Geriatric Depression Scale (Yesavage et al., 1983)		X					X	X		
Hamilton Anxiety Rating Scale (M. Hamilton, 1959)	X					X				X
Hamilton Rating Scale for Depression (M. Hamilton, 1960)		X				X				X
Minnesota Multiphasic Personality Inventory–Second Edition (Butcher, Dahlstrom, & Graham, 1989)			X				X	X		
Multidimensional Anxiety Questionnaire (W. Reynolds, 1999)	X						X	X		
Reynolds Depression Screening Inventory (Reynolds & Kobak, 1998)			X				X		X	
Measures originally developed for neurogenic patients										
Cornell Scale for Depression in Dementia (Alexopolous, Abrams, Young, & Shamoian, 1988)		X				X	X	X		
Dementia Mood Assessment Scale (Sunderland et al., 1988)		X				X				X

(continues)

TABLE 5-3 (continued)

	SYMPTOMS ASSESSED					FORMAT		LINGUISTIC DEMANDS		
	Anxiety	Depression	Multi-dimensional	Irritability	Self-esteem	Observer-rated	Self-rated	Sentence-level	Word-level	N/A
Frontal Behavioral Inventory (Kertesz, Davidson, & Fox, 1997)			x			x				x
Frontal Systems Behavior Scale (Grace & Malloy, 2001)			x			x	x	x		
National Taiwan University Irritability Scale (C. Yang et al., 2011)				x		x	x	x		
Neurobehavioral Functioning Inventory (Kreutzer, Seel, & Marwitz, 1999)			x			x	x	x		
Neuropsychiatric Inventory (NPI; Cummings et al., 1994) or NPI-Q (Kaufer et al., 2000)			x			x				x
Patient Health Questionnaire 9 (Kroenke, Spitzer, & Williams, 2001)		x					x	x		
Post-Stroke Depression Rating Scale (Gainotti et al., 1997)		x				x				x
Rating Anxiety in Dementia (Shankar, Walker, Frost, & Orrell, 1999)	x					x				x
Stroke and Aphasia Depression Scale (Smollan & Penn, 1997)		x					x		x	
Stroke Aphasic Depression Questionnaire (SADQH; Sutcliffe & Lincoln, 1998) or SADQH-10 (Cobley et al., 2011)		x				x				x
Visual Analogue Self-Esteem Scale (Brumfitt & Sheeran, 1999)					x		x		x	
Visual Analogue Mood Scales (Stern, 1998)			x				x		x	

N/A = not applicable.

These tests are more appropriate because they have taken into consideration the above-discussed testing confounds. For example, many of these tests (e.g., *National Taiwan University Irritability Scale*, which was developed for TBI patients; Yang et al., 2011) incorporate both self- and observer ratings to examine for the possible influence of patient self-awareness deficits. Including both self- and observer ratings is also important given that researchers have raised some concerns related to relying on just observer or proxy ratings (Berg, Lonnqvist, Palmoaki, & Kaste, 2009; E. Miller et al., 2010). That is, there is a tendency for proxies to rate patients as having more severe symptoms than the patients would rate themselves. Additionally, proxies' ratings can be influenced by their own emotional or psychiatric status (e.g., a proxy will be more likely to rate a patient as depressed if she herself is depressed).

There are now some assessment protocols, such as the *Stroke and Aphasia Depression Scale* (SADS; Smollan & Penn, 1997), *Stroke Aphasic Depression Questionnaire* (SADQH; Sutcliffe & Lincoln, 1998), SADQH-10 (Cobley et al., 2011), *Visual Analog Mood Scales* (VAMS; Stern, 1998), and *Visual Analogue Self-Esteem Scale* (VASES; Brumfitt & Sheeran, 1999), that have no or minimal linguistic and cognitive demands. The SADS, VAMS, and VASES utilize visual analog scales that are anchored by both picture and printed-word stimuli. Therefore, even patients with severe linguistic impairments have been shown to be able to indicate accurately and reliably their self-perceptions of their current emotional status. The SADQH and its shorter version, the SADQH-10, involve caregiver ratings of items such as "Did he/she have weeping spells?" and "Did he/she refuse to participate in social activities?" (Cobley et al., 2011, p. 378).

Even if clinicians do not administer formal tests to identify psychiatric problems in their patients, they should, at the very least, ensure that their patients' psychiatric well-being is evaluated in some fashion and on a regular basis. Clinicians must be aware of symptoms and behaviors that are indicative of psychiatric problems so that appropriate referrals for psychological or psychiatric assessment and/or treatment can be made when necessary.

Come On... How Can I Know All of This Before I Assess the Patient?

There is no question that it would be ideal for confounding deficits in sensation, perception, and motor control and for psychiatric issues to be identified prior to assessment of language and cognition. In the "real world," this may not happen for a number of reasons. For example, in acute care, it would be extremely unlikely that patients with common neurologic diagnoses (e.g., stroke, traumatic brain injury) would be assessed by an audiologist or psychiatrist prior to being evaluated by a speech-language pathologist. Moreover, you may have only 20 minutes with the patient, and it could take that much time to administer even the simplest of appropriate standardized tests. When formal assessment of these potential confounds is unfeasible, the clinician can draw on other sources of information that may identify or signal the presence of relevant deficits.

Many times patients will simply tell us, "I can't hear worth a hoot" or "I can't read that without my glasses." Neurologists routinely assess visual fields and praxis, reporting their findings in their notes. Critical observation of the patient's behaviors is also needed. If the patient consistently points to items pictured on the right but "doesn't know" any of the items on the left, visual or perceptual deficits should be strongly suspected. Family members can be another potentially rich source of relevant information, often commenting that patients "haven't been themselves."

Whether or not formal assessment of these important factors is carried out prior to assessment of cognition and/or language, the clinician must be sensitive to how such impairments impact performance and be prepared to make appropriate referrals for additional assessment.

Summary

Neurogenic disorders of language and cognition frequently co-occur with a variety of sensory, motoric, perceptual, and emotional or psychiatric disorders. Because these disorders may directly contribute to patients' communicative and cognitive difficulties (e.g., negative effects of dysarthria on spoken language skills or of dominant hand paresis on writing) or, at the very least, confound patients' performance of language and cognitive tests (e.g., hearing loss may result in errors on a repetition subtest of an aphasia battery), it is imperative that the presence and severity of these disorders be established prior to proceeding with formal or informal language or cognitive assessment procedures.

It is unlikely that speech-language clinicians would be solely responsible for identifying the variety of confounding conditions reviewed in this chapter, as a variety of health-care team members are involved in this component of the assessment process. Speech-language clinicians must, however, maintain an understanding of these potential complicating conditions and be prepared to make appropriate referrals if they lack the appropriate training to administer and interpret the procedures necessary to quantify and qualify such conditions.

Discussion Questions

1. Create a battery of formal and/or informal test procedures that would allow you to screen for sensory, motoric, perceptual, and psychiatric problems that are common in patients who have suffered right hemisphere brain damage. How would this battery differ if you were evaluating a patient with aphasia?
2. Select a test battery for evaluating memory abilities (see Chapter 7). On which subtests might a visual deficit (e.g., visual field cut) confound performance? On which subtests might a hearing deficit confound performance?
3. Identify factors that might make it difficult to identify depression in a patient with Parkinson's disease and dementia.

Assessment of Body Structure and Function: Quantifying and Qualifying Linguistic Disorders

chapter 6

Learning Objectives

After reading this chapter, you should be able to:

- Specify why observations must precede formal language testing procedures
- Identify clinical situations in which screening of language abilities is appropriate
- Compare and contrast test batteries designed for patients with aphasia with those designed for patients with dementia, or cognitive-communicative disorders associated with right hemisphere brain damage or traumatic brain injury
- List the pros and cons of aphasia classification systems
- Identify patient populations for whom testing of specific language functions is typically essential
- Describe tests that evaluate specific linguistic abilities, including comprehension and production of phonology and orthography, lexical-semantics, morphosyntax, and pragmatics and discourse
- Identify tests that evaluate gesture and drawing abilities
- Explain the cognitive neuropsychological and neurolinguistic approaches to linguistic assessment
- Explain factors that may confound the administration or interpretation of language tests
- Describe biographic, medical, and cognitive variables that should be considered when making prognoses about linguistic outcomes

Key Terms

- ageism
- canonical
- circumlocution
- cohesion
- derivational affix
- discourse genre
- inflectional affix
- informativeness
- neologism
- paraphasia
- relational or closed class words
- segmental versus suprasegmental phonology
- speech acts
- substantive or open class words

Introduction

As reviewed in Chapter 1, language consists of a number of linguistic functions, each of which may be compromised by acquired brain damage or disease. Because the nature of the brain damage (e.g., focal vs. diffuse, static vs. progressive) and location of the brain damage (e.g., cortical vs. subcortical, right vs. left hemisphere, frontal vs. posterior) varies among the different neurogenic patient populations, clinicians must be able to assess and treat a variety of circumscribed (i.e., impairment of one specific linguistic process) and broad (i.e., impairment of several linguistic processes) linguistic deficits. For example, a patient who suffers a small, focal stroke to the left parietal lobe might present with only one linguistic symptom: a reading deficit due to impaired access to the orthographic input lexicon (see the model illustrated in Figure 1-3). In contrast, a patient who suffers a severe traumatic brain injury (TBI) and diffuse cortical and subcortical damage to both hemispheres might present with not only this same reading deficit, but additional semantic problems that affect his comprehension and production abilities in other language modalities.

The purpose of this chapter, therefore, is to describe assessment procedures specific to evaluating the linguistic components of neurogenic language disorders, with an emphasis on procedures and tools that allow quantifying and qualifying linguistic symptoms at the body structure and function level of the International Classification of Functioning, Disability, and Health (ICF) framework (World Health Organization; WHO, 2001). First, procedures pertaining to the initial steps of a language assessment—that is, collecting case history and completing unstructured observations—are described. Next, more formal or structured methods for quantifying and qualifying language skills at the ICF level of body function are reviewed, including the administration of test batteries designed to evaluate general language ability and tests that assess more circumscribed linguistic functions. Lastly, factors that should be considered when making prognoses regarding linguistic outcomes are reviewed.

General Assessment Procedures

Although the exact format of a language assessment will vary depending on the clinical setting (e.g., acute-care hospital vs. skilled nursing facility vs. outpatient rehabilitation) and on the patient's current needs and abilities, language evaluations designed to quantify and qualify problems at the ICF level of body function and structure generally begin with the completion of a case history and informal observations, followed by more formal or structured assessment procedures. The structured component of a language assessment may consist of one or more of the following: (a) a test that only screens general language abilities, (b) a test battery that evaluates a number of language processes and modalities, and/or (c) a test that examines in detail only one or two specific linguistic functions. Regardless of what procedures are selected, clinicians must remain flexible, as each step of the assessment process may reveal new patient strengths and weaknesses that will either negate the use of certain tests and procedures or highlight the need for additional tests and procedures. Likewise, even once the initial evaluation is completed, plans for further assessment are typically necessary to document treatment progress.

Case History and Observations

The collection of case history information is the first essential step of the assessment process, as it aids clinicians in their subsequent selection of informal procedures as well as structured tests. In addition to reviewing medical charts or files, clinicians need to obtain further information from patients and, ideally, their caregivers and other healthcare team members (see Chapter 4 for suggestions regarding what case history information should be accumulated). This information can be acquired by asking patients and caregivers to complete questionnaires or, if time permits, by interviewing them in person. The latter method is preferable, as observations pertaining to patients' communicative strengths and weaknesses as well as their caregivers' communication styles and strategies also can be attained. Figure 6-1 provides an example of a case history or patient intake form that clinicians might adapt for their clinical setting.

Clinicians also may consult published tools such as the *Caregiver-Administered Communication Inventory* (Tanner & Culbertson, 1999a), the *Neurobehavioral Functioning Inventory* (Kreutzer, Seel, & Marwitz, 1999), or the *La Trobe Communication Questionnaire* (J. Douglas, O'Flaherty, & Snow, 2000; Struchen et al., 2008b), which require patients and/or caregivers to rate the occurrence or frequency of common cognitive and communicative disorders. Additionally, guidelines for structuring interviews of patients with aphasia and their caregivers can be found in *Conversation Analysis Profile for People With Aphasia* (Whitworth, Perkins, & Lesser, 1997) or in a study by Luck and Rose (2007); for patients with cognitive impairments, the *Conversation Analysis Profile for People With Cognitive Impairment* (Perkins, Whitworth, & Lesser, 1997) can be consulted.

Regardless of how case history information is acquired, clinicians should ensure that some observation of their patients is completed prior to selecting and administering any formal tests. These observations should focus on documenting patients' positive and negative communicative behaviors, as well as the conditions (e.g., environmental conditions, communicative partners, time of day, conversational topic, language modality) under which language successes and failures occur. Clinicians should not limit their observations to just patients' language behaviors, but should also take note of how caregivers interact with the patients. For example, clinicians may watch for whether caregivers utilize strategies that facilitate the patients' language abilities (e.g., use short, simple commands, reduce ambient noise to enhance the patient's auditory comprehension) or impede them (e.g., correct the patient's output, ask for multiple repetitions that lead to patient frustration).

Observations are particularly important in certain clinical settings and for assessing certain patient populations. For example, in acute-care facilities, patients with neurogenic conditions are often unable to complete structured or formal language tests because of their physical limitations and/or emotional reactions to the onset of their neurological insult and subsequent symptoms (A. Holland & Fridriksson, 2001; R. Marshall,

(text continues on p. 171)

Patient Intake Form

DEMOGRAPHIC/BACKGROUND INFORMATION

1. Name: _____ 2. Birthplace: _____
3. Address: _____ 4. Birthdate: _____
5. Phone Number: _____ 6. Date of Report: _____
7. Patient's native language(s): _____

   If not English, at what age did the patient learn English? _____ What other languages does the patient speak, read, and/or write? _____

   In what daily activities does the patient use English, and which language abilities (e.g., reading, writing, listening) are needed for these activities? _____
   _____

   In what daily activities does the patient use his or her other language(s), and which language abilities (e.g., reading, writing, listening) are needed for these activities? _____
   _____

8. Patient's ethnocultural background: _____
9. Patient's highest level of education: _____
10. Patient's current (or if retired, previous) primary occupation: _____
11. List patient's interests or favorite activities: _____
    _____
    _____

12. Marital status: Single ☐   Widowed ☐   Separated ☐
                     Married ☐   Divorced ☐   Remarried ☐

13. List patient's primary caregiver and/or immediate family members:

Name	Age	Relationship	Phone Number	Email
_____	_____	_____	_____	_____
_____	_____	_____	_____	_____
_____	_____	_____	_____	_____
_____	_____	_____	_____	_____
_____	_____	_____	_____	_____
_____	_____	_____	_____	_____

MEDICAL HISTORY

Date of injury or onset of symptoms: _____
Patient's handedness (before stroke or disease onset):   Right ☐   Left ☐   Ambidextrous ☐
Does the patient wear glasses? _____ See well enough to read? _____ Have any other visual problems, such as right/left visual field cut, cataracts, or macular degeneration? _____
Does the patient have a hearing loss? _____ Wear a hearing aid? _____ If yes, in the right ear _____, left ear _____, or both _____?

(continues)

Figure 6-1. Example of a case history or patient intake form.

Describe the patient's general health: _____

_____

List the patient's current medications and dosages: _____

_____

Has the patient had or does the patient currently have any of the following?

                                                         Onset Date and Current Status

- Stroke   Yes ☐   No ☐   _____
- Aphasia   Yes ☐   No ☐   _____
- Other Communication Disorder   Yes ☐   No ☐   _____
- Right- or Left-Sided Weakness   Yes ☐   No ☐   _____
- Neglect   Yes ☐   No ☐   _____
- Dementia   Yes ☐   No ☐   _____
- Memory Impairment   Yes ☐   No ☐   _____
- Other Neurological Disease   Yes ☐   No ☐   _____
- Head Injury   Yes ☐   No ☐   _____
- Seizure Disorder   Yes ☐   No ☐   _____
- Clinical Depression   Yes ☐   No ☐   _____
- Other Psychiatric Problems   Yes ☐   No ☐   _____
- Alcohol Abuse/Problems   Yes ☐   No ☐   _____
- Other Substance Abuse   Yes ☐   No ☐   _____
- Other Major Illness   Yes ☐   No ☐   _____

COMMUNICATION AND COGNITIVE STATUS AND NEEDS

1. Patient's current or suspected communication and/or cognitive problems: _____

_____

2. What communication and/or cognitive problems, if any, are of concern to the patient and caregiver? _____

_____

_____

3. Cause of current or suspected communication and/or cognitive problems: _____

_____

4. Date of onset of communication and/or cognitive problems: _____

5. Describe the patient's ability to communicate:

   Preferred output language modality _____

   Most successful output language modality _____

   Preferred input language modality _____

   Most successful input language modality _____

   Pragmatic/social communication strengths/weaknesses _____

_____

(continues)

Figure 6-1. *(continued)*

6. Current communication strategies used by:
   Patient _____
   _____
   Caregivers _____
   _____

7. Describe the patient's cognitive status:
   Attention _____
   _____
   Memory _____
   _____
   Executive Functioning (e.g., problem solving, planning): _____
   _____

8. Has the patient received previous:

	Dates	Agency	Address
a. Speech-language therapy	_____	_____	_____
b. Audiology	_____	_____	_____
c. Cognitive assessment	_____	_____	_____
d. Cognitive therapy	_____	_____	_____

NOTES

Figure 6-1. (*continued*)

1997). Observations also may be the primary means for assessing patients who present with a broad range of severe impairments (e.g., severe hemiparesis, aphasia, apraxia, and cognitive deficits), as most formal language tests will be beyond their ability level, resulting in basal level test performances (i.e., at or near 0% accuracy) (Beaumont, Marjoribanks, Flury, & Lintern, 1999; Threats, 2009). Likewise, patients whose language problems are primarily reflective of high level cognitive deficits typically perform well on structured tasks and in controlled environments (Bernicot & Dardier, 2001; Coelho, Ylvisaker, & Turkstra et al., 2005; Murray & Ramage, 2000); therefore, failure to observe their language behaviors in less predictable settings may result in an overestimation of their language skills. Accordingly, for at least some patients, observation may provide the most valid, reliable, and thus informative means of qualifying a neurogenic language disorder.

Screening or Bedside Procedures

Typically, screening tests are used in acute health-care settings, or when there is little time available for assessment and only general information concerning a patient's linguistic abilities is needed (e.g., Is the patient aphasic or not aphasic?). The purposes of screening or bedside tests are to establish efficiently the presence or absence of language disorders and to identify language skills in need of further assessment or that will be the focus of initial treatment (Flamand-Roze et al., 2011; Gaber, Parsons, & Guatam, 2011; Salter, Jutai, Foley, Hellings, & Teasell, 2006). Additionally, a few screening measures have been designed with simple administration and scoring procedures so that a variety of health-care professionals (e.g., physicians, nurses) may use them to determine if a referral for a speech-language pathology evaluation is needed. Because of these tests' short length and tendency to sample only a narrow range of language functions, clinicians must keep in mind that screening tests do not provide a complete depiction of patients' language profiles and thus are inadequate for planning treatment (Berthier, 2005; Salter et al., 2006). Instead, they are useful when (a) in the early and acute stages of recovery from stroke, TBI, or other abrupt-onset neurological disorder, patients are too ill or fatigued to undergo a lengthy evaluation (Laska, Bartfai, Hellblom, Murray, & Kahan, 2007); (b) the patients' length of stay in the clinical facility is brief; or (c) cost containment dictates immediate clinical information without extensive testing.

Clinicians have two options for screening language abilities: (a) They may create their own screening or bedside tools or (b) they can utilize commercially available tests. Those interested in developing their own screening protocol should consult Holland and Fridriksson (2001). These researchers provided suggestions for developing brief as well as functional diagnostic activities such as (a) having patients read their "get well" cards to evaluate reading aloud and/or comprehension skills; (b) making mistakes such as calling the patient by the wrong name to determine if the error is caught and, if so, how is it addressed (i.e., does the patient respond in a pragmatically appropriate manner?); and (c) encouraging patients to complete their daily hospital menu (e.g., reading meal choices and indicating their food preferences) to assess reading and basic writing abilities. A strength of informal protocols is that they can be developed to reflect the specific needs of the primary patient profile. For example, items on a protocol designed to screen patients being admitted to an Alzheimer's disease unit would most likely differ from those on a protocol for screening patients being admitted to a stroke rehabilitation unit. A weakness of informal protocols is that often the validity and reliability of the data gleaned from these measures cannot be determined because clinicians have not established observation or measurement consistency within and across clinicians or over time (Peach, 2001).

Because of their convenience and typically stronger psychometric properties (Davis, 2007), many clinicians utilize published screening tests versus informal protocols. As shown in Table 6-1, most language screening instruments that are commercially available or described in the research literature have been specifically developed for patients with aphasia, and they screen language abilities in several or all modalities. These vary in terms of length and number of language processes and modalities screened. For example, the *Language Screening Test* (Flamand-Roze et al., 2011) consists of 15 items,

TABLE 6-1
Screening or Bedside Tests of Linguistic Disorders

INSTRUMENT	SOURCE
Acute Aphasia Screening Protocol	Crary, Haak, & Malinsky (1989)
Addenbrooke's Cognitive Examination-Revised: Language Component	Gaber, Parsons, & Gautam et al. (2011); Mioshi, Dawson, Mitchell, Arnold, & Hodges (2006)
Aphasia Screening Test-3	R. Whurr (2011)
Bedside Evaluation Screening Test-Second Edition	West et al. (1998)
Cognistat	Kiernan et al. (2011)
Frenchay Aphasia Screening Test	Enderby, Wood, Wade, & Langton Hewer (1997)
In-Patient Functional Communication Interview	McCooey et al. (2000)
Language Screening Test	Flamand-Roze et al. (2011)
Mississippi Aphasia Screening Test	Nakase-Thompson (2004)
ScreeLing	Doesborgh et al. (2003)
Shortened Porch Index of Communicative Ability	Holtzapple et al. (1989)
Quick Assessment for Aphasia	Tanner & Culbertson (1999)

whereas the *ScreeLing* (Doesborgh et al., 2003) has 72 items. Published tools typically have stronger psychometric characteristics compared with those developed by clinicians or facilities or with neurological screening tests (which typically have a very limited set of language or aphasia items) (Laska et al., 2007). It is important, however, to keep in mind that researchers have raised concerns regarding the measurement properties of most language screening tests (Flamand-Roze et al., 2011; Salter et al., 2006). Accordingly, clinicians need to be aware of those psychometric weaknesses when selecting a language screening tool, and when interpreting the data yielded by these measures.

As a more detailed example of a language screening tool, the *Bedside Evaluation Screening Test of Aphasia–Second Edition* (BEST-2; West, Sands, & Ross-Swain, 1998) was designed to evaluate in 20 minutes or less the listening, speaking, and reading skills of both high- and low-level aphasic patients. BEST-2 was standardized on approximately 200 patients, has acceptable reliability and validity, and provides two sets of norms: those for patients less than 75 years of age and those for patients over the age of 75. Because BEST-2 does not assess writing, clinicians may instead select the *Mississippi Aphasia Screening Test* (MAST; Nakase-Thompson, 2004; Nakase-Thompson et al., 2005), as this screening test examines all language modalities (i.e., speaking, listening, reading, and writing) and in fact, includes a broader range of language tasks (e.g., verbal fluency, automatic speech, reading instructions) than other aphasia screening measures (Salter et al., 2006). Although the psychometric properties of the English version of the MAST have not yet been fully described (Salter et al., 2006), studies examining a Spanish (Romero et al., 2011) and a Czech version (Kostalova et al., 2008) reported good validity (convergent, construct), including high sensitivity and specificity, and acceptable reliability (test–retest, inter-rater) (see Chapter 4 for a review of these psychometric constructs).

Another option for screening language is using shortened versions of more comprehensive language test batteries. For instance, shorter versions of several aphasia test batteries, including the *Porch Index of Communicative Ability* (Holtzapple, Pohlman, LaPointe, & Graham, 1989), can be found in the research literature. Likewise, truncated versions of the *Boston Diagnostic Aphasia Examination–Third Edition* (BDAE-3; Goodglass et al., 2001) and the *Western Aphasia Battery–Revised* (WAB-R; Kertesz, 2006) are commercially available.

Whereas there are many test options available for screening for the presence of aphasia or basic language impairments, there remains a need to develop tools that are appropriate for identifying the high-level and social language difficulties (e.g., impaired comprehension of implied information; inefficient or disorganized discourse production) that are characteristic of patients with TBI, with right hemisphere brain damage (RHD), or who are in the early stages of certain dementing illnesses such as Parkinson's disease or the behavioral variant of frontotemporal lobar degeneration (Pakhomov et al., 2010; Struchen et al., 2008b; Turkstra et al., 2005). Even screening instruments such as *Cognistat* (Kiernan, Mueller, & Langston, 2011), which were standardized on patients representing a broad spectrum of neurogenic disorders, focus on assessing only lower level language abilities.

An exception is the *La Trobe Communication Questionnaire* (J. Douglas et al., 2000), which measures the perceptions of patients with TBI and their caregivers regarding the patients' communicative abilities. It consists of two forms, one for the patient and one for the caregiver to complete. Each form has the same 30 items that are rated on a four-point scale to indicate whether the discourse-level cognitive-communicative problems occur *never or rarely, sometimes, often,* or *usually or always.* Sample items include "Go over and over the same ground in conversation," "Switch to a different topic of conversation too quickly," "Carry on talking about things for too long in your conversations," "Keep track of the main details of conversations," and "Answer without taking time to think about what the other person has said." Importantly, since this test's initial publication in the research literature, additional studies have been completed to establish its reliability and validity in broad samples of TBI patients and caregivers (e.g., diverse ages, ethnicities, and education levels; a range of TBI severities and time post-onset; J. Douglas, Bracy, & Snow, 2007; Struchen et al., 2008b). Although this questionnaire has been found appropriate for evaluating the perceived communicative abilities of TBI survivors, its suitability for individuals with high-level or social communication problems related to other etiologies (e.g., RHD, dementing diseases) has not yet been established. Accordingly, when clinicians suspect, and want to document, the presence of high-level language difficulties in patients with these latter types of etiology, they will need either to establish normative data for the patient population of interest or to rely on observations or informal protocols that allow quantifying and qualifying their patients' interactions in a variety of contexts and with a number of conversational partners.

> ### Screening: A Good Place to Start but a Bad Place to End
>
> Clinicians must always keep in mind that a pass on a screening test does not invariably signify that the patient has intact linguistic abilities. For example, Mr. Russell suffered a left hemisphere stroke that affected small portions of his parietal and occipital lobes. At two days poststroke, he accurately completed the BEST-2. Although his clinician noted that some of his test responses were slow, she attributed this to fatigue, as Mr. Russell had complained of feeling extremely tired since his stroke. Because no one—including Mr. Russell, his family, and other healthcare team members—voiced any concerns regarding Mr. Russell's communication abilities, the clinician concluded that further speech-language therapy services were not needed. Unfortunately, upon discharge to home, Mr. Russell began to experience significant communication problems, including word retrieval difficulties, problems reading the newspaper, and difficulties completing daily email and online chat room activities. Had his clinician extended Mr. Russell's initial language assessment to include observation of him discussing controversial issues or talking in noisy environments, his word finding difficulties would have been evident. Likewise, had the clinician included reading and writing tasks reflective of his daily reading and writing needs in his screening, his written word retrieval difficulties and visual scanning problems would have been exposed.

Test Batteries

In rehabilitation and long-term health-care settings or when more assessment time is available and patients have adequate stamina, clinicians may begin a language assessment by administering a test battery specific to their patient's documented or presumed neurogenic language diagnosis. For instance, a clinician would administer an aphasia battery to a patient who has already been diagnosed with aphasia or who she suspects has aphasia based on initial assessment data. Whereas aphasia test batteries have been around for over 50 years, the development of test batteries for patient populations with RHD, TBI, and dementia has only occurred over the last 25 years; consequently, fewer test battery options are available for these patient populations (see Table 6-2). When utilizing test batteries, clinicians must keep in mind that even though these tools provide more comprehensive data than screening tests, their primary functions are to identify the presence and severity of a language disorder and to highlight language functions that may be compromised. In most cases, they are not designed to indicate the specific linguistic or cognitive locus of the identified language disorder. Consequently, test battery results should ideally be supplemented by findings from tests of specific linguistic and/or cognitive functions and qualitative assessment procedures (e.g., analyzing error types, exploring stimulability) prior to specifying treatment goals and procedures (L. Murray & Coppens, 2011).

Aphasia Test Batteries

Aphasia test batteries consist primarily of tasks designed to assess basic language functions (e.g., semantics, syntax) in each communication modality (i.e., speaking, listening, reading, writing, and gesturing). As shown in Table 6-2, a number of batteries are currently available, each having its own distinct strengths and weaknesses. As examples, two of the more frequently used batteries in clinics and research (R. Katz et al., 2000; Simmons-Mackie, Kearns, & Potechin, 2005) are described below.

Popular aphasia batteries evaluate all language modalities and were designed to categorize patients' language profiles into connectionist aphasia syndromes (e.g., Broca's, Wernicke's, transcortical motor). For example, the WAB-R (Kertesz, 2006) assesses spoken and written language production, construction, praxis, and calculation skills. Aphasia types are assigned on the basis of specific test scores, and three summary scores can be calculated to quantify WAB performances: (1) the Aphasia Quotient, based on scores from the oral language subtests, which can be used to qualify aphasia severity; (2) the Language Quotient, based on scores from the oral, reading, and writing subtests (for specific instruction for calculating this score, see Shewan & Kertesz, 1984); and (3) the Cortical Quotient, based on scores from all subtests. As previously mentioned, the WAB-R has a Bedside version designed to identify (in approximately 15 minutes) the presence and type of aphasia in acute-care settings. Supplemental tasks are also included to assist in determining type of reading disorder (e.g., surface vs. deep dyslexia; see Chapter 2). Several language versions of the WAB are available (e.g., a Korean version called the K-WAB; H. Kim & Na, 2004). Whereas Kertesz (1982; Shewan & Kertesz,

TABLE 6-2
Test Batteries for Specific Neurogenic Language Disorders

INSTRUMENT	SOURCE	Aphasia	Right hemisphere disorders	Traumatic brain injury	Dementia
Arizona Battery for Communication Disorders of Dementia	Bayles & Tomoeda (1993)				X
Assessment of Communicative Effectiveness in Severe Aphasia	Cunningham et al. (1995)	X			
Assessment of Language-Related Functional Activities	Baines et al. (1999)	X	X	X	X
Bilingual Aphasia Test	Paradis & Libben (1987)	X			
Boston Assessment of Severe Aphasia	Helm-Estabrooks et al. (1989)	X			
Boston Diagnostic Aphasia Examination–Third Edition	Goodglass et al. (2001)	X			
Brief Test of Head Injury	Helm-Estabrooks & Hotz (1991)			X	
Burns Brief Inventory of Communication and Cognition:	Burns (1997)				
• Complex Neuropathology Inventory				X	X
• Left Hemisphere Inventory		X			
• Right Hemisphere Inventory			X		
Comprehensive Aphasia Test	Swinburn, Swinburn, Porter, & Howard (2004)	X			
Examining for Aphasia–Fourth Edition	LaPointe & Eisenson (2008)	X			
Functional Linguistic Communication Inventory	Bayles & Tomoeda (1994)				X
Mini Inventory of Right Brain Injury–Second Edition	Pimental & Knight (2000)		X		
Neuropsychological Assessment Battery–Language Module	Stern & White (2003)	X			
Oral and Written Language Scales–Second Edition	Carrow-Woolfolk (2012)			X	
Pediatric Test of Brain Injury	Hotz et al. (2010)			X	
Porch Index of Communicative Ability–Revised	Porch (2001)	X			
Repeatable Battery for the Assessment of Neuropsychological Status Update	Randolph (2012)		X	X	X

TABLE 6-2 (continued)

		TARGET NEUROGENIC DISORDER(S)			
INSTRUMENT	SOURCE	Aphasia	Right hemisphere disorders	Traumatic brain injury	Dementia
RIC Evaluation of Communication Problems in Right Hemisphere Dysfunction-Revised	Halper, Cherney, Burns, et al. (1996)		X		
Right Hemisphere Language Battery-Second Edition	Bryan (1995)		X		
Scales of Cognitive and Communicative Ability for Neurorehabilitation	Milman & Holland (2012)	X	X	X	X
Severe Impairment Battery	Saxton et al. (1993)				X
Western Aphasia Battery-Revised	Kertesz (2006)	X			

1980) reported that the WAB possesses strong psychometric properties in terms of both reliability and validity, K. Ross and Wertz (2001) identified significant correlations between age and Aphasia and Cortical Quotients. These findings indicate that additional assessment data must be acquired to assist in interpreting the WAB outcomes of elderly patients, and to avoid underestimating their language abilities. This is particularly important to keep in mind because the standardization sample of the WAB-R only goes up to age 89. A description of some additional psychometric concerns pertaining to certain WAB scores and items can be found in Hula, Donovan, Kendall, and Gonzalez-Rothi (2010a).

The BDAE-3 (Goodglass et al., 2001) represents an updated and expanded version of Goodglass and Kaplan's (1983) earlier and extremely popular BDAE. The Standard Test of the BDAE-3 has many of the same subtests found in earlier BDAE editions for evaluating conversational and narrative speech (e.g., description of the Cookie Theft Picture), auditory and reading comprehension (e.g., Commands), oral and written expression (e.g., Responsive Naming), and repetition; the Standard Test also utilizes similar rating scales and scoring procedures to determine aphasia severity and type. Like its predecessors, the BDAE-3 manual describes supplementary tests to examine nonverbal skills, such as drawing to command and finger agnosia. Most new subtests are part of the BDAE-3's Extended Test and include retelling of Aesop's Fables, Word Comprehension by Categories, Semantic Probe (i.e., comprehension of semantic features of target nouns), Syntactic Processing (i.e., comprehension of semantically reversible and complex syntactic forms), Naming in Categories, Lexical Decision, Phonics (e.g., identifying homophones), Derivational and Grammatical Morphology, spelling Nonsense Words, and Limb/Hand and Bucco-Facial/Respiratory Praxis. These Extended subtests allow clinicians to form more precise linguistic explanations of their patients' communication difficulties. There also is a BDAE-3 Short Form that may be utilized when time or patient factors such as fatigue necessitate only screening patients' language abilities. Another addition is the Language Competency Index, which can be calculated if the Standard Test and the *Boston Naming Test–Second Edition* (Kaplan, Goodglass, & Weintraub, 2001) have been given. This index is calculated from percentile scores from expressive syntax, auditory comprehension, and naming measures, and was designed to provide a quantitative indicator of the severity of patients' language impairment, although guidelines regarding the interpretation of this index are not provided. Despite many improvements (e.g., choice of administering Standard, Extended, or Short Test Forms, addition of new subtests), the psychometric properties of the BDAE-3 remain weak. For example, its standardization sample is relatively small, ranging from 85 to only 33 aphasic subjects across subtests, and demographic characteristics of the standardization sample are not provided. Likewise, the test manual provides no information pertaining to intra- or inter-rater or test–retest reliability, or construct validity.

In addition to the above frequently used aphasia batteries, there are comprehensive tests for special populations of patients with aphasia. For example, when assessing patients who do not speak English or who speak it as a second language, clinicians may choose from aphasia tests created in another language (e.g., *Aachen Aphasia Battery*; Huber, Poeck, Weniger, & Willmes, 1983; Huber, Poeck, & Willmes, 1984), translated versions of aphasia tests originally developed in English (e.g., Hua, Chang, & Chen, 1997; Mazaux & Orgozo, 1981), or aphasia tests that offer several language versions that are functionally and culturally equivalent in content (vs. simply direct translations), such as the *Bilingual Aphasia Test* (BAT; Paradis, 2011; Paradis & Libben, 1987, 1993) or the *Multilingual Aphasia Examination* (A. Benton et al., 2001; Rey, Sivan, & Benton, 1991). Of these options, the first and last are preferred, as direct translations of English tests do not take into consideration language and/or cultural differences. For example, items on a naming subtest may vary from high to low word frequency in English, but when translated to another language, only represent low-frequency words. Clinicians might find the BAT a particularly attractive option given that it has versions for numerous common languages (e.g., Spanish, Chinese) and uncommon languages (e.g., Rarotongan, Friulian), has been used with aphasic as well as other populations with language impairments (e.g., Alzheimer's and Parkinson's diseases, mild cognitive impairment), and is available free of charge at www.mcgill.ca/linguistics/research/bat/ (Paradis, 2011).

Aphasia test batteries specific to patients with severe language impairments, including the *Boston Assessment of Severe Aphasia* (BASA; Helm-Estabrooks, Ramsberger, Morgan, & Nicholas, 1989) and the *Assessment of Communicative Effectiveness in Severe Aphasia* (Cunningham, Farrow, Davies, & Lincoln, 1995), also are available. These tests tend to probe simpler language functions and have more liberal response requirements so that patients with severe aphasia do not simply receive basal-level scores (as they typically do on the more common aphasia batteries, such as the BDAE-3 or WAB; Threats, 2009); basal-level scores are problematic because they fail to provide insight into language areas of relative strength and only indicate areas of weakness. For instance, whereas on other aphasia batteries, only verbal responses are scored as correct or incorrect, on the BASA, *both* gestural and verbal responses are scored in terms of whether they are *partially* or *fully* communicative, and clinicians also record refusals, perseverations, and affective responses. Therefore, more qualitative and quantitative information regarding the language abilities of patients with severe aphasia can be obtained using these special tests versus traditional aphasia batteries.

Aphasia Classification: Pros and Cons

As just described, many aphasia test batteries (e.g., WAB, BDAE-3), in addition to identifying the presence and severity of language impairments, help clinicians categorize their patients' language profiles into aphasia types (see also Chapter 2). The most common classification system to which most aphasia test batteries adhere is anatomically based and includes Broca's, Wernicke's, conduction, anomic, transcortical motor, transcortical sensory, transcortical mixed, and global aphasia types. Even when the test battery does not assist with aphasia classification (e.g., *Burns Brief Inventory of Communication and Cognition;* Burns, 1997), clinicians often will still qualify their patients' language symptoms using the dichotomous classifications of fluent versus nonfluent aphasia (some physicians also still use the dichotomous categories of receptive vs. expressive aphasia).

As touched upon in Chapter 2, however, there are several negatives associated with these aphasia classification systems (D. Caplan, 1993; J. Gordon, 1998; J. Marshall, 2010; Varney, 1998). First, as many practicing clinicians can attest, many patients' language symptoms do not neatly fit into just one aphasia type, with some clinicians and researchers estimating that they have difficulty assigning an aphasia classification to up to 70% of their patients. Second, the language symptoms of patients within a given aphasia type are not truly homogenous (e.g., some patients with Wernicke's aphasia have greater reading than auditory comprehension deficits, whereas other Wernicke's patients show the inverse profile). Third, dichotomous classification systems (e.g., receptive vs. expressive; sensory vs. motor) are often misleading, as both language comprehension and production are impaired, at least to some degree, in most patients with aphasia. Fourth, aphasia classification may be influenced by which aphasia test battery is used (e.g., the aphasia type assigned to a given patient may differ depending on whether the WAB-R or BDAE-3 was used). Fifth, aphasia classifications do not specify the nature of patients' underlying linguistic problems (e.g., a semantic vs. lexical access problem), and consequently do not provide a sufficient basis for selecting treatment goals and procedures.

Despite these limitations, the use of classification systems will likely persist in both clinical practice and research because, for at least some patients, an aphasia type succinctly describes their language syndrome to other clinicians or researchers (J. Marshall, 2010). That is, when other clinicians or researchers read this label in the medical chart, clinical report, or published study, they will have a good general idea of what specific language symptoms to expect in the patient.

Right Hemisphere Test Batteries

A few standardized test batteries are available for assessing cognitive-communicative disorders associated with RHD (see Table 6-2), although each has weaknesses related to its theoretical rationale and psychometric properties (Cote et al., 2007; Myers & Blake, 2008; Tompkins & Lehman, 1997). RHD test batteries contrast with aphasia batteries in two significant ways. First, RHD batteries assess not only language abilities but also cognitive functions (e.g., attention) that are commonly compromised by RHD. Second, whereas aphasia batteries evaluate basic language processes, RHD batteries examine higher-level language processes (e.g., interpretation of figurative language) and pragmatic skills that are more frequently affected by RHD. Accordingly, clinicians should avoid administering aphasia test batteries to their RHD patients, as most RHD patients will either ceiling out on the language tasks (perform at or near 100% accuracy) or display difficulties that are cognitively versus linguistically based. For example, a patient with RHD who errs on matching spoken words to pictures, a common task on aphasia test batteries, might be making mistakes because of visual neglect or visuoperceptual deficits rather than poor auditory comprehension.

The *Mini Inventory of Right Brain Injury* (MIRBI; Pimental & Kingsbury, 1989) and its updated version, MIRBI-II (Pimental & Knight, 2000), were designed to identify quickly patients with RHD between the ages of 20 and 90 who are having difficulties in one or more of the following areas: visuoperception, neglect, affect, orientation, memory, behavior, and language. MIRBI-II test items are arranged into the following 10 sections: visual scanning, integrity of gnosis, integrity of body image, visuoverbal processing (i.e., reading and writing), visuosymbolic processing, integrity of visuomotor praxis (i.e., drawing), higher-level language skills (e.g., interpretation of humor), expressing emotion, general affect, and general behavior. Because only a few items are dedicated to assessing each section, this test is actually more similar to a screening test than a comprehensive test battery and typically can be completed in less than 30 minutes. The integrity of body image, general affect, and general behavioral processing sections are based on clinicians' ratings versus patients' performance of specific test procedures. For example, to quantify general affect, a plus/minus rating is used to indicate whether or not patients display flat effect (i.e., decreased intonation, little variation in facial expression). Total raw scores on the MIRBI-II can be converted to standardized scores, percentiles, and an overall severity rating that ranges from *normal* to *profound impairment*. The psychometric properties of the MIRBI-II exceed those of the original version in terms of reliability, validity, and size and description of the RHD normative sample (e.g., 128 vs. 30 RHD subjects for the MIRBI-II vs. MIRBI). In summary, MIRBI findings may be used to determine the presence and general severity of RHD-related cognitive-communicative problems but, with no exceptions, must be supplemented by additional observational and test findings before treatment goals and procedures should be specified.

The *Burns Brief Inventory of Communication and Cognition* (Burns, 1997) consists of three sections: (1) a Left Hemisphere Inventory for patients with aphasia, (2) a

Complex Neuropathology Inventory for patients with TBI or dementia, and (3) a Right Hemisphere Inventory for patients with RHD. The Right Hemisphere Inventory is designed to identify attention, visuospatial perception and construction, and communicative impairments, and consists of 12 tasks, such as visual scanning, clock drawing, and recognizing familiar faces, to assess attention and visuospatial skills, and interpreting implied information and idioms to assess abstract language abilities. Scores for each task are plotted on a grid to indicate whether for that particular skill, the patient has a severe deficit (i.e., impaired to a degree that rapid improvement in treatment is unlikely), moderate deficit (i.e., impaired but likely to respond to treatment), mild deficit (i.e., unlikely to be an immediate treatment priority), or no deficit (i.e., perfect score on the task). The test manual also provides standard error of measurement for each task so that meaningful changes in patients' performances across repeated testings can be determined. Like the other *Burns* inventories, the Right Hemisphere Inventory takes approximately 30 minutes to administer and is suitable for patients between the ages of 18 and 80. The *Burns* was validated on a sample of 333 individuals representing a spectrum of neurogenic disorders (i.e., left or right stroke, TBI, and dementia) and reports acceptable levels of reliability and validity. Because most tasks consist of only five items, follow-up testing, as with the MIRBI, is essential to qualify and quantify problem areas.

Although there are at least four test batteries currently available that were developed specifically for assessing the cognitive-communicative abilities of patients with RHD (see Table 6-2), all have content and/or standardization weaknesses that limit their usefulness (Cote et al., 2007; Myers & Blake, 2008). As Tompkins and Lehman (1997) cautioned: "Theoretical foundations for these measures are often underdeveloped and out-of-date"; "Standardization samples are typically small and poorly characterized"; and "Reliability and validity data also are diluted by questionable evidence and methods for deriving them" (pp. 282–283). Whereas some tests have been revised to address, at least in part, some of Tompkins and Lehman's critique (e.g., MIRBI-II), clinicians should avoid relying solely on the results of these test batteries when attempting to quantify and qualify cognitive-communicative disorders related to RHD. Instead, tests of more specific linguistic and/or cognitive functions should be selected from those described below or in Chapter 7, respectively, and/or battery protocols described in the research might be used (e.g., Cote et al., 2007).

Traumatic Brain Injury Test Batteries

To date, a limited number of test batteries have been developed to assess the presence and severity of cognitive-communicative deficits associated with TBI (see Table 6-2). In fact, prior to the 1990s, clinicians relied on tests developed for other patient populations (particularly aphasia tests) or utilized their own informal assessment protocols (R. Schwartz, 1989). Aphasia tests, however, are only appropriate for the minority of TBI patients who present with frank language deficits (Demir et al., 2006; Vukovic et al., 2008), as they were not designed to assess the types of high-level language and discourse problems that are a more common consequence of TBI (Coelho et al., 2005; Turkstra et al., 2005; M. Wong et al., 2010). Generally, TBI test batteries evaluate not only high-level language abilities but also a range of basic cognitive functions, as these too are commonly compromised by head injury and may contribute to these patients' communicative difficulties (e.g., McDonald & Flanagan, 2004; Turkstra & Holland, 1998).

In 1992, an initial TBI test option became available, the *Scales of Cognitive Assessment for Traumatic Brain Injury* (SCATBI; Adamovich & Henderson, 1992). However, the SCATBI has not been updated and thus its tasks, stimuli, and standardization data are now outdated. Furthermore, significant concerns regarding its psychometric properties have been raised (Turkstra et al., 2005).

Another older option, but with stronger psychometric characteristics, is the *Brief Test of Head Injury* (BTHI; Helm-Estabrooks & Hotz, 1991). It was developed for patients with TBI who have more severe or acute injuries. The BTHI takes approximately 30 minutes to administer and assesses orientation/attention, auditory comprehension (e.g., following commands) and reading comprehension, spoken language production (e.g., naming, picture description), memory (e.g., word recall), and visuospatial abilities (e.g., matching of abstract designs). Stimuli and response demands were designed to be suitable for patients with concomitant motor symptoms or visual neglect. In terms of scoring, either verbal or gestural responses can receive full credit on several test items, again indicating the suitability of this test for more severely impaired patients. BTHI performances can be converted into cluster standard scores (i.e., scores for each cognitive-communicative domain) or a total standard score. The total test score can also be interpreted as a Severity Score (i.e., Severe, Moderate, Mild, Borderline Normal). Confidence intervals can be plotted, making the BTHI suitable for repeated testings. It was standardized on a relatively large sample of patients with TBI ($n = 265$) and small sample of healthy controls ($n = 29$), most of whom were less than 50 years old and male. Acceptable levels of several forms of reliability and validity are reported in the test manuals, although specific statistical data for some psychometric properties (e.g., inter-rater reliability) are not provided. Additionally, given that the test was published over 20 years ago, the normative sample and stimuli now require updating.

The most recently developed TBI test battery focuses on children, *The Pediatric Test of Brain Injury* (PTBI; Hotz, Helm-Estabrooks, Nelson, & Plante, 2010). This test is suitable for children ages 6 to 16 and, in approximately 30 minutes via 10 subtests, evaluates attention, memory, executive functioning, and language abilities. Both language comprehension and production skills are assessed at the word (e.g., Naming) through discourse (e.g., Story Retelling) levels. The PTBI yields criterion ability scores to help the clinician determine if the child's performance of each subtest should be considered *very low, low, moderate,* or *high*. Detailed description of the psychometric characteristics of the PTBI is provided in the test manual.

Another option, particularly for younger patients who have TBI, is comprehensive language test batteries, such as the *Test of Adolescent and Adult Language–Fourth Edition* (TOAL-4; Hammill, Brown, Larsen, & Wiederholt, 2007) or the *Clinical Evaluation of Language Fundamentals–Fifth Edition* (CELF-5; Semel, Wiig, & Secord, 2013). The TOAL-4 evaluates semantic and morphosyntactic aspects of speaking (i.e., generating an opposite to a word spoken by the clinician; completing a sentence spoken by the clinician with the correct derivative of a target word [e.g., for the target word "laugh," complete this sentence: "The play was very funny. The people broke out . . ."]; completing a partial analogous sentence spoken by the clinician with a spoken word [e.g., "*Birds* are to *sing* as *dogs* are to . . . ?"]) and writing skills (i.e., generating a written synonym for a printed word presented by the clinician, combining two or more sentences into one written sentence, writing sentences to dictation with correct words and punctuation). Test items and tasks have been selected to minimize floor and ceiling effects so that the test will be an appropriate choice for a broad spectrum of clients (ranging from having severe to above-average language abilities). Composite standard scores for speaking, writing, and overall general language ability can be calculated. To help determine areas of strength and weakness for a given individual client, difference scores can be determined so that the clinician can identify meaningful differences among the various subtest and composite scores. The TOAL-4 was standardized on an extensive sample of individuals up to the age of 24 years 11 months, and the test manual reports strong psychometric properties.

Despite the current availability of test batteries specifically designed for populations of patients with TBI, survey data indicate that many clinicians continue to utilize tests standardized on other patient populations (Turkstra et al., 2005). For example, Frank and Barrineau (1996); Duff, Proctor, and Haley (2002); and Turkstra et al. (2005) all found that the BDAE was one of the most frequently utilized test batteries when clinicians were assessing cognitive-communicative disorders associated with TBI. This is unfortunate given that (a) the BDAE was standardized only on patients with aphasia (i.e., primarily left hemisphere stroke patients), (b) this test does not evaluate the types of cognitive-communicative problems that patients with TBI frequently endure (i.e., pragmatic communication deficits), and (c) more appropriate test batteries are now available. As Duff et al. (2002) warned, clinicians using aphasia tests "will not have clinically valid information on the individual [with TBI] and the extent of his/her deficits. Ultimately, this may prevent detection and administration of proper information and treatment referrals" (p. 782).

Dementia Test Batteries

Similar to RHD and TBI test batteries, dementia test batteries are limited in number and evaluate language as well as cognitive skills (see Table 6-2). They contrast with RHD and TBI batteries, however, in that the content of their language subtests often focuses more on basic rather than high-level language skills. Clinicians should note that because Alzheimer's disease is the most frequent cause of dementia, most dementia test batteries were designed to identify and quantify the types of language and cognitive impairments associated with this dementing disease. This means that these tests may not be suitable for patients with other forms of dementia, as the types and progression of language and cognitive symptoms are not uniform across all dementing illnesses (see Chapters 2 and 3). For example, an aphasia battery may be more appropriate for patients in the early stages of the nonfluent progressive aphasia variant of frontotemporal lobar degeneration, as many of their initial symptoms are language-based, including problems with syntax (Reilly et al., 2010; Rousseaux, Seve, et al., 2010), a deficit that would not be quantified by current dementia test batteries. This point highlights the need for clinicians always to ensure that the demographic and clinical characteristics of their patients match those of the subject sample on which the tests they use were developed and standardized.

The *Arizona Battery for Communication Disorders of Dementia* (ABCD; Bayles & Tomoeda, 1993) represents the first commercially available test battery for assessing communication disorders associated with dementing diseases. The ABCD has 14 subtests that assess language comprehension (e.g., Following Commands, Comparative Questions, Reading Comprehension subtests), language production (e.g., Repetition, Confrontation Naming, Object Description subtests), memory (e.g., Mental Status, Story Retelling Immediate and Delayed, Word Learning subtests), and visuoconstruction abilities (e.g., Generative Drawing, Figure Copying subtests), and that take between 45 and 90 minutes to complete, depending on the severity of the patient's dementia. ABCD performances can be interpreted in terms of individual subtests, construct scores (i.e., Mental Status, Episodic Memory, Linguistic Expression, Linguistic Comprehension, Visuospatial Construction), or overall total test score. The ABCD was standardized on patients with Alzheimer's disease, patients with Parkinson's disease (the majority of whom did not have dementia), and young and age-matched healthy adults. According to the test authors, young adults were included in the control group because this test also may be suitable for some patients with TBI. Although certain forms of reliability and validity appear adequate, others, such as inter-rater reliability, are not discussed at all in the test manual. Given that this test is now almost 20 years old, test stimuli and procedures as well as the normative sample require updating. For example, several new variants of dementia have been identified since the ABCD was developed, and those dementia types should be included in the normative sample (e.g., frontotemporal dementia; dementia with Lewy bodies).

Test batteries such as the *Functional Linguistic Communication Inventory* (FLCI; Bayles & Tomoeda, 1994) and *Severe Impairment Battery* (SIB; Saxton, Swihart, & Boller, 1993) also are available, but for a specific dementia patient population—those with moderate to severe dementia. These tests were developed because patients in the later stages of dementia are often too impaired to complete the ABCD or other standard tests of language and cognition. For example, to assess more basic communication skills, the FLCI consists of 10 subtests, including Greeting and Naming, Comprehension of Signs (e.g., stop sign, exit sign), Object-to-Picture Matching, Word Reading and Comprehension, Following Commands, and Pantomime. Subtest scores and the total test score can be compared to the standardization sample's scores to determine a severity level. The FLCI is shorter than the ABCD, taking between 20 and 30 minutes to complete. Although acceptable test–retest reliability and criterion validity are reported, other forms of reliability and validity are not addressed in the test manual, and the standardization was limited to a relatively small sample of 40 patients, all of whom had Alzheimer's disease. Recent studies have utilized the SIB and offer data pertaining to its use with a variety of patient populations and in languages other than English (e.g., Bergh, Sebaek, & Engedal, 2008; Hutchinson & Oakes, 2011). In contrast, current standardization data reflecting the broader dementia population remain lacking for the FLCI.

Test Batteries for a Variety of Neurogenic Language or Cognitive Disorders

A few test batteries have been designed so that they can identify problems in a broad array of neurogenic patients (see Table 6-2). These batteries typically include *both* language and cognitive subtests and have more than one type of neurogenic language or cognitive disorder represented in their standardization sample. For example, the *Scales of Cognitive and Communicative Ability for Neurorehabilitation* (SCCAN; Milman & Holland, 2012) was designed to identify the presence and severity of neurogenic language and cognitive disorders in patients in rehabilitation and long-term-care settings. It includes 13 subtests that assess spoken and written language comprehension and production, as well as aspects of attention, memory, and executive functioning, with tasks designed to reflect daily activities to provide information about the ICF levels of body structure and function, and activities. Test administration includes use of basal and ceiling points to reduce testing time, with a total estimated administration time of 30 minutes. The SCCAN was normed on adults aged 18 to 91, including small samples of patients reflecting a variety of neurogenic disorders (i.e., aphasia, RHD, dementia, TBI), and has acceptable levels of reliability and validity.

Another option for assessing the overall cognitive-communicative abilities of patients with dementia, RHD, or TBI is the *Repeatable Battery for the Assessment of Neuropsychological Status Update* (RBANS; Randolph, 2012). It has 12 subtests designed to evaluate visuospatial (e.g., Figure Copy subtest), memory (e.g., Story Memory and Recall subtests), attention (e.g., Digit Span), and language (e.g., Picture Naming) abilities in approximately 30 minutes in patients between the ages of 12 and 89 years. Compared to the other batteries reviewed above, the RBANS provides a less comprehensive examination of language abilities. It does, however, have strong psychometric properties, has a Spanish version, and offers parallel test forms, which make it more appropriate for repeated testing and thus for monitoring patient ability over time. Additionally, updates pertaining to the interpretation of RBANS scores and summaries of clinical validation studies can be found on the publisher's website.

Tests of Specific Linguistic Functions

As listed in Table 6-3, there are many test options available for evaluating the integrity of specific language functions in patients with neurogenic disorders. For most patients, these tests are needed to delineate the nature of language difficulties identified during

(text continues on p. 190)

TABLE 6-3
Tests of Specific Language Functions

INSTRUMENT	Gesture Comprehension and/or Production	Lexical-Semantics: Comprehension	Lexical-Semantics: Production	Phonology/Orthography: Reading	Phonology/Orthography: Writing	Phonology/Orthography: Phonemic Perception	Phonology/Orthography: Suprasegmental Phonology	Pragmatics and/or Discourse*: Comprehension	Pragmatic and/or Discourse*: Production	Syntax: Comprehension	Syntax: Production	SOURCE
Apraxia Battery for Adults–Second Edition	X											Dabul (2000)
Aprosodia Battery							X					Ross, Thompson, & Yenkosky (1997)
Assessment Battery of Communication								X	X			Sacco et al. (2008)
Auditory Comprehension Test for Sentences										X		Shewan (1979)
Auditory Naming Test			X									Hamberger & Seidel (2003)
Boston Naming Test-Second Edition			X									Kaplan et al. (2001)
Comprehensive Receptive and Expressive Vocabulary Test-Third Edition		X	X									Wallace & Hammill (2013)
Controlled Oral Word Association Test			X									Benton et al. (2001)
Conversation Analysis Profile for People With Cognitive Impairment									X			Perkins et al. (1997)
Discourse Comprehension Test								X				Brookshire & Nicholas (1997)
Delis-Kaplan Executive Function System: Word Context Subtest								X				Delis et al. (2001)
Expressive One-Word Picture Vocabulary Test-Fourth Edition			X									N. Martin & Brownell (2011a)
Expressive Vocabulary Test-Second Edition			X									K. Williams (2007)
Facial Expression Stimuli and Test								X				A. Young et al. (2002)
Florida Affect Battery							X					Blonder et al. (1991)
Functional Assessment of Verbal Reasoning and Executive Strategies								X	X			MacDonald (2005)

TABLE 6-3 (continued)

INSTRUMENT	Gesture Comprehension and/or Production	Lexical-Semantics: Comprehension	Lexical-Semantics: Production	Phonology/Orthography: Orthography/Reading	Phonology/Orthography: Orthography/Writing	Phonology/Orthography: Phonemic Perception	Phonology/Orthography: Suprasegmental Phonology	Pragmatics and/or Discourse*: Comprehension	Pragmatic and/or Discourse*: Production	Syntax: Comprehension	Syntax: Production	SOURCE
Gray Diagnostic Reading Tests–Second Edition		X		X				X				Bryant et al. (2004)
Gray Oral Reading Tests–Fifth Edition		X						X				Wiederholt & Bryant (2012)
Gray Silent Reading Test		X						X				Wiederholt & Blalock (2001)
Johns Hopkins University Dysgraphia Battery**			X		X							Goodman & Caramazza (1986a)
Johns Hopkins University Dyslexia Battery**		X		X								Goodman & Caramazza (1986b)
Listening Comprehension Test-Adolescent			X					X				Bowers et al. (2009)
NAB Naming Test			X			X						Stern & White (2009b)
NAB Writing Test									X		X	Stern & White (2010)
Northwestern Syntax Screening Test											X	L. Lee (1971)
Oral and Written Language Scales (OWLS-2)		X			X					X		Carrow-Woolfolk (2012)
OWLS-2 Written Expression Scale			X		X				X		X	Carrow-Woolfolk (2012)
Pantomime Recognition Test	X											Benton et al. (1993)
Peabody Individual Achievement Test–Revised Edition		X		X	X							Markwardt (1997)
Peabody Picture Vocabulary Test–Fourth Edition		X										L. Dunn & Dunn (2007)
Psycholinguistic Assessments of Language Processing in Aphasia		X	X	X		X				X		Kay et al. (1997)
Putney Auditory Comprehension Screening Test		X								X		Beaumont et al. (2002)
Pyramids and Palm Trees		X										D. Howard & Patterson (1992)

(continues)

TABLE 6-3 (continued)

INSTRUMENT	Gesture Comprehension and/or Production	Lexical-Semantics: Comprehension	Lexical-Semantics: Production	Phonology/Orthography: Orthography/Reading	Phonology/Orthography: Orthography/Writing	Phonology/Orthography: Phonemic Perception	Phonology/Orthography: Suprasegmental Phonology	Pragmatics and/or Discourse*: Comprehension	Pragmatic and/or Discourse*: Production	Syntax: Comprehension	Syntax: Production	SOURCE
Reading Comprehension Battery for Aphasia–Second Edition		X		X								LaPointe & Horner (1998)
Receptive One-Word Picture Vocabulary Test–Fourth Edition		X										Martin & Brownell (2011b)
Revised Token Test		X								X		McNeil & Prescott (1978)
Seashore Tonal Memory Test							X					Seashore et al. (1960)
Social Language Development Test: Adolescent								X	X			Bowers et al. (2010)
Tennessee Test of Rhythm and Intonation Patterns							X					Koike & Asp (1981)
Test for Reception of Grammar–Second Edition										X		Bishop (2003)
Test of Adolescent and Adult Word-Finding			X									German (1990)
Test of Language Competence–Expanded								X	X			Wiig & Secord (1989)
Test of Oral and Limb Apraxia	X											Helm-Estabrooks (1991)
Test of Pragmatic Language–Second Edition								X	X			Phelps-Terasaki & Phelps-Gunn (2007)
Test of Problem Solving-2: Adolescent								X				Bowers et al. (2007)
Test of Reading Comprehension–Fourth Edition		X						X				V. Brown et al. (2009)
Test of Silent Reading Efficiency and Comprehension								X				Wagner et al. (2010)
Test of Upper Limb Apraxia	X											Vanbellingen et al. (2010)
Test of Word Knowledge		X	X									Wiig & Secord (1992)
Test of Word Reading Efficiency–Second Edition		X		X								Torgesen et al. (2012)

TABLE 6-3 (continued)

INSTRUMENT	Gesture Comprehension and/or Production	Lexical-Semantics: Comprehension	Lexical-Semantics: Production	Phonology/Orthography: Orthography/Reading	Phonology/Orthography: Orthography/Writing	Phonology/Orthography: Phonemic Perception	Phonology/Orthography: Suprasegmental Phonology	Pragmatics and/or Discourse*: Comprehension	Pragmatic and/or Discourse*: Production	Syntax: Comprehension	Syntax: Production	SOURCE
Test of Written Language–Fourth Edition			X		X				X			Hammill & Larson (2009)
The Awareness of Social Inference Test–Revised	X							X				McDonald et al. (2011)
The Liles Communication Test									X			Rousseaux et al. (2001)
The Naming Test			X									M. Williams (1996)
The Reporter's Test			X								X	DeRenzi & Ferrari (1978)
The Word Test 2-Adolescent		X	X									Bowers et al. (2005)
Thurstone Word Fluency Test			X									Thurstone & Thurstone (1962)
Verb and Sentence Test		X	X							X	X	Bastiaanse et al. (2002)
Wide Range Achievement Test–Fourth Edition		X		X	X							G. Wilkinson & Robertson (2006)
Woodcock Reading Mastery Tests–Third Edition		X		X		X						Woodcock (2011)

*These pragmatic and discourse-level tests assess multiple linguistic and cognitive functions, including syntactic and semantic processing as well as attention, memory, and high-level cognitive skills such as inferencing.

**A complete listing of these Johns Hopkins tests' stimuli and tasks can be found in Beeson and Henry (2008).

earlier steps of the assessment process (e.g., observations, screening test, language test battery). Use of these tests will be particularly important when evaluating patients with mild language impairments, as they often perform at ceiling levels on test batteries (K. Ross & Wertz, 2003, 2004; M. Wong et al., 2010). Because test batteries for RHD are generally psychometrically weak (Cote et al., 2007; Tompkins & Lehman, 1997), tests of specific linguistic (and cognitive) functions also should be included when evaluating patients with cognitive-communicative disorders related to RHD. Likewise, assessment beyond the use of test batteries is essential when pragmatic and discourse-level deficits are suspected, because these language abilities are frequently not evaluated or receive only cursory attention on language test batteries (e.g., MIRBI-II, Burns Complex Neuropathology Inventory, ABCD) (Coelho et al., 2005; Rousseaux, Daveluy, et al., 2010a; Rousseaux, Seve, et al., 2010; Turkstra et al., 2005). Finally, as a caveat, clinicians must keep in mind that many tests designed to evaluate specific language functions actually assess additional perceptual, linguistic, and cognitive functions (L. Murray, 2012a). For example, a test designed to evaluate comprehension of complex syntactic structures that involves matching spoken sentences to pictures will require, in addition to syntactic processing, verbal memory skills (i.e., temporarily retaining the sentence while scanning the picture stimuli), lexical-semantic skills (i.e., understanding the vocabulary in the target sentence), and visuoperceptual skills (i.e., discriminating visual differences between the picture stimuli). Therefore, before utilizing one of these tests with a given patient, clinicians must determine what demands the test makes on other linguistic and cognitive abilities, as well as have an understanding of whether these additional linguistic and cognitive abilities are problematic for their patient.

Phonological and Orthographic Processes

Further assessment of phonological and orthographic processes is typically only necessary when evaluating patients with aphasia. Whereas other neurogenic patient populations may display difficulties with these levels of language processing, these difficulties are usually cognitively or motorically based, or will not be a treatment priority. For example, although patients with RHD can have difficulties identifying or producing letters, these difficulties are unlikely to reflect problems in selecting or using graphemes, but rather reflect visuospatial or attentional deficits (e.g., neglect dyslexia or dysgraphia, spatial dysgraphia) (Kortte & Hillis, 2011; Lindell, 2006). Likewise, in patients with TBI, phonological and orthographic deficits are possible, but treatments for these deficits are typically inappropriate as remediation of other language impairments (i.e., pragmatic problems), cognitive impairments (e.g., memory, attention), and behavioral impairments (e.g., disinhibition) will have a greater impact on their daily functioning.

Phonology

Both **segmental** (i.e., processing the sound elements of words or syllables) and **suprasegmental** (i.e., processing intonation, stress, and pauses) aspects of phonology may be compromised in patients with aphasia, particularly those with concomitant dysarthria and/or apraxia of speech (Alexander & Hillis, 2008; Blumstein, 1998). Although some aphasia test batteries include subtests to evaluate segmental phonology in terms of production of syllables or the influence of the phonological composition of words on repetition skills (e.g., BDAE-3), there are no commercial tests available for examining just this component of language in adults. Clinicians may, however, use the following procedures to quantify and qualify segmental phonology production difficulties (L. Murray & Chapey, 2001): (a) identify phonemic errors in discourse samples and on word retrieval tests and attend to the phonological context of those errors, (b) utilize stimulability testing to determine what contexts and cueing variables may assist patients' production of error phonemes, and (c) identify problems with patients' peripheral speech mechanism that may be contributing to their phonology difficulties.

Difficulties with phonemic perception are also possible in neurogenic language disorders (Alexander & Hillis, 2008; Corsten, Mende, Cholewa, & Huber, 2007). To identify problems processing language at this level, tasks that involve discriminating nonword and/or word minimal pairs may be used. Such tasks can be found on the *Psycholinguistic Assessments of Language Processing in Aphasia* (PALPA; Kay, Lesser, & Coltheart, 1997). As the name indicates, this test is based on a psycholinguistic model of aphasia (similar to that depicted in Figure 1-3) and consists of 60 tasks divided into 4 sections (i.e., Auditory Processing, Reading and Spelling, Word and Picture Semantics, Sentence Processing) and designed to identify what level or levels of the model are impaired and affecting production or comprehension of spoken and written language. It was not intended to be given in its entirety; rather, based on other assessment data, clinicians should select only certain subtests to delineate further their patients' language impairment. A major limitation of the PALPA is that there has been scant exploration of the reliability or validity of its subtests. When validity has been explored, insufficiencies have been identified (e.g., Cole-Virtue & Nickels, 2004). Furthermore, normative data are limited to the means and standard deviations of a small group (i.e., $n = 32$) of non–brain-damaged adults of unspecified age, education, or ethnocultural background, and are provided only for certain subtests. Although Nickels and Cole-Virtue (2004) conducted a study to establish normative accuracy and response time data for some PALPA subtests that lacked this information, they, too, included a relatively small sample and included predominantly young participants. Indeed a recent study examining the use of the PALPA in research and clinical practice noted that although the test remains quite popular in use, particularly in Europe, both researchers and clinicians have raised concerns regarding the PALPA's standardization as well as the need for updated stimuli (S. Bate, Kay, Code, Haslam, & Hallowell, 2010). Collectively, these psychometric weaknesses make interpretation of PALPA subtest performances difficult.

Phonemic perception subtests can also be found as part of some reading test batteries, given that phonemic perception and awareness are important skills that contribute to reading proficiency (Beeson & Henry, 2008; Hillis, 2008). For instance, the *Woodcock Reading Mastery Tests–Third Edition* (WRMT-III; Woodcock, 2011) includes five tasks within its Phonemic Awareness subtest: first sound mapping, last sound mapping, rhyme production, blending, and deletion. This most recent edition of the WRMT also includes parallel forms and normative data for individuals ranging in age from 4.5 to 80 years.

Research has documented that several neurogenic disorders, such as RHD and Parkinson's and Alzheimer's diseases, may negatively affect processing of suprasegmental components of phonology (Bruck, Wildgruber, Kreifelts, Kruger, & Wachter, 2011; Cote et al., 2007; Rodriguez, 2009; Tosto, Gasparini, Lenzi, & Bruno, 2011). As in aphasia, however, problems producing suprasegmentals subsequent to the onset of these other neurogenic disorders may, at least in part, reflect concomitant dysarthria or other motor issues (Alexander & Hillis, 2008; Rodriguez, 2009). Likewise, researchers have questioned whether problems perceiving suprasegmentals following onset of brain damage or disease are truly linguistic in nature (Bruck et al., 2011; Tompkins & Flowers, 1985). That is, evidence has accumulated to suggest that lower-level auditory sensory or perceptual problems as well as cognitive limitations may underlie difficulties on prosodic comprehension tasks for patients with neurogenic disorders. Additionally, if impaired production of prosody or suprasegmentals is suspected, clinicians must attempt to ensure that they have an adequate description of their patients' premorbid suprasegmental abilities (Cote et al., 2007). For instance, patients might have always spoken with flat intonation and excessive pausing; thus, failure to determine this information at the outset would lead to unnecessary assessment procedures.

In terms of assessment, some RHD test batteries have items dedicated to evaluating comprehension and production of certain aspects of suprasegmental phonology (e.g., production of various emotional intonations on the MIRBI-2), although the reliability of these tasks is suspect. There also are some specific tests for examining this aspect of language, most of which are described in the research literature (see Table 6-3). For example, the *Florida Affect Battery* (Blonder, Bowers, & Heilman, 1991) evaluates skills such as discriminating facial emotions, emotional and nonemotional (e.g., statement vs. question intonation) prosody, and matching facial emotions with spoken emotional prosody. To ensure that other impairments are not confounding performance of these tests, however, motor speech and cognitive assessment results must be considered before final decisions regarding the presence of suprasegmental phonology difficulties are made.

Orthographic Processing

Orthographic or graphemic processing problems can result in deficits of reading, writing, or both, and do occur in a number of neurogenic language disorders (e.g., aphasia, dementia). Patients with difficulties at this level of language processing have problems converting graphemes to phonemes (i.e., letter to sound) or phonemes to graphemes (i.e., sound to letter) for reading or writing, respectively.

Several tests are available to help determine whether patients' reading or writing difficulties reflect problems with graphemic decoding, phonemic-to-graphemic conversion, and/or lexical–semantic access (e.g., whole word reading) (see Table 6-3). Typically, these tests include tasks that involve writing, reading aloud, or identifying nonwords (e.g., "plif," "forgel"), as nonword stimuli can only be decoded using grapheme-to-phoneme conversion or written using phoneme-to-grapheme conversion. For example, the *Test of Word Reading Efficiency–Second Edition* (Torgesen, Wagner, & Rashotte, 2012) has two subtests: Sight Word Efficiency, which assesses the number of real words an individual can identify within 45 seconds, and Phonemic Decoding Efficiency, which assesses the ability to read aloud nonwords in a brief time period (45 s). Four equivalent forms for each subtest are available to help control for practice effects when repeated administrations are necessary. Although the test only has norms for individuals up to the age of 25, it may still be useful for older patients, as clinicians may interpret their performances in terms of grade equivalent scores. Some core and supplemental subtests of the *Reading Comprehension Battery for Aphasia–Second Edition* (RCBA-2; LaPointe & Horner, 1998) also evaluate whether patients display graphemic and/or lexical–semantic reading difficulties, although no reliability or validity studies have been completed on the supplemental subtests (see the "Lexical–Semantic Processes" section of this chapter for a further description of the RCBA-2).

For writing, several subtests of the PALPA (e.g., Nonword Spelling, Letter Length Spelling) allow assessment at the grapheme level (Kay et al., 1997); as previously mentioned, because of undocumented psychometric properties and limited normative data, interpreting PALPA findings can be difficult, particularly if clinicians fail to obtain information regarding their patients' premorbid spelling abilities.

Lexical–Semantic Processes

As reviewed in Chapter 1 and depicted in Figure 1-3, lexical–semantic processing involves the phonological input and output lexicons (i.e., the stores of previously heard or produced spoken word forms), the orthographic input and output lexicons (i.e., the stores of previously read or written word forms), and the semantic system. Problems with lexical–semantic processing are universal in aphasia and frequent in other neurogenic language or cognitive disorders as well (J. Douglas, 2010; Lindell, 2006; L. Murray, 2000; J. Reilly et al., 2010). Accordingly, numerous test choices are available to evaluate the integrity of lexical–semantic comprehension or production abilities (see Table 6-3). These tests vary in terms of which language modalities (i.e., speaking, listening, reading, and/or writing) and contexts (i.e., isolated words vs. sentence level vs. discourse level) are evaluated. Although test batteries for each neurogenic patient population will typically include lexical–semantic subtests (e.g., WAB-R, ABCD, RBANS), specific tests will often delineate the effects of influential variables on patients' lexical–semantic comprehension and production skills (see Table 6-4); the direction (e.g., positive vs. negative influence) and magnitude of these effects are important when selecting treatment stimuli and procedures. Examples of commercially published tests and research protocols for assessing lexical–semantic skills are described below.

Lexical–Semantic Comprehension

Common procedures for evaluating patients' understanding of lexical–semantic information at the word level include having them identify real or pictured objects, actions, attributes, categories, or relationships that match or are associated with a spoken or written word or another pictured object, action, or attribute. For example, to determine

TABLE 6-4
Variables That May Influence Lexical-Semantic Processing Abilities

VARIABLE	RELATIONSHIP TO LEXICAL-SEMANTIC ABILITIES*	SOURCE EXAMPLES
Length of linguistic stimulus	Negative	Middleton & Schwartz (2010); Nickels & Howard (1995)
Semantic similarity of response choices	Negative	Breese & Hillis (2004); J. Duffy & Watkins (1984)
Word frequency	Positive	Edmonds & Donovan (2012); Hoffman, Rogers, & Lambon Ralph (2011)
Phonological/orthographic neighborhood density (i.e., number of words that sound/look like the target word)	Positive for production; negative for comprehension	Goldrick, Folk, & Rapp (2010); Lindell (2006); Middleton & Schwartz (2010)
Distance of semantic neighbors (e.g., "dog" has mostly near neighbors vs. "camel" has mostly distant neighbors)	Positive	Mirman (2011); Mirman & Magnuson (2008)
Exemplar typicality (within a given semantic category)	Positive	Kiran, Ntourou, & Eubank (2007); Kiran & Thompson (2003)
Imageability	Positive	Jefferies, Patterson, Jones, & Lambon Ralph (2009); Mätzig et al. (2009)
Concreteness	Positive	Lindell (2006); Nickels (1995)
Age of acquisition	Negative	Edmonds & Donovan (2012); Kremin et al. (2001)
Salience (i.e., main idea vs. detail)	Positive	L. Murray & Stout (1999); Nicholas & Brookshire (1995a)
Semantic diversity (i.e., number of senses, meanings, and use contexts associated with a given word)	Variable	Hoffman et al. (2011)
Part of speech (e.g., nouns vs. verbs)	Variable**	De Bleser & Kauschke (2003); Mätzig et al. (2009)
Semantic category	Variable	Laiacona, Luzzatti, Zonca, Guarnaschelli, & Capitani (2001); Martinaud, Opolczynski, Gaillard, & Hannequin (2009)
Stimulus modality (e.g., visual vs. auditory)	Variable	Barca et al. (2009); Hamberger & Seidel (2003)
Sentence constraint	Positive	Corbett et al. (2008); L. Murray (2000a)
Cognitive demands of the task (e.g., attention, memory)	Negative	Hodgson & Lambon Ralph (2008); L. Murray (2000a)

TABLE 6-4 (*continued*)

VARIABLE	RELATIONSHIP TO LEXICAL-SEMANTIC ABILITIES*	SOURCE EXAMPLES
Stimulus presentation and/or response rate	Negative	Blumstein, Katz, Goodglass, Shrier, & Dworetsky (1985); Hodgson & Lambon Ralph (2008)
Visual complexity of picture stimuli	Negative	Heuer & Hallowell (2007); Mätzig et al. (2009)
Personal relevance of and degree of contextualized information in the stimuli	Positive	Krackenfels Jones, Pierce, Mahoney, & Smeach (2007); McKelvey, Hux, Dietz, & Beukelman (2010)

* Clinicians must keep in mind that these relationships were established via group studies, in which significant effects were not observed for all subjects. Therefore, it remains possible that a given patient's lexical–semantic skills may not be influenced by these variables or even may be inversely affected (Hoffman et al., 2011; Laiacona et al., 2001).

** Most research has focused only on noun vs. verb processing comparisons, with little exploration of other parts of speech (e.g., noun vs. adjective). In aphasia, however, noun processing is typically more intact than verb processing is (Mätzig et al., 2009).

whether patients have a general semantic or modality-specific impairment, clinicians may utilize *Pyramids and Palm Trees* (D. Howard & Patterson, 1992). By manipulating whether stimulus and response modalities involve pictures or written or spoken words, six versions of this test are possible. The basic task involves presenting patients with three stimuli, one of which they need to match with one of the others in terms of the strongest or closest semantic association. For example, for the stimuli "pyramid," "pine tree," and "palm tree," the best match for "pyramid" is "palm tree." A number of semantic relationships, such as function and location, are assessed. Because of its forced-choice response format, the test has proven appropriate for a spectrum of patient severity levels. Guidelines for identifying performance patterns indicative of semantic- versus lexical-level impairments are provided in the test manual. No normative data for patient populations are available, but the test manual does indicate that scores of 90% correct or better should be considered indicative of adequate semantic processing, at least on this test; cutoff scores for chance-level performance also are provided. Recent studies provide additional information pertaining to the psychometric status of and normative data for *Pyramids and Palm Trees* (e.g., L. Klein & Buchanan, 2009; Rami et al., 2008).

Because many test batteries (e.g., MIRBI-2, ABCD) include only a cursory evaluation of reading abilities, additional testing to quantify and qualify lexical–semantic aspects of reading comprehension is often necessary. If problems at the word level are suspected, clinicians might select the *Reading Comprehension Battery for Aphasia–Second Edition* (RCBA-2; LaPointe & Horner, 1998), as it has 17 subtests that require silent or oral reading, 8 of which evaluate reading at the word level (e.g., Synonyms) and the remainder of which evaluate reading at the letter (e.g., Letter Naming), sentence (e.g., Sentence Comprehension), or paragraph level (e.g., Paragraph—Factual Comprehension). Raw scores for each subtest and the total test score can be converted to percentiles. The limited information in the test manual pertaining to the RCBA-2's psychometric properties consists of brief descriptions of previous studies utilizing the original version of this test. Therefore, interpreting RCBA-2 findings will be difficult for clinicians who are unable to access copies of these earlier studies; futhermore, this test now requires updating, given its publication date. Other tests that evaluate reading at the word level include the *Test of Word Reading Efficiency–Second Edition* (Torgesen et al., 2012) and the WRMT-III (Woodcock, 2011), the latter of which includes normative data for a broad age range (i.e., young children through adults 80 years of age).

Some tests evaluate lexical–semantic understanding at the sentence or discourse levels versus receptive vocabulary or word level abilities. Because of the length and complexity of stimuli on many of these tests, however, clinicians must keep in mind that test completion may stress other linguistic (e.g., morphosyntax) and cognitive (e.g., memory) functions, in addition to lexical–semantic comprehension. For instance, the *Revised Token Test* (RTT; McNeil & Prescott, 1978) requires patients to complete auditory commands that vary in terms of length and syntactic complexity with a set of tokens of various shapes, sizes, and colors. A strength of this test is its 15-point multidimensional scoring system that provides qualitative as well as quantitative information pertaining to the accuracy, completeness, promptness, and motoric efficiency of patients' responses, as well as patients' need for stimulus repetitions or cues. The RTT has normative data for healthy adults and patients who have had a left or right hemisphere stroke, and also reports acceptable levels of reliability and validity. Although an update to the commercially available RTT remains needed, further information about its psychometric properties (e.g., Hula, Doyle, McNeil, & Mikolic, 2006) and the development and use of a computerized version (e.g., Sung et al., 2009) can be found in the empirical literature.

Another option is the *Putney Auditory Comprehension Screening Test* (Beaumont et al., 1999; Marjoribanks, Flury, & Lintern, 2002), which was specifically developed for patients with severe motor and/or visual problems who are unable to complete the response requirements of more traditional comprehension tests (e.g., manipulating and pointing to objects, as on the RTT; completing commands with body parts, on the BDAE-3). This test is designed to determine an optimal language complexity level for maximizing patients' auditory comprehension by utilizing 60 yes/no questions (e.g., "Do judges earn less than milkmen?"; "Is orange a color and a fruit?"), which patients are allowed to answer via whatever modality they can handle (e.g., verbally, buzzer, pointing, eye movements). Additionally, stimuli have been developed to minimize orientation and memory demands. Accordingly, this test would be appropriate for a number of neurogenic patient populations, particularly those with severe motoric or visual impairments (e.g., Huntington's disease, brain stem stroke, TBI).

Lexical-Semantic Production

Numerous tests are available for evaluating spoken and written production of lexical–semantic information, including the ability to retrieve and produce labels or names of objects, actions, events, attributes and relationships, or categories (see Table 6-3). Most of these tests use highly structured tasks to evaluate word retrieval skills, including confrontation naming (i.e., providing the name of a real or pictured stimulus), providing definitions, superordinate or category naming, verbal fluency (e.g., name as many exemplars of a semantic category or that start with a certain letter as possible in a short time period), phrase completion or closure, production of rote or overlearned material (e.g., naming the months of the year, reciting the Pledge of Allegiance), repetition or copying, and recognition naming (i.e., choosing the correct label from a small set of stimuli).

Without question, the *Boston Naming Test* (BNT; Kaplan, Goodglass, & Weintraub, 1983) is the most frequently used test for evaluating word finding in both clinical and research settings (e.g., R. Katz et al., 2000). It consists of 60 black-and-white drawings that depict nouns, which decrease in familiarity as the test progresses. If patients are unable to name a picture, the test examiner provides a semantic or function cue and then, if the target is still not named, a phonemic cue. In 2001, a revised edition of the BNT was published (Kaplan, Goodglass, & Weintraub, 2001). This newer version differs from the original BNT in that it includes a Short Form to screen naming abilities and it allows for providing multiple-choice cues after semantic and phonemic cues have been given, when patients are having difficulty naming an item.

Close examination of the content and statistical qualities of both versions of the BNT raises several concerns and questions about their popularity. First, both BNT editions examine only noun retrieval, even though production of other parts of speech (e.g., verbs, adverbs, adjectives) is frequently problematic in neurogenic language and cognitive disorders (M. Kim & Thompson, 2004; Mätzig, Druks, Masterson, & Vigliocco, 2009). Second, neither BNT manual provides information regarding any aspect of reliability, which is particularly problematic given that there is insufficient description of how to administer and score either test. Finally, the normative data listed in the first version's manual are outdated and extend up to the age of only 59 years. This last weakness can be mitigated by consulting more recently published norms in the research literature that take into consideration a number of influential demographic variables (e.g., education, residence) and cultural variables, and provide data for a larger age range (Barker-Collo, 2001, 2007; Tombaugh & Hubley, 1997). Updated norms for adults between the ages of 18 and 79 years are provided in the new edition of the BNT, but a description of this normative sample is limited to education level only. It should be noted that versions of the BNT have been developed for several other languages, including Greek (Patricacou, Psallida, Pring, & Dipper, 2007), Spanish (Peña-Casanova et al., 2009; Rami et al., 2008), and Cantonese (Cheung et al., 2004). Several short forms have also been described and evaluated in the research literature (del Toro et al., 2011; Tombaugh & Hubley, 1997).

Compared to the BNT, several other commercially available word-finding tests have stronger psychometric characteristics. For example, the *Comprehensive Receptive and Expressive Vocabulary Test–Third Edition* (CREVT-III; Wallace & Hammill, 2013) has two subtests—one that evaluates vocabulary comprehension via a picture-pointing task and one that assesses vocabulary production via a definition task. A variety of word types, including nouns, verbs, and adjectives, serve as stimuli for the receptive subtest and can be elicited on the expressive subtest because of its task format (i.e., providing definitions of nouns and verbs vs. simply labeling pictures of objects). This test is suitable for a wide variety of patients, as its test items have been found unbiased for gender and ethnicity, its norms extend from age 4 through 90 years, and it has strong reliability and validity. Furthermore, it has two equivalent forms so that repeated testing can be conducted to monitor patient progress over time. Similarly, both the *NAB Naming Test* (Stern & White, 2009b) and the *Expressive Vocabulary Test–Second Edition* (K. T. Williams, 2007) offer equivalent forms and have been standardized on individuals ranging in age from 18 to 97 years and 2.5 to over 90, respectively. Interestingly, the *NAB Naming Test* utilizes digital photographs, in contrast to older naming tests that tend to use line drawings (e.g., the BNT).

Because many language test batteries do not include a comprehensive assessment of writing abilities (e.g., *Burns,* WAB-R, ABCD), additional evaluation of written lexical–semantic skills is frequently needed. The Spelling subtests of the *Wide Range Achievement Test–Fourth Edition* (G. Wilkinson & Robertson, 2006) require patients to write the names of pictures, as well as individual letters and words from dictation. The strengths of this test include that (a) it offers equivalent forms and thus is appropriate for documenting changes in writing over time, (b) it has computer software to facilitate scoring, and (c) its normative data extend up to age 94.

For patients in whom more abstract aspects of semantic processing are compromised, tests such as *The WORD Test–Second Edition: Adolescent* (TWT; Bowers, Huisingh, LoGiudice, & Orman, 2005) might be used. The TWT allows evaluating a broad spectrum of word finding skills, including the ability to generate synonyms, antonyms, definitions, or multiple meanings. This test underwent extensive standardization and has strong psychometric properties. Although the TWT was developed only for children up to age 18, the test's authors acknowledge that this assessment tool may additionally provide valuable information regarding the word retrieval abilities of adults. Indeed, Turkstra and colleagues (2005) also recommended use of this test when evaluating language abilities subsequent to TBI, and based on that recommendation, Wong et al. (2010) more recently found it sensitive to high-level language problems subsequent to mild TBI.

Language Sampling. Whereas the above tests utilize structured tasks to evaluate lexical–semantic abilities at primarily the single-word level, other assessment tools involve less controlled activities to examine lexical–semantic aspects of patients' connected language. Ensuring that language assessments include the examination of spontaneous, connected language output is necessary because for many patients there is only a weak relationship between their word- and discourse-level lexical–semantic abilities (Coelho et al., 2005; Herbert, Hickin, Howard, Osborne, & Best, 2008; Mayer & Murray, 2003). Although picture description tasks are most frequently used to elicit spoken and written language samples, clinicians might also use conversation, story-retelling, role playing, video-narration, procedural description (e.g., "How do you make scrambled eggs?"), or explaining picture sequences (Bracy & Drummond, 1993; Cherney, 1998; Coelho et al., 2005; McNeil et al., 2007). Use of these other elicitation methods instead of or in addition to picture descriptions is recommended because picture description tasks can elicit labeling behavior, which in turn restricts the number and variety of lexical–semantic, syntactic, and discourse behaviors in the language sample and thus, sensitivity to language production deficits (Beeke, Maxim, & Wilkinson, 2008; Coelho et al., 2005; Shadden, 1998). Additionally, language samples should be minimally 300 to 400 words in length to ensure adequate test–retest stability of whatever measures are being used to quantify and qualify language output (Brookshire & Nicholas, 1994).

There are a number of approaches to analyzing lexical–semantic content in spoken or written language samples. One of the most frequently used approaches quantifies how informative samples are using measures such as "content units" (Yorkston & Beukelman, 1980), "discourse clarity measures or disruptors" (Sherratt & Penn, 1990; Sherratt & Bryan, 2012), "main concepts" (A. Kong, 2011; Nicholas & Brookshire, 1995b), and "correct information units" (CIUs; Nicholas & Brookshire, 1993). For example, Nicholas and Brookshire (1993) described a series of rules for calculating and comparing the number of words and CIUs, which are words that are "accurate, relevant and informative relative to the eliciting stimulus" (p. 340). To determine the **informativeness** and efficiency of patients' language samples, Nicholas and Brookshire advised clinicians to determine the number of words per minute as well as the percentage of CIUs (i.e., number of CIUs/number of words). Subsequent research has supported the use and reliability of CIU analysis for quantifying communicative informativeness and efficiency on a variety of discourse tasks and in a variety of patient populations (Carlomagno et al., 2011; L. Murray, 2010; L. Murray, Holland, & Beeson, 1998), and indicates that CIUs and other content measures predict well how unfamiliar listeners will rate the informativeness of the verbal output of patients with aphasia (Doyle, Tsironas, Goda, & Kalinyak, 1996) and socially relevant changes therein (B. Jacobs, 2001; K. Ross & Wertz, 1999). A study by Oelschlaeger and Thorne (1999), however, indicated that the reliability of the CIU approach may be inadequate for analyzing samples of "naturally occurring conversation" (p. 636); these researchers suggested that there are insufficient guidelines for using CIU analysis with conversational samples (vs. narrative or picture description samples) and recommended obtaining additional training with this measurement technique before applying it to naturally occurring conversation.

Lexical–Semantic Production Error Analyses. In addition to documenting lexical–semantic retrieval accuracy, clinicians should evaluate the nature and pattern of content errors, or **paraphasias**, made by patients in their verbal or written output (L. Murray & Coppens, 2011). For example, word retrieval errors can be classified as (a) **phonemic**

or literal paraphasias**, which contain substitutions, additions, omissions, and/or rearrangements of target word phonemes; (b) **semantic paraphasias**, which are substitutions of words that are semantically related to the target words; (c) **phonemically related paraphasias**, which are whole-word substitutions that are phonemically, but not semantically, related to the target; (d) **random paraphasias**, which are substitutions of words that lack apparent semantic relations to the target words; (e) **circumlocutions**, which involve the use of descriptions or definitions for the target words; (f) **neologisms**, which involve the use of nonsense versus target words; (g) **indefinite substitutions**, which involve the use of nonspecific words or descriptions for target words; (h) perseverations, which are inappropriate recurrences of previous responses for the target words; and (i) **no responses**.

Additionally, clinicians may monitor for other word finding difficulties in the spoken and written discourse of their patients, including the use of fillers (e.g., "um," "well," "you know"); part-word, word, or phrase repetitions; silent pauses; false starts; abandoned utterances; and metalinguistic comments about the task or language ability (e.g., "I know it, but I can't say it") (Brookshire & Nicholas, 1995; Sherratt & Bryan, 2012; Tingley, Kyte, Johnson, & Beitchman, 2003) (see Table 6-5 for further examples). Tingley et al. (2003) cautioned, however, that these disruptions may reflect not

TABLE 6-5
Examples of Types of Paraphasias and Discourse-Level Symptoms of Word Finding Difficulty

ERROR OR SYMPTOM TYPE	EXAMPLES
Phonemic/literal paraphasia	"Canadan" for "Canadian"; "picinica" for "picnic"
Semantic paraphasia	"puppy" for "cat"; "train" for "bus"
Phonemically related paraphasia	"percolator" for "calculator"
Random paraphasia	"September" for "hungry"; "jumping" for "washing"
Circumlocution	"It's red and grows on trees" for "cherry"
Indefinite substitution	"there" for "my house"; "thing" for "clock"
Neologism	"tember" for "happy"; "banertine" for "soccer"
No response	
Nonword, word, or phrase fillers	"I lost my, um … uh … wallet." "I lost my … you know … wallet."
Part-word, word, or phrase repetitions	"She went to the … the … the … islands."
Silent pauses	"My … friend gave it to me."
False starts	"He had … the girl had the wrong number."
Abandoned utterances	"Dylan was practicing for …"
Metalinguistic comments	"I just can't think of it."

only lexical–semantic retrieval difficulties but also problems with syntactic or pragmatic aspects of discourse production or even the patients' emotional status or knowledge of the discourse topic.

Cognitive Neuropsychological and Neurolinguistic Approaches

Cognitive neuropsychological and neurolinguistic approaches to evaluating lexical–semantic processing abilities aim to identify which component or components of language models (see Chapter 1 and Figure 1-3) have been compromised (Beeson & Henry, 2008; M. Schwartz, Dell, Martin, Gahl, & Sobel, 2006; Whitworth, Webster, & Howard, 2005). For example, lexical–semantic comprehension problems could emerge from impaired access to or organization of the phonological or graphemic input lexicon and/or the semantic system. To identify the locus or loci of impairment, clinicians can use the PALPA (Kay et al., 1997), one of the first commercially available tests based solely on psycholinguistic theory; even though this is a published test, information pertaining to its psychometric properties is currently unavailable, minimal normative data are provided, and stimuli are becoming outdated. Another option is to consult assessment protocols described in the literature (e.g., N. Martin, Schwartz, & Kohen, 2006; Raymer & Rothi, 2001; Whitworth et al., 2005). These protocols often involve a set of tasks that differ in terms of input modality (e.g., spoken word vs. written word vs. picture) and mode of response (e.g., repetition vs. written naming vs. pointing to a picture), and one set of target and foil stimuli that have been carefully selected to control or examine a number of linguistic factors (e.g., word frequency, length, semantic category, spelling regularity, phonological similarity). Patients' performances of these various comprehension tasks (e.g., semantically related picture matching; spoken word-to-picture matching; synonym judgment) and production tasks (e.g., writing to dictation, naming to spoken definitions) are then contrasted to identify the level(s) of impairment. The consistency of patients' errors across modalities, tasks, and sessions also is evaluated, as access deficits are associated with inconsistent errors, whereas loss of linguistic representations is associated with consistent errors.

Overwhelmed?

If you are studying adult language assessment for the first time, you might be overwhelmed by the breadth, depth, and complexity of factors that can be considered during assessment. Rest assured that you will not likely assess every factor affecting language performance for even one patient, much less every patient. Instead, your clinical questions will drive the tools and processes you select for any given assessment. For example, if a primary question is whether the individual's communication difficulty reflects primarily linguistic versus cognitive impairment, you might select batteries that are more sensitive to these areas of impairment in the broad sense. If you already have a good sense for the broad nature of the problem, then you might instead be focusing on treatment targets, in which case you might select tools that identify specific impairments, the level at which breakdowns occur, and the types of cues that facilitate accuracy. If the primary purpose of a given assessment is to document change, either in response to treatment or in the context of disease progression, then you will likely select tools that have demonstrated sensitivity to meaningful aspects of performance. The detailed information in this chapter will help you select tools and techniques once you have established your clinical questions (as discussed in Chapter 4) and will also serve as a reminder, once all of this is "old hat," of the complexity of the questions you will be addressing for each individual patient.

Morphological and Syntactic Processes

Further assessment of morphological and syntactic skills is most frequently necessary when evaluating the language abilities of patients with aphasia or TBI who have suffered focal dominant hemisphere lesions, as morphosyntactic impairments are common in these patient populations. A more detailed morphosyntactic evaluation also may be informative when trying to determine dementia type, as certain dementing illnesses can be distinguished, at least in part, by their differential effects on morphosyntax. For example, an agrammatic language profile is common in the nonfluent progressive aphasia variant of frontotemporal dementia, but rare in Alzheimer's disease (e.g., J. Reilly et al., 2010).

Morphosyntactic Comprehension

Comprehension of morphosyntactic processes may be evaluated at both word and discourse levels. At the word level, understanding of **substantive or open class words** (e.g., verbs, nouns, adjectives, adverbs) and **relational or closed class words** (e.g., prepositions, pronouns, determiners, conjunctions) should be evaluated. Because comprehension of nouns is invariably evaluated on test batteries for aphasia, RHD, TBI, and dementia, further assessment is typically only necessary to evaluate other substantive and relational words. Likewise, few test batteries examine patients' comprehension of grammatical morphemes, including **derivational affixes** (i.e., morphemes that transform words into different types of form words; e.g., "sleep" into "sleepy") or **inflectional affixes** (i.e., morphemes that provide syntactic information; e.g., "s" on "sleeps" indicates subject–verb agreement).

There is only a limited choice of commercial tests for examining understanding of form words (beyond nouns) or derivational and inflectional morphemes (Table 6-3). The *Verb and Sentence Test* (VAST; Bastiaanse, Edwards, & Rispens, 2002) has one subtest dedicated to evaluating auditory comprehension of 40 verbs that vary in transitivity (i.e., whether or not the verb may take an object), word frequency, and name relatedness with a noun. Another option, the PALPA (Kay et al., 1997), has a few listening and reading subtests for assessing understanding of verbs, adjectives, and locative prepositions (e.g., Written Comprehension of Locative Relations) and recognizing a variety of grammatical morphemes (e.g., Auditory Lexical Decision: Morphological Endings). Although the BDAE-3 (Goodglass et al., 2001) also has a few Extended Subtests that evaluate recognition of written form words (e.g., prepositions, auxiliary verbs) and words with derivational or inflectional affixes, only a limited number of items are included, and thus further testing is often necessary. Another possibility is research protocols described in the literature. For example, D. Caplan and Bub (1990) created a test that includes lexical decision, word–picture matching, and similarity judgment tasks to evaluate recognition and comprehension of morphologically complex words.

Assessing morphosyntactic comprehension at the sentence level primarily involves identifying problems in understanding a range of simple (e.g., active) and complex (e.g., passives, object-relative clauses) sentence forms. For example, the VAST (Bastiaanse et al., 2002) has two subtests, Grammaticality Judgment and Sentence Comprehension, which examine the recognition and understanding of spoken **canonical** (e.g., active sentences) and **noncanonical** (e.g., passives) sentence types. This test also assesses morphosyntactic production abilities at the word (i.e., Verb Production) and sentence levels. The sentence level subtests include Sentence Construction, Sentence Anagrams with and without Pictures, and *Wh*-Anagrams subtests, which require patients to produce grammatically complete declarative and interrogative sentences. The anagram tasks involve more complex sentence forms than are typically elicited by picture description tasks. For these anagram subtests, patients are given a set of word and phrase cards and are asked to create a sentence (e.g., "the bike," "is fixed by," "the man" cards to form a target passive sentence); in the Sentence Anagrams with Pictures and *Wh*-Anagrams subtests, the sentence that they form should match the target picture that they are given. Although administration of the entire VAST may take as long as two to three hours, clinicians can opt to give only two to four subtests, which should require only approximately 30 minutes. Because this test was developed and standardized in Europe, there may be certain items that need to be adapted to reflect American English vocabulary.

Other structured tests available for examining syntax comprehension include the *Revised Token Test* (McNeil & Prescott, 1978), PALPA (Kay et al., 1997), and *Test for Reception of Grammar–Second Edition* (Bishop, 2003). Some of these tests, however, have been criticized because they do not assess a broad enough range of sentence types, do not allow distinguishing between syntax comprehension and working memory problems, or both (D. Caplan, 1993; Thompson, 2008). Clinicians may therefore choose to utilize protocols described in the literature (e.g., D. Caplan & Bub, 1990; D. Caplan, Waters, & Hildebrandt, 1997; Thompson, 2008). These tests typically involve sentence–picture matching (e.g., Thompson, 2008) or object manipulation or acting out (e.g., D. Caplan et al., 1997) tasks, and evaluate a variety of morphosyntactic forms that vary in sentence canonicity (e.g., active sentences with subject-verb-object order vs. passives with noncanonical, object-verb-subject order), and number of verbs and propositions (e.g., active vs. conjoined sentences). Additionally, to ensure that patients are not using lexical-semantic processing or world knowledge to interpret the sentences, semantically reversible stimuli are preferable (e.g., "The woman was served by the man" vs. "The customer was served by the waiter").

Morphosyntactic Production

Morphosyntactic production abilities can be evaluated using structured or constrained tasks, by analyzing samples of patients' spoken and written language, or both. As with word-level comprehension tests, most formal tests of word level, morphosyntactic production abilities evaluate retrieval of nouns more than other word forms. Exceptions include the VAST (Bastiaanse et al., 2002), which assesses verb production, and the CREVT-III (Wallace & Hammill, 2013), *Test of Adolescent and Adult Word-Finding* (German, 1990), and PALPA (Kay et al., 1997), which require production of a range of form words, including verbs, adjectives, and prepositions. The PALPA additionally includes repetition, reading aloud, and spelling subtests that evaluate production of a variety of grammatical morphemes. A few research protocols also are available that use sentence completion and pictures to evaluate production of a range of form words or inflectional and derivational affixes (D. Caplan & Bub, 1990; Shankweiler et al., 2010; Thompson, 2008).

There are only a few structured tests for assessing sentence level morphosyntactic abilities. For example, the VAST (Bastiaanse et al., 2002), as previously described (see the "Morphosyntactic Comprehension" section earlier in this chapter), includes three subtests for evaluating production of declarative and interrogative sentence forms. For identifying morphosyntactic problems in patients' written output, clinicians may select the Written Expression Scale of the *Oral and Written Language Scales–Second Edition* (OWLS-2; Carrow-Woolfolk, 2012), which was designed for individuals between the ages of 5 and 22 years and evaluates word level (e.g., spelling, punctuation), syntactic level (e.g., phrase and sentence structure, modifiers), and discourse level writing abilities (e.g., cohesion, organization). Oral, written, and pictorial prompts are used to elicit the writing samples, and the entire test takes about 15 to 25 minutes to administer. This test was standardized on a large sample (i.e., $n = 2,123$), has strong psychometric properties, and offers a parallel form. Although normative data are limited to young adults, this OWLS-2 scale may still prove informative for older patients, as their performances can be converted to age- and grade-based standard scores. Another option is to consult assessment protocols described in the research literature (e.g., Shankweiler et al., 2010; Thompson, 2008).

Given that performance of structured tests does not always relate to patients' morphosyntactic abilities during unstructured tasks (Beeke et al., 2008; Shankweiler et al., 2010), another approach to evaluating morphosyntactic production is to analyze the accuracy, types, and frequency of form words, grammatical morphemes, and syntactic structures used by patients in their spoken and/or written discourse. Numerous scoring systems are available for this purpose in the research literature (Edwards, 1995; Menn, Ramsberger, & Helm-Estabrooks, 1994; Rochon, Saffran, Berndt, & Schwartz, 2000; Thompson et al., 1995). Because some of these systems were created to quantify and qualify agrammatic output (e.g., Rochon et al., 2000; Thompson et al., 1995) and others for fluent or paragrammatic output (e.g., Edwards, 1995), the types of structural forms analyzed across these systems can vary. Most systems, however, include sufficient description of language sample collection and analysis procedures, and thus have been associated with acceptable levels of intra- and inter-rater reliability (Prins & Bastiaanse, 2004).

In addition to determining what morphosyntactic forms patients are producing, clinicians should examine what types of errors are being made (L. Murray & Coppens, 2011). That is, clinicians should document whether their patients are omitting certain form words, grammatical morphemes, or sentence forms (e.g., leave out auxiliary verbs); substituting incorrect form words, grammatical morphemes, or sentence forms (e.g., use "she" for all subject pronouns); or both. Likewise, the consistency of morphosyntactic errors should be determined. If patients are inconsistently making errors, clinicians should additionally explore whether or not linguistic variables (e.g., vocabulary familiarity), patient variables (e.g., fatigue), or task variables (e.g., story retelling vs. unconstrained conversation) are influencing their patients' language output.

Pragmatics and Discourse Skills

Assessing pragmatics and discourse abilities is essential when evaluating the language abilities of patients with RHD, TBI, and certain types of dementia (e.g., frontotemporal lobar degeneration), given that these aspects of language are frequently compromised in these patient populations (Carlomagno et al., 2011; L. Murray, 2010; Rousseaux, Daveluy, et al., 2010; L. Williams et al., 2010), but inadequately addressed by RHD batteries (e.g., MIRBI-2), TBI batteries (e.g., BTHI), or dementia test batteries (e.g., ABCD). Although in aphasia pragmatic skills are often assumed to be an area of relative strength, pragmatic difficulties and discourse deficits may occur (A. Holland, 1996; Rousseaux, Daveluy, et al., 2010). Accordingly, a comprehensive language assessment of any neurogenic patient should include pragmatic and discourse-level tasks. Furthermore, it is important to keep in mind the complex nature of these language areas; that is, deficits in other linguistic (e.g., lexical–semantic processing), emotional (e.g., depression), and cognitive (e.g., attention, memory, social cognition) functions may underlie or contribute to pragmatic and discourse impairments (Douglas, 2010; R. Griffin et al., 2006; L. Murray, 2010; Sherratt & Bryan, 2012; Williams et al., 2010). Therefore, assessment of these other areas is necessary before making conclusions about the presence and nature of pragmatic and discourse difficulties.

Pragmatic and Discourse Comprehension

As shown in Table 6-3, several commercially available tests evaluate patients' understanding of pragmatic and discourse rules and conventions. Most of these tests examine one or more of the following: (a) whether patients can glean main ideas from spoken or written discourse, (b) whether patients can process main ideas as well as detailed information in spoken or written discourse, and (c) whether patients can make inferences, interpret figurative language, resolve ambiguities or discrepancies, or revise interpretations based on the spoken or written text to which they were exposed, contextual cues (e.g., communication partner's facial expression), and/or their general world knowledge.

For example, the *Discourse Comprehension Test* (DCT; Brookshire & Nicholas, 1997) was developed to evaluate comprehension of spoken or written discourse in patients with aphasia, RHD, or TBI. Patients listen to or read story passages, and then after each story answer a set of yes/no questions that evaluate their understanding and retention of directly stated or implied main ideas and details. The stories and questions are audiotaped to allow for reliable test administration; furthermore, the speaker's rate and prosody on the audiotapes were controlled to maximize auditory processing in patients with aphasia. Unfortunately, the DCT's standardization sample is quite limited, consisting of only 40 adults with no brain damage and 60 adults with brain damage (i.e., 20 with aphasia, 20 with TBI, and 20 with RHD); reliability and standard error data were established on an even smaller sample size (i.e., 14 adults with aphasia and 7 with RHD). Data regarding the DCT performances of patients in the early or middle stages of Alzheimer's disease (Welland, Lubinski, & Higginbotham, 2002), patients with Parkinson's or Huntington's disease (L. Murray & Stout, 1999), adolescents with autism (Asberg & Sandberg, 2010), and larger samples of RHD patients (Tompkins, Meigh, Scott, & Lederer, 2009; Tompkins, Scharp, Meigh, & Fassbinder, 2008) can be found in the research literature, but again these participant samples are relatively small (i.e., $n < 40$) compared to the normative samples of other commercially available tests.

Another formal test option is the *Test of Language Competence–Expanded Edition* (TLC-E; Wiig & Secord, 1989). Although the TLC-E was developed for adolescents, it has proven suitable in several research studies aimed at quantifying and qualifying high-level language comprehension and production problems in adults with a variety of disorders, including Alzheimer's disease, depression, multiple sclerosis, TBI, RHD, Parkinson's disease, and Huntington's disease (N. Belanger, Baum, & Titone, 2009; Chenery, Copland, & Murdoch, 2002; McKinlay, Dalrymple-Alford, Grace, & Roger, 2009; L. Murray, 2002b, 2010; Wong et al., 2010). The TLC-E consists of three comprehension subtests—Ambiguous Sentences, Making Inferences, and Figurative Language—which evaluate understanding of lexical and structural ambiguities, alternative inferences, and metaphors, respectively. It also has one expressive subtest—Recreating Sentences—which requires the generation of sentences that are appropriate to the pictured context and that contain a prescribed set of words. The TLC-E was standardized on a large sample of students ($n = 1,796$) between the ages of 9 and 19, and has acceptable levels of validity and reliability. Depending on their patients' ages and premorbid abilities, clinicians may choose to interpret their patients' TLC-E performances in terms of standard scores for the oldest normative group on the test, age-equivalent scores, or data reported for healthy, older adults in the research literature (e.g., L. Murray, 2010).

Several recently published tests evaluate aspects of discourse comprehension similar to those assessed in the DCT (e.g., *Listening Comprehension Test–Adolescent*; Bowers, Huisingh, & LoGiudice, 2009) or aspects of high-level language comprehension and production similar to those assessed in the TLC-E (e.g., *Social Language Development Test–Adolescent*; Bowers, Huisingh, & LoGiudice, 2010). Like the TLC-E, however, these too were designed for adolescents (i.e., normative data only go up to age 18). Because these tests are relatively new, the empirical literature does not yet contain research pertaining to their use with older adults or a variety of neurogenic patient populations. Until such data are available, clinicians may opt to interpret their older patients' performances on these new tools in a manner similar to that described for the TLC-E above.

Some cognitive test batteries have subtests that are suitable for evaluating pragmatic or discourse comprehension skills. For example, the *Delis-Kaplan Executive Function System* (D-KEFS; Delis, Kaplan, & Kramer, 2001), a battery of executive function tests, includes a Word Context subtest that assesses comprehension of language in context. On this subtest, patients are told that they need to figure out the meaning of some words from a "different language" (the words are actually nonsense words) and then are given sentence clues to help them generate an answer. For example, for the item "gesh," clues include "You *gesh* a space," "Loud music can *gesh* a room," and "You *gesh* a bucket with water." Bardo, Delis, and Kaplan, (2002) found that this subtest better discriminated patients with frontal lobe lesions from their healthy peers than the D-KEFS Proverb Interpretation subtest, and concluded that the Word Context subtest requires a greater degree and more realistic integration of information than proverb interpretation tasks.

If problems with reading connected text are suspected, clinicians should opt to use reading tests developed for academic purposes, as those developed for neurogenic patient populations are often too easy, tend to evaluate only understanding of basic language forms and explicitly stated information, or have content weaknesses. For example, patients whose reading difficulties are restricted to the discourse level typically perform at ceiling levels on the RCBA-2, perhaps in part because the most difficult paragraph falls below a seventh-grade reading difficulty level. Likewise, paragraph-level reading subtests on aphasia test batteries have been found to have relatively low passage dependency, meaning that patients can correctly respond to questions about these paragraphs *without* reading the paragraphs (Nicholas, MacLennan, & Brookshire, 1986).

Accordingly, tests such as the *Test of Silent Reading Efficiency and Comprehension* (R. Wagner, Torgesen, & Rashotte, 2010), WRMT-III (Woodcock, 2011), or *Gray Oral Reading Tests–Fifth Edition* (GORT-5; Wiederholt & Bryant, 2012), which have more acceptable levels of passage dependency and offer a broader range of reading complexity/grade levels, are more appropriate test choices for patients whose reading abilities break down beyond the sentence level. For example, the GORT-5 evaluates comprehension of passages that increase in complexity, oral reading rate, and oral reading accuracy. Comprehension of each reading passage is assessed via five questions pertaining to main ideas, details, and possible inferences. Strengths of the GORT-5 include its strong psychometric properties, including an absence of gender or ethnocultural bias; that the comprehension questions have been evaluated to assure they are passage dependent, and that the test offers parallel forms so that changes in reading ability over time can be monitored. Although the GORT-5 was standardized only on individuals up to the age of 24, clinicians assessing older adults may still be able to establish the presence and severity of a reading disorder through the calculation of grade- or age-equivalent scores.

The Awareness of Social Interference Test–Revised (TASIT; McDonald, Flanagan, & Rollins, 2011) represents one of the few tests available to identify problems with processing pragmatic or social contextual information (McDonald, 2012). This test consists of three subtests, Emotion Evaluation, Social Inference–Minimal, and Social Inference–Enriched, that use videotaped vignettes and standardized response probes to examine patients' perceptions of basic visual and vocal emotional demeanors (e.g., fear, anger, happiness) and more subtle ones (e.g., sincerity, sarcasm, deception). TASIT includes alternate forms of each subtest to allow reliable repeated testing. McDonald (2012) recently reviewed the psychometric characteristics of the TASIT, including a summary of studies that have utilized this test with a number of neurogenic language and cognitive disorders (e.g., TBI, frontotemporal dementia, Alzheimer's disease, RHD) and documented its sensitivity to social perception impairments.

In addition to or instead of the above formal tests, clinicians could develop their own probe tasks based on activities described in the literature to evaluate patients' understanding of other pragmatic and discourse functions (e.g., Hartley, 1995; Rousseaux, Delacourt, Wyrzykowski, & Lefeuvre, 2001; Tompkins, 1995). For example, the general format of these probes could involve patients listening to or reading different types of discourse samples (e.g., procedural, conversational, news editorial), and then requiring them to complete one or more of the following: (a) answering a series of yes/no questions that probe understanding of main ideas versus details and/or explicitly versus implicitly stated information; (b) summarizing the main idea by providing a title for the sample; (c) ranking statements from the sample in terms of importance to the main idea; (d) identifying factual versus opinion statements; and/or (e) providing a plausible conclusion to an incomplete sample. A variety of variables may be manipulated to increase or decrease the difficulty level of these probe tasks, including length of discourse sample, topic, context, vocabulary familiarity, number or density of propositions, extent of semantic redundancy, and ratio of essential to nonessential propositions (for a comprehensive description of influential variables and development of probe tasks, see Tompkins, 1995).

Pragmatic and Discourse Production

Although extensive research has been dedicated to characterizing pragmatic and discourse production in a variety of neurogenic language disorders (Carlomagno et al., 2011; Cocks, Hird, & Kirsner, 2007; Cote et al., 2007; McNeil et al., 2007; L. Murray, 2010; L. Williams et al., 2010), scant resources have been devoted to developing standardized procedures for assessing these language skills. Accordingly, only a limited number of commercial tests and discourse analysis procedures are listed in Table 6-3. For instance, there are a few academically based tests, such as the *Test of Written Language–Fourth Edition* (TOWL-4; Hammill & Larsen, 2009), that can evaluate both the word- and discourse-level writing skills of patients who are expected to ceiling out on more basic writing tasks, like those found on aphasia test batteries. The TOWL-4 was developed for children up to the age of 18 but may be used with adults, as raw scores can be converted to grade and age equivalents in addition to percentiles and standard scores. A Story Construction subtest provides information regarding discourse-level writing (e.g., plot, character development, general composition), whereas other subtests (e.g., Vocabulary, Spelling, and Logical Sentences) assess writing at the word and sentence levels. Equivalent forms also are available for repeated testing.

Other tests designed for children, such as the *Test of Pragmatic Language–Second Edition* (TOPL-2; Phelps-Terasaki & Phelps-Gunn, 2007) and the *Social Language Development Test–Adolescent* (Bowers et al., 2010), focus on evaluating the ability to generate socially appropriate responses. For example, the TOPL-2, which was standardized on children ages 6 to 19, involves presenting short stories accompanied by a drawing of the social situations taking place in the stories and followed by a question pertaining to the target social situation. The TOPL-2 evaluates several aspects of pragmatics, including consideration of the physical setting, audience, language topic, purpose (i.e., speech acts), visual and gestural cues, and abstract language interpretation. As with other tests developed for children but used with patients who are adults, clinicians could interpret their adult patients' performances on these two pragmatic tests in reference to age-equivalent scores (rather than the standard scores or percentiles).

Given this limited choice of commercially available tools, clinicians will also or instead need to exploit procedures described in the research literature to evaluate the pragmatic and discourse production abilities of their patients. A plethora of tasks and analysis procedures (e.g., using local and global coherence ratings; identifying participants' speaking roles when conversing with individuals with communication impairments; calculating the number and length of conversational turns) have been developed reflecting the broad range of abilities that are encompassed by these areas of language processing (e.g., Douglas et al., 2007; Ferguson & Harper, 2010; Lock et al., 2008; Rousseaux, Daveluy, et al., 2010; Sherratt & Bryan, 2012; Simmons-Mackie & Damico, 1996; Togher, 2001). Because a description of assessment activities for each area of pragmatic and discourse production is beyond the scope of this textbook, only a few example areas deemed to apply to a variety of neurogenic language and cognitive disorders that have ecological importance and have been used frequently in previous empirical studies will be addressed (for more comprehensive reviews see E. Armstrong, 2012; E. Armstrong et al., 2011; Cherney, Shadden, & Coelho, 1998; McDonald, Togher, & Code, 1999). Specifically, procedures for collecting discourse samples and assessing cohesion, speech acts, and discourse and topic management strategies will be reviewed briefly.

Collecting Discourse Samples. As mentioned previously in the "Lexical–Semantic Production" section of this chapter, formal test batteries and, thus, clinicians tend to utilize primarily picture description tasks to elicit spoken and written discourse samples. As several researchers have warned, however, relying solely on descriptive discourse samples will result in a skewed assessment of patients' abilities, given that only a limited range of pragmatic and discourse behaviors are being elicited (Cocks et al., 2007; Coelho et al., 2005; Sherratt & Bryan, 2012). Instead, language samples collected from a variety of **discourse genres,** or types of discourse, should be analyzed to identify patients' pragmatic and discourse strengths and weaknesses. These genres include the more traditional narrative (i.e., storytelling or story retelling), procedural (i.e., explaining how to complete a procedure, such as changing a tire), and expository (e.g., "Where were you when President Kennedy was assassinated?" or "Why are you in the hospital?") discourse types, as well as more recently advocated and perhaps ecologically valid service encounters (e.g., making telephone calls to get information on a product or service), expert interviews (e.g., being interviewed by student clinicians about the consequences of RHD), gossiping, and other conversational (e.g., having a discussion with the clinician on a topic provided by the clinician) discourse tasks (Coelho et al., 2005; McNeil et al., 2007; Rousseau, Daveluy, et al., 2010,; Rousseau, Seve, et al,, 2010; Tu, Togher, & Power, 2011).

Likewise, incorporating different communication partners (e.g., familiar vs. unfamiliar, authority figure vs. peer) into discourse tasks will also allow examining patients' flexibility in adapting their pragmatic and discourse output to different contexts (Togher, 2001; Tu et al., 2011). To assist with including communication partners in the assessment process, clinicians might consult the *Supporting Partners of People With Aphasia in Relationships and Conversation* program developed by Lock and colleagues (2008). This program describes the steps to preparing, recording, transcribing, and analyzing conversations between individuals with aphasia and their communication partners. Although designed for aphasia, the guidelines for assessment procedures are helpful when clinicians are collecting conversation samples from other neurogenic patient populations.

Language Sampling: The Benefits of Going Beyond Picture Description

Collecting and analyzing only one discourse sample can easily result in an inaccurate characterization of a patient's discourse production abilities. For example, Mr. Leggat is a patient with moderate nonfluent aphasia who has been attending our clinic's aphasia support group for several years. In conversation, he is a rather passive participant in that he primarily only responds to questions and rarely initiates new topics or provides elaborated responses. His picture description samples are similar in that he provides very limited output that primarily consists of labeling objects and people in the picture, rather than providing a story about what is going on in the picture. In contrast, if Mr. Leggat is asked to describe his vocational history or hobbies, the mean length of his utterances, the informativeness of his verbal output, and his use of discourse repair strategies increase significantly. Accordingly, if a clinician had only included a picture description or conversation sample as part of Mr. Leggat's initial assessment, his spoken discourse skills would have been appreciably underestimated.

Cohesion Analysis

Cohesion refers to the linguistic means by which words and sentences are meaningfully linked to each other within a text or spoken discourse sample. A variety of cohesive devices have been identified, including (Coelho, 1999; Glosser & Deser, 1990) (a) reference markers such as personal pronouns (e.g., "he," "our," "us") and demonstrative pronouns (e.g., "these," "here," "that") that refer to preceding or shortly following unambiguous antecedents; (b) lexical markers, such as reiteration (e.g., repeating exact words, using synonyms or superordinates to tie to previously stated or written vocabulary); (c) conjunctive devices, such as causal (e.g., "because," "otherwise"), temporal (e.g., "then," "while"), and additive (e.g., "and," "likewise," "additionally") conjunctions; and (d) ellipsis, in which previously stated or written words are omitted because they can be presupposed from the preceding text (e.g., in response to "Where did Dylan leave his lunchbox?," answering "At the front door" is acceptable even though "He left his lunchbox" was omitted from the response).

When analyzing discourse samples for cohesion, clinicians should identify not only the types of cohesive devices that patients are using but also the extent and adequacy of their use. That is, use of cohesive markers can be quantified by calculating the number of cohesion ties per utterance, and qualified by determining whether these ties were appropriately used and complete (e.g., unambiguous and easily determined antecedent), inappropriately used and incomplete (e.g., antecedent is missing), or inaccurate (e.g., ambiguous or incorrect antecedent) (for more specific information about cohesion analysis, see Cherney et al., 1998; C. Ellis, Rosenbek, Rittman, & Boylstein, 2005). Coelho and colleagues (2005) reported that calculating cohesive adequacy by dividing the number of complete cohesive ties by the number of cohesive ties used has been associated with acceptable inter-rater reliability, at least when used to analyze discourse in individuals with TBI.

Speech Acts. **Speech acts** refer to theoretical units of communication that encompass "what the message-sender means, what the message (or other linguistic elements) means, what the message-sender intends, what the message-receiver intends, what the message-receiver understands, and what the rules governing the linguistic utterance are" (Murray & Chapey, 2001, p. 94). Several classification systems have been developed to describe the range of intentions available (Dore, 1974; Halliday, 1994; Searle, 1969). Some intents encountered most frequently on a daily basis include requests for information or goods and services, greetings, responses, protests, and assertions. Although called "speech acts," these communication units can be expressed through any modality (e.g., facial expressions, intonation, body movements). Accordingly, because our words alone do not always express intent, some speech acts are "indirect," as they require processing of not only linguistic information but also contextual cues.

A few discourse analysis systems described in the literature involve tallying and/or rating patients' use of speech acts (e.g., Angeleri et al., 2008; Penn, 1988; Prutting & Kirchner, 1987; Terrell & Ripich, 1989). For instance, to use the Pragmatic Protocol (Prutting & Kirchner, 1987), clinicians collect a 15-minute, unstructured conversational sample between the patient and a familiar communication partner, and then rate the appropriateness of 30 pragmatic parameters that encompass a number of speech acts, as well as discourse and topic management skills (e.g., topic initiation and maintenance). The adequacy of nonverbal (e.g., body language, or kinesics) and paralinguistic (e.g., prosody) behaviors also are rated. To summarize Protocol findings, the proportion of appropriate to inappropriate pragmatic behaviors is calculated. High inter-rater reliability has been reported, but only when raters received between 8 and 10 hours of training with the Protocol. Prins and Bastiaanse (2004) raised additional concerns with the Pragmatic Protocol, including the lack of information regarding its validity and test–retest reliability and that each pragmatic parameter is rated on only a two-point scale (i.e., *appropriate* vs. *inappropriate*). Additionally, Coelho et al. (2005) noted that the Pragmatic Protocol, as well as other discourse rating systems, typically lack sufficient normative data (making it difficult to determine if a given patient's scores should be considered problematic).

Discourse and Topic Management Strategies. Effective use of each discourse or genre type (e.g., narrative, procedural, expository, casual conversation) requires an understanding of and adherence to a set of discourse rules or format regularities. For example, successful storytelling or narrative discourse requires organizing and producing one or more story episodes, each of which should at minimum specify the setting (i.e., characters, location, time), an initiating event (that leads a character to develop a plan), an action, and an outcome (related to the character's plan) (Le et al., 2011; N. Stein & Glenn, 1979). Likewise, successful conversations and other **discourse genres** (e.g., service encounters) require effective use of behaviors such as (a) topic initiation, including topic selection, introduction, and switching; (b) topic maintenance, which is achieved through turn-taking (i.e., appropriate use and comprehension of verbal and nonverbal cues to indicate the beginning and end of a conversational turn) and elaborations; and (c) repair and/or revision strategies, including use of repetitions, simplifications, and other forms of revision, and requests for repetitions or revisions (Angeleri et al., 2008; Mentis & Prutting, 1991; Terrell & Ripich, 1989).

A number of rating scales and analysis protocols have been commercially published or described in the research literature to assist clinicians in quantifying and qualifying their patients' use of these various discourse and topic management behaviors (e.g., Angeleri et al., 2008; Le et al., 2011; L. Murray, 2010; Sherratt & Bryan, 2012; Rousseaux et al., 2001). For example, the *Liles Communication Test* (Rousseaux et al., 2001) examines how well patients manage their spoken discourse during three tasks: directed conversation, discussion of a set topic, and a *Promoting Aphasics' Communicative Effectiveness* (PACE; Davis & Wilcox, 1985) activity (see Chapter 12 for a description of PACE). A scoring system is used to rate a number of receptive and expressive communication behaviors and to quantify patients' overall communication participation (e.g., greeting behaviors, degree of interaction engagement), verbal communication (e.g., topic introduction and maintenance, logical organization of discourse), and nonverbal communication (e.g., understanding gestures related to physical or emotional state, use of facial expressions and eye contact). Rousseaux and colleagues (Rousseaux, Daveluy, et al., 2010; Rousseaux, Seve, et al., 2010) have used the *Liles* to describe spoken discourse characteristics in individuals with aphasia, RHD, and various types of dementing diseases (i.e., Alzheimer's disease, frontotemporal dementia, dementia with Lewy bodies).

Before adopting one of these analysis tools, clinicians should determine how much training is necessary to achieve acceptable levels of intra- and inter-rater reliability, or alternatively whether or not the tool's authors even reported any measures of reliability. Likewise, because many analysis protocols were developed for select patient populations (e.g., Sherratt & Bryan's [2012] system was devised to analyze discourse samples of patients with RHD), it is possible that one protocol will be unable to characterize sufficiently the discourse and topic management strengths and weaknesses associated with the spectrum of neurogenic language and cognitive disorders.

Gesture and Drawing

Assessing whether gesture and drawing are viable communication modalities is necessary when patients have severe language deficits that significantly restrict their spoken and written language abilities (Lyon & Helm-Estabrooks, 1987; Threats, 2009; Ward-Lonergan & Nicholas, 1995). Gesture might also be assessed when examining the integrity of nonverbal pragmatic abilities (Angeleri et al., 2008; Cocks et al., 2007; Rousseaux, Daveluy, et al., 2010; Rousseaux, Seve, et al., 2010). In terms of gestures, research indicates that iconic gestures (i.e., gestures having a relatively direct correspondence with the concepts that they represent, such as pantomiming the function of objects) and AmerInd signs (i.e., a modified version of American Indian Hand-Talk; see also Chapter 12) are easier to perceive and produce than American Sign Language by naïve viewers or users, respectively; consequently, these types of gestures are more appropriate assessment and treatment stimuli if the end goal is to encourage gesture use as part of a multimodality communication intervention (C. Campbell & Jackson, 1995; Daniloff, Fritelli, Buckingham, Hoffman, & Daniloff, 1986; Rao, 2001).

The *Assessment of Nonverbal Communication* (R. Duffy & Duffy, 1984) evaluates gestural recognition and production abilities; however, this test is no longer available from the publisher, so only clinicians who already have access to this test will be able to make use of it. Furthermore, although some aphasia test batteries include gesture subtests, these typically do not evaluate comprehension skills and have only a limited number of test items to evaluate production abilities (e.g., BDAE-3). Accordingly, many clinicians will need to rely on tests and experimental tasks described in the research literature (e.g., Angeleri et al., 2008; Rothi et al., 1997; Rousseaux, Daveluy, et al., 2010; Rousseaux et al., 2001; Rousseaux, Seve, et al., 2010), or develop their own probe tasks. A typical gesture-comprehension task will involve presenting gestures, either live or in the more reliable videotaped format, and then requiring patients to point to the correct picture in a multiple-choice format that matches the gesture stimulus. It also may be informative to assess the influence of gestural information on patients' auditory comprehension abilities (Records, 1994). In this case, the clinician could complete the following additional versions of the above probe task: Present just an auditory stimulus (i.e., evaluate spoken-word-to-picture matching), and present both the auditory and gestural versions of the stimulus. For assessing gesture production, apraxia tests such as Dabul's (2000) *Apraxia Battery for Adults–Second Edition* or the *Test of Upper Limb Apraxia* (Vanbellingen et al., 2010) can provide some information. Likewise, clinicians could present real or pictured objects and ask patients to produce or imitate gestures for these objects.

To determine if drawing may be a suitable means of communication, Helm-Estabrooks and colleagues (Helm-Estabrooks & Albert, 2004; Lyon & Helm-Estabrooks, 1987) recommended first establishing that patients have the following: (a) relatively intact visuosemantic processing skills, at least for the concepts to be drawn; (b) sufficient access to symbols within their visuosemantic system; (c) adequate visual attention; (d) sufficient motor and praxic skills for holding a writing implement and drawing; (e) skill at revising and augmenting drawing to facilitate communication interactions; and (f) a willingness to use drawing as a means of communication. Accordingly, a drawing assessment should evaluate not only patients' ability to depict a variety of concepts and events but also their ability to copy, draw from memory, and perform hand and limb motoric and praxic skills. Although several RHD and dementia batteries include drawing subtests, these tasks were designed to evaluate primarily visuoperceptual and visuoconstruction abilities and thus should be augmented by an evaluation of more advanced drawing abilities, such as the Event Drawing Task (Sacchett & Black, 2011) or the Daily Mishaps Test (Helm-Estabrooks & Albert, 1991). For instance, the Daily Mishaps Test examines how well patients draw enacted scenarios that contain one- to three-part scenes; because standardized scoring criteria are not provided, clinicians must either create their own or use procedures described in the research literature (e.g., L. Murray, 1998).

Test Confounds

Clinicians must be cognizant of a number of factors that may confound the interpretation of language test results. Two particularly influential factors are age and education. That is, because strong negative effects of age and education on language abilities have been found (MacKenzie, 2000; P. Roberts & Doucet, 2011; Salter et al., 2006), clinicians must always try to ensure that the normative samples of the language tests they use match the age and education backgrounds of their patients closely. The normative data of many language tests, however, are based on population samples that fail to represent a broad enough age or education range to be suitable for all patients. Furthermore, in some cases, particularly among aphasia screening measures, the influence of age or education is neither reported nor considered when providing cutoffs to identify a deficit (Salter et al., 2006). In terms of age, normative samples often do not extend to represent the oldest age group; and in terms of education, those with low education levels are often underrepresented (Hawkins & Bender, 2002; MacKenzie, 2000; Salter et al., 2006). This is particularly important when assessing high-level language abilities (e.g., proverb explanation, understanding of implied information), as age and education effects are most apparent on tests of these language skills. Most frequently, the failure to identify tests with suitable normative data results in the misdiagnosis of impaired language abilities.

The premorbid literacy level of patients must also be determined when collecting case history information. Research indicates that individuals who are illiterate or who have poor literacy proficiency do more poorly than their literate peers not only on tests that require reading or writing but also on tests with phonological awareness demands, including auditory discrimination, auditory comprehension, and repetition subtests found on aphasia batteries (Coppens, Parente, & Lecours, 1998; Tsegaye, de Bleser, & Iribarren, 2011).

Another important factor to consider when assessing language skills, in particular pragmatic and discourse abilities, is ethnocultural background (C. Ellis, 2009; Kennepohl et al., 2004). A growing literature has documented that the variety and frequency of discourse and topic management strategies used by adults varies as a function of their ethnocultural background (e.g., Molrine & Pierce, 2002; Ulatowska, Olness, Hill, Roberts, & Keebler, 2000). Failure to consider these ethnocultural differences could result in (a) inappropriate interpretation of certain discourse behaviors as linguistic symptoms or (b) failure to document compromised usage of certain discourse behaviors.

If the normative sample of a given test or discourse analysis procedure does not match the demographic background of a given patient, clinicians should consult the research literature to determine if (a) additional normative information is available for the test or procedure or (b) culturally equivalent or language-equivalent forms of that test or procedure have been developed. Often, for commercially available tests (as well as those described in the research literature), extended normative data and versions for languages other than English become available subsequent to the tests' initial publication as investigators explore the tests' suitability for additional patient populations (e.g., Edmonds & Donovan, 2012; Kim & Na, 2004; Kostalova et al., 2008; P. Roberts & Doucet, 2011).

Prognostic Factors for Linguistic Outcomes

Once language assessment procedures have been completed and assessment findings interpreted, speech-language pathologists must be prepared to make prognoses about their patients' language recovery. Not only will patients, their caregivers, and other health team members be interested in expected language outcomes, but so too will medical insurance companies, which utilize this information to approve treatment services (see Chapter 13). Rather than providing generic "will get better" or "won't get better" prognoses, clinicians should try to be as specific as possible (e.g., the patient will be able to tolerate intensive treatment at this time; the patient will require at least two months of biweekly outpatient treatment to show meaningful gains on the WAB-R; the patient will be able to return to independent-living conditions). To do so, a number of the prognostic indicators must be taken into consideration. The various predictor variables identified in the research literature include those related to biographical, medical, and linguistic and cognitive factors, each of which are described below and summarized in Table 6-6.

TABLE 6-6
Prognostic Indicators for Language Recovery

FACTORS SUGGESTING BETTER PROGNOSIS	FACTORS SUGGESTING POORER PROGNOSIS	NONPREDICTIVE FACTORS
Younger age (TBI only)	Etiology:	Age (etiologies other than TBI)
High premorbid intellectual ability	• Stroke (vs. TBI)	Gender
Adequate patient motivation	• Ischemic stroke	Education level
Appropriate family and caregiver attitudes	• Progressive disease	
Premorbid high physical activity level	Fast- (vs. slow-) growing tumor	
Communication symptoms:	Lesion location:	
• Awareness of deficits	• Dominant hemisphere	
• Less severe language impairment	• Multiple lesions	
• Anomic or conduction aphasia	• Bilateral lesions	
• Stimulability and self-cueing ability	• Cortical (vs. subcortical)	
	• Frontal lobe (in TBI)	
	• Arcuate fasciculus lesion	
	Amount of brain damage:	
	• TBI severity	
	• Large regions of ischemia	
	• Previous stroke	
	Concomitant medical, physical, or psychiatric problems:	
	• Apraxia of speech	
	• Depression	
	• History of sedentary lifestyle	
	Medications:	
	• Those that cause confusion or fatigue	
	• Those with communication side effects	
	Communication symptoms:	
	• Auditory comprehension deficits	
	• Global or severe Wernicke's aphasia	
	Cognitive deficits:	
	• Anosognosia	
	• Memory impairments	
	• Neglect	

Note. TBI = traumatic brain injury.

Biographical Factors

Biographical factors that clinicians should consider include the patient's age, gender, education, premorbid intelligence, personality, support systems, usual or daily activities, and level and type of life participation. A significant negative relationship between age and treatment outcomes has been observed for patients with TBI (Cifu et al., 1996; Sendroy-Terrill et al., 2010). Although older adults are at greater risk of becoming aphasic after their first stroke than younger adults are (Engelter et al., 2006), mixed findings have been reported for aphasic and dementia patient populations' language recovery or rate of language deterioration, respectively (de Riesthal & Wertz, 2004; Maas et al., 2010; Plowman et al., 2011; Rountree, Chan, Pavlik, Darby, & Doody, 2012). These equivocal results no doubt reflect that many variables, such as personal attitude, general medical health, and level and type of daily activities and social participation, may confound the influence of age on recovery (Haslam et al., 2008; L. Murray & Chapey, 2001; Sendroy-Terrill et al., 2010; Tompkins, Jackson, & Schulz, 1990). Therefore, final prognoses should never be based solely upon a patient's age (Sendroy-Terrill et al., 2010). This is particularly important to keep in mind, given that **ageism**, the systematic stereotyping and discrimination of people on the basis of their age, is still pervasive in health care (Searl & Gabel, 2003).

> **Even Old People Like to Get Better!**
>
> In our university clinics, we continue to receive requests for assessment, treatment, or both from patients who have received no or minimal services from a variety of health-care facilities (e.g., acute care, long-term care, home health). Unfortunately, patient age often appears to underlie why these patients never received a speech-language pathology referral or were provided an inadequate course of speech-language therapy. For example, we recently worked with Mrs. Stroffolino, who in her mid-80s suffered a closed head injury from a fall. She was admitted and treated in an acute-care hospital for her orthopedic injuries. Although she reported to her doctor difficulties thinking of words and remembering recent events, she was never given a speech-language pathology or neuropsychological evaluation during her hospital stay. Her doctor instead told Mrs. Stroffolino and her family that these problems were typical for someone of Mrs. Stroffolino's age and that no rehabilitation services were therefore necessary. Fortunately, Mrs. Stroffolino and her family were not satisfied with this doctor's feedback and sought additional information from our clinic.

The influence of gender on language outcomes also remains unresolved (Lazar & Antoniello, 2008; Plowman et al., 2011). In some studies, gender and outcome are linked with better recovery or slower disease progression in males (A. Holland, Greenhouse,

Fromm, & Swindell, 1989), whereas in other studies, females are favored (Pizzamiglio, Mammucari, & Razzano, 1985; Rountree et al., 2012). In still other studies, no significant differences in the language deficit severity or recovery or, in the case of progressive diseases, rate of language deterioration of female versus male patients have been observed (Bayles et al., 1999; Engelter et al., 2006; Maas et al., 2010). Given these mixed findings, gender does not appear to be a particularly influential prognostic variable.

Although education level can affect patients' performances of language tests (Hawkins & Bender, 2002; Kawano et al., 2010; P. Roberts & Doucet, 2011), it is not clear whether it affects the degree or rate of their language recovery or, in dementing diseases, their rate of language deterioration (de Riesthal & Wertz, 2004; Laska, Kahan, Hellblom, Murray, & von Arbin, 2011; Plowman et al., 2011; Rountree et al., 2012). Instead, clinicians should consider patients' overall premorbid intellectual ability, which appears to have more predictive power than education level (Leritz, McGlinchey, Lundgren, Grande, & Milberg, 2008; Pavlik, Doody, Massman, & Chan, 2006; Tompkins et al., 1990). To obtain estimates of premorbid intelligence, clinicians can use easy-to-calculate equations published in the research literature that are based on statistical weightings of patients' age, education, gender, occupation, race, and other demographic information (Barona, Reynolds, & Chastain, 1984; R. Wilson, Rosenbaum, & Brown, 1979). For patients without reading deficits, oral word reading tests may also be used to predict premorbid intelligence (e.g., Wechsler, 2001); for patients with reading deficits, the *Lexical Orthographic Familiarity Test* has been developed and validated by Leritz et al. (2008).

Research indicates that personality variables and levels of social support are strongly associated with overall health, morbidity, mortality, and treatment prognosis in many health conditions, including stroke and head injury (Andersson & Fridlund, 2002; Fraas & Calvert, 2009; Haslam et al., 2008). For instance, patients' motivation, desire, and determination to improve will clearly influence the course and outcomes of their treatment (Fraas & Calvert, 2009; Wressle, Eeg-Olofsson, Marcusson, & Henriksson, 2002). As van Harskamp and Visch-Brink (1991) noted, "the patient's motivation is of utmost importance: patients need to exert themselves to make progress" (p. 533). Likewise, family or caregiver attitudes regarding patients' improvement potential and treatment program, as well as their emotional well-being and level of support for the neurogenic patient, will affect intervention outcomes (Fraas & Calvert, 2009; Freed, 2004; E. Miller et al., 2010; Mittelman, Haley, Clay, & Roth, 2006). Accordingly, to foster patients' and caregivers' willingness to participate actively in treatment, clinicians must ensure that patients and their caregivers are well educated about the patients' symptoms, have the opportunity to contribute to treatment planning, and are provided support to minimize negative emotional reactions (E. Miller et al., 2010; Wressle et al., 2002).

Medical Factors

Influential medical factors that should be considered when making prognoses include the etiology and duration of the neurogenic language disorder, the site and extent of brain damage, and the presence and severity of concomitant physical and mental health problems.

Different language outcomes are associated with the different neurological etiologies. For example, there is better recovery from aphasia subsequent to TBI than aphasia subsequent to stroke or other vascular disorders (Gil, Cohen, Korn, & Groswasser, 1996; M. Sarno, Buonaguro, & Levin, 1986; Vukovic et al., 2008). Better communication outcomes and less frequent onset of language deficits also may be expected if a patient survives a hemorrhagic rather than an ischemic (i.e., thrombotic or embolic) stroke, because hemorrhages tend to produce less permanent brain damage, particularly within cortical areas (Berthier, 2005; Engelter et al., 2006; Ferro, Mariano, & Madureira, 1999). Patients with slow-growing tumors demonstrate better language recovery following treatment of their tumor than patients with rapidly growing tumors (Thiel et al., 2001, 2005). With respect to dementia, certain dementing illnesses are associated with greater compromise of language abilities than others. For instance, initial symptoms of Alzheimer's disease, vascular dementia, and certain variants of frontotemporal dementia are often language-based, whereas in Huntington's, Parkinson's, and dementia with Lewy bodies, cognitive symptoms often precede and are more severe than language symptoms (Kempler & Goral, 2008; J. Reilly et al., 2010; Sutton-Brown & Suchowersky, 2003).

For stroke, TBI, and other nonprogressive neurological disorders, the greatest language recovery rate is most frequently observed during the first few months postonset, a time line that overlaps with spontaneous physiological recovery processes such as the resorption of edema (Engelter et al., 2006; Katz, Polyak, Coughlan, Nichols, & Roche, 2009; Lazar & Antoniello, 2008; Maas et al., 2010; Sinanovic, 2010). Patients and caregivers, however, must be reminded that patients with static neurological disorders can continue to demonstrate significant progress for years beyond the period of spontaneous recovery (Katz et al., 2009; Marsh & Hillis, 2006; Moss & Nicholas, 2006). Similarly, with treatment, patients with progressive neurological disorders can slow the rate and extent of their disease progression for many years following symptom onset (Arkin & Mahendra, 2001; Mittelman et al., 2006).

The site and extent of brain damage also may influence language outcomes. Generally, poor language prognosis, in terms of amount and rate of recovery (or in the case of progressive diseases, rate of deterioration), is often associated with large dominant-hemisphere lesions or multiple lesions (Maas et al., 2010; Mosch, Max, & Tranel, 2005; Plowman et al., 2011), or relatedly, severe TBI (Chabok, Kapourchali, Leili, Saberi, & Mohtasham-Amiri, 2012; Katz et al., 2009); that is, the larger the lesion, the poorer the language outcome. More specifically, severe or more enduring aphasia may be expected if brain damage (a) encompasses the central core of the dominant-hemisphere language area subserved by the middle cerebral artery (Kang et al., 2010; Maas et al., 2010; F. Oliveira & Damasceno, 2011); (b) affects dominant-hemisphere temporobasal areas (Goldenberg & Spatt, 1994; Naeser & Palumbo, 1994); (c) extends deep into underlying white matter pathways or other subcortical structures of the dominant hemisphere (de Boissezon et al., 2009; Ferro et al., 1999); (d) with respect to spoken language deficits, significantly compromises the arcuate fasciculus (Marchina et al., 2011); or (e) involves bilateral lesions (Naeser et al., 1998). In RHD, communicative disorders are more likely if patients suffer cortical versus subcortical brain damage (Joanette et al., 1990), whereas in TBI, they are more frequent and significant following a moderate or severe frontotemporal or closed head injury (Chabok et al., 2012; Chapman et al., 1992, 1994; Struchen et al., 2008b).

An extensive literature documents that patients suffering from concomitant medical, physical, or psychiatric complications are more likely to have longer hospital stays and less likely to achieve the same extent or rate of recovery as that obtained by patients without these conditions (Liman et al., 2011; Maas et al., 2010; Safaz, Alaca, Yasar, Tok, & Yilmaz, 2008). For example, patients with TBI who develop a hardening of connective tissue, called "heterotopic ossification," have been found to have longer inpatient rehabilitation stays, poorer functional outcomes by discharge, and less frequent discharges to home, compared with patients with TBI who had similar severities of head injury but no heterotopic ossification (Johns, Cifu, Keyser-Marcus, Jolles, & Fratkin, 1999; Safaz et al., 2008). Likewise, aphasia recovery is compromised by the presence of motor speech disorders such as apraxia of speech (Ogrezeanu, Voinescu, Mihailescu, & Jipescu, 1994), and patients with poor premorbid physical health (e.g., history of a sedentary lifestyle) tend to experience less aphasia recovery (Maas et al., 2010). Patients with neurogenic disorders who have depression, anxiety, or other psychological problems also are at risk for poorer rehabilitation outcomes than their cohorts without these mental health problems (Ben-Yishay & Daniels-Zide, 2000; Fucetola et al., 2006; King & Kirwilliam, 2011; E. Miller et al., 2010). It is important to note, however, that this risk of poorer outcome can be reduced if depression is diagnosed and treated as soon as possible (E. Miller et al., 2010; Oliveira & Damasceno, 2011).

Medications also may negatively affect patients' communicative functioning. For example, the side effects of some antidepressant, cancer, antipsychotic, and anticonvulsant drugs include dysarthria, aphasia, and stuttering (Atri, 2011; de Boissezon, Peran, de Boysson, & Demonet, 2007; O'Sullivan & Fagan, 1998). Furthermore, a number of medications frequently prescribed to neurogenic patients, including anticonvulsants, sedatives, and antihypertensives, may cause confusion, depression, fatigue, and decreased arousal or alertness, which in turn can affect patients' ability to complete language activities, and more generally can reduce their rate of recovery (Hoppe & Elger, 2011; S. Small, 2002; Vogel et al., 2000). Accordingly, clinicians should review what medications their patients are taking to ascertain whether these drugs have the potential to inhibit or enhance their patients' current communication abilities.

Linguistic and Cognitive Factors

A number of linguistic and cognitive factors should be considered when attempting to provide prognostic information. In terms of language, variables such as language stimulability and severity and type of aphasia have been found influential. For instance, several studies have found initial severity of aphasia to be a strong predictor of language recovery (Berthier, 2005; Laska et al., 2007; Maas et al., 2010; Pedersen et al., 2004; Plowman et al., 2011): More severe initial language impairments are associated with less positive language outcomes. Relatedly, TBI survivors with aphasia have been found to have poorer cognitive and functional outcomes compared with TBI survivors without aphasia (Demir et al., 2006). It is important to keep in mind that patients with significant language impairments still demonstrate recovery but do not recover to the level of language functioning achieved by those who have initially less severe language problems. Furthermore, patients with severe auditory recognition and comprehension problems tend to demonstrate not only less language recovery than those with less severe impairments in this language modality (de Boissezon et al., 2009; Demir et al., 2006; Gialanella, 2011) but also poorer overall functional recovery (Gialanella, 2011).

Links between aphasia type and the extent of recovery or the residual pattern of language impairment have also been reported (Bakheit, Shaw, Carrington, & Griffiths, 2007; Lazar & Antoniello, 2008). Generally, patients with anomic, Broca's, or conduction aphasia have the best language prognosis, and those with global or severe Wernicke's have the worst prognosis (Bakheit et al., 2007; Ferro et al., 1999; F. Oliveira & Damasceno, 2011); given the previous discussion of the relationship between aphasia severity and language prognosis, this pattern of outcomes might be predicted, as anomic and conduction aphasias produce less severe language symptoms than global and severe Wernicke's aphasias. Whereas even patient survival is negatively affected by global aphasia in acute stroke (F. Oliveira & Damasceno, 2011), patients who continue to present with global aphasia beyond three months postonset are at greatest risk for poor language outcomes (Kang et al., 2010; Kertesz, 1979). In addition to making predictions regarding the extent of language improvement, clinicians may also make predictions regarding changes in aphasia type (Ferro et al., 1999; Lazar & Antoniello, 2008; Ogrezeanu et al., 1994). With recovery, Broca's, Wernicke's, conduction, or transcortical (sensory, motor, or mixed) aphasia types often evolve toward anomic aphasia; global aphasia frequently resolves toward Broca's aphasia, although recovery to both fluent and nonfluent aphasia types has been reported.

The extent to which patients may profit from cues, that is, the extent to which the patients are stimulable, should also be considered when making language outcome predictions. Some research has indicated that patients with aphasia who are initially responsive to prompts and cues have better recovery of language production abilities than patients for whom cueing is unproductive (Beeson et al., 2003; Keenan & Brassell, 1974). Likewise, several researchers have hypothesized that patients who can learn to cue themselves will display better language outcomes, as well as maintenance and generalization of trained language skills, than patients who must rely on others for cues (L. Murray & Chapey, 2001; Singer & Bashir, 1999).

Generally the presence of cognitive deficits is associated with greater levels of disability and higher rates of institutionalization (Gialanella & Ferlucci, 2010; Jehkonen et al., 2006). More specifically, there is growing evidence to support the contention that language recovery and rehabilitation outcomes, including generalization of trained skills or compensatory strategies, may be negatively affected by the presence of concomitant cognitive impairments (Lambon Ralph et al., 2010; Murray, Ballard, & Karcher, 2004; Vukovic et al., 2008). For example, the executive functions of self-awareness and self-monitoring appear closely linked to language outcomes and therapy progress, as patients with poor awareness of their language or other symptoms, or of situations that enhance and degrade their language skills, have a poorer prognosis than patients without these cognitive deficits (Cocchini, Gregg, Beschin, Dean, & Della Sala, 2010; Nicholas et al., 2011; Starkstein et al., 2010). Patients with aphasia who have bilateral lesions or damage to temporobasal regions, and concomitant impairments of memory and/or executive functioning, also are less successful in speech-language therapy than patients whose brain damage did not affect these areas (Goldenberg & Spatt, 1994; Naeser et al., 1998). Likewise, stroke patients with neglect, anosognosia, or both have longer hospitalizations and less favorable rehabilitation outcomes than those without these cognitive symptoms (Jehkonen et al., 2006; Wee & Hopman, 2008). Finally, significant associations between the discourse problems of patients with RHD or TBI and deficits of working memory or executive functioning (Champagne-Lavau & Joanette, 2009; Douglas, 2010; Eslinger et al., 2011; Tompkins et al., 1994) also indicate that the integrity of cognitive abilities should be considered when making prognoses regarding language outcomes.

Summary

Over the past several decades, advances in our understanding of linguistic impairments associated with aphasia, RHD, TBI, and dementia have led to the development of numerous approaches and procedures for evaluating neurogenic language disorders at the ICF level of body structure and function. A key to managing this broad spectrum of test options is acknowledging that the evaluation of linguistic abilities is a multistep process that cannot be completed via the administration of a single language test. Instead, the assessment process must begin with the collection of case history information and completion of observations. On the basis of those data, clinicians next select and administer tests of general and specific linguistic functioning. The last step of the assessment process involves interpreting linguistic test findings in light of cognitive test results (see Chapter 7), findings from participation and activity evaluations (see Chapter 8), and the consideration of certain influential biographic and medical variables. Only when all of these assessment procedures have been completed should final recommendations regarding linguistic outcomes and treatment goals and procedures be made.

Discussion Questions

1. Devise a case history/interview form to obtain information about language functioning from an outpatient with chronic aphasia. How might this case history form differ from that used to obtain language information about an inpatient with acute traumatic brain injury?
2. What modifications could be made to a picture-naming test to provide qualitative information about the word finding abilities of patients with (a) aphasia, (b) right hemisphere brain damage, (c) traumatic brain injury, or (d) dementia related to Alzheimer's disease? Generate at least two modifications for each patient population based on your knowledge of that patient group's language and concomitant symptom profile.
3. Why is it typically inappropriate to use aphasia test batteries to document the presence and severity of language impairments in patients with right hemisphere brain damage or traumatic brain injury?
4. What steps would be necessary to adapt a test of pragmatic language abilities originally developed for English-speaking adolescents for use with Spanish-English bilingual adults for whom English is their second language?
5. Why is analyzing a spoken language sample based on a picture description inadequate for identifying discourse deficits in adults with neurogenic language or cognitive disorders?

Assessment of Body Structure and Function: Quantifying and Qualifying Cognitive Disorders

chapter 7

Learning Objectives

After reading this chapter, you should be able to:

- Provide a rationale for assessing the cognitive abilities of patients with neurogenic language disorders
- Identify formal and informal procedures that may be used to help collect case history information pertaining to a cognitive assessment
- Describe the purpose and format of cognitive screening tests
- Differentiate between test batteries for evaluating general cognitive abilities and those for assessing attention, memory, or executive functioning
- Describe tests that evaluate specific attention, memory, or executive function abilities at the ICF level of body structure and function
- Identify test batteries and tests of specific cognitive functions that are suitable for patients with concomitant language disorders
- Explain factors that may confound the administration or interpretation of cognitive tests
- Describe biographic, medical, and cognitive variables that should be considered when making prognoses about cognitive outcomes

Key Terms

- cognitive flexibility
- divided attention
- inhibition
- orientation
- selective or focused attention
- sustained attention
- working memory

Introduction

It is well established that patients with neurogenic language disorders frequently, if not always, have concomitant cognitive impairments, including deficits of attention, memory, and/or executive functioning (e.g., Barker-Collo et al., 2010; Cook et al., 2011; L. Murray, 2012b; Park et al., 2011; see also Chapter 2). Additionally, caregivers and neurogenic patients who are cognizant of the severity and breadth of their symptoms typically voice most concern over cognitive problems associated with the onset of brain damage or disease (Marsh, Kersel, Havill, & Sleigh, 2002; Visser-Keizer et al., 2002). As discussed in Chapter 2, cognitive impairments also may be the sole cause of communication problems (as is commonly the case in patients who have suffered a traumatic brain injury or right hemisphere brain damage), or may exacerbate linguistic problems (as may occur in patients with aphasia or certain forms of dementia) (Bittner & Crowe, 2006; Kempler & Goral, 2008; Lehman Blake, 2007; L. Murray, 2004a).

In addition to their negative influences on communication, cognitive deficits may have dire effects on the rehabilitation process. For example, patients with concomitant cognitive deficits are less likely to benefit from behavioral treatments and, accordingly, have a slower recovery or poorer functional outcomes compared with their peers without these coexisting problems (Ginstfeld & Emanuelson, 2010; Kortte & Hillis, 2011; Lambon Ralph et al., 2010; Morton & Barker, 2010). More specifically, patients with anosognosia tend to do poorly in rehabilitation because they fail, at least acutely, to recognize their need for therapy, their expectations for treatment outcomes far exceed their true potential, or both (Jehkonen et al., 2006; Kortte & Hillis, 2011). Likewise, one group of researchers found that attention-test performance was a strong predictor of brain-injured patients' use of memory aids (Evans et al., 2003).

Just as rehabilitation can be negatively affected by cognitive problems, so too can social and vocational outcomes. For instance, several studies have found a negative relationship between neglect and the social and vocational outcomes of stroke and TBI (traumatic brain injury) patients (Appelros, Karlsson, Seiger, & Nydevik, 2002; Shames, Treger, Ring, & Giaquinto, 2007), and an older investigation reported that attentional abilities were most influential on the ability of patients with aphasia to return to work—even more so than their language abilities (Ramsing, Blomstrand, & Sullivan, 1991). Finally, there is evidence supporting a positive association between neglect or executive function deficits and caregiver burden (Al-Aloucy et al., 2011; Appelros et al., 2002; Marsh et al., 2002; Rymer et al., 2002). Consequently, including a cognitive assessment aimed at the ICF level of body function may result in improved estimations of the extent and type of treatment needed by patients with neurogenic language disorders, as well as the type of support and training needed by their caregivers.

Whereas it is clear that most patients with neurogenic language disorders will benefit from a comprehensive cognitive evaluation, it is less clear which health-care professional should complete that evaluation. That is, the scopes of practice for several disciplines currently encompass assessing at least some cognitive functions. For example, in hospital and rehabilitation settings, occupational therapists, neuropsychologists, and speech-language pathologists may all be capable of assessing cognitive skills. Likewise, in school settings, resource teachers or learning specialists, speech-language pathologists, and school psychologists all may have been trained to complete cognitive testing. Accordingly, an essential first step to a cognitive evaluation is to determine whether cognitive skills will be assessed by one or several health-care-team members: Failing to predetermine team member responsibilities could result in redundant or, conversely, inadequate testing.

As mentioned in Chapter 4, it also is important to review state and national professional association guidelines to determine what assessment tools each health-care team member is allowed to administer. For example, in some states and provinces, only psychologists are licensed to use and interpret the results of certain cognitive tests, particularly those that evaluate memory and executive functioning. Even in the presence of these professional restrictions, a speech-language pathologist's input is recommended, especially when patients have language impairments that may confound standardized assessment administration and scoring procedures. Speech-language pathologists have the most professional training related to assessing and treating language disorders, and thus often have the greatest insight regarding how best to adapt testing procedures, interpret test findings, or both when assessing the cognitive abilities of patients with neurogenic disorders.

Dementia Due to Inaccurate Test Results Versus Impaired Cognition

The failure to acknowledge the influence of communication impairments on the outcomes of cognitive tests can result in inaccurate interpretation of test results. For example, during an initial speech-language diagnostic session with a patient presenting with a degenerative cerebellar disorder, the patient's wife, Mrs. Ashcroft, was interviewed to determine the previous services that Mr. Ashcroft had received. She was asked whether or not Mr. Ashcroft had received any prior cognitive testing, and about the outcome of that testing. Mrs. Ashcroft replied that Mr. Ashcroft's neurologist had completed a short cognitive test on several occasions, but she did not know the name of the test. She did know, however, that the neurologist had concluded that Mr. Ashcroft was presenting with dementia, based on the results of that cognitive testing. Following further questioning, we were able to determine that Mr. Ashcroft had received the *Mini-Mental State Examination–Second Edition* (MMSE-2; Folstein & Folstein, 2010; see the "Cognitive Status and Dementia Screening Tools" section of this chapter for further description of this test). This was alarming to us, given that Mr. Ashcroft had been presenting with severe ataxia, severe ataxic dysarthria, and mild anomia for some time, and, consequently, his performance on the MMSE-2 would no doubt have been confounded by these motor and communication problems. That is, basing a diagnosis of dementia only on MMSE-2 results was inappropriate, as it is difficult to determine whether or not Mr. Ashcroft's verbal and written MMSE-2 responses were inaccurate because of possible cognitive problems or because of his severe motor and communication difficulties.

Regardless of whether speech-language pathologists fulfill a direct or indirect role in evaluating cognitive skills, they must be knowledgeable about cognitive tests and assessment procedures to ensure an appropriate understanding of their patients' cognitive strengths and limitations. Accordingly, the purpose of this chapter is to overview the components of a cognitive evaluation and to provide an introduction to the multitude of commercially available tests and research protocols that are currently available to quantify and qualify the cognitive abilities of patients with neurogenic disorders at the

ICF (International Classification of Functioning, Disability, and Health; WHO, 2001) level of body structure and function.

Assessment Procedures

Cognitive evaluations should follow the same format as that utilized to complete language evaluations: Begin with the compilation of case history and observational data. Then, based on that information, select and administer formal or structured tests of cognition. Recall that assessment must be considered a continual process, as initial tests may reveal new areas of cognitive strength or weakness, or patients' cognitive profiles or functional needs may change as a result of spontaneous recovery or treatment.

Case History and Observations

Prior to giving structured or formal tests of cognition, an imperative first step to assessment is the assemblage of case history and observational information to help make decisions regarding test selection, as well as subsequent interpretation of test results. Interviewing patients and their caregivers to collect the case history can be particularly valuable when completing a cognitive evaluation. For instance, a comparison of patient and caregiver responses can provide information regarding the patient's long-term memory limitations (e.g., is the patient able to recall accurately information encoded prior to the onset of the brain damage or disease?). Likewise, executive problems such as anosognosia can be identified by noting whether or not patients specify the same types and severities of problems that their caregivers do. Indeed, research indicates that compared with their significant others, patients who have suffered a traumatic brain injury, regardless of head injury severity, underreport cognitive, emotional, and behavioral symptoms (Sbordone, Seyranian, & Ruff, 1998; K. Wilson, Donders, & Nguyen, 2011). Information pertaining to other cognitive abilities also can be accrued during the patient interview. For example, the clinician might suspect attention problems if the patient appears distractible and requires continuous prompts to stay on task. For a listing of more information to accrue during the case history, refer to Chapter 4.

Several confounds necessitate that cognitive assessments include direct observations of patients in a variety of contexts. First, the external structure of formal test procedures may minimize or even completely obscure certain cognitive problems (Constantinidou et al., 2012; Murray & Ramage, 2000; Schmitter-Edgecombe et al., 2011). For example, formal assessments are typically conducted in a quiet environment (e.g., a testing room with just the examiner and patient present) and thus are accommodating for patients with attention problems. Likewise, patients often are provided supports, such as the repetition of task instructions and cues to stay on task or to switch to the next task, which can help some patients compensate for memory impairments or disinhibition and other executive function deficits. Accordingly, failing to observe patients in informal and unstructured environments may lead to an overestimation of their cognitive abilities. Inversely, formal testing situations may negatively affect the performance of patients who are unfamiliar with such procedures, such as those with little formal education or from certain ethnocultural backgrounds, as well as elderly populations (Bender, Garcia, & Barr, 2010; R. Morris, Worsley, & Matthews, 2000; Nussbaum, 1998); in these cases, omitting the observational aspect of the assessment may lead to overestimation of the presence and/or severity of cognitive problems. Finally, it is also important to keep in mind that some patients with neurogenic language or cognitive disorders, especially those with severe impairments, with many concomitant sensory and motoric problems, or who are dealing with significant medical challenges (e.g., a patient in the acute recovery phase), may be unable to complete structured tests.

Clinicians may consult protocols in the research literature or commercially available tools to help interview patients and caregivers, and to assist in collecting, organizing, and summarizing observational data pertaining to patients' cognitive abilities. There are tools aimed at assisting in the evaluation of deficits in just one specific cognitive domain, such as the Mental Slowness Questionnaire (Winkens, VanHeugten, Fasotti, et al., 2009) or the *Moss Attention Rating Scale* (Whyte, Hart, Ellis, & Chervoneva, 2008), as well those aimed at identifying more global problems across several cognitive domains, such as the AD8 Dementia Screening Interview (Galvin, Roe, Coats, & Morris, 2007).

As an example of these tools, the Dysexecutive Questionnaire of the *Behavioral Assessment of Dysexecutive Syndrome* (BADS; Wilson, Alderman, Burgess, Emslie, & Evans, 1996) consists of 20 items (e.g., "She/he loses his/her temper at the slightest thing"; "She/he has difficulty thinking ahead or planning for the future"). Each item is rated on a scale from 0 (*never*) to 4 (*very often*) to determine the frequency with which common symptoms of executive dysfunction occur (e.g., personality changes such as aggressiveness, behavior problems such as impulsivity, cognitive impairments such as planning difficulties). There are two versions, one to be used with patients and one for caregivers, so that clinicians can compare patients' self-ratings to those of their caregivers. Importantly, high correlations between the Dysexecutive Questionnaire ratings of caregivers and the performances of their brain-damaged relatives on formal tests of executive functioning have been reported (Burgess, Alderman, Evans, Emslie, & Wilson, 1998). However, it is also important to keep in mind that data from self- and caregiver-report rating scales and questionnaires may be compromised by reporter bias (Schmitter-Edgecombe et al., 2011; Tate, 2010). Indeed, Barker, Morton, Morrison, and McGuire (2011) found only moderate correlations between the Dysexecutive Questionnaire ratings of different caregivers for a given patient (i.e., more than one caregiver rated each patient in the study). Accordingly, it is important to interpret questionnaire and rating data cautiously and in concert with findings gleaned from other cognitive assessment procedures.

Cognitive Status and Dementia Screening Tools

Following completion of the case history, interviews, and observations, formal or structured test procedures can be implemented. Formal testing often begins with administration of a bedside or screening test, particularly when patients are in an acute-care setting. The purposes of these tools are to determine the presence or absence of cognitive impairments or dementia, and to identify cognitive functions in need of further evaluation. As shown in Table 7-1, many bedside or screening tests are currently available, each of which invariably includes a limited number of items to assess a variety of cognitive functions, including **orientation** (e.g., oriented to time, person, and place), visuoperception and visuoconstruction, verbal and nonverbal memory, language, attention, and some executive functions (for a more comprehensive listing, see Tate, 2010). Because these tests are short in length and only sample a limited number of cognitive

TABLE 7-1
Bedside and Screening Tests of Cognitive Disorders

INSTRUMENT	SOURCE
Addenbrooke's Cognitive Examination–Revised	Mioshi et al. (2006)
Alzheimer's Disease Caregiver's Questionnaire	Solomon (2002)
Alzheimer's Quick Test	Wiig et al. (2002)
Clock Drawing	Freedman et al. (1994)
Cognistat	Kiernan, Mueller, & Langston (2011)
Cognitive Linguistic Quick Test	Helm-Estabrooks (2001)
Community Screening Interview for Dementia	Hall et al. (1996)
Dementia Rating Scale–Second Edition	Mattis (2001)
Frontal Assessment Battery	Dubois et al. (2000)
Galveston Orientation and Amnesia Test	Levin, O'Donnell, & Grossman (1979)
Informant Questionnaire of Cognitive Decline in the Elderly	Sikkes et al. (2011)
Julia Farr Services Post-Traumatic Amnesia Scale	Forrester & Geffen (1995)
Kaufman Brief Intelligence Test–Second Edition	Kaufman & Kaufman (2004)
Middlesex Elderly Assessment of Mental State	E. Golding (1989)
Mini-Mental State Examination–Second Edition	Folstein et al. (2010)
Minnesota Cognitive Acuity Screen	Knopman, Knudson, Yoes, & Weiss (2000)
Montreal Cognitive Assessment	Nasreddine et al. (2005)
Orientation Log	W. Jackson et al. (1998)
Parkinson's Disease-Cognitive Rating Scale	Pagonabarraga et al. (2008)
Philadelphia Brief Assessment of Cognition	Libon et al. (2011)
Rancho Los Amigos Levels of Cognitive Functioning	Hagen (1981)
Repeatable Battery for the Assessment of Neuropsychological Status	Randolph (2012)
Rowland Universal Dementia Assessment Scale	Storey et al. (2004)
Telephone Interview for Cognitive Status	Brandt & Folstein (2003)

functions, their results have limited usefulness in terms of planning treatment or evaluating treatment effects (Tate, 2010).

The *Mini-Mental State Examination* (MMSE; Folstein, Folstein, & McHugh, 2001) is perhaps the most widely used and researched cognitive screening tool. It consists of a brief set of questions and tasks designed to assess orientation to time and place (e.g., what is the year?), mental calculation (e.g., subtract 7 from 100 and then keep subtracting by 7), verbal short-term memory (i.e., recall three words after a short delay), language (e.g., write a sentence), and visuoconstruction skills (i.e., copy a design). A cutoff score of 23 out of a maximum of 30 is recommended to indicate impaired cognitive status. To help classify the severity of cognitive impairment, Folstein et al. (2001) have provided score ranges in which normal = 27–30, mild impairment = 21–26, moderate impairment = 11–20, and severe impairment = 0–10.

In 2010, a major revision of the MMSE was published, the MMSE-2 (Folstein & Folstein, 2010). Although the MMSE-2 still contains the original form described above (i.e., the Standard Version), it also includes a Brief Version (i.e., a 5-minute screening) and an Expanded Version (i.e., one 20 minutes in length). The Expanded Version is more difficult and has been found to be sensitive to subcortical dementia and normal age-related cognitive changes; in contrast, the original MMSE had been shown to miss early cognitive decline associated with subcortical and vascular disease (Godefroy et al., 2011; LeBlanc et al., 2006). Other advantages of the MMSE-2 (Folstein & Folstein, 2010) are that it offers (a) alternate forms; (b) norms stratified by age and education; (c) cutoff scores for the Brief, Standard, and Expanded Versions; (d) reliable change scores to assist in interpreting data from serial assessments; and (e) versions in over 70 languages (e.g., Arabic, French, Hebrew, Japanese, Russian, Thai). Both the MMSE and MMSE-2 are also now available as an application so that they can be administered and scored via a smartphone or computer tablet.

Although numerous studies attest to the reliability and validity of the MMSE (e.g., Harvan & Cotter, 2006; for a review see Tombaugh & McIntyre, 1992), its use with certain patient populations should be avoided, or at the very least its scores must be interpreted cautiously. For example, because of their heavy language and motor speech demands, the MMSE and MMSE-2 are inappropriate for many patients with neurogenic communication disorders, as poor performance might reflect aphasia, dysarthria, and/or apraxia rather than cognitive problems (Golper, Rau, Erskins, Langhans, & Houlihan, 1987; Osher, Wicklund, Rademaker, Johnson, & Weintraub, 2008). Likewise, research suggests that the MMSE is insensitive to cognitive symptoms associated with right hemisphere brain damage, particularly in acute patients (A. Nelson, Fogel, & Faust, 1986; Nys et al., 2005a). Therefore, clinicians should consider other screening tests that are commercially available or in the research literature that have been developed for these patient populations (e.g., *Cognitive-Linguistic Quick Test*; Helm-Estabrooks, 2001).

The additional tools listed in Table 7-1 are similar to the MMSE or MMSE-2 but in some cases are more suitable for identifying cognitive problems in a broader spectrum of patients. For example, the *Telephone Interview for Cognitive Status* (TICS; Brandt & Folstein, 2003) is similar in length and content to the MMSE, but was developed for administration over the phone to individuals with motoric, emotional, or financial limitations that may impede their ability to attend an in-person assessment; similarly, caregivers can complete the *Alzheimer's Disease Caregiver's Questionnaire* (Solomon, 2002) online. Tools such as the *Rowland Universal Dementia Assessment Scale* (Storey, Rowland, Conforti, & Dickson, 2004) and *Community Screening Interview for Dementia* (K. S. Hall, Ogunniyi, Hendrie, & Brittain, 1996) were developed for administration to patients representing diverse ethnocultural and educational backgrounds. Finally, some of the newer cognitive screening tests are available in several languages, including the *Dementia Rating Scale–Second Edition* (Mattis, 2001) and MMSE-2 (as described above), to meet the needs of the ever-growing bilingual and multilingual population.

A few cognitive screening tools have been developed for specific patient populations. For instance, the *Orientation Log* (W. Jackson, Novack, & Dowler, 1998) was designed to evaluate orientation in individuals with TBI, the *Frontal Assessment Battery* (Dubois, Slachevsky, Litvan, & Pillon, 2000) was validated for patients with neurogenic disorders associated with frontal lobe dysfunction (e.g., Parkinson's disease, frontotemporal lobar degeneration, progressive supranuclear palsy), the *Parkinson's Disease–Cognitive Rating Scale* (Pagonabarraga et al., 2008) was developed to identify cognitive deficits in early to late stages of Parkinson's disease, the *Cognitive Change Checklist* (Schinka et al., 2010) quantifies cognitive change in mild cognitive impairment and the early stage of dementing diseases such as Alzheimer's, and the *Philadelphia Brief Assessment of Cognition* (Libon et al., 2011) helps distinguish dementia related to Alzheimer's disease from that related to frontotemporal lobar degeneration.

As a more detailed example of these more specific screening tools, the *Alzheimer's Quick Test* (Wiig, Nielsen, Minthon, & Warkentin, 2002) consists of five sets of timed naming tasks (i.e., Color–Form, Color–Number, Color–Letter, Color–Animal, and Color–Object Naming). Based on previous research, these tasks have been shown effective at identifying the presence of mild to moderate parietal lobe dysfunction, which, as mentioned in Chapters 2 and 3, is associated with Alzheimer's disease, even early in the disease process. Each naming task is completed three times: once to name each single dimension of the visual stimuli, and once to name both dimensions of the visual stimuli. For instance, on the Color–Form task, patients first name as quickly and accurately as possible the color of each shape stimulus depicted on the test page. Next, they name as quickly and accurately as possible the name of each shape stimulus; finally, they are required to name as quickly and accurately as possible both the color and shape of each stimulus. Both naming accuracy and response time are evaluated to determine if patients are performing within a normal range, slower- or less-accurate-than-normal range, or non-normal or pathological range. These performance ranges are based on a standardization sample that represents a fairly broad range of ages (i.e., 15 to 72 years) and ethnocultural backgrounds. Although the test manual states that the same criterion ranges of naming accuracy and response time can be used for individuals "between 15 and 75+ years," use of the test with individuals over the age of 72 appears inappropriate, as adults over that age did not participate in the standardization process. However, further normative data for older patients, as well as those who speak languages other than English, can be found in the empirical literature (e.g., Nielsen & Wiig, 2006) and on the website of the test's publisher.

Finally, a cognitive screening tool that is one of the quickest and easiest to administer is *Clock Drawing* (Freedman et al., 1994) (see Figure 7-1). Although it was initially developed to assess visuoconstructional abilities, subsequent research has found that it also evaluates attention, memory, and executive function abilities and is sensitive to general cognitive decline, including dementia (Nair et al., 2010; Royall, Cordes, & Polk, 1998). Several versions of the clock-drawing task and scoring are available (for reviews see Barrie, 2002; Pinto & Peters, 2009). For example, the task can be administered as a free-drawn condition in which patients are asked to "draw a clock, put in all the numbers, and set the hands to . . ." or a predrawn condition in which they are given a piece of paper with a pre-drawn circle representing a clock and asked to write in the numbers and set the hands to a specified time (usually "ten past eleven"). While patients complete the task, clinicians can observe the patients' planning strategies (e.g., placing anchor numbers—12, 3, 6, and 9—before placing other numbers), areas of difficulty (as evidenced by overwriting or latencies), and whether repetition of instructions is necessary (suggesting possible memory problems). Clock-drawing performance correlates well with other cognitive screening tools, including the MMSE, and has been shown to be more suitable than the MMSE for patients who are not native English speakers or who have low education levels (Barrie, 2002; Royall et al., 2003). Concerns, however, have been raised regarding the sensitivity of clock drawing to mild dementia or mild cognitive impairment (Pinto & Peters, 2009).

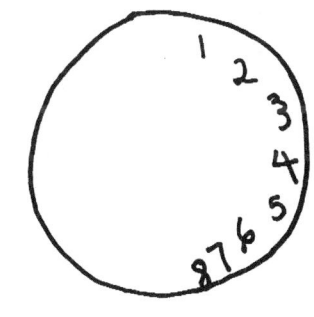

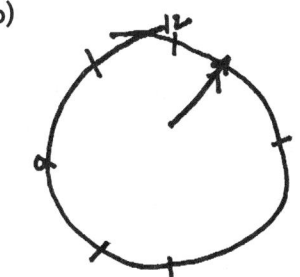

Figure 7-1. Examples of clock drawings by (a) a patient with left neglect and perseveration (i.e., extra loops on "3") and (b) a patient with Alzheimer's disease and visuoconstruction problems. In both examples, patients were asked to set the clock to 1:45.

In summary, a variety of screening tests are available to establish the presence or absence of cognitive impairment. For patients whose screening test outcomes indicate cognitive problems, the next step of the evaluation may be completing a more in-depth and/or comprehensive cognitive test battery or tests of specific cognitive functions. Alternately, in cases in which the clinician has ample assessment time available and the patient has already been determined to have cognitive difficulties, the screening step of the evaluation may be skipped, with the clinician instead opting to begin with one of the cognitive test batteries described below.

For Screening Purposes Only—Even When It Comes to Dementia!

Although the developers of screening measures, along with textbook authors (e.g., Tate, 2010), consistently remind clinicians that screening measures should only be used to identify the need for more extensive testing, our clinical experiences and those of our students indicate that this reminder is not being regularly remembered.

A former undergraduate student recently emailed me to share one of her recent cases. She was working as a health-care aide providing in-home services to a 94-year-old gentleman. She had noticed the onset of some symptoms possibly indicative of dementia (e.g., orientation problems), so she recommended that he see his primary care physician. At his doctor's appointment, the only test given was the MMSE (e.g., no blood-work tests). Based on this screening test, the physician put him on a cholinergic agonist (see Chapter 11) typically prescribed for Alzheimer's disease and told him to come back in six weeks, at which time the MMSE would be readministered to see if the medication was helping. Clearly, the physician in this case needs to revisit the purpose of screening tools as well as the comprehensive assessment procedures recommended to determine the presence and etiology of dementia!

Test Batteries

Administration of a test battery is frequently the next step of a cognitive evaluation if the cognitive screening or other initial assessment procedures suggest impaired cognitive functioning. Two basic types of cognitive test batteries are available: those designed to evaluate a range of cognitive functions and thus provide an overview of patients' general cognitive abilities or intelligence, and those designed to evaluate a range of cognitive behaviors within only one domain of cognition (e.g., a memory battery that assesses short- and long-term memory skills). Examples of each of these types of test batteries are described below.

General Cognitive Functioning Test Batteries

A number of general cognitive test batteries are currently available (see Table 7-2). Speech-language pathologists should check with other health-care-team members and state requirements before utilizing these tools, as administration of these batteries often falls under the purview of psychology or neuropsychology. Typically, speech-language pathologists utilize these test batteries only when neuropsychology services are unavailable (which is the case in many rural communities and nursing homes), and even then, they typically only give certain subtests rather than the entire battery. Regardless of whether speech-language pathologists play a direct or indirect role in administering these batteries, they should be familiar with them so that they can accurately interpret neuropsychology reports and, if need be, appropriately select and utilize specific subtests.

The most widely applied battery of overall cognitive functioning is the *Wechsler Adult Intelligence Scales*, which is currently in its fourth edition (i.e., WAIS-IV; Wechsler, 2008). Although the WAIS-IV is a common component of psychology and neuropsychology evaluations, it is infrequently included in speech-language pathology assessments, in part due to the licensure and educational requirements (e.g., doctoral degree) for purchase of this test. The WAIS-IV consists of 10 core and 5 supplemental subtests that evaluate a range of verbal and nonverbal, or "performance," skills, including language (e.g., Vocabulary), auditory verbal memory (e.g., Digit Span), visuoconstruction (e.g., Block Design), and executive function (e.g., Matrix Reasoning) abilities. Compared with its earlier versions, the WAIS-IV provides more extensive norms covering ages 16 through 91; updated tasks, items, and visual stimuli (e.g., visual stimuli were enlarged to facilitate administration to older adults and patients with impaired visual acuity); and on several subtests, extended floors and shortened discontinue rules to provide a more informative and efficient assessment of patients with severe cognitive impairments. The entire test takes approximately 60 to 90 minutes to complete and allows calculation of a Full Intelligence quotient, five index scores (i.e., General Ability, Verbal Comprehension, Perceptual Reasoning, Working Memory, and Processing Speed), and scaled scores for individual subtests. Of greatest interest for identifying more specific areas of strength and weakness are individual subtest scores, patterns of performance across subtests, and index scores, rather than the intelligence quotient outcomes.

One of the more recently developed cognitive test batteries is the *Neuropsychological Assessment Battery* (NAB; Stern & White, 2003). It consists of 33 subtests grouped into six modules: Screening (e.g., Screening Mazes, Screening Word Generation), Attention (e.g., Digits Forward, Driving Scenes), Language (e.g., Oral Production, Writing), Memory (e.g., List Learning, Story Learning), Spatial (e.g., Visual Discrimination, Figure Drawing), and Executive Functions (e.g., Judgment, Categories). Importantly, each module, with the exception of the Screening module, contains one subtest that is more functional in nature. For example, the Daily Living Memory subtest requires patients to learn and then recall and recognize information such as medication instructions,

(text continues on p. 238)

TABLE 7-2
Cognitive Test Batteries

INSTRUMENT	SOURCE	GENERAL COGNITIVE FUNCTIONING	ATTENTION	MEMORY	EXECUTIVE FUNCTIONING
Barkley Deficits in Executive Functioning Scale	Barkley (2011)				X
Behavior Rating Inventory of Executive Function–Adult Version	Roth et al. (2005)				X
Behavioral Assessment of the Dysexecutive Syndrome	B. Wilson et al. (1996)				X
Birmingham Cognitive Screen	Humphreys, Bickerton, Samson, & Riddoch (2012)	X			
Delis-Kaplan Executive Function System	Delis et al. (2001)				X
Executive Control Battery	Goldberg, Podell, Bilder, & Jaeger (2000)				X
Executive Interview (EXIT)	Royall, Mahurin, & Gray (1992)				X
Functional Cognitive Assessment Scale	Kounti, Tsolaki, & Kiosseoglou (2006)				X
Halstead-Reitan Neuropsychological Test Battery	Reitan & Wolfson (1993)	X			
Kaplan Baycrest Neurocognitive Assessment	Kaplan, Leach, Rewilak, Richards, & Proulx (2000)	X			
Neuropsychological Assessment Battery	Stern & White (2003)	X			
Rivermead Behavioral Memory Test–Third Edition	B. Wilson et al. (2008)			X	
Ross Information Processing Assessment–Second Edition	Ross-Swain (1996)	X			
Ross Information Processing Assessment–Geriatric: 2	Ross-Swain & Fogle (2012)	X			
Scales of Cognitive and Communicative Ability for Neurorehabilitation	Milman & Holland (2012)	X			
Severe Impairment Battery	Saxton et al. (1993)	X			
Test of Everyday Attention	Robertson et al. (1994)		X		

TABLE 7-2 (continued)

INSTRUMENT	SOURCE	GENERAL COGNITIVE FUNCTIONING	ATTENTION	MEMORY	EXECUTIVE FUNCTIONING
Test of Memory and Learning–Second Edition	Reynolds & Voress (2007)			X	
Test of Memory and Learning–Senior Edition	Reynolds & Voress (2012)			X	
Wechsler Adult Intelligence Scale–Fourth Edition	Wechsler (2008)	X			
Wechsler Memory Scale–Fourth Edition	Wechsler (2009)			X	
Wessex Head Injury Matrix	Shiel et al. (2000)	X			
Wide Range Assessment of Memory and Learning–Second Edition	Adams & Sheslow (2003)			X	

an address, and a phone number. It takes approximately four hours to administer the entire battery, but the NAB was developed so that clinicians may choose to administer individual modules or subtests. The NAB provides two alternative forms to reduce practice effects, has excellent psychometric properties, was extensively standardized (i.e., $n = 1,448$) on a broad age range (18 to 97 years), and offers two sets of norms: (1) Demographically Corrected Norms that allow comparison of a patient's score to that of age-, sex-, and education-matched peers, and (2) U.S. Census–Matched Norms that allow comparison of a patient's score to that of an age-matched group representative of the current U.S. population in terms of education levels, ethnocultural background, and geographic region. Given that it costs approximately \$3,000 to purchase the entire NAB, the publisher has more recently allowed purchase of each of the individual modules described above, as well as certain NAB subtests. When the modules or subtests are purchased separately, they come with a manual that includes research published since the NAB's original publication (e.g., *NAB Mazes Test*; Stern & White, 2009a).

Based on our clinical experiences and on previous research conducted by Frank and Barrineau (1996), the *Ross Information Processing Assessment* (RIPA; D. Ross, 1986) appears to be the cognitive test battery most frequently utilized by speech-language pathologists, particularly when assessing the cognitive status of patients with TBI. In addition to the original RIPA, a revised version, RIPA-2 (Ross-Swain, 1996), as well as an updated version for geriatric inpatient populations, RIPA-Geriatric:2 (RIPA-G:2; Ross-Swain & Fogle, 2012), are currently available. All versions of the RIPA evaluate orientation, short- and long-term verbal memory, auditory comprehension, and some executive functioning skills (i.e., problem solving and verbal fluency tasks). Clinicians should avoid use of the original RIPA because of its psychometric weaknesses. And though the RIPA-2 has better reliability and validity qualities than its earlier version, it too has psychometric limitations, including construct validity problems. The RIPA-2 test manual stated that it is appropriate for patients up to age 90, but the oldest participants in the standardization sample were only 72 years of age; therefore, calculating standard scores and percentiles for patients over the age of 72 may be inappropriate. Instead, clinicians should use the RIPA-G:2 when evaluating elderly patients, as it has norms for adults ages 55 to 97 who represented a variety of neurogenic patient populations (i.e., mild cognitive impairment, Alzheimer's disease, right hemisphere brain damage [RHD], and TBI).

Some general cognitive test batteries have been designed for specific patient populations. For example, the *Wessex Head Injury Matrix* (Shiel, Wilson, McLellan, Horn, & Watson, 2000) represents one of the few assessment options available to document initial status, as well as slow and subtle progress, in patients with severe brain injuries. This test requires a health-care team member to rate patients on 62 items to monitor the integrity of cognitive skills, as well as communicative and social skills. These items can be rated by just observing or by testing the patient on certain tasks that involve everyday objects.

Other cognitive test batteries have been developed primarily for patients with dementia. For instance, the *Severe Impairment Battery* (SIB; Saxton et al., 1993) was designed for patients with severe cognitive and behavioral impairments associated with dementia. Versions of the SIB in languages other than English are also available (e.g., French version; Verny et al., 1999). Like other cognitive test batteries, the SIB evaluates attention, orientation, memory, and other cognitive skills; it differs, however, from other batteries in that SIB items are easier, and clinicians are allowed to give gestural cues. Furthermore, patients may receive credit for partial or gestural responses to help avoid a test performance profile referred to as a **basement** or **floor effect**, in which patients predominantly receive scores of zero. Consequently, researchers quantifying the effects of medications for advanced dementia often utilize the SIB (e.g., Tariot et al., 2004).

Test Batteries for Specific Cognitive Domains

When it is clear, based on observation, interview, and screening data, that the patient is displaying difficulty in only one or two cognitive domains, clinicians may opt to utilize test batteries that comprehensively assess only one cognitive domain. For example, if early assessment findings suggest that a patient has primarily memory problems, a memory test battery that evaluates a number of memory functions (e.g., verbal working memory, nonverbal short-term memory, episodic memory) might be selected rather than a general cognitive test battery that evaluates all cognitive domains. Batteries for specific cognitive domains typically consist of subtests that represent shorter versions of a collection of specific cognitive function tests. For instance, the *Delis-Kaplan Executive Function System* (D-KEFS; Delis et al., 2001) consists of nine tests, most of which were or are available as separate tests (e.g., Trail Making, Color–Word Interference [similar to the Stroop test], Proverb). The strength of cognitive domain batteries is that they evaluate a number of skills within one cognitive area (e.g., separate subtests for sustained, focused, and divided attention skills) and thus provide the clinician with detailed information regarding strengths and weaknesses within that cognitive domain, which in turn will help identify specific treatment goals and procedures.

Attention Test Batteries

Presently, clinicians have a limited choice of attention test batteries (see Table 7-2). Of those available, the *Test of Everyday Attention* (TEA; Robertson, Ward, Ridgeway, & Nimmo-Smith, 1994) has been the most frequently used and evaluated in the research literature (e.g., A. Bate, Mathias, & Crawford, 2001; Murray, 2012b) and has gained acceptance in both speech-language pathology and neuropsychology clinical practice (e.g., Kinsella, 1998; L. Murray, 2002a). The TEA consists of eight subtests designed to evaluate a number of attention functions in adults 16 to 80 years of age (Robertson et al., 1994). Example subtests are as follows: (a) To assess attention switching, the Visual Elevator subtest requires patients to switch between counting forward and backward to figure out at which floor an elevator arrives; (b) to assess sustained attention, the Lottery subtest requires patients to listen for a target lottery number among a long list of numbers; (c) to assess focused attention, the Elevator Counting With Distraction subtest requires patients to count one type of tone stimulus and ignore another to figure out at which floor an elevator arrives; and (d) to assess divided attention abilities, the Telephone Search While Counting subtest requires patients to complete a counting and a visual scanning task at the same time. In contrast to most other attention tests, the TEA utilizes everyday life materials and tasks and, accordingly, has been found to have good ecological validity. For example, the Map Search subtest, which evaluates visual selective attention, requires patients to scan a large map of a city to locate all the symbols indicative of a restaurant. Other strengths of the TEA are that it provides parallel forms to facilitate measuring changes in attention abilities over time, and it has been standardized on adults with hearing impairments (Robertson et al., 1994), as well as patients representing a range of neurological disorders, including stroke, head injury, and progressive dementing diseases (Robertson, Ward, Ridgeway, & Nimmo-Smith, 1996). It has also been used recently in empirical studies evaluating attention abilities in patients with mild to moderately severe aphasia (Murray, 2012b).

Memory Test Batteries. Of the various memory batteries currently available, the *Wechsler Memory Scale*, now in its fourth edition (i.e., WMS-IV; Wechsler, 2009), is certainly the most frequently used. The WMS-IV evaluates auditory and visual learning, and auditory and visual short- and long-term memory functions. An example auditory memory subtest is Logical Memory, which requires patients to retell a story immediately and then after a 25- to 35-minute delay. One of the visual memory subtests is Spatial Addition, for which patients indicate the location of blue dots, which were shown on two previous grids; the task involves ignoring red dots while also determining which blue dots were shown on only one prior grid versus those that were shown on both prior grids. Several memory indices can be calculated (i.e., Immediate and Delayed Memory Indices, Auditory and Visual Indices, and Visual Working Memory), along with contrast scores (e.g., Immediate vs. Delayed Memory) to describe the memory strengths and weaknesses of a given patient. Compared to its earlier versions, WMS-IV improvements include the development of separate batteries for younger adults (i.e., Adult Battery for ages 16 to 69) and older adults (i.e., Older Adult Battery for ages 65 to 91); although these batteries are similar, they each include some unique stimuli, and test administration and scoring procedures are adapted to meet the needs of these two age groups. WMS-IV software to assist with scoring and report writing is also available. Like the WAIS-IV, the WMS-IV is most frequently administered by psychologists and neuropsychologists due to the licensure and education purchase restrictions listed by the publisher.

In an attempt to develop a memory test with ecological validity, Wilson and colleagues created the *Rivermead Behavioral Memory Test*, which is now in its third edition (RBMT-III; B. Wilson et al., 2008). This memory battery utilizes tasks analogous to everyday memory activities (such as remembering a short route, the name of a person, or that an appointment needs to be made) or learning a new skill. Consequently, performances of these types of tasks have been found to predict accurately functional independence and employment outcomes in many cultures and countries (Fraser, Glass, & Leathem, 1999; Man & Li, 2001). The RBMT-III can be administered fairly quickly (in about 25 to 30 minutes) and provides normative data on individuals varying from age

16 to 96 years. This test provides alternate forms so that it can be administered repeatedly to monitor treatment effects and avoid practice effects.

Executive Functioning Test Batteries. Executive function test batteries are particularly useful because, as Delis and colleagues (2001) noted, "the single-score method is especially problematic with executive-function tasks because such tests typically tap a host of fundamental and higher-level cognitive skills. Patients perform poorly on executive-function tests for vastly different reasons, and the single score provided by most of the existing instruments often fails to provide useful data for capturing the neurocognitive mechanisms of the impairment" (pp. 4–5). That is, relying on just one test of executive functioning might result in over- or underestimating the integrity of a given patient's executive function abilities (Constantinidou et al., 2012; Pickens, Ostwald, Murphy-Pace, & Bergstrom, 2010). For example, overestimation may result because only one or a limited number of executive skills were evaluated, and those executive skills were not those that are problematic for the patient. Underestimation may occur when a patient displays difficulty on an executive function test, not because of a deficit in that executive skill but rather because of impairments in other, more basic cognitive abilities, such as attention; likewise, many other executive function abilities may be relatively intact in that patient, but if these were not evaluated, the clinician remains unaware of these areas of strength.

Accordingly, clinicians should consider administering an executive function test battery (or a number of executive function tests) so that a range of executive skills is assessed. MacNeill Horton, Soper, and Reynolds (2010) recommended that the array of executive function measures used should vary not only in terms of which executive function or functions are assessed but also in terms of the measures' task demands (e.g., high vs. low motor demands; high vs. low language demands). Clinicians also should ensure that tests of more basic cognitive abilities have already been administered so that performances on executive function tests can be interpreted in the light of these other cognitive test results.

A number of executive function test batteries are available (Table 7-2). The *Delis-Kaplan Executive Function System* (D-KEFS; Delis et al., 2001) has nine subtests that can be used alone or in combination with other D-KEFS subtests and that are designed to evaluate a number of verbal and nonverbal executive function abilities, such as cognitive flexibility, inhibition, and problem solving. Specific subtests include the Trail Making, Verbal and Design Fluency, Color–Word Interference, Sorting, Twenty Questions, Word Context, Tower, and Proverb tests. Several of these subtests represent versions of tests that were previously available separately, either commercially or in the research literature. For example, the D-KEFS's Sorting Test was previously known as the California Card Sorting Test (Delis, Squire, Bihrle, & Massman, 1992). The advantages of using the D-KEFS versus individual executive function tests include the following: (a) To improve the reliability of repeated testing, the D-KEFS provides alternate forms for three subtests: Sorting, Twenty Questions, and Verbal Fluency; (b) the D-KEFS's normative data encompass ages 8 through 89 years; and (c) in terms of severity, the D-KEFS is sensitive to the full spectrum of executive function deficits. In terms of scoring, many D-KEFS subtests provide several measures to reflect the variety of basic and complex cognitive abilities assessed by these subtests. Clinicians also may calculate indices for key executive function abilities, including initiation, verbal concept formation, nonverbal concept formation, cognitive flexibility, and behavioral response flexibility based on performance of a number of subtests. Use of the contrast scores (which allow identifying discrepancies among the key executive abilities), however, is not recommended because of inadequate reliability levels (Pickens et al., 2010).

The seven subtests of the *Behavioral Assessment of Dysexecutive Syndrome* (BADS; Wilson et al., 1996) were designed to evaluate executive functioning via tasks that are more similar to daily activities than those of the D-KEFS. For example, the Key Search Test assesses planning and self-monitoring by asking patients to draw the route they would take to find a lost set of keys in a large field (illustrated by a square on a piece of paper). The Zoo Map Test examines planning and **cognitive flexibility** by requiring patients to draw the route they would take to visit a number of prescribed locations on a map of a zoo while also following a set of stipulations, such as traveling on certain paths only once. The BADS is suitable for a broad range of patients and provides normative data for healthy adults 16 to 87 years of age and individuals with brain damage 19 to 76 years of age. Additionally, certain BADS subtests have been shown to be useful in other languages and cultures (e.g., R. Chan & Manly, 2002).

More recently, virtual reality technology has been exploited to allow evaluating executive functioning in environments that simulate real-world settings. For example, the Virtual Library Task (VLT; Renison, Ponsford, Testa, Richardson, & Brownfield, 2008) examines a number of executive abilities by requiring patients to complete several tasks in a virtual library. The virtual library is achieved via a computer, software, and an Xbox or PlayStation hand controller. Example tasks include determining the best order in which to complete tasks on a to-do list (evaluates planning), figuring out how to cool the library when the patient learns the library air conditioner is broken (evaluates problem solving), and inhibiting answering the telephone (evaluates inhibition). The test takes between 9 and 20 minutes to complete, depending on the patient's abilities. The VLT has been shown to be ecologically valid and compared with other executive function tests, more sensitive to executive function problems subsequent to TBI (Renison, Ponsford, Testa, Richardson, & Brownfield, 2012).

Other executive function measures require patients to complete activities in real-world settings (e.g., Multiple Errands Test; Burgess et al., 2006). Given the complexity of most daily tasks, as well as the less predictable nature of daily environments, these measures allow evaluating a number of executive functions and, like the virtual reality tests described above, are ecologically valid. As an example, Chevignard and colleagues (2008) developed a cooking task that requires the patient to make a chocolate cake and an omelette for two people. Instructions to complete the task are relatively open-ended in that the patient is only oriented to where items necessary to complete that task are located (the task was designed to be completed in the kitchen typically located in the occupational therapy unit of rehabilitation departments), told what must be made, and instructed to leave the kitchen in the same condition as it was prior to starting the task. Thus, this task involves a number of executive skills, including planning, problem solving, cognitive flexibility, and inhibition. A detailed scoring system has been developed so that both quantitative data (e.g., time to complete the task, number of errors) and qualitative data (e.g., whether the food was edible, types of errors) can be recorded. Importantly, these ecologically valid tasks identify executive function deficits that are not captured on more structured cognitive tests (Burgess et al., 2006; Chevignard et al., 2008; Constantinidou et al., 2012; Schmitter-Edgecombe et al., 2011).

In contrast to the above executive function tests that require patients to complete a set of tasks, a few executive function measures, such as the *Barkley Deficits in Executive Functioning Scale* (BDEFS; Barkley, 2011) and the *Behavior Rating Inventory of Executive Function–Adult Version* (BRIEF-A; Roth, Isquith, & Gioia, 2005), collect self- and/or caregiver-report data. For instance, the BRIEF-A evaluates the perceptions of patients and informants (i.e., individuals who are familiar with the patients' everyday, functional status) regarding the patients' executive functioning in daily environments. It was normed on a broad age range (adults 18 to 90 years), has been validated with a number of clinical populations (e.g., with multiple sclerosis, with TBI), and is available in over 20 languages (e.g., French, German, Spanish, Korean). There are two forms, one for the patient to complete and one for the informant to complete. Both forms contain 75 items that examine a number of executive functions, including inhibition, self-monitoring, initiation, and planning. The BRIEF-A yields scores pertaining to the broad indices of Behavioral Regulation and Metacognition, which when combined provide a composite score of overall executive functioning. Given that both the BDEFS and BRIEF-A allow examining and comparing patient and informant ratings, they may be particularly helpful in identifying anosognosia.

Tests of Specific Cognitive Functions

There are numerous choices available when clinicians are looking for tests to assess specific attention, memory, or executive function abilities. Table 7-3 contains only a small sample of tests that can be found commercially or in the research literature that are appropriate for one or more neurogenic patient populations. Clinicians should base their test selections on previous observation, interview, or test battery findings, and on patients' concomitant symptoms. For example, when attempting to assess a patient with reduced visual acuity, the clinician should rely on tests that utilize auditory stimuli. Likewise, clinicians assessing cognitive abilities in patients with severe aphasia may choose tests with relatively low language demands, in terms of both test stimuli and response requirements. Clinicians also must keep in mind that many well-established measures purported to evaluate a specific cognitive function actually are multifactorial in nature. This means that several cognitive skills are needed to complete (and thus are assessed by) these tests (Lezak et al., 2004; L. Murray & Ramage, 2000; Stuss, 2011). For example, several attention tests, such as the *Paced Auditory Serial Addition Test* (Gronwall, 1977)

(text continues on p. 248)

TABLE 7-3
Measures of Specific Cognitive Functions

INSTRUMENT	SOURCE	ATTENTION	EXECUTIVE FUNCTIONS	NEGLECT	NONVERBAL MEMORY	VERBAL MEMORY
Auditory-Verbal Working Memory Test	Tompkins et al. (1994)					X
Balloons Test*	Edgeworth et al. (1998)			X		
Behavioral Inattention Test*	B. Wilson et al. (1987)			X		
Benton Visual Retention Test*	Sivan (1991)				X	
Beta III*	Kellogg & Morton (1999)		X			
Booklet Category Test-Second Edition	DeFilippis & McCampbell (1997)		X			
Brief Test of Attention	Schretlen (1997)	X				
Brief Visuospatial Memory Test-Revised*	Benedict (1997)				X	
Burning House Test	J. C. Marshall & Halligan (1988)			X		
Butt Non-Verbal Reasoning Test*	Butt & Bucks (2004)		X			
Calibrated Ideational Fluency Assessment	Schretlen & Vannorsdall, (2011)		X			
California Verbal Learning Test-Second Edition	Delis et al. (2000)					X
Cambridge Prospective Memory Test*	B. Wilson et al. (2005)				X	X
Catherine Bergego Scale*	Azouvi et al. (2003, 2006)			X		
Color Trails Test*	D'Elia et al. (1996)	X	X			
Comb and Razor Test*	McIntosh et al. (2000)			X		
Common Objects Memory Test	Kempler et al. (2010)					X
Comprehensive Test of Nonverbal Intelligence-Second Edition*	Hammill et al. (2009)		X			

TABLE 7-3 (continued)

INSTRUMENT	SOURCE	ATTENTION	EXECUTIVE FUNCTIONS	NEGLECT	NONVERBAL MEMORY	VERBAL MEMORY
Comprehensive Trail-Making Test	Reynolds (2002)	X				
Conners' Continuous Performance Test–Third Edition	Conners (2013)	X				
Contextual Memory Test	Toglia (1993)					X
Continuous Visual Memory Test	Trahan & Larrabee (1988)				X	
Criterion-Oriented Test of Attention	M. Williams (1994b)	X				
d2 Test of Attention*	Brickenkamp & Zillmer (1998)	X				
Doors and People*	Baddeley, Emslie, & Nimmo-Smith (1994)				X	X
Executive Function Route-Finding Task	Boyd & Sauter (1994)		X			
Expanded Trail Making Test	Stanczak et al. (1998)	X				
FAS/Controlled Oral Word Association Test	Benton et al. (2001)		X			
Functional Assessment of Verbal Reasoning and Executive Strategies	MacDonald (2005)		X			
Hopkins Verbal Learning Test–Revised	Brandt & Benedict (2001)					X
Indented Paragraph Test	B. Caplan (1987)			X		
Kicking Test	Grossi et al. (2001)			X		
Location Learning Test*	Bucks et al. (2000)				X	
Memory for Intentions Test	D. Raskin & Buckheit (2010)				X	X
Modified Wisconsin Card Sorting Test*	Schretlen (2011)		X			
NAB Mazes Test*	Stern & White (2009a)		X			
Paced Auditory Serial Addition Test	Gronwall (1977)	X				X

(continues)

TABLE 7-3 (continued)

INSTRUMENT	SOURCE	ATTENTION	EXECUTIVE FUNCTIONS	NEGLECT	NONVERBAL MEMORY	VERBAL MEMORY
Photocopy Tasks	Crepeau et al. (1997)		X			
Porteus Maze Test*	Porteus (1965)		X			
Rapid Assessment of Problem Solving	R. Marshall et al. (2003); R. Marshall & Karow (2008)		X			
Raven's Progressive Matrices*	Raven (2003)		X			
Recognition Memory Test*	Warrington (1999)				X	X
Rey Complex Figure Test and Recognition Trial*	Meyers & Meyers (1995)				X	
Ruff Figural Fluency Test*	Ruff (1996)		X			
SCAN-3: A Test for Auditory Processing Disorders in Adolescents and Adults	Keith (2009)	X				
Selective Reminding Test	Buschke (1973)					X
Sentence Repetition Test	Spreen & Strauss (2006); Meyers et al. (2000)					X
Stroop Color and Word Test	Golden (2002)	X	X			
Stroop Neuropsychological Screening Test	Trenerry et al. (1989)	X	X			
Tasks of Executive Control	Isquith et al. (2010)		X			
Test of Nonverbal Intelligence–Fourth Edition*	L. Brown et al. (2010)		X			
Test of Problem Solving–Second Edition: Adolescent	Bowers et al. (2007)		X			
Test of Variables of Attention, Version 8	Greenberg (2011)	X				
Test of Verbal Conceptualization and Fluency	Reynolds & Horton (2007)		X			
Test of Visual Field Attention*	M. Williams (1994c)			X		
The Category Test*	M. Williams (1994a)		X			
Tinkertoy Test	Lezak et al. (2004)		X			

TABLE 7-3 (continued)

INSTRUMENT	SOURCE	ATTENTION	EXECUTIVE FUNCTIONS	NEGLECT	NONVERBAL MEMORY	VERBAL MEMORY
Tower of Hanoi*	Simon (1975)		X			
Tower of London DX–Second Edition*	Culbertson & Zillmer (2012)		X			
Trail Making Test	Reitan & Wolfson (1985)	X				
Verbal and Nonverbal Cancellation Test*	Weintraub & Mesulam (1985)			X		
Vigil Continuous Performance Test	The Psychological Corporation (1996)	X				
Visual Patterns Test*	Della Sala, Gray, Baddeley, & Wilson (1997)					X
Visual Search and Attention Test	Trenerry, Crosson, DeBoe, & Leber (1990)			X		
Wechsler Test of Adult Reading	Wechsler (2001)					X
Wheelbarrow Test	O. Butler et al. (1989)		X			
Williams Inhibition Test*	Williams (1994d)		X			

*Indicates that subtests or entire test may be suitable for patients with language production and/or comprehension impairments.

and the *Criterion-Oriented Test of Attention* (M. Williams, 1994b), exploit not only attention but also complex language and math skills for completion; therefore, before using these tests' findings to make final conclusions regarding the integrity of attention, clinicians also must have accrued additional assessment data concerning the integrity of these other skills.

Test of Specific Attention Functions

Given that attention encompasses a number of cognitive skills, including sustained attention, focused or selective attention, attention switching, and divided attention, tests that assess one or a few specific attention functions in the modality of audition, vision, or both are available (see Table 7-3). Examples of tests that evaluate these different attention functions are described below. Because it is difficult to isolate specific cognitive skills, however, clinicians are reminded that some attention tests assess additional cognitive abilities. This is why certain tests are listed as both attention and executive function tests in Table 7-3.

Sustained attention tests typically involve completing mundane tasks (e.g., monitoring for a visual or auditory target in the absence or presence of foils) for extended time periods. Many currently available sustained attention tests, such as the *Test of Variables of Attention–8* (Greenberg, 2011), *Conners' Continuous Performance Test III* (Conners, 2013), and *Vigil Continuous Performance Test* (The Psychological Cooperation, 1996), are computer-based. For example, the *Vigil Continuous Performance Test* provides computerized administration and scoring of several sustained attention tasks, each of which takes about eight minutes to complete. These tests can be varied in terms of complexity (e.g., rate of stimulus presentation) and stimulus type (e.g., verbal vs. nonverbal targets) and are suitable for a broad age range of 6 to 90 years. Whatever test is used to evaluate sustained attention, the clinician should monitor not only the amount of time patients are on task but also whether they can maintain performance quality over time.

Focused or selective attention tests are similar to complex sustained attention tasks in that they require identifying target stimuli while rejecting irrelevant stimuli. One of the long-standing tests used to evaluate focused attention, as well as attention switching, is the *Trail Making Test* (Reitan & Wolfson, 1993). This test has normative data for elderly patients (Spreen & Strauss, 2006) and has been found sensitive to even subtle deficits associated with mild acquired brain damage (Brooks, Fos, Greve, & Hammond, 1999; C. Reynolds & Horton, 2007). Currently several versions of this test are available, including the *Color Trails Test* (D'Elia, Satz, Uchiyama, & White, 1996), the *Comprehensive Trail-Making Test* (C. Reynolds, 2002), and the *Expanded Trail Making Test* (Stanczak, Lynch, McNeil, & Brown, 1998). Basically, *Trails* tests involve connecting a series of stimuli (e.g., numbers written as numerals or, in words, letters) in a set order as quickly as possible. In one condition, patients typically are asked to connect one stimulus series, whereas in the other, more complex condition, they must switch between connecting a stimulus from one series with that from the other. For example, in the simpler condition, patients might be required to connect numbers in increasing order, whereas in the more complex condition, they would have to connect numbers and letters in increasing order by alternating between the numbers and letters (e.g., 1 – A – 2 – B – 3 – C, etc.). The *Color* (D'Elia et al., 1996) and *Expanded* (Stanczak et al., 1998) versions were developed for patient populations who have communication disorders that may confound their performance of the original test, which requires connecting letters and numbers. For example, in the *Expanded* version, patients connect a series of clock faces drawn with clock hands and tick marks, rather than numbers in ascending time order (e.g., 12:00, 12:15, 12:30) or a series of black dots in order of increasing size. Because of its low language demands, this version of the *Trails* would be appropriate for patients with number- or letter-recognition problems.

Few test options are available for assessing **divided attention.** Dual-task procedures are typically used because divided attention refers to the ability to complete more than one task at the same time (L. Murray, 2002a). Although several dual-task protocols are described in the research literature (e.g., Holtzer, Burright, & Donovick, 2004; L. Murray, 2000a), currently only a limited number of commercially available dual-task tests are available. One option is the Telephone Search While Counting subtest of the TEA (Robertson et al., 1994). On this subtest, patients must, at the same time, count strings of audiotaped tones and search a replica of a page from a telephone book for pre-specified target businesses; their dual-task performances are then quantified in terms of accuracy and total response time. There remains a clear need to develop more tests of divided attention, particularly those with minimal language demands, as only patients with mild to moderate aphasia may be able to perform this TEA subtest without their language deficits significantly impeding their performance (L. Murray, 2012b).

Neglect Tests. As neglect is considered a disorder of attention (Kortte & Hillis, 2011; see also Chapter 2), tests for identifying the presence and severity of neglect are discussed here. Even though patients with neglect can often have relatively intact speech, language, and memory skills, they still have a much poorer prognosis for an independent outcome compared to patients without neglect (de Haan et al., 2006; Jehkonen et al., 2000; Kortte & Hillis, 2011). Consequently, it is important not only to document the presence of neglect but also to determine which environmental conditions exacerbate or ameliorate neglect symptoms. Clinicians also are reminded that although neglect is most frequently associated with right hemisphere brain damage (Kortte & Hillis, 2011), it also can occur following left hemisphere damage, and thus may be a possible symptom in a variety of neurogenic disorders, including aphasia (Wee & Hopman, 2008), dementia (Oda et al., 2008), and cognitive-communicative impairments associated with traumatic brain injury (Cocchini et al., 2002).

A number of tests and research protocols are available to identify the presence of neglect. These assessment tools frequently involve one or more of the following tasks (Azouvi et al., 2006; Cherney, 2002; Golisz, 1998; Vallar, 2007): (a) line bisection, in which patients try to divide a line in half (patients with neglect will mark the line toward their ipsilesional side); (b) cancellation tasks, in which patients cross out or identify a target letter, number, object, or shape among an array of stimuli (patients with neglect will fail to cross out more stimuli on their contralesional vs. ipsilesional side);

(c) drawing or copying of symmetrical objects or shapes, or preferably asymmetrical stimuli, as these have been found to be more sensitive to subtle forms of neglect (patients with neglect will leave out more details on the contralesional vs. ipsilesional side of their drawing); and (d) reading aloud or copying of words, sentences, and/or paragraphs (patients with neglect may omit or make substitution errors when reading or writing letters, syllables, or words on their contralesional side). Clinicians can manipulate a number of variables to increase or decrease the complexity of neglect tasks (Table 7-4). Complexity should be increased when mild neglect problems are suspected (Rabuffetti et al., 2012). Due to the variable sensitivity of the above-mentioned neglect tasks, as well as patient variability in completing these tasks, it is recommended that several neglect measures be administered (Azouvi et al., 2006; R. Hamilton et al., 2008; Shiraishi, Yamakawa, Itou, Muraki, & Asada, 2008).

Commercially available tests of neglect vary in length and, consequently, comprehensiveness (see Table 7-3). For example, for a quick visual neglect screening tool, clinicians might consider the *Balloons Test* (Edgeworth, Robertson, & MacMillan, 1998). This cancellation task takes only about six minutes to administer. Its first subtest requires canceling out line drawings of balloons from among line drawings of circles; the second

TABLE 7-4
Variables to Manipulate the Complexity of Neglect Tests

TYPE OF TASK	VARIABLES TO INCREASE TASK COMPLEXITY	VARIABLES TO DECREASE TASK COMPLEXITY
Cancellation tasks	• Similar targets and foils • Scattered distribution of stimuli • Complex stimuli (e.g., letters) • Dense stimulus presentation • Many foils	• Dissimilar targets and foils • Arranged display of stimuli (e.g., rows, columns) • Simple stimuli (e.g., basic shapes) • Dispersed stimulus presentation • Few foils
Line bisection	• Long line • Extrapersonal space (e.g., on wall with light pointer) • Vertical or radial line orientation • No anchor	• Short line • Peripersonal space (e.g., tabletop) • Horizontal line orientation • Anchor placed at neglected end of line
Drawing/ copying	• Asymmetrical stimulus • Spatially separated (e.g., two objects)	• Symmetrical stimulus • Spatially integrated or meaningful scene (e.g., two men shaking hands)
Writing	• Pseudowords	• Real words
Reading aloud	• Long text (e.g., passage containing several paragraphs) • Irregular margins (e.g., margins for first line of text are 1 inch, margins for second line of text are 2 inches, margins for third line of text are .25 inches)	• Short text (e.g., single sentence) • Consistent left and right margins

subtest is a more complex, inverse version of the first subtest and involves canceling out the circles (which perceptually do not "pop out" as much) from among the balloons.

On the other end of the length spectrum is the *Behavioral Inattention Test* (BIT; B. Wilson, Cockburn, & Halligan, 1987), which consists of (a) six conventional paper-and-pencil subtests (such as line bisection, drawing, and figure copying) that take about 10 minutes to complete and (b) several more functional or "behavioral" subtests (such as telephone dialing, menu and article reading, telling and setting the time, and map navigation) that take about 45 minutes to complete. Patients' scores on the conventional and behavioral portions are calculated, and cutoff scores are provided to determine the presence of unilateral visual neglect. Research indicates that the conventional and behavioral portions of the BIT are significantly correlated (Cassidy, Lewis, & Gray, 1998; Cherney & Halper, 2001), suggesting that administering only the conventional portion may be adequate if clinicians are faced with significant assessment time constraints. More recently, Nurmi and colleagues (2010) reported that mild visual neglect could be identified on the BIT if clinicians monitored how patients complete the BIT cancellation tasks; that is, these researchers found that starting more than one cancellation task on the right side of the page was indicative of neglect (regardless of whether or not all targets are cancelled out).

Whereas the above tests document response accuracy, a few tests also allow collecting reaction times, which in turn may provide a more sensitive measure of neglect. For example, M. Williams's (1994c) *Test of Visual Field Attention* is a software program through which patients indicate via a mouse-press response whenever they see a simple visual stimulus on the computer screen. The visual stimuli are presented at random locations, so that by the end of the test, the patients' accuracy and response times for stimuli presented to each visual quadrant or central versus peripheral fields can be determined. Similarly, researchers have developed computerized methods for administering standard visual neglect tasks, such as line bisection and cancellation (Potter et al., 2000; Rabuffetti et al., 2012). Rabuffetti and colleagues used touch screen technology for administration of letter and shape cancellation tasks. Their software permits documenting not only cancellation accuracy (e.g., how many targets were not cancelled; how many distracters were cancelled) but also quantification of how the cancellation task was completed (e.g., length of time to detect each target; distance between targets cancelled to characterize search pattern; lateral vs. horizontal search direction). The researchers found that their computerized task identified individuals with brain damage and visual neglect (i.e., significant differences between the group with neglect and non–brain-damaged controls), as well as individuals with brain damage without neglect but with spatial exploration deficits (e.g., significantly slower search compared to non–brain-damaged controls); these findings underscore the sensitivity of their protocol to subtle neglect and visuospatial perceptual symptoms.

Although several test options are available for assessing the presence and severity of neglect, few of these go beyond evaluating visuospatial neglect and thus may overlook other neglect symptoms, such as sensory extinction, auditory neglect (although for an example of an auditory neglect task, see Eramudugolla & Mattingley, 2008), or hemiakinesia (Azouvi et al., 2002, 2006; see also Chapter 2). Most neglect tests, especially those that are commercially available, have normative data that require updating (e.g., BIT was published 25 years ago). Another criticism of most neglect tests is their questionable ecological validity and test–retest reliability (Azouvi et al., 2003, 2006; Kortte & Hillis, 2009; Rabuffetti et al., 2012). That is, patients who perform within the normal range on many of these paper-and-pencil tests may still display or report significant neglect problems in their daily environments. Accordingly, more recently developed neglect measures described in the research literature involve observing patients as they complete more functional, daily tasks (e.g., using a wheelchair [Turton et al., 2009]; following a path while kicking small obstacles out of the way [Grossi et al., 2001]) or using virtual environments (achieved via computer software), which allow documenting search patterns, eye gaze and postural changes, along with other accuracy and response-time measures while patients complete orientation and search tasks (Tsirlin, Dupierrix, Chokron, Coquillart, & Ohlmann, 2009).

Tests of Specific Memory Functions

There are a myriad of memory tests available, some that focus more on evaluating verbal memory skills and others that aim to evaluate nonverbal or visual memory skills. Selection from these should be based on specific assessment goals, time availability, and, depending on the patient's communication and physical abilities, test adaptability. For example, patients with neurogenic language or motor speech disorders often are given nonverbal or visual memory tests that use drawings and objects versus linguistic stimuli in an attempt to circumvent these patients' communicative problems and, consequently, to allow an unconfounded view of their memory abilities. Healthy adults, however, often exploit their verbal skills (e.g., subvocalization of object names) to aid their performance on these "nonverbal," visual tests; consequently, clinicians must be vigilant in determining whether the poor visual memory test performances of patients with communication disorders reflect impaired language, a true memory deficit, or perhaps a combination of both.

Verbal Memory Tests. One of the more frequently administered tests of verbal memory is the *California Verbal Learning Test–Second Edition* (CVLT-2; Delis, Kramer, Kaplan, & Ober, 2000). This test, as well as those similar to it, such as the *Hopkins Verbal Learning Test–Revised* (Brandt & Benedict, 2001), is popular because it provides information regarding a number of auditory verbal memory functions, including recall and recognition accuracy, encoding strategies (e.g., ability to use semantic clustering), learning rates, and error types (e.g., perseverative responses, false-positive errors). Basically, the CVLT requires patients to learn, recall, and recognize a 16-item "shopping list" of words that represent four semantic categories (e.g., clothes, fruits) (Delis et al., 2000). Over five consecutive trials, patients listen to the list read by the examiner and then immediately try to recall as many items as possible. After these trials, a new "shopping list" of 16 items is read aloud for patients to recall; this second list allows the clinician to evaluate proactive interference, in which patients use words from the first list while trying to recall the second list, and retroactive interference, in which patients use words from the second list while trying to recall the first list during subsequent delayed trials. Next, patients are instructed to recall as many items as possible from the first list, followed by a cued recall task in which they are given category cues for items that they fail to recall; these free and cued recall tasks are then repeated 25 minutes later to evaluate unstructured and structured retrieval, respectively, from long-term memory. The final step of the CVLT is a recognition task in which clients listen to a word list and indicate which items are from the first shopping list. This test also provides a short form that may be useful when there are time constraints or the patient fatigues easily. Finally, the CVLT may be used with commercially available software to aid in scoring and in comparing test performances to normative data.

Other verbal memory tests are less comprehensive and examine only a subset of the memory abilities evaluated by the CVLT. For example, there are a variety of span tasks available that only assess immediate verbal memory span. These span tasks are sometimes categorized as tests of basic attention ability, as span performance can be affected negatively by concentration problems (Butters, Delis, & Lucas, 1995; Lezak et al., 2004). Verbal span tasks can be found on several test batteries, as well as in the research literature, and typically require the patient to repeat back a series of digits (e.g., Digit Span of the WAIS-IV), syllables (see Lezak et al., 2004 for examples), phrases (e.g., Repetition subtest of the *Arizona Battery of Communication Disorders of Dementia* [ABCD]; Bayles & Tomoeda, 1993), or sentences (e.g., *Sentence Repetition Test*; Spreen & Strauss, 2006; Meyers, Volkert, & Diep, 2000) in the same order as the clinician presented them. A more functional span task is the Telephone Test, which requires patients to recall 7- and 10-digit strings that are presented visually in a format akin to telephone numbers (Crook, Ferris, McCarthy, & Rae, 1980). Generally, forward span measures by themselves are not informative, as many neurogenic patient populations adequately perform these tasks, particularly if they have suffered only mild to moderate degrees of brain damage or are in the early to middle stages of a dementing disease (Lezak et al., 2004; L. Murray, 2002b; Vakil, 2005).

Verbal **working memory** tests are similar to span tasks in that they require the temporary storage and then recall of verbal information. They differ from span tasks, however, in that they also impose some form of interference on patients while those patients are trying to hold that information temporarily (A. Conway et al., 2005; H. Wright & Fergadiotis, 2012). For example, backward span tasks, such as the Digits Backwards subtest of the WAIS-IV, are proposed to assess working memory because not only must patients temporarily retain a list of items but then they also must switch the order of those items before responding (Vakil, 2005). Another example of a complex span task is Tompkins and colleagues' (1994) auditory-verbal working memory test, in which patients listen to sets of audiotaped sentences that increase over time in terms of the number of sentences within a set (see Figure 7-2). For each sentence set, patients must try to recall the last word of each sentence *and* indicate whether each sentence is true or false (i.e., the interference component of the task). Clinicians then tally the number of word recall and true/false errors and can compare their patients' performances to those

2-Sentences Set	
You sit on a **chair**.	True
Trains can **fly**.	False
3-Sentences Set	
Sugar is **sweet**.	True
Florida is next to **Ohio**.	False
Horses run in the **sky**.	False
4-Sentences Set	
Twelve equals one **dozen**.	True
Bicycles are slower than **cars**.	True
A book can **play**.	False
Feathers can **tickle**.	True
5-Sentences Set	
Carrots can **dance**.	False
Fish swim in **water**.	True
You sleep on a **bed**.	True
You eat breakfast at **night**.	False
People have **eyes**.	True

Figure 7-2. Sample stimulus items from Tompkins and colleagues' (1994) auditory-verbal working memory test. *Note.* Bolded words are those that must be recalled after each sentence in the set has been presented.

reported for healthy adults or individuals with left or right hemisphere brain damage by Tompkins and colleagues (Lehman & Tompkins, 1998; Tompkins et al., 1994).

As an alternative to complex span tasks, *n*-back tasks may also be used to evaluate verbal working memory (Mayer & Murray, 2013; H. Wright & Fergadiotis, 2012). *N*-back tasks require the patient to recall whether each stimulus in a series of stimuli was previously shown *n* items ago; *n* represents the number, typically varying from 1 to 3. An example *n*-back task is shown in Figure 7-3. Such tasks involve temporarily storing stimuli, determining possible stimuli matches, and consistently updating working memory contents. *N*-back tasks are typically computerized so that both response accuracy (e.g., hits, misses, false alarms) and speed can be recorded.

Other working memory tests can be found in the research literature (e.g., Conway et al., 2005) or as subtests on cognitive or memory test batteries (e.g., WAIS-IV Letter-Number Sequencing). Establishing the integrity of working memory in patients with neurogenic language disorders is important because a growing research literature has documented a positive relationship between working memory and language abilities in a number of neurogenic patient populations (Bayles, 2003; Bittner & Crowe, 2006; Hochstadt et al., 2006; Sung et al., 2009).

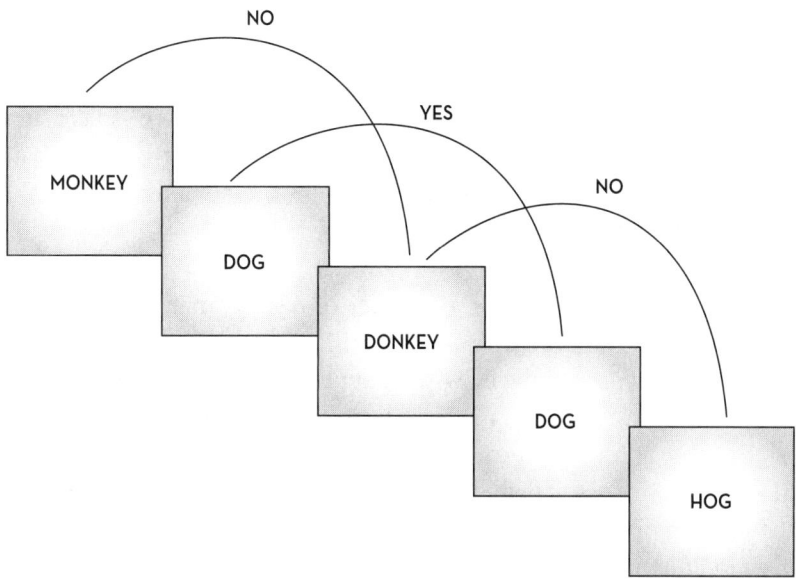

Figure 7-3. Example of an *n*-back task used to evaluate verbal working memory. In this figure, a 2-back task is shown in which the patient is first shown the word "monkey" on the computer screen; this word disappears when the next word, "dog," appears. The patient must determine for subsequent words whether the word shown matches that shown two stimuli back, hitting the YES key if it is a match and the NO key if it is not. Therefore, when the word "donkey" appears, the patient hits the NO key because it does not match the word shown 2 back (i.e., "monkey").

Story retelling tasks also are used to evaluate immediate and delayed verbal memory. In many cases, these tasks are preferable to span tests because they represent a more realistic daily memory activity (Lezak et al., 2004). In these tasks, patients are asked to retell—word for word, if possible—a story immediately after they have heard it. After a 20- to 30-minute delay, patients are again asked to recall the story word for word, if possible. Patients' responses are then typically analyzed in terms of the number of correctly recalled story "ideas" versus words. Patterns of recall also may be evaluated, such as presence of a primacy effect, in which patients recall more ideas from the beginning of the story, or a recency effect, in which patients recall more from the end of the story. Interference effects also may be examined if patients are required to recall more than one story. The Logical Memory Immediate and Delayed subtests of the WMS-IV are perhaps the most frequently used story retelling tasks. Additional story retelling tasks may be found in the research literature (e.g., Mapou, Kramer, & Blusewicz, 1989) or other test batteries, such as the Story Retelling subtests of the ABCD.

Recently, tests such as the *Cambridge Prospective Memory Test* (B. Wilson et al., 2005) and the *Memory for Intentions Test* (MIST; Raskin & Buckheit, 2010) that allow evaluating prospective memory have been published. For example, the MIST assesses both time- and event-based prospective memory via a set of eight time-delayed real-world tasks, some of which require verbal responses and some of which require an action response. A number of error types can be analyzed, such as (a) a loss of content error, in which the patient recalls the correct time at which to complete a task but can't remember what task to complete or completes the wrong task, or (b) a task substitution error, in which the patient gives a verbal response rather than performing an action (or vice versa). The MIST is suitable for adults age 18 to 95 and has alternate forms available to avoid practice effects if repeated testing is required.

Nonverbal Memory Tests. There are a number of tests available to assess nonverbal or spatial memory abilities (see Table 7-3). Familiarity with these tests is particularly important if clinicians work primarily with patients with aphasia whose linguistic deficits contraindicate the use of verbal memory tests; that is, when patients with linguistic deficits perform poorly on verbal memory tests, it is difficult to distinguish whether poor verbal memory, linguistic deficits, or both underlie this poor performance. Nonverbal or spatial memory tests also are a valuable component of an RHD evaluation, as this memory modality is commonly compromised by RHD (Rosen & Viskontas, 2008; Vallar, 2007).

Many nonverbal memory tests parallel those already described with respect to assessing verbal memory abilities, except that they require the recall of object locations, symbols, or matrix patterns specifically designed to minimize verbal coding, and thus minimize use of verbal memory skills. For example, there are a few visual span tasks, such as the Symbol Span subtest of the WMS-IV, that are akin to the previously described verbal span tasks, except that rather than recalling verbal stimuli, patients point to a series of visual designs in a specified order. Likewise, *Rey's Visual Design Learning Test* (RVDLT; Spreen & Straus, 2006) approximates the CVLT by requiring patients to learn a series of 15 visual designs over several trials, and by providing information regarding visual learning and recall.

Several nonverbal or visual memory tests, including the RVDLT, require drawn responses. Another example is the Complex Figure Test, on which patients first copy, then recall immediately after a 30-second to 3-minute delay, and finally recall after a 20- to 30-minute delay, a complex, abstract design; the copy task provides information about visuoperceptual and construction skills, whereas the latter two tasks yield information pertaining to immediate and delayed visual memory abilities, respectively. Several versions of this test are available commercially, such as the *Rey-Osterrieth Complex Figure Test* (Meyers & Meyers, 1995), and in the research literature, such as the scoring system of Stern et al. (1999), which vary in terms of task and scoring procedures, and normative data. To identify the most appropriate version for a given client, clinicians might consult the entire book dedicated to reviewing different complex figure protocols and scoring systems as well as clinical and research applications of this test (J. Knight & Kaplan, 2003). Importantly, clinicians must ensure that the task instructions and procedures they use match those on which their selected scoring system and normative data were based.

If patients' motoric deficits negate the use of a drawing task, another test option is the *Continuous Visual Memory Test* (CVMT; Trahan & Larrabee, 1988). This test examines immediate and delayed visual memory by requiring patients to view a series of complex, abstract designs and indicate for each design whether it is a "new" design that they have not yet been shown during the test, or an "old" design that they have already seen during the test. Once patients have viewed all of the 112 designs, there is a 30-minute delay, and then patients are asked to identify which designs they had previously viewed several times (i.e., which are the "old" designs). There also is a visual discrimination subtest to ensure that visuoperceptual difficulties were not affecting patients' performances negatively. The CVMT comes with a new manual supplement that provides updated norms for individuals 7 through 80 years of age.

The *Location Learning Test* (Bucks, Willison, & Byrne, 2000) utilizes a more functional nonverbal memory task to assess visuospatial learning and recall. In this test, patients are shown an array of pictures depicting everyday objects that are commonly misplaced (e.g., glasses, keys, a purse) and are asked to learn the location of each object. The pictures are then removed, and patients are asked to replace the pictures in their appropriate location. There also is a recognition task to determine if visual perceptual problems are confounding test results. Scoring documents the degree of displacement error, not just the number of correctly placed pictures. This test was specifically designed for older adults, particularly those with suspected dementia, and has normative data for the ages of 50 through 96 years. The WMS-IV contains a similar task, the Design Memory Subtest, but utilizes picture cards with abstract designs versus everyday objects.

Test of Specific Executive Functions

Because the cognitive domain of executive functioning is considered a multidimensional construct, it is most appropriate to administer several tests that assess a number of executive functions (MacNeill Horton et al., 2010; Murray & Ramage, 2000; Pickens et al., 2010). Before administering these tests, however, clinicians must consider the following caveats (Constantinidou et al., 2012; Murray & Ramage, 2000; Pickens et al., 2010; Testa, Bennett, & Ponsford, 2012). First, clinicians must recognize that completing any executive function test will invariably evoke a combination of basic (e.g., attention, perception, language) and high-level cognitive abilities (e.g., planning, inhibition). Consequently, poor performance on an executive function test could be indicative of problems at any cognitive processing level. It is therefore highly inappropriate to administer executive function tests without having previously administered tests of other linguistic and cognitive functions. Second, clinicians must keep in mind that most executive function tests have poor test–retest reliability. This is not necessarily a fault of the test developers, but rather reflects the nature of executive functioning. That is, many executive function tests examine how well patients can cope with novel or unusual situations or problems. Therefore, after they have completed these tests once, performing these tests again will not necessarily be as informative, as the tests' situations or problems will no longer be novel. To avoid this problem, clinicians should select, when possible, executive function tests that include alternate or equivalent forms. Finally, clinicians are reminded that there is little agreement regarding either the vernacular or composition of the domain of executive functioning.

Therefore, to help clinicians become familiar with the variety of executive function tests currently available (see Table 7-3), we have adopted the following categorization of executive function tests, acknowledging that these categories are not completely distinct, that some tests could be applied to more than one category, and that other authors may describe different categories or domains of executive functioning: (a) planning tests, which evaluate formulation of strategies and sequencing of strategy steps to meet intended goals; (b) organization tests, which assess structuring or categorizing of external stimuli and one's own responses; (c) **inhibition** tests, which evaluate control over automatic, habitual, or irrelevant processing or responding; (d) cognitive flexibility tests, which examine the ability to change or revise one's own responses in the event of failure; (e) problem-solving tests, which assess problem identification as well as generation and selection of possible solutions; and (f) self-monitoring tests, which examine the evaluation and regulation of one's own performance, including the identification of one's own strengths and weaknesses.

Planning Tests. Planning tasks include maze completion, tower tests, and clock drawing (described in the Cognitive Status and Dementia Screening Tools section of this chapter). To complete these tasks efficiently, patients must plan the sequence of their responses before executing those responses. For example, maze completion tests, which are similar to maze tasks found in children's activity books, require patients to solve a series of mazes that increase in complexity (e.g., more incorrect path options, longer path between the beginning and the end of the maze). Because of their minimal language demands, these tasks are suitable for patients with neurogenic language disorders. Both accuracy and completion time can be recorded to quantify and qualify patients' performances. Two frequently used maze tests are the *Porteus Maze Test* (Porteus, 1965) and the Maze subtest of the *Cognitive Linguistic Quick Test* (CLQT; Helm-Estabrooks, 2001). More recently, the *NAB Mazes Test* (Stern & White, 2009a) has been published, which has advantages over other maze tests in terms of more recent and broader normative data (e.g., suitable for ages 18 to 97), its suitability for a range of impairment severity, and alternate forms that reduce practice effects when repeated testing is needed.

A number of tower tests are available both commercially (e.g., *Tower of London DX: Research Version* [TOL:RV; Culbertson & Zillmer, 1999]) and in the research literature (e.g., *Tower of Hanoi*; Simon, 1975). These tests require patients to develop an efficient plan in order to use the fewest moves to complete a spatial arrangement task. For example, on the TOL:RV, which provides norms for both children and adults, patients must rearrange colored wooden beads from their initial position on two of three upright rods, or "towers," to a target configuration on another rod using as few moves as possible. Trial difficulty is manipulated by increasing the number and complexity of steps necessary to reconfigure the beads, and test performance can be evaluated in terms of the number of moves necessary to achieve a solution, and the number of task trials that were solved. Tower tests described in the research literature offer a number of procedural and scoring options to manipulate task complexity and provide more test measures, respectively (Denney, Hughes, Owens, & Lynch, 2012; Kafer & Hunter, 1997). For example, the tower test can be made more difficult by increasing the number of towers and beads, or can be made easier by requiring patients to estimate the minimum numbers of moves they would need to solve the task prior to completing the task (i.e., cueing patients to plan their solution ahead of time to help minimize trial-and-error moves). Likewise, additional data can be collected, such as how long patients take to plan their solution and implement their solution.

A more functional planning test is the *Executive Function Route-Finding Task* (Boyd & Sautter, 1994). This test requires patients to find their way from a starting point to a target location, such as an unfamiliar office within the building in which testing is taking place. No specific instructions regarding how patients should find their final location are provided, other than they are asked to find the destination as quickly and efficiently as possible and are told they cannot ask the clinician any questions. The clinician accompanies the patient throughout the test so that the patient can be rated on a four-point scale in the following areas: (a) task understanding (e.g., does not ask clinician questions, begins task spontaneously), (b) incorporation of information seeking (e.g., asks building staff for directions, looks for signs), (c) retaining directions (e.g., takes notes to remember directions), (d) error detection (e.g., checks signs to assure that directions are being followed correctly), (e) error correction (e.g., realizes when an error has been made and attempts to self-correct independently), and (f) on-task behavior (e.g., avoids chatting with familiar staff or patients to complete task as quickly as possible). If necessary, the clinician may provide nonspecific cues such as "What should you be doing?" or specific cues such as "Maybe you should ask someone for help." Whatever cues are provided, clinicians should make note of what level of assistance was necessary for the patient to complete the test. Whereas this test provides qualitative information about patients' planning skills, quantitative interpretation (i.e., severity of impairment) is not possible, as normative data are unavailable.

The *Functional Assessment of Verbal Reasoning and Executive Strategies* (FAVRES; MacDonald, 2005) evaluates planning, along with other executive functions and language skills. Standardized on adults ages 18 to 79 with and without TBI, the FAVRES requires patients to complete a series of functional and complex tasks (e.g., planning an event, scheduling a workday). To complete each task successfully, patients must read a page of text, determine what information is needed to complete the task, shift their attention to accompanying documents (e.g., to-do lists), and consider other people's perspectives. The FAVRES has acceptable psychometric properties, and a version for adolescents is currently being developed (MacDonald, in press).

Organization Tests. One of the most popular organization tests is the *Wisconsin Card Sorting Test* (WCST; Grant & Berg, 1993), no doubt in part because it has relatively low language demands and thus is suitable for a variety of neurogenic patient populations.

Although often referred to as an "organization task" or a "categorization task," the WCST actually evaluates a number of executive functions, including whether a patient can develop a strategy to sort or categorize a deck of cards (i.e., organization or categorization), maintain that strategy (i.e., inhibition of impulsive responses), and switch to a new strategy when feedback indicates to do so (i.e., cognitive flexibility). Cards in the WCST deck vary in terms of the symbols on them (e.g., circles vs. stars), the color of the symbols (e.g., red vs. green circles), and/or the number of symbols (e.g., one vs. four circles), and thus can be sorted by form, color, or number. Based on the clinician's limited feedback of "correct" or "incorrect," patients must figure out how to sort the cards, one-by-one, under the three stimulus or key cards that represent each of the possible categories. Following 10 consecutive correct sorts, the target category is switched so that patients must deduce the new correct sorting strategy, again based on only the clinician's feedback.

Because the WCST can be exceedingly frustrating and time consuming for neurogenic patients (Nussbaum, 1998), several modified versions have been developed that use fewer cards, ease the requirements for task discontinuation, or remove cards that share more than one stimulus characteristic with the key cards to reduce confusion and make discerning the correct sorting strategy easier (e.g., Haaland, Vranes, Goodwin, & Garry, 1987). In fact, the most recently developed commercially available version, the *Modified Wisconsin Card Sorting Test* (M-WCST; Schretlen, 2011), involves two of these modifications: It has only 48 cards (vs. 128 in the original version) because cards sharing more than one stimulus characteristic have been removed. The M-WCST has age- (18 to over 90 years of age), education-, and gender-based norms, and has been shown to be sensitive to categorization impairments and perseveration in a number of neurogenic patient populations (e.g., mild cognitive impairment, Parkinson's disease).

Other examples of organization or categorization tests include the *Booklet Category Test–Second Edition* (DeFilippis & McCampbell, 1997), the computerized *Category Test* (M. Williams, 1994a), and the *Object Sorting Test* (K. Goldstein & Scheerer, 1953). The latter test differs from the WCST and many other organization tests in that it utilizes a set of 30 common objects, and thus, unlike the abstract visual stimuli found on other tests, these stimuli should be familiar to most patients. To complete the task, patients are asked to sort these objects and then explain their strategy. Next, they are asked to group the objects again, but in a different way. This process can be repeated several times, given that the objects can be classified according to a number of features, including object function, color, composition, and location, or where the object would normally be found. An advantage to this test is that clinicians can adapt the basic sorting task to elicit other responses. For instance, the clinician could (a) group a subset of objects and ask the patient to figure out the clinician's sorting strategy, (b) select one object and ask the patient to find other objects similar to it, or (c) dictate by which category the patient should sort the objects. Regardless of which response format is utilized, clinicians should require patients to give verbal explanations of their actions to provide more insight into the patients' organization strategies.

Inhibition Tests. Inhibition tests evaluate patients' ability to disregard irrelevant information, to avoid automatic response tendencies, or to prevent use of previously acceptable responses (L. Murray & Ramage, 2000). Most frequently, Stroop tasks (e.g., Golden, 2002; Trenerry, Crosson, DeBoe, & Leber, 1989; Wiig et al., 2002) are used to assess these forms of inhibition. These tests typically consist of at least two timed tasks, one in which patients read aloud color names, and another in which they name the color of ink in which the word is written (for a grayscale version, see Figure 7-4). The second task should take patients longer to complete because they must inhibit the more frequent response of reading words aloud; they should experience the greatest interference when the written word and color conflict. To quantify how well patients deal with this interference, their response accuracies and speed on the two tasks are compared: The greater the difference between the two trials, the more interference and thus greater problems with inhibition the patient experienced. Of the various commercially available Stroop tasks, Golden (2002) provided the most extensive normative data for patients ranging in age from 15 to 90 years. Although most Stroop tasks are visual in nature, auditory versions have been developed and are described in the research literature (e.g., T. Christensen, Lockwood, Almryde, & Plante, 2011).

Because of its high speech and language demands, the Stroop task is highly inappropriate for many patients with dysarthria, aphasia, or both. For these patients, clinicians must look for inhibition test protocols in the research literature. For example, Guitton, Buchtel, and Douglas (1985) developed an antisaccade inhibition task that has minimal speech or language demands. Their task requires patients to focus on a center fixation point on a computer. Visual cues are then randomly flashed to the right or left of the fixation point, and patients are asked to direct their eyes in the direction opposite to the cue. Inhibition is tested, as the automatic response of looking in the same direction as the cue (i.e., saccade) must be avoided (i.e., antisaccade). Performance is quantified by determining the patient's percentage of incorrect saccades. Another option is the computerized *Tasks of Executive Control* (Isquith, Roth, & Gioia, 2010), which in-

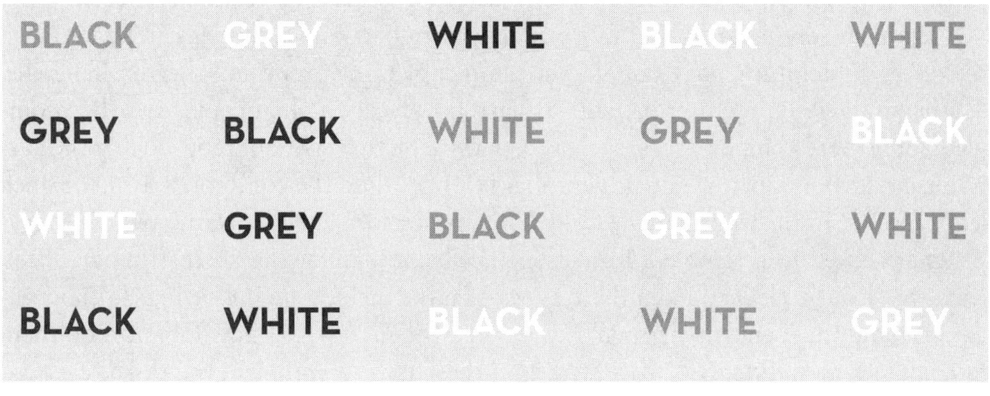

Figure 7-4. Example of a grayscale Stroop-like test.

cludes a go/no-go test involving visual stimuli (i.e., involves only a key press response). Although this test has equivalent forms and fairly strong psychometric properties, it includes normative data only for individuals up to the age of 18.

Cognitive Flexibility Tests. Cognitive flexibility is closely related to the cognitive functions of attention switching and inhibition, as it refers to how well patients can shift from one task to another when internal or external feedback indicates the need to change. Consequently, many tests traditionally described as cognitive flexibility tasks, such as the *Trail Making Test*, have already been described in other sections of this chapter. Additional cognitive flexibility tasks, such as copying alternating figures or letters (e.g., alternate between writing cursive "n" then "m") and repetitive sequential hand movements (e.g., quickly switching among a fist, edge, and palm hand positions), are included as subtests in cognitive test batteries such as the *Dementia Rating Scale–Second Edition* (Mattis, 2001), or can be found in research studies (e.g., Rende, 2000) or textbooks (e.g., Lezak et al., 2004; Strauss, Sherman, & Spreen, 2006).

Problem-Solving Tests. There are many test options available to evaluate problem-solving skills, including the *Test of Problem Solving–Adolescent: Second Edition* (Bowers, Huisingh, & LoGiudice, 2007), Tinkertoy Test (Lezak et al., 2004) and *Rapid Assessment of Problem Solving* (R. Marshall, Karow, Morelli, Iden, & Dixon, 2003). Several tests have limited language demands and thus are appropriate for a broad range of neurogenic patient populations. For example, tests such as *Raven's Progressive Matrices* (Raven, 2003), the *Test of Nonverbal Intelligence–Fourth Edition* (TONI-4; Brown, Sherbenou, & Johnsen, 2010), and the *Comprehensive Test of Nonverbal Intelligence–Second Edition* (CTONI-2; Hammill, Pearson, & Wiederholt, 2009) involve showing patients a design or series of designs with a piece of the design or design series missing. Patients then must determine which symbol or design from an array of possibilities best completes the design or design series. All of these tests provide extensive norms for children and adults (e.g., the TONI-4 and the CTONI-2 were standardized on adults up to age 90). Both the *Raven's* and the TONI-4 also have equivalent forms, which make them useful when multiple test administrations are needed for monitoring treatment effects.

Problem-solving tasks that more closely resemble daily activities can be found in the research literature. For example, the photocopy task (Crepeau, Scherzer, Belleville, & Desmarais, 1997) requires patients to learn how to use a photocopier and then complete some more complex tasks, such as copying a picture without reproducing the surrounding text or copying a document that is longer than the common 8.5 × 11.5-inch letter format. In the wheelbarrow test (Butler, Anderson, Furst, & Namerow, 1989), patients are asked to assemble a full-scale wheelbarrow following an instruction sheet. Data that can be gleaned from these types of tasks include the following: (a) how accurately and independently patients completed the task(s), (b) how long it took them to complete the task(s), (c) what strategies they used to complete the tasks (e.g., did they ask the clinician or others for assistance?), (d) whether they self-corrected, and/or

(e) whether clinician cues were required, and if so, how many and what kind (e.g., general or specific cues).

Self-Monitoring Tests. Fluency tasks are frequently considered measures of self-monitoring because they require patients to provide responses on a continuous basis while keeping track of responses they have already produced, as well as those they are not allowed to produce. Fluency tasks that require verbal or nonverbal responses are available. For example, many aphasia and dementia test batteries, such as the *Western Aphasia Battery–Revised* (Kertesz, 2006) and ABCD, respectively, have a verbal fluency subtest on which patients list as many exemplars as possible in one or two minutes, without repeating themselves, from a prescribed semantic category (e.g., animals, means of transportation). Verbal fluency tasks also may require the generation of words that begin with a certain letter. For instance, the FAS or *Controlled Oral Word Association Test* (Benton et al., 2001), which has been widely used and standardized, requires patients to name as many words as possible beginning with the letter *F*, then *A*, and then *S*, given one minute for each letter. Not only must patients avoid repeating themselves on this test, but they also must avoid listing proper names or numbers. The *Test of Verbal Conceptualization and Fluency* (TVCF; C. Reynolds & Horton, 2007) includes both category and letter fluency tasks, along with two subtests similar to executive function tests, described earlier: a version of the *Trail Making Test* (i.e., shifting between Arabic numerals and the printed words for those numerals) and a version of the WCST. The TVCF was normed on a broad age range (i.e., ages 8 to 89) and can be administered in both individual and group settings.

Regardless of which verbal fluency task is administered, verbal fluency performance is most often quantified in terms of how many correct exemplars were generated. Clinicians, however, also may examine whether or not patients utilized any organization strategies, such as semantic clustering (e.g., first naming domestic animals, then naming zoo animals) or a phonemic strategy (e.g., first naming words that start with "fa," then naming words that start with "fe"), to aid their performance. Therefore, additional variables to measure could include number of semantic or phonemic clusters, as well as the length of those clusters. Fluency performance can also be qualified by examining error types (e.g., perseverative errors; proper nouns). The TVCF does incorporate some of these other measures of verbal fluency.

If the patients' speech or language deficits preclude the use of a verbal fluency task, clinicians can instead administer a test such as the *Ruff Figural Fluency Test* (RFFT; Ruff, 1996), which has minimal verbal demands. To complete the RFFT, patients must create as many unique designs as possible in a minute on a sheet of paper with a grid of 35 squares, each of which contains five dots. Patients are instructed to make a design in each square by using straight lines to connect at least two dots. Five trials are completed with different dot configurations, some of which include predrawn lines so that the effects of interference can be evaluated. Scoring consists of calculating the number of novel patterns and perseverative errors. Clinicians also can examine whether patients utilized any strategies such as pattern rotation. Although the RFFT is standardized, the normative sample is somewhat limited, as age norms only extend up to 70 years.

The most recently published fluency test, the *Calibrated Ideational Fluency Assessment* (CIFA; Schrelten & Vannorsdall, 2011), includes both verbal and nonverbal fluency subtests and offers normative data for a broad age range (18 to over 90). The Verbal Fluency subtest includes both semantic and phonemic fluency tasks, whereas the Design Fluency subtest is similar to that just described for the RFFT. Ideally, both subtests would be administered, but just the Design Fluency subtest could be used and scored if the patient's language deficits contraindicated the Verbal Fluency subtest.

Related to self-monitoring is the awareness of one's own strengths and weaknesses. As mentioned in Chapter 2, many patients with neurogenic language or cognitive disorders have anosognosia, or an impaired awareness of the nature, severity, and/or consequences of their physical, behavioral, linguistic, and/or cognitive symptoms. Accordingly, clinicians may need to quantify and qualify awareness disorders. Although there are no standardized measures available for assessing awareness, clinicians can obtain information pertaining to the integrity of their patients' self-awareness via interviews, rating scales, and observations. For example, as mentioned in the Case History and Observations section of this chapter, interviewing or giving questionnaires or rating scales to both patients and their caregivers will allow the clinician to compare responses for any disparities in perceptions of the patients' weaknesses and strengths.

In addition to the previously mentioned and commercially available BADS Dysexecutive Questionnaire, BRIEF-A, and BDEFS, there are several questionnaire and interview protocols in the research literature to help clinicians structure this aspect of an executive function assessment (for a review of several of these, see Starkstein et al., 2010). For example, the Self-Awareness of Deficits Interview (Bogod, Mateer, & McDonald, 2003; Fleming, Strong, & Ashton, 1996) provides questions regarding three areas of awareness: self-awareness of deficits, self-awareness of the functional implications of one's deficits, and the ability to set realistic goals. The clinician then rates responses using a four-point scale on which zero represents appropriate awareness and four indicates impaired awareness. Another new option when evaluating patients with aphasia is the *Visual-Analogue Test Assessing Anosognosia for Language* (VATA-L; Cocchini et al., 2010). This measure consists of a set of drawings to illustrate daily tasks that involve language production, comprehension, or both. Patients as well as their caregivers rate how well the patients can carry out these daily communication tasks using a 4-point visual-analogue scale (ranging from 0 [*no problem*] to 3 [*major problem* in carrying out the task]). The VATA-L yields a discrepancy score, with a positive value indicating that the patient has overestimated his or her language ability during these daily tasks. Clinicians can also compare scores to examine awareness of language comprehension versus expression abilities.

A caveat to relying on just the comparison of patient and caregiver reports to quantify and qualify self-awareness is that caregivers, like patients, can provide unreliable responses (Schmitter-Edgecombe et al., 2011; Tate, 2010). For instance, factors such as caregivers' stress levels, personality, and personal involvement, or the patients' time postonset may influence the accuracy of caregivers' responses (Bogod et al., 2003). The validity of these questionnaire and rating scales has also been minimally explored (Starkstein et al., 2010; Tate, 2010). Accordingly, clinicians should augment interview/questionnaire responses with data collected from other awareness assessment strategies, and in fact, it is recommended that several assessment procedures be used when evaluating self-awareness and self-monitoring (Chiou, Carlson, Arnett, Cosentino, & Hillary, 2011). Therefore, in addition to questionnaire and rating scale measures, clinicians could have patients make predictions regarding their performance of standardized tests (sometimes called "retrospective confidence judgments") and then compare patients' predicted and actual test scores (Chiou et al., 2011; Fischer, Trexler, & Gauggel, 2004; Markova & Berrios, 2006). These judgments could be elicited after every test item, after completion of a subtest or entire test, or even prior to completing an item or task; additionally, patients could be asked to judge their predicted accuracy, response speed, or both. Poor awareness is indicated when patients frequently overestimate their performance. Another option is to watch for certain behaviors indicative of anosognosia throughout the cognitive assessment (Sohlberg, 2000). These behaviors include minimal or no self-correcting behaviors, failure to use compensatory strategies, and poor motivation or lack of cooperation during structured assessment tasks because the patient does not see the need for an assessment.

Test Confounds

Although numerous cognitive test choices are available, not all of these will be appropriate for all patients with neurogenic language or cognitive disorders. Consequently, clinicians must carefully read test manuals to determine if the tests they are considering using were standardized on a normative sample that is representative of their patients. In particular, clinicians should always check for the age, education, ethnocultural, and language backgrounds of tests' normative samples, as these variables have been found to influence outcomes on formal cognitive tests (Agranovich et al., 2011; Ardila, 2005; Kennepohl et al., 2004). Unfortunately, because of relatively narrow normative samples, many tests, particularly those published 15 or more years ago, have limited use for patients who are elderly, have low education, speak English as a second language, or represent an ethnocultural minority. To avoid this confound, some newer tests provide standardized versions for individuals who speak English as a second language (e.g., *Cognitive Linguistic Quick Test*, MMSE-2), provide instructions in common non-English languages used in the United States (e.g., CTONI-2), were developed for one or several languages other than or including English (e.g., Common Objects Memory Test, which was developed for English, Vietnamese, and several dialects of Spanish and Chinese; Kempler, Teng, Taussig, & Dick, 2010), and/or have normative data that are stratified by age and education (e.g., NAB). Likewise, although the normative data in many tests' manuals may be restrictive, extended norms often are available in research studies conducted subsequent to these tests' initial publication (e.g., Kessels, Nys, Brands, van den Berg, & Van Zandvoort, 2006; Messinis Malegiannaki, Christodoulou, Panagiotopoulos, & Papthanasopoulos, 2011).

Clinicians also must ensure that the instructions and response demands of cognitive tests are compatible with the physical, sensory, and language abilities of their patients. For example, cognitive tests that require understanding of long, complex task instructions would be inappropriate for many patients with language comprehension difficulties due to aphasia or dementia. Likewise, cognitive tests that require drawing complex designs may be unsuitable for patients with hemiparesis, who must use their nondominant hand to draw or write, or for patients with visual impairments (e.g., blast injury survivors). The use of tests that exceed patients' physical, sensory, and/or language skills will produce invalid results, as the clinician will be unsure whether poor performance on these tests was reflective of a true cognitive deficit, or was rather the product of these other symptoms.

Clinicians must also keep in mind that the testing environment may affect their patients' performances on cognitive tests (Constantinidou et al., 2012). For instance, given that formal testing is usually conducted in a relatively distraction-free environment, the effects of focused attention deficits on the real-world functioning of many patients are likely underestimated. Similarly, the structure provided by formal testing procedures and environments can mask executive function impairments that may be easier to identify in less predictable settings. These environmental confounds underscore the contributions of observations and other informal and qualitative approaches to assessment.

Qualitative Assessment Considerations

If time limitations or other confounds obstruct administering formal cognitive tests, clinicians should keep in mind that information regarding the integrity of their patients' cognitive abilities can be gleaned informally while completing language assessment procedures. More specifically, cognitive abilities may be informally evaluated by observing the presence of certain behaviors indicative of cognitive problems, and by administering language tests in formats that vary the cognitive demands of the language tasks or assessment environment. Furthermore, use of the following qualitative assessment procedures may provide additional information, even when formal cognitive testing is completed.

Clinicians may monitor for possible cognitive problems while completing their initial observations and interviews, or while administering formal language tests. For example, attention impairments might be suspected if patients appear easily distracted (i.e., sustained and/or selective attention problems), the quality of their performance quickly deteriorates (i.e., sustained attention problems), they have difficulty switching between language tasks (i.e., attention-shifting problems), or their performance breaks down when they attempt to process more than one modality or information source or to complete more than one task at a time (i.e., divided attention problems). Signs of memory problems include the need for frequent reminders about task instructions, or when patients' comprehension abilities appear to be more influenced by the length of the material rather than by linguistic factors such as grammatical complexity or vocabulary familiarity. Likewise, clinicians should consider the possibility of impaired executive functioning when patients appear impulsive, inappropriate, perseverative, concrete, or unaware of their deficits, the extent of their deficits, or the implications of their deficits.

Another option is to adapt language tests so that the cognitive demands of the language tasks are varied. For example, a reading comprehension test could be administered both in quiet and in noisy, distracting environments to determine whether focused attention demands negatively affect patients' reading rate or comprehension accuracy. To evaluate the effects of increased memory demands on the repetition abilities of patients with aphasia, patients could be instructed to repeat immediately after the clinician on some items, to repeat only after a five-second delay on other items, and to count to five and then repeat on still other items (i.e., filled delay condition). Whatever manipulations are introduced to evaluate the effects of high and low cognitive demands on language task performance, clinicians must remember to keep the linguistic complexity of the stimuli similar across the various task conditions; for instance, for the repetition test example, the repetition items for the immediate, delayed, and filled delay response conditions must be similar in length and phonological, syntactic, and semantic complexity. Failure to do so will result in ambiguous findings, as clinicians will not be able to determine whether their patients' poor performances were a product of linguistic or cognitive factors.

Prognostic Factors for Cognitive Outcomes

A final step of assessment is to formulate prognoses regarding patients' rehabilitation potential, recovery rate, or eventual outcome. Several of the biographical, medical, and cognitive prognostic factors noted in Chapter 6 to influence language outcomes also may relate to cognitive outcomes (see Tables 6-6 and 7-5). Clinicians are reminded that predictions regarding patients' recovery patterns or outcomes must be based on the consideration of many prognostic variables, as by themselves these variables provide only weak and thus possibly inaccurate approximations of patients' future cognitive status.

In terms of biographical variables, age appears to be a strong cognitive outcome predictor, as many studies have found that older patients with neurogenic disorders tend to have more severe cognitive problems and poorer functional outcomes than their younger counterparts (Kortte & Hillis, 2009; Liman et al., 2011; Mailles et al., 2012; Sendroy-Terrill et al., 2010). Some researchers contend, however, that normal age-related

TABLE 7-5
Prognostic Indicators for Rehabilitative Outcome Related to Cognitive Impairments

FACTORS SUGGESTING BETTER PROGNOSIS	FACTORS SUGGESTING POORER PROGNOSIS
Younger age Good premorbid physical health High premorbid intelligence Regular exercise Cognitively active Socially active	Lesion variables: • Lesion severity (as evidenced by coma length, duration of post-traumatic amnesia) • Large lesions • Frontal lobe involvement • Early right hemisphere involvement in Parkinson's disease • Left hemisphere cortical lesions in stroke
	Concomitant medical, physical, or psychiatric problems: • Diabetes • Depression • Apathy • Anxiety
	Presence of certain linguistic/cognitive deficits: • Anosognosia • Neglect • Early language symptoms in Alzheimer's disease and frontotemporal dementia • Aphasia in stroke and traumatic brain injury

changes in cognition may contribute, at least in part, to poor neuropsychological outcomes among elderly patients (Johnstone, Childers, & Hoerner, 1998). A potent relationship between premorbid intelligence and cognitive outcomes has been reported in static, as well as progressive, neurogenic disorders (Anson & Ponsford, 2006; Pavlik et al., 2006). Controversy persists, however, regarding the relationship between education and cognitive outcomes: Some studies report that well-educated adults show fewer, less progressive, or delayed onset of cognitive impairments than their less-educated peers (Paradise, Cooper, & Livingston, 2009; Sigurdardottir, Andelic, Roe, & Schanke, 2009) or better cognitive outcome (Mailles et al., 2012), whereas other studies find no significant association between education and cognitive outcomes (Gilleard, 1997; Pavlik et al., 2006). H. Christensen et al. (2001) noted that in many investigations in which a strong relationship between education and cognitive changes was identified, researchers failed to control for practice or retest effects. This is particularly problematic because adults' test-taking skills are linked to their education level, and thus highly educated adults tend to show larger practice effects when completing multiple administrations of the same tests. As with language outcomes, gender does not appear to be a useful predictor of cognitive or functional recovery (Renner et al., 2012).

Medical variables also should be considered, as patients who have one or more medical, physical, or psychiatric complications are at risk for poorer outcomes compared with patients without these concomitant conditions (Denti, Agosti, & Franceschini, 2008; Mailles et al., 2012). For instance, diabetes should be considered a complicating factor, as patients with diabetes are more likely to have cognitive impairments subsequent to stroke than those who don't have diabetes (Liman et al., 2011), and they also have been reported to have slower recovery rates (Lukovits, Mazzone, & Gorelick, 1999; Newman, Bang, Hussain, & Toole, 2007); slower recovery in these patients may be related to severe hypoglycemic episodes or to daily fluctuations in glucose levels, both of which can negatively affect attention and other cognitive abilities (Fujioka et al., 1997; Zammitt, Warren, Deary, & Frier 2008). In contrast, patients who had good premorbid physical health, and who exercise regularly subsequent to the onset of their brain damage or disease, are more likely to have positive cognitive, emotional, and/or overall functional outcomes than their out-of-shape peers (Bassey, 2000; Denti et al., 2008; Krarup et al., 2008). Relatedly, a higher level of daily physical activity can lower one's risk of developing diseases that cause cognitive impairments (e.g., Alzheimer's disease, stroke) (Buchman et al., 2012; Roger et al., 2011). Social activity and support levels also appear influential in that better functional outcomes or less cognitive decline are observed among individuals who have a social support system or are able to maintain their social activity level and group memberships (Denti et al., 2008; Haslam et al., 2008; James, Wilson, Barnes, & Bennett, 2011). Emotional or psychiatric health also is an influential prognostic indicator, as patients with psychiatric disorders (e.g., depression, apathy, anxiety) or who adopt negative coping strategies (e.g., denial or avoidance) tend to have less success in rehabilitation, poorer cognitive or functional outcomes, or greater cognitive impairments than patients without psychiatric problems or those who utilize positive coping strategies (e.g., problem-oriented coping strategies or seeking education about their symptoms or disease) (Anson & Ponsford, 2006; Eslinger, Moore, Antani, Anderson, & Grossman, 2012; Hama et al., 2007). Relatedly, certain drugs for psychiatric disorders, particularly antipsychotic medications, have been found to increase the rate of cognitive decline among individuals with dementia (Vigen et al., 2011).

Lesion variables also appear influential. In TBI, the greater the severity of the brain injury, as indexed by length of coma and duration of post-traumatic amnesia or confusion, as well as extent of brain damage, the more likely it is that the patient will experience slow cognitive recovery or enduring cognitive impairments (Babikian & Asarnow, 2009; Howard, 2008). More generally, regardless of etiology, large brain lesions and frontal lobe involvement are most detrimental to overall cognitive abilities and outcomes (Duering et al., 2011; Liman et al., 2011; Mosch et al., 2005; Robertson & Murre, 1999). Links between lesion location and presence or recovery of general, as well as specific, cognitive deficits also have been reported. For example, neglect recovery is more likely if frontoparietal or, more generally, cortical areas are spared (Hier, Mondlock, & Caplan, 1983; Kortte & Hillis, 2009). In Parkinson's disease, patients who demonstrate initial left-sided motor symptoms and thus early right hemisphere involvement tend to present with more diverse and severe cognitive problems than patients who initially experience right-sided motor symptoms and thus early left hemisphere involvement (A. Lee, Harris, Atkinson, & Fowler, 2001; Riederer & Sian-Hülsmann, 2012). In contrast, Newman and colleagues (2007) reported that left hemisphere cortical lesions predicted poorer cognitive recovery among a large and diverse sample of stroke patients. As with language recovery, the greatest and most rapid cognitive improvements are observed within the first several months postonset of nonprogressive brain damage (A. Benton & Tranel, 2000; B. Christensen et al., 2008), but importantly, cognitive recovery can persist, albeit at a slower rate, for years postonset (Liman et al., 2011).

In general, the presence of any cognitive deficit may compromise patient recovery, response to treatment, and subsequent functional outcome (Denti et al., 2008; Lambon Ralph et al., 2010; Nicholas et al., 2011; Ones et al., 2009), and more severe initial cognitive deficits are associated with slower recovery and poorer outcomes (One, Yalçinkaya, Toklu, & Cağlar, 2009; Sigurdardottir et al., 2009). Certain cognitive deficits, however, appear to be more detrimental to long-term outcomes. For example, findings from several studies indicate that patients with neglect and/or executive dysfunctioning, particularly impaired self-awareness, will have poorer overall cognitive recovery and rehabilitation outcomes than patients without these cognitive symptoms (Chiou et al., 2011; Gialanella & Ferlucci, 2010; Gialanella, Monguzzi, Santoro, & Rocchi, 2005; Starkstein et al., 2010; Wee & Hopman, 2008). Similarly, in progressive diseases, early and more marked demonstration of executive deficits is associated with rapid cognitive deterioration (Butters, Lopez, & Becker, 1996; Musicco et al., 2010). There also appears to be a link between language skills and cognitive or rehabilitation outcomes. In Alzheimer's disease and frontotemporal dementia, patients who demonstrate language deficits (e.g., confrontation naming problems or impaired semantic categorization abilities) as an early or initial symptom show faster cognitive deterioration and poorer prognosis than patients without these language problems (A. Chan, Salmon, Butters, & Johnson, 1995; Garcin et al., 2009); in TBI and stroke, patients with aphasia, particularly those with comprehension deficits, often have more severe cognitive impairments than their non-aphasic peers (Demir et al., 2006; Gialanella, 2011; Gialanella & Ferlucci, 2010).

Summary

A growing body of research indicates that patients with neurogenic disorders often present with concomitant deficits of attention, memory, and executive functioning, and that these deficits may negatively affect not only their communication abilities but also their rehabilitation and functional outcomes. Accordingly, this chapter reviewed the basic format of a cognitive evaluation by describing a number of informal and formal procedures and tests that may be used to assess general (as well as specific) cognitive abilities. Currently, the role of speech-language pathology in assessing and treating neurogenic cognitive disorders continues to evolve and varies depending on the clinical setting. Regardless, however, clinicians must be prepared to evaluate the cognitive abilities of their patients or, even if they are not directly involved in the cognitive assessment, be able to interpret the results of cognitive evaluations in order to plan and provide effective treatment of their patients' cognitive and linguistic disorders.

Discussion Questions

1. What expertise do speech-language pathologists bring to the assessment of cognitive function? How does this complement the expertise of other professionals?
2. Which medical or education professions in your state are licensed to administer tests of attention, memory, and/or executive functioning?
3. How are cognitive screening tools used in the assessment of neurogenic language and cognitive function?
4. How would you determine when to employ an assessment battery versus a series of tests targeting specific cognitive functions?
5. How can clinicians minimize confounds affecting performance during tasks targeting cognitive functions?

Assessment of Activity, Participation, and Quality of Life

chapter 8

Learning Objectives

After reading this chapter, you should be able to:

- List the purposes of assessing functional performance, participation, and quality of life
- Define *functional measures* and describe how they are used
- Describe informal ways to assess function
- Define *participation measures* and describe how they are used
- Describe informal ways to assess participation
- Define *quality-of-life measures* and describe how they are used
- Describe informal ways to assess quality of life
- Discuss how authentic assessment strategies inform assessment of function, participation, and quality of life
- Compare and contrast assessment tools designed for general populations, disease-specific populations, and communicatively disordered populations

Key Terms

- authentic assessment
- functional measures
- measures of participation
- measures of quality of life
- outcomes
- process measures

Introduction

In Chapters 6 and 7, strategies for assessing the underlying impairments contributing to cognitive and communicative limitations were described. These assessment techniques allow the clinician to describe the nature of language and cognitive-communicative disorders, as well as design treatment programs that target these aspects of language and/or cognitive function. In addition to understanding the underlying impairments and function or structure limitations experienced by our patients, we also need to appreciate the impact of these conditions on their ability to participate in desired activities, as well as on their overall quality of life. Assessment of participation and quality of life serves two main purposes. First, understanding the impact of communication and cognitive deficits on real-life activities informs treatment planning. That is, patients who experience significant participation restrictions related to their neurogenic language or cognitive disorder may be more likely to pursue treatment than patients whose participation and quality of life have been impacted minimally by their impairments. Furthermore, understanding the types of interactions that the patient is seeking or feels unable to conduct provides very specific treatment targets that will be most meaningful to the patient.

Second, the assessment procedures described in Chapters 6 and 7 typically seek to isolate the specific language and cognitive impairments, respectively, contributing to an individual's communicative and cognitive functions. To do so, measures are constructed with a goal of minimizing "confounding" factors beyond underlying language/cognitive skills that influence performance. This is necessary and important, yet these same confounds can be quite relevant in determining the most appropriate interventions that can lead to meaningful improvements in activity, participation, and quality of life. Thus, the tools described in this chapter typically include items that either directly identify important personal or environmental factors impacting an individual or characterize the ways participation and quality of life are affected by these factors (Geyh, Cieza, Kollerits, Grimby, & Stucki, 2007).

Finally, participation and quality-of-life measures are critical when determining treatment effectiveness. Although improvements on impairment-level measures suggest that treatment has been beneficial, only when we demonstrate that treatment has had a positive effect on the patient's functional performance, societal participation, and/or quality of life can we be sure treatment has been truly effective. More complete discussions of issues related to treatment efficacy are included in Chapter 1. In this chapter, we will highlight strategies for assessing functional performance, societal participation, and quality of life for the purposes of planning treatment and evaluating treatment efficacy.

Defining Terms

The tools described in this chapter are variably termed **functional measures**, **measures of participation**, or **measures of quality of life**. In some literature, these terms are used interchangeably, but in this chapter, each term will be used to denote a specific aspect of "real-life" performance.

Functional measures of performance are used in all areas of rehabilitation and typically target real-life activities such as self-care and ambulation. With respect to communication, "functional assessment" refers to describing a "person's ability to communicate despite the presence of impairments, such as aphasia, dysarthria, or hearing loss" (Frattali, 1994, p. 306). For example, a functional measure may assess a patient's success in communicating with a family member. Within this framework, functional measures assess the International Classification of Functioning, Disability, and Health (ICF) level of activity limitations (as defined in Chapter 1; WHO, 2001) and address communication in ways unlike those targeted by the impairment-level measures (i.e., ICF level of body structure and function) described in Chapters 6 and 7. Whereas those measures help describe underlying impairments of language and other cognitive domains, as well as communication behaviors during structured tasks, functional measures attempt to describe communication and cognitive behaviors during daily life activities. In this respect, functional measures are similar to participation-level measures.

Measures of participation are those that assess the degree to which individuals participate in the activities characteristic of their daily lives. For example, the measure may assess whether a patient attends sporting events, performs job duties, or participates in social activities. The focus of participation measures *is* participation. Other measures address how the individuals *feel* about their participation (Hirsch & Holland, 2000). Such **quality-of-life measures** target factors beyond participation and include issues of feelings, attitudes, and beliefs related to the ability to enjoy life. Quality-of-life measures often include items such as "I am generally happy" or "My life is satisfying."

All three of these assessment targets (i.e., functional communication, participation, and quality of life) contribute to our understanding of how a neurogenic language or cognitive disorder impacts the well-being of any given patient. Furthermore, by addressing these factors, we are better able to make recommendations regarding the need for treatment and potential treatment procedures, and to evaluate the effectiveness of the treatment that is provided. Table 8-1 lists the measures reviewed in this chapter, as well as additional measures available through the research literature.

Other Assessment Frameworks

We selected the ICF as the organizing framework for this book, with this chapter additionally considering quality of life. However, the ICF is not the only framework developed to characterize the many ways in which health conditions affect individual patients. *Living With Aphasia: Framework for Outcome Measurement* (A-FROM; Kagan et al., 2008) was developed to help clinicians identify and assess the "impact of aphasia on life areas deemed important by people with aphasia and their families" (p. 1). The central focus of A-FROM is the experience of living with aphasia, and it incorporates four broad domains: (1) severity of aphasia; (2) personal identity, attitudes, and feelings; (3) participation in life situations; and (4) communication and language environment. These domains are not unlike the constructs of the ICF, with the added explicit acknowledgement of quality of life. The authors of A-FROM identified examples of assessment tools that address each of the domains and developed a comprehensive assessment instrument (the *Assessment for Living With Aphasia* [Aphasia Institute, 2010], discussed later in this chapter) that addresses each of the domains. Although the framework was created to address the experience of individuals with aphasia, it is easy to see how the domains could be applied to the assessment of cognitive and communicative functions associated with traumatic brain injury, right hemisphere disorders, or dementia.

(text continues on p. 278)

TABLE 8-1
Measures of Communication and Cognitive Function, Participation, and Quality of Life

INSTRUMENT	SOURCE	General measures (for all populations)	For specific populations	For individuals with communication disorders
Affect Balance Scale (ABS)	Bradburn (1969)	X		
Craig Handicap Assessment and Reporting Technique (CHART)	Whiteneck et al. (1992)	X		
Dartmouth COOP Functional Assessment Charts	Nelson et al. (1987)	X		
Functional Independence Measure (FIM)	State University of New York (1993)	X		
Functional Life Scale (FLS)	Sarno et al. (1973)	X		
Psychosocial Well-Being Index (PWI)	Lyon et al. (1997)	X		
Ryff Scales of Psychological Well-Being	Ryff et al. (1989)	X		
Satisfaction With Life Scale (SWLS)	Diener et al. (1985)	X		
Sickness Impact Profile (SIP)	Bergner et al. (1981)	X		
Burden of Stroke Scale (BOSS)	Doyle et al. (2004)		X	
Community Integration Questionnaire (CIQ)	Willer et al. (1993)		X	
DEMQOL	Smith et al. (2007)		X	
Quality of Life after Brain Injury (QUOLIBRI)	von Steinbüchel et al. (2010)		X	
Quality of Life in Alzheimer's Disease (QOL-AD)	Logsdon, Gibbons, McCurrey, & Teri (1999, 2002)		X	
Stroke and Aphasia Quality of Life Scale-39 (SAQLS-39)	Hilari, Byng, Lamping, & Smith (2003)		X	X
Stroke Impact Scale (SIS 3.0)	Duncan, Bode, Min Lai, & Perera (2003)		X	
Stroke-Specific Quality of Life Scale (SS-QOL)	Williams, Weinberger, Harris, Clark, & Biller (1999)		X	

TABLE 8-1 (continued)

INSTRUMENT	SOURCE	General measures (for all populations)	For specific populations	For individuals with communication disorders
Amsterdam-Nijmegen Everyday Language Test (ANELT)	Blomert et al. (1987, 1994)			X
ASHA Functional Assessment of Communication (ASHA FACS)	Frattali et al. (1995)			X
ASHA Functional Communication Measures ASHA Quality of Communication Life (CQL)	Paul-Brown, Frattali, Holland, Thompson, Caperton, & Slater (2004)			X
Cognitive-Communicative Abilities Following Brain Injury	Hartley (1995)			X
Communication Confidence Rating Scale for Aphasia (CCRSA)	Babbitt & Cherney (2010)			X
Communication Disability Profile (CDP)	Swinbourne & Byng (2006)			X
Communication Profile	Gurland et al. (1982)			X
Communication Profile: Functional Skills Survey	Payne (1994)			X
Communicative Activities of Daily Living–Second Edition (CADL-2)	Holland et al (1999)			X
Communicative Effectiveness Index (CETI)	Lomas et al. (1989)			X
Communicative/Competence Evaluation Instrument	Houghton et al. (1982)			X
Communicative Participation Item Bank	Yorkston et al. (2008); Yorkston & Baylor (2010)			X
Functional Communication Profile (FCP)	Sarno (1969)			X
LaTrobe Communication Questionnaire (LCQ)	Douglas, Bracy, & Snow (2007)			X
Pragmatic Protocol	Prutting & Kirchner (1987)			X

Issues to Consider When Measuring Functional Communication, Participation, and Quality of Life

As will be clear from the detailed discussion below, assessing functional communication, participation, and quality of life often differs from assessing cognitive and language ability (Chapters 6 and 7) with respect to the degree to which behaviors of interest are directly observed. The measures discussed in this chapter often rely on patient self-report or family report (Eadie et al., 2006). These reports can be relatively objective (e.g., identifying the number of social gatherings attended during the previous week) or subjective (e.g., rating the degree of effort associated with a given activity). Regardless of whether an item requires an objective or subjective response, the item may require some degree of interpretation from the responder (Dijkers, 2010). For example, consider an item such as "I am a parent," which targets participation in social institutions and/or interpersonal relationships. Imagine the difficulty you might have responding to this item if you had borne children but were no longer actively parenting, perhaps because your children have grown, because you have never had custody of the children, or because you no longer have custody because of functional deficits (e.g., a father who has severe aphasia that restricts his spoken and written output to a couple of stereotypical responses is no longer able to partake in parenting activities, such as reprimanding or counseling). This question might be equally challenging for an individual who is actively parenting but now parents in a different way because of changes in his or her functional abilities. It is important to recognize the subtle differences among legal status, identity, and role-fulfillment and to allow patients or other responders (e.g., family members, friends) to qualify their responses as necessary.

A second issue to consider is that most of the measures described in this chapter are not "normed" in the sense that an individual's performance can be compared with the range of performance of individuals without a brain disease or disorder. This is due in part to the assumption that many items addressing functional communication and cognition, participation, and quality of life will pose no difficulty to healthy individuals. Equally relevant is the recognition that what is "normal" for one person may not be true for another. As we discussed in Chapter 1, each individual has unique communication and cognitive needs, as well as environment and personal factors influencing his or her experience of a neurogenic language or cognitive disorder. It would be inappropriate to compare the participation restrictions reported by a broadcast journalist to those described by an individual with less "extraordinary" daily communication demands (Yorkston & Baylor, 2011). In recognition that normative sampling of the target constructs may not be particularly meaningful to interpretation, measures of functional communication and cognition, participation, and quality of life more commonly report the range of responses reported by individuals with varying functional impairments (e.g., limb weakness), etiologies (e.g., traumatic brain injury), or communicative demands (e.g., those made of teachers).

Finally, it is important to acknowledge that although we have organized this chapter by discussing measures of functional communication and cognition, participation, and quality of life in separate sections, these constructs are very closely related. Not only do many of the standardized instruments address more than one construct (Perenboom & Chorus, 2003) but also there can be disagreement about which construct a specific item targets (Dijkers, 2010; Eadie et al., 2006; Noonan, Kopec, Noreau, Singer, & Dvorak, 2009). We will revisit the discussion of the relationships among these measures in the conclusion of this chapter.

Functional Measures

Of the measures to be discussed in this chapter, functional measures have the longest history in health-care settings and are likely the most widely used by speech-language pathologists. Functional measures are typically used for two main purposes (Brookshire, 2007). These measures are more commonly used to document program effectiveness. The second purpose, which is of greater importance to this discussion, is to assess changes in the performance of individual patients.

Functional Measures Designed for Program Evaluation

Most rehabilitation programs conduct ongoing evaluation of program effectiveness. Often termed "continuous quality improvement," the process of systematically evaluating program effectiveness is required by accreditation agencies (e.g., Joint Council for the Accreditation of Healthcare Organizations). Historically, programs could document quality by verifying that established policies and procedures were monitored and administered consistently (i.e., **process measures**). Process measures were convenient for administrators because performance data (e.g., average delay between the time a referral was received and when the evaluation was completed) were readily obtained, and thus improvements in quality could be documented easily. Unfortunately, process measures are insensitive to important indicators of program quality, such as improved patient function or reduced treatment costs. In recognition of these limitations, accrediting agencies began requesting that programs document quality **outcomes**.

> ### Process Measures in Acute Care: An Example
>
> Evaluating quality through the use of process measures can be very helpful in some situations. In an acute-care setting, we wanted to verify that hospital staff members were following speech-language pathology's recommendations for maximizing communication with individual patients. To study this, we asked each staff member involved with the patient to initial a form indicating that he or she understood not only the unique needs of this patient but also what procedures to use to communicate best with this patient. When we analyzed the documentation

collected from many patients over time, we found that a good proportion of the staff initialed the forms. Our process measure indicated that the procedures we had in place were appropriate for our goal of facilitating effective communication between our patients with neurogenic language and cognitive disorders and their hospital care providers.

What we were unable to determine from our data, however, was whether the patients *actually communicated* more effectively when hospital staff members were made aware of the patients' unique communication needs. Information about this aspect requires outcome measures.

"Outcomes," as the term suggests, refer to the end results of program efforts—specifically, changes in patients' communicative and cognitive functioning. Whereas impairment-level measures such as those discussed in Chapters 6 and 7 might serve to document outcomes, such measures do not serve well for program evaluation for one main reason: Not all patients exhibit the same impairments. To demonstrate that a *program* is effective, the measure used should be appropriate for all patients who participate in the program. To this end, the most frequently used functional measures for program evaluation (i.e., outcome measures) are very general so as to be applicable to all patients regardless of their medical diagnosis or type of neurogenic language and cognitive disorder. Additionally, these functional measures tend to be brief and simple, allowing them to be administered to patients as they enter a program and again at discharge, ideally by any member of the health-care team. What follows is a description of some of the outcome measures most frequently utilized in today's health-care systems.

Perhaps the most well-known and widely used functional outcome measure is the *Functional Independence Measure* (FIM; State University of New York at Buffalo Research Foundation, 1993). Developed specifically to document rehabilitation outcomes, it consists of a seven-point scale for evaluating six performance domains: self-care, sphincter control, mobility, locomotion, communication, and social cognition. Each domain includes two or more specific performance areas (e.g., locomotion includes walking and stairs) that are rated according to level of independence. The communication domain consists of two performance areas: comprehension and expression. Social interaction, problem solving, and memory are the three behaviors included in the social cognition domain. It is clear that these performance areas are broad enough to be applicable to all patients with neurogenic language and cognitive disorders. Unfortunately, because the behaviors are so broadly defined, and because the independence rating scale is neither particularly sensitive nor reliable (Adamovich, 1990; Odell et al., 2005; Warren, 1992), the FIM has not been widely acclaimed by speech-language pathologists. Despite the limitations of the FIM, however, its application to multiple facets of rehabilitation makes it a popular outcome measure for program evaluation.

In recognition of the FIM's limitations in identifying changes in functional performance in the areas of communication, the American Speech-Language-Hearing Association (ASHA) developed a functional measure specifically for communication. The *ASHA Functional Assessment of Communication Skills for Adults* (ASHA FACS; Frattali, Thompson, Holland, Wohl, & Ferketic, 1995) is similar to the FIM in several ways. First, it includes a seven-point rating scale assessing level of independence. Additionally, the ASHA FACS targets several specific behaviors grouped into related domains: social communication (e.g., uses names of familiar people), communication of basic needs (e.g., recognizes familiar faces/voices), daily planning (e.g., dials telephone numbers), and reading/writing/number concepts (e.g., follows written directions). However, unlike the FIM, the ASHA FACS assesses independence in 33 cognitive-communicative behaviors, making it potentially more sensitive to changes in communicative skill. Additionally, the ASHA FACS allows examiners to assess performance qualitatively in each domain, in terms of adequacy, appropriateness, promptness, and communicative sharing. Finally, the ASHA FACS has been standardized for patients with left hemisphere damage, as well as those with TBI; more recently, de Carvalho and Mansur (2008) provided data to support the use of the ASHA FACS when evaluating communication in patients with dementia. There remains a need, however, for data specific to patients with communication disorders related to right hemisphere damage.

Because the ASHA FACS and the FIM provide similar independence scores, some speech-language pathology programs may choose to use the ASHA FACS instead of the FIM to evaluate program effectiveness. Moreover, the ASHA FACS scores reported by the speech-language pathology program can be compared to those submitted by other rehabilitation programs. The high number of items assessed and the complex qualitative scoring system, however, dictate that only trained individuals administer the tool.

ASHA's *National Outcomes Measurement System* (NOMS; ASHA, 2003) is a data collection system developed to help speech-language pathologists and audiologists demonstrate the effectiveness of the services they provide. Included in the NOMS are 15 *Functional Communication Measures* (FCMs), which are disorder-specific rating scales, designed to track changes in functional communication and swallowing behaviors. Six of these scales target behaviors relevant to neurogenic language and cognitive disorders (see Table 8-2).

Participants in the NOMS project rate relevant scales at the beginning of treatment and at discharge, contributing these data to the nationwide NOMS database. Clinicians, facilities, and even integrated health-care delivery systems can then compare their outcomes to the national average. The FCM scales are available to the general population through the ASHA website. However, only facilities that contribute data to the NOMS project have access to the database and program-level outcome analyses provided.

Although program evaluation is a common component of institutional oversight, it may also be mandated by external entities, such as third-party payers and accrediting bodies. In some cases, the external entities specify the tools/measures that must be used to document program effectiveness. An example is the Minimum Data Set (MDS) designed by the United States federal government for use by skilled or long-term nursing facilities that receive funding through Medicare (health insurance for individuals over age 65) or Medicaid (health insurance for individuals with low income). The MDS

TABLE 8-2
ASHA's Functional Communication Measures (FCMs) Relevant to Assessment of Neurogenic Language and Cognitive Disorders

SCALE	EXAMPLE LEVEL
Attention	**Level 5.** The individual maintains attention within simple living activities with occasional minimal cues within distracting environments. The individual requires increased cueing to start, continue, and change attention during complex activities.
Memory	**Level 2.** The individual consistently requires maximal verbal cues or uses external aids to recall personal information (e.g., family members, biographical information, physical location) in structured environments.
Spoken Language Comprehension	**Level 1.** The individual is alert, but unable to follow simple directions or respond to yes/no questions, even with cues.
Spoken Language Expression	**Level 7.** The individual's ability to successfully and independently participate in vocational, avocational, and social activities is not limited by spoken language skills. Independent functioning may occasionally include use of self-cueing.
Reading	**Level 3.** The individual reads single letters and common words, and with consistent moderate cueing, can read some words that are less familiar, longer, and more complex.
Writing	**Level 6.** The individual is successfully able to write most material, but some limitations in writing are still apparent in vocational, avocational, and social activities. The individual rarely requires minimal cueing to write complex material. The individual usually uses compensatory strategies when encountering difficulty.

Note. From ASHA (2003) *National Outcomes Measurement System* (NOMS): *Adult Speech-Language Pathology User's Guide*, Rockville, MD: Author. Copyright 2003 by ASHA. Reprinted with permission. Information about ASHA's *National Outcomes Measurement System* can be found at http://www.asha.org/members/research/noms/

includes, among others, sections for rating cognitive and communicative behavior patterns, psychosocial well-being, and participation in activities. The items targeting cognitive and communicative patterns are best characterized as functional measures, with each item incorporating unique rating scales. For example, the item targeting recall ability is rated according to whether the patient can recall the current season, the location of his or her room, staff names/faces, that he or she lives in a nursing home, or none of those. Other items are rated along a continuum of severity, such as the item targeting speech clarity, which is rated as *clear speech*, *unclear speech*, or *no speech*. In addition to the sections targeting functional behaviors (the ICF level of activity), the MDS sections on psychosocial well-being and participation target the ICF level of participation. Example items include establishing one's own goals and general activity preferences (e.g., games, sports, gardening).

Like the FIM, the MDS can be completed by speech-language pathologists and other health-care team members. In fact, even if the speech-language pathologist is not responsible for administering the MDS, he or she may be involved in educating other health-care team members before they use this tool; that is, the newest version of the MDS mandates that those administering the tool must be educated about communication (including hearing) and cognition problems, as well as techniques that can be used to facilitate communication when assessing a patient with communication or cognitive disorders (Wisely, 2010). Because the MDS targets a broader range and yields a more detailed assessment of relevant behaviors than many tools used for program assessment, it may also be used for individual patient evaluation, similar to the tools described in the next section.

Functional Measures Designed for Patient Evaluation

Measures designed for program evaluation may not be particularly useful when applied to individual patients. That is, measures such as the FIM do not readily inform treatment planning, nor are they necessarily sensitive to treatment-related changes. Therefore, when the purpose is to assess the functional communication or cognitive skills of individual patients, other tools may be more appropriate. Although a number of scales have been described in the research literature (see Table 8-1), the discussion here will be limited to the most well-known and widely applied functional measures.

Because the ASHA FACS describes in detail patient behaviors across a variety of domains, it may be used to evaluate patient performance, as well as program effectiveness. When used for patient evaluation, the qualitative rating scale assessing adequacy, appropriateness, promptness, and communicative sharing is employed to a greater extent than for program evaluation. The independence rating scale may be used for both patient and program evaluation, but the qualitative scale may provide information more valuable for planning treatment and evaluating treatment effectiveness.

The FCMs designed for ASHA's NOMS may also be used to characterize the functional abilities of individual patients. In fact, the six FCMs listed in Table 8-2, as well as two others targeting dysphagia and motor speech disorders, have been approved by the Centers for Medicare and Medicaid Services for documenting patient progress. Moreover, several of the scales include "risk adjustments" that suggest appropriate outcome goals given a particular starting functional level, medical diagnosis, and/or the proportion of treatment addressing that goal. For example, for patients whose memory function is rated at an initial level of 4 or 5, the risk adjustment suggests a target goal of level 7, if at least 50% of treatment time is spent addressing memory and if the memory deficits are not due to TBI. If the memory deficits are due to TBI, the recommended target level is 6. Clinicians can refer to these guidelines as they develop treatment plans and again when decisions regarding discontinuation of treatment are being made. The use of the FCMs is expanding, due in part to the adoption of these scales by Medicare as the means of documenting treatment effectiveness (Skrine & Brown, 2011).

The functional assessment tools developed by ASHA are not, however, the only (or even the first) measures developed specifically for the assessment of functional communication and cognitive abilities. The *Functional Communication Profile* (FCP; M. Sarno, 1969) is one of the earliest measures of functional communication. The FCP includes a rating scale targeting several performance domains. The clinician rates the patient's ability to perform specific tasks in the areas of movement (e.g., ability to imitate oral movements), speaking (e.g., saying noun-verb combinations), understanding (e.g., understanding television), reading (e.g., reading newspaper headlines), and other cognitive and communicative areas (e.g., writing name, calculation, money skills). The FCP's rating system is scored not according to level of independence but rather as the proportion of the patient's ability to perform the tasks prior to neurological injury or disease onset. This scoring method may be challenging because clinicians may not be fully aware of patients' premorbid abilities. Other measures address this limitation.

Lomas and her colleagues (1989) developed a functional measure of communication that differs from those described above in that the rating scales of their *Communicative Effectiveness Index* (CETI) may be scored by the spouse or caregiver of the individual with the neurogenic language and cognitive disorder. Like the FCP, the CETI is based on comparing the patient's current communicative performance with his or her premorbid abilities. Because caregivers likely have greater knowledge than the clinician does about premorbid abilities, as well as more opportunities to observe patients in their current functional communication situations, CETI ratings might be expected to be particularly valid for assessing functional communication skills. Patients with adequate comprehension skills at the sentence level may be able to complete the CETI rating scales themselves. In these cases, the clinician may wish to have the caregivers, as well as the patient, complete the CETI to identify any differences in perceptions regarding treatment effectiveness.

Rating scales such as those described above typically do not specify a particular protocol for eliciting or observing the behaviors in question. Indeed, clinicians frequently complete the rating scales based on behaviors observed during a variety of communicative tasks and situations. Another method of assessing functional skills is by directly eliciting target behaviors. The *Communicative Activities of Daily Living–Second Edition* (CADL-2; A. Holland, Frattali, & Fromm, 1999), a standardized test for patients with aphasia or right hemisphere damage due to stroke or TBI, was designed to elicit communicative behaviors in structured yet functional interactions. It includes items targeting divergent, contextual, and nonverbal communication, social interaction, and other functional skills, such as sequential relationships and humor. Whereas several items utilize scenarios to elicit communicative behaviors (e.g., "You need shoelaces, but you can't find them. If a clerk asked, 'May I help you?' what would you say?"), others elicit responses in a more spontaneous way (e.g., asking the patient to complete a form, but not offering a writing utensil, to determine if the patient notices the anomaly and attempts to correct it). An earlier version of the CADL (A. Holland, 1980) included role-playing tasks that simulated functional communication interactions, which is yet another way to assess functional skills.

Another tool that directly elicits functional behaviors is the *Assessment of Language-Related Functional Activities* (ALFA; Baines, Martin, & Heeringa, 1999). Addressing a diverse array of activities involving the use of language (e.g., telling time, counting money, using a calendar, understanding medicine labels), ALFA items were designed to incorporate scenarios representative of functional activities. For example, one item requires the patient to write a check for a specific bill, being sure to include the current date. The ALFA yields an independent functioning rating that estimates the probability the patient will exhibit independent functioning. Clinicians may consider the independent functioning rating when developing treatment goals and prognoses.

A strength of the ALFA is that the standardization sample was relatively large (i.e., $n = 495$ patients and 150 normal controls) and diverse, including patients with stroke, TBI, and dementia. Thus, the ALFA may be appropriate for patients demonstrating neurogenic language and cognitive disorders resulting from a variety of etiologies. However, an update to the standardization sample and assessment materials is needed for both the ALFA and CADL-2, as each approaches 15 years since its publication.

Informal Measures of Functional Communication

Clinicians may take advantage of the fact that "functional communication" often occurs spontaneously during interactions among the patient, family members, healthcare providers, and other patients. How such interactions are assessed may vary from the primarily subjective (e.g., successful, inefficient) to systematic and objective (e.g., conversational analysis; Crockford & Lesser, 1994). Tools assessing discourse effectiveness (see Chapter 6) might be employed to assist in the description and analysis of functional communication samples. There is some evidence that informal assessment strategies are helpful in revealing changes in functional communication, and that they also hold the potential benefit of revealing the functional communication strengths and weaknesses of patients' communication partners (S. Barnes & Armstrong, 2010; Beeke, Maxim, & Wilkinson, 2007; Crockford & Lesser, 1994).

Selecting Functional Measures for Patients With Neurogenic Language and Cognitive Disorders

Before leaving the discussion of functional measures, it is important to note that we have highlighted the use of these tools to address neurogenic language and cognitive disorders. Some tools, however, may be more or less suited for documenting functional skills in patients with different communication disorders. For example, the highly generic items on the FIM may be appropriate for patients with aphasia, apraxia of speech, or dysarthria, but less sensitive to changes in patients with disorders such as right hemisphere damage (Odell et al., 2005) or TBI (K. M. Hall et al., 2001). Both the ASHA FACS and FIM are heavily weighted with items most appropriate for individuals with aphasia, including only a few items relevant to motor speech or cognitive disorders (e.g., "saying own name" and "using writing instead of speech"). The CETI predominately includes items that address communication limitations commonly experienced by patients with either aphasia or motor speech disorders (e.g., "giving 'yes' and 'no' answers appropriately"), although a few key items (e.g., "describing or discussing something at length") are appropriate for individuals with cognitive-communicative disorders as well. In contrast, the *La Trobe Communication Questionnaire* was designed to capture perceptions of social communication abilities subsequent to TBI (Douglas et al., 2007); that is, for this functional measure, individuals with TBI and their communication partners provide ratings of items related to social and discourse skills frequently compromised by TBI (e.g., "When talking to others do you: Say or do things others might consider rude or embarrassing? Give information that is completely accurate? Switch to a different topic of conversation too quickly?"). The FCM provides separate scales for each of the functional behaviors targeted, allowing clinicians to select the appropriate scale or scales for individual patients. Given these differences across functional communication measures, clinicians should carefully consider both the patient's impairments and the features of the outcome measure, to determine the most appropriate match.

Participation Measures

A common characteristic of functional communication measures is that they attempt to assess communication skills as they are observed in activities outside of the therapeutic setting. A related, but separate, strategy is to assess the degree to which individuals with neurogenic language and cognitive disorders participate in typical daily activities. Historically, participation measures have not been used as frequently as functional measures during initial assessment or to evaluate treatment effectiveness, but they can offer the clinician unique insight into the impact of an individual's communication or cognitive limitations. Whereas functional communication and cognitive measures attempt to characterize communicative and cognitive behaviors during relevant tasks, participation measures may be more general in assessing an individual's level of participation irrespective of the specific functional limitations he or she may be experiencing (Baylor, Burns, Eadie, Britton, & Yorkston, 2011; Hula, Doyle, & Austermann-Hula, 2010).

Consequently, many participation measures were not designed specifically for patients with neurogenic language and cognitive disorders; rather, they target activities for which participation might be restricted due to any number of conditions. For example, the *Craig Handicap Assessment and Reporting Technique* (CHART; Whiteneck, Charlifue, Gerhart, Overholser, & Richardson, 1992) includes, among others, items related to economic self-sufficiency. Clearly, this factor might be affected by limited communication or cognitive skills, as well as other impairments, such as reduced mobility. The CHART has been found to be sensitive to the effects of social communication deficits on occupational and social participation in patients with TBI (Struchen et al., 2008a).

In contrast to the CHART, the *Community Integration Questionnaire* (CIQ; Willer, Rosenthal, Kreutzer, Gordon, & Rempel, 1993) is an example of a participation measure targeting a specific diagnostic group: in this case, patients with TBI. Although both the CHART and CIQ provide information about an individual's degree of participation in standard daily activities and have also been used as rehabilitation outcome measures (e.g., L. Zhang et al., 2002), they have been criticized for being more sensitive to participation restrictions related to physical rather than communication limitations (Hirsch & Holland, 2000).

The *Stroke Impact Scale* (SIS 3.0; Duncan, Bode, Min Lai, & Perera, 2003) is another instrument designed for a specific population. Patients rate their perceived difficulty completing tasks in various domains (e.g., hand function, communication, memory/thinking, participation). Relatively few of the items on the SIS specifically target participation in general, with even fewer targeting communicative participation specifically. Nonetheless, a key advantage of the SIS is its validation in a population of individuals frequently demonstrating communicative or cognitive impairments.

Although not designed to address the participation restrictions of any specific patient group, the *Functional Life Scale* (FLS) developed by J. Sarno, Sarno, and Levita (1973) has been shown to be sensitive to changes in performance as a result of speech-language treatment (M. Sarno, 1997). This tool targets several activity domains, including cognition (e.g., orientation to time, shifts from one task to another with relative ease), activities of daily living (e.g., feeds self, dresses self), activities in the home (e.g., performs light housekeeping chores, uses television), outside activities (e.g., goes shopping for food, uses public transportation alone), and social interaction (e.g., participates in games with other people, attends social functions outside of home). Items within each activity domain are rated along the four dimensions of self-initiation, frequency, speed, and overall efficiency. Using the FLS, M. Sarno (1997) reported that individuals with aphasia participating in a rehabilitation program showed improvement in several domains (e.g., cognition and outside activities), as well as with respect to quality of activity performance (e.g., speed and efficiency). Whereas the complex nature of the rating scale enhances the FLS's sensitivity to changes as a result of treatment, it also increases the amount of time and skill required to administer the instrument and score it reliably. That is, clinicians will require training and should determine the consistency of their ratings prior to using this tool independently.

Participation measures developed either for general populations or for specific populations often include items that are frequently affected by communication and cognitive impairments. Nonetheless, through a systematic review of the literature, Eadie et al. (2006) determined that no existing self-report measures exclusively addressed communicative participation. Moreover, these authors judged the majority of items as targeting general communicative function (similar to what has been operationally defined in this chapter as functional communication), with less than one fourth of items assessing communication during leisure, during work, and within the context of personal relationships (i.e., participation).

In recognition that tools that exclusively target communicative participation are lacking, efforts are under way to develop the *Communicative Participation Item Bank* (Yorkston et al., 2008; Yorkston & Baylor, 2011). Initial investigations have examined the usefulness of the items for characterizing participation restrictions reported by individuals whose communication disorders resulted from spasmodic dysphonia, multiple sclerosis, stroke, Parkinson's disease, amyotrophic lateral sclerosis, and laryngectomy

(Baylor et al., 2011). As study of this item bank continues, additional information will become available regarding the aspects of communication participation restrictions most commonly reported by individuals with neurogenic language and cognitive disorders.

Informal Measures of Participation

Many clinicians will find it advantageous to include informal measures of participation as part of the complete evaluation process. A distinct advantage of informal measures is that the clinician can tailor the content and form to meet the unique presentation of each patient. For example, if a clinician is aware of a patient's premorbid interests and activities, assessment activities can be devised that carefully document that patient's participation in these specific areas.

Informal assessment of participation might include asking the patient, family members, or both about participation in typical activities. Many questions utilized in the formal measures described above might serve as a model for the types of questions clinicians could include in an informal interview. For example, Swigert (1997) described a four-question interview to address participation. In this approach, patients are asked to identify situations in which communication is most difficult and to describe how communication difficulties have impacted interactions with friends and family and at work. A unique item asks the patient, "Do you avoid situations because of your speech?" (p. 59). These questions could easily be incorporated into the clinical interview.

Additionally, useful information regarding participation can be gained through direct observation of the patient during typical activities. Ideally, these observations would take place in naturalistic settings, such as social events, vocational activities, or other activities the patient had been involved in premorbidly. A clear advantage of direct observation is that the clinician may gain valuable insights into the interactions between the patient and the communication or cognitive situation. That is, many times it will become clear that the key factor limiting a patient's participation in a particular activity is not the communication or cognitive disorder, but rather the environment (i.e., the contextual factors component of the ICF model). For instance, factors such as background noise and the pacing of the activity, which may have a strong influence on the success with which patients with neurogenic language and cognitive disorders participate in activities, are often difficult to ascertain from an interview alone (see Chapter 4 for further discussion of the benefits of including observation into assessment procedures).

Quality-of-Life Measures

Although participation measures contribute unique information to our understanding of the impact of neurogenic language and cognitive disorders on our patients' lives, they do not address a key component of treatment effectiveness: quality of life. That is, the inability to balance the checkbook or select items at a grocery store (i.e., participation measures) may have little or no impact on the quality of life of a patient who has never been responsible for these tasks or perhaps never enjoyed or valued being responsible for these tasks. Similarly, some patients may participate in highly unique activities that are not addressed by standardized participation measures (e.g., participation in a foreign language club). Quality-of-life measures allow clinicians to assess more directly the impact of communication and cognitive limitations on patients' overall well-being.

Just as overlap exists among measures of function and participation, the same is true for measures of participation and quality of life. The unique aspect of quality of life measures is the attempt to characterize patients' emotional response to disruptions in function and participation. Quality of life and well-being may be assessed both formally and informally (see Table 8-1). We will first review some formal measures targeting quality of life.

Quality of Life: The Patient's Priority

Assessing both participation and quality of life may reveal patient experiences that are surprising, yet quite relevant to the clinical process. Ray is a 64-year-old man with severe aphasia characterized by limited auditory comprehension and fluent, empty speech. He presented for outpatient evaluation approximately one year after his left hemisphere stroke. Through interviews with Ray's neighbor, who graciously accompanied Ray to the evaluation, we learned that following his stroke, Ray had been committed to a psychiatric hospital by his (now) ex-wife, who had then proceeded to obtain authority over Ray's finances.

We further learned that even though Ray continued to participate in nearly all the activities he enjoyed, his quality of life was limited by the loss of his driver's license resulting from his inappropriate committal and his inability to adequately defend his legal rights. Ray's goals for therapy were very specific: to pass the written test to regain his driver's license, and to develop strategies for effectively communicating with his ex-wife and legal representatives.

General Quality-of-Life Measures

Many measures have been devised to assess quality of life. In this section, we first discuss a select sample of such general measures that have been used to assess quality of life in individuals with neurogenic language and cognitive disorders. Second, a sample of quality-of-life measures developed specifically for individuals experiencing communication disorders will be presented.

The *Sickness Impact Profile* (SIP; Bergner, Bobbitt, Carter, & Gibson, 1981) includes items describing activities in 12 categories of daily living: sleep and rest, emotional behavior, body care and movement, home management, mobility, social interaction, ambulation, alertness behavior, communication, work, recreation and pastimes, and eating. Patients identify each of the 136 items that are impacted by their health. Based on the overall number as well as the type of items identified, the SIP provides scores representing overall dysfunction, dysfunction in each activity category, and dysfunction in psychosocial and physical domains. Shorter versions of the SIP have also been developed to facilitate its use in both clinical and research settings (e.g., the SIP68, with 68 items; Nanda, McLendon, Andresen, & Armbrecht, 2003).

The SIP may be self-scored by the patient or administered as an interview. The items are heavily weighted with respect to daily activities, making the SIP very similar to functional communication and participation measures. However, the items related to emotional behavior may provide some insight into patient well-being. Hirsch and Holland (2000) recommended supplementing the SIP with additional questions addressing life satisfaction.

A measure similar to the SIP but having the advantage of incorporating fewer items is the *Dartmouth COOP Functional Assessment Charts* (Nelson et al., 1986). In this measure, patients respond to a single question on each of nine charts that target physical fitness, feelings, daily activities, social activities, pain, changes in health, overall health, social support, and quality of life. For each chart, the patient is asked to respond by rating the question along a five-point scale that is depicted both verbally and visually, which may facilitate the responses of individuals with communication limitations. As is the case with many of the instruments described in this chapter, this tool targets ratings of participation as well as quality of life.

Whereas rating scales often directly ask patients about the impact of impairments on their quality of life, another strategy for assessing qualify of life is to ask patients to respond to items that indirectly reflect well-being. One measure utilizing this strategy is the *Affect Balance Scale* (ABS; Bradburn, 1969). Similar in length to the Dartmouth Charts, the ABS requires patients to respond to 10 questions regarding their experience of a variety of feelings during the past few weeks. For example, one item asks, "During the past few weeks did you ever feel depressed or very unhappy?" The patient responds with a simple "yes" or "no" answer. Because ABS questions do not specify that health issues are necessarily the cause of positive or negative feelings, the scale can be used for a variety of purposes outside of rehabilitation. When the ABS has been employed in studies examining the effectiveness of communication treatment, it has failed to reveal differences in ratings as a result of aphasia treatment (Lyon et al., 1997) or between young adults with or without a history of specific language impairment (Records, Tomblin, & Freese, 1992). Therefore, although the ABS may provide the clinician with some insight into the patient's current state of well-being, additional evidence is needed to support the use of this tool for documenting treatment outcomes.

The *Satisfaction With Life Scale* (SWLS; Diener, Emmons, Larsen, & Griffin, 1985) involves even fewer items than the Dartmouth Charts or the ABS. The SWLS requires patients to respond to five items using a seven-point rating scale. The items are quite general and, like the ABS, do not relate specifically to medical issues. For example, one item is "In most ways, my life is close to my ideal." Hirsch and Holland (2000) proposed that the ABS and SWLS might complement each other in the assessment of overall quality of life, given that the ABS focuses on affect, whereas the SWLS focuses on satisfaction.

Using General Quality-of-Life Measures for Patients With Neurogenic Language and Cognitive Disorders

Limited information is available regarding which quality-of-life measures may be most appropriate for individuals with neurogenic language and cognitive disorders. Hirsch and Holland (1999) attempted to identify the strengths and weaknesses of several tools for addressing the quality of life of individuals with aphasia. These authors examined five measures: the *Dartmouth COOP Charts*; the *Affect Balance Scale* (ABS); the Behavior, Emotion, Attitude, and Communication questionnaire (BEAC); the *Sickness Impact Profile* (SIP); and the OneQ, an informal measure of quality of life that involves only one question.

Of the measures studied, the SIP had the longest administration time (average 36 minutes) and the OneQ had the shortest (average 1 minute). The three remaining measures had average administration times of less than 13 minutes. The examiners rated the OneQ and ABS the most favorably with respect to item wording. The SIP and BEAC were rated the least favorably, with items that were long, complex, and/or ambiguous. With respect to response format, the BEAC was rated least favorably by the examiners. Patients completing the OneQ and ABS required less assistance than when completing the remaining measures. These two measures were also rated most favorably with respect to overall appropriateness, with the OneQ rated above the ABS. The factors affecting ratings of overall appropriateness included ease of administration, reliability of subject responses, appropriateness of content, and face validity. When all examiner ratings were summed, the OneQ measure was rated most favorably and the SIP least favorably.

The patients judged the various measures to be no different from one another with respect to item wording, validity, or like/dislike. Even when all patient ratings were summed, no differences among measures were identified. These findings suggest that whereas patients may not prefer any measure to another, examiners reported a strong preference for the OneQ. Speech-language pathologists might consider these findings when selecting a tool for assessing the quality of life of patients with neurogenic language and cognitive disorders.

Communication-Related Quality of Life

The scales described above are considered "general" in that they were not explicitly designed for populations likely to demonstrate cognitive or linguistic impairments. In this section, we review tools designed for individuals with communicative impairments or conditions commonly accompanied by communicative or cognitive impairments. The clear advantage of these tools over general quality-of-life measures is that each has published psychometric data supporting their use with patients who have communication disorders.

The *Stroke-Specific Quality of Life Scale* (SS-QOL; Williams, Weinberger, Harris, Clark, & Biller, 1999) and its shorter version, *Stroke and Aphasia Quality of Life Scale–39* (SAQOL-39; Hilari, Byng, Lamping, & Smith, 2003; Hilari et al., 2007), are two scales designed to address the unique needs of individuals experiencing aphasia following stroke. Although described as quality-of-life measures, these tools involve patient ratings of function (e.g., trouble with preparing food, trouble with speaking), participation (e.g., going out less, doing hobbies less), and quality of life (e.g., feeling discouraged). The SS-QOL and SAQOL-39 include items related to physical (e.g., trouble with walking), psychosocial (e.g., feeling irritable), communication (e.g., trouble with finding words), and energy (e.g., feeling tired often) domains. Notably, versions of the SAQOL-39 in languages other than English (e.g., Italian, Spanish, Greek), along with some description of the psychometric properties of these translated versions, can be found in the empirical literature (e.g., Lata-Caneda et al., 2009; Posteraro et al., 2006).

A quality-of-life measure very similar to the SS-QOL and SAQLS-39 is the *Burden of Stroke Scale* (BOSS; Doyle et al., 2004). Like the SS-QOL and SAQLS-39, the BOSS incorporates items addressing function, participation, and quality of life. Its psychometric properties have also been documented (e.g., Hula, Doyle, et al., 2010). The BOSS is unique, however, in the way its items are combined to address each level of description. For example, in the communication domain, the examiner asks, "Because of your stroke, how difficult is it for you to talk with a group of people?" The patient then responds according to a five-point scale (i.e., *not at all, a little, moderately, very, cannot do*). If the patient indicates difficulty with that particular area of function, follow-up probes addressing participation and quality of life are administered (e.g., "You indicated that you have some difficulties communicating. How often do difficulties communicating cause you to feel anxious, unhappy, or frustrated?" and "How much do difficulties communicating prevent you from doing the things in life that are important to you?").

The BOSS includes items in the domains of mobility (e.g., balance), self-care (e.g., dressing), communication (e.g., writing a letter), cognition (e.g., concentrating), swallowing (e.g., swallowing liquids), social relations (e.g., maintaining family roles), energy and sleep (e.g., staying awake through the day), negative mood (e.g., loneliness), and positive mood (e.g., confidence). Similar to the SS-QOL and SAQLS-39, these domains are relevant to patients experiencing cognitive or communication disorders resulting from etiologies other than stroke, but additional research is needed to evaluate their application to these other patient groups.

The *Quality of Life After Brain Injury* (QOLIBRI; von Steinbuchel et al., 2010) instrument is one of the first scales developed specifically to address the quality of life of individuals recovering from brain injury. The QOLIBRI includes six scales; the Cognition, Self, Daily Life and Autonomy, and Social Relationships scales are framed with respect to satisfaction, whereas the Emotions and Physical Problems scales address the extent to which an individual feels "bothered." Initial evidence suggests the QOLIBRI is sensitive to aspects of quality of life targeted in intervention, such as accommodation and work participation (Truelle et al., 2010).

Similar disease-specific tools have been developed to assess quality of life for individuals with dementia. The DEMQOL (Smith et al., 2007) is an example of an instrument that can be administered to the patient or to a caregiver (DEMQOL-Proxy). An update of the *Dementia Quality of Life Questionnaire* (DQOL; Brod et al., 1999), the DEMQOL, includes items addressing feelings generally (e.g., loneliness, enjoyment) and feelings of worry about memory and everyday activities, including communication. A similar tool is the *Quality of Life in Alzheimer's Disease* (QOL-AD; Logsdon, Gibbons, McCurry, & Teri, 1999, 2002). This instrument includes a relatively small number of items and may be more appropriate than the DEMQOL for individuals with severe cognitive impairments (Moyle, Gracia, Murfield, Griffiths, & Venturato, 2011). The Dementia Outcomes Measurement Suite (DOMS; Sansoni et al., 2007) provides a website that further reviews tools for assessing quality of life in individuals with dementia: http://www.dementia-assessment.com.au.

The scales reviewed above were designed for specific patient populations that frequently experience communication difficulties. Such scales may be particularly useful for patients who exhibit a number of impairments impacting mobility, cognition, and communication, all of which interact to influence overall quality of life. Another approach is to consider how the disruption of communication ability, regardless of etiology, impacts quality of life. To address this issue, the American Speech-Language-Hearing Association developed the *Quality of Communication Life Scale* (ASHA QCL; Paul-Brown et al., 2004). The ASHA QCL consists of 18 statements for which patients are asked to state their agreement. Unlike other quality-of-life scales, patients are instructed that the statements are specifically concerned with communication. For example, the clinician instructs, "Think about how you feel now. For each statement, first ask yourself: 'Even though I have difficulty communicating...', then read the statement" (p. 35). Several items address participation issues (e.g., "I stay in touch with family and friends," "People include me in conversations"), whereas others address well-being and quality of life (e.g., "I am confident that I can communicate," "I like myself"). Patients indicate their agreement with each statement by placing a mark on a five-point printed vertical scale (i.e., the top of the scale indicates the statement describes the patient well). The clinician then calculates the average rating, excluding the final item, "In general, my quality of life is good," to provide an overall estimate of patients' quality of communication life.

The ASHA QCL can be administered in less than 20 minutes, with patients completing the scale either independently or with clinician assistance. Although the standardization sample was relatively small ($n = 57$), patients with aphasia, cognitive-communicative disorders, or dysarthria were included, suggesting that the ASHA QCL may be appropriate for a variety of patients.

Informal Measures of Quality of Life

Informal measures of quality of life will most likely take the form of an interview focusing on the patient's emotional response to impairments, activity limitations, and participation restrictions. The informal measure shown below asks patients to rate the impact of their disorder on various aspects of their life. Alternatively, clinicians might assess quality of life using a single, carefully worded question such as, "Overall, how would you rate your current lifestyle?" (Hinckley, 1998). Regardless of the precise format, informal measures of quality of life should aid the clinician in determining the unique impact of communication and cognitive limitations for each individual patient.

> **EXAMPLE OF INFORMAL ASSESSMENT OF QUALITY OF LIFE**
>
> Have your communication/cognitive difficulties affected your:
>
> - Ability to work?
> - Interactions with friends and family?
> - Ability to participate in social activities?
> - Overall sense of well-being?

Relationships Among Measures of Impairment, Function, Participation, and Quality of Life

As pointed out in the introduction to this chapter, the tools available to facilitate assessment of functional communication and cognition, participation, and quality of life often address two or more of those constructs. This phenomenon likely reflects, at least partially, the lack of agreement about how various behaviors should be categorized, and leads to the question of whether these various tools actually measure different underlying constructs (Hula, Doyle, et al., 2010; Irwin et al., 2002). Surprisingly few studies have explored the relationships among measures of impairment, activity, and participation/quality of life. Additionally, such studies addressing neurogenic language and cognitive impairments in adults have focused on aphasia more than cognitive-communicative disorders associated with right hemisphere brain damage, TBI, or dementing diseases.

The nature of the relationships among various levels of measurement has varied across studies, as has the interpretation of the findings. Ross and Wertz (2002) investigated relationships among two language impairment tests (*Western Aphasia Battery, Porch Index of Communicative Ability*—see Chapter 6), two tests of functional communication (CADL-2, ASHA FACS), and two measures of quality of life (neither were reviewed in this chapter but were similar in nature to those summarized in the preceding sections). For a group of individuals with aphasia, no significant relationships were observed between language impairment and quality of life, or between functional communication and quality of life. The authors interpreted these findings to suggest that because quality of life was not related to language impairment or functional communication, language therapy targeting quality of life could not be justified. Alternately, the findings might suggest that each level of description is unique, so it is therefore worthwhile to address each construct during assessment and potentially during treatment.

Two additional studies (Aftonomos, Steele, Appelbaum, & Harris, 2001; Irwin et al., 2002) examining relationships among similar instruments reported significant correlations between scores on impairment-level (e.g., *Western Aphasia Battery*) and activity-level tools (e.g., CETI). Aftonomos and colleagues (2001) further reported, however, that the changes in scores over time were not the same across measurements, supporting the clinical value of including measures of impairment and function when reporting patient response to treatment.

Nonetheless, as Irwin et al. (2002) recommended, additional research utilizing appropriate statistical methods is needed to describe more clearly the relationships among the measures targeting the various ICF constructs, as well as quality of life. Our understanding of these issues will be further strengthened as measures of impairment and function in patients with cognitive-communicative disorders (e.g., Fromm & Holland, 1989) are included in such studies. Finally, given that performance on measures of language impairment, functional communication, and quality of life has been shown to be influenced by the patient's age, gender, and/or educational level (Ross & Wertz, 2001), it is likely that additional research will identify further factors that influence the relationship among the constructs of impairment, activity, participation, and quality of life.

Recognizing that issues of functional communication, participation, and quality of life are not only closely related but also influenced by environmental and personal factors, the developers of the *Assessment for Living With Aphasia* (ALA; Aphasia Institute, 2010) incorporated items directly addressing these factors. The ALA was developed out of the A-FROM model introduced at the beginning of this chapter (Kagan et al., 2008). This instrument uses an interview format to elicit ratings from the patient with aphasia regarding the domains of communication performance, participation, aspects of the environment, and the personal experience of aphasia. A relatively unique feature of the ALA is the use of visual rating scales augmented with images to facilitate comprehension and expression (see Figure 8-1). The instrument yields scores for each domain, as well as an overall total. Moreover, responses to individual items may lead to the development of specific targets for intervention. To date, the ALA has been studied only in the context of aphasia and is arguably most appropriate for this population, in that several items refer explicitly to aphasia. Nonetheless, it is likely that responses provided by individuals with cognitive impairments would also be meaningful in characterizing the impact on communicative effectiveness and participation, as well as environmental and personal factors influencing these issues.

Authentic Assessment and Ethnography

The final section of this chapter addresses a method of assessing communication function, life participation, and quality of life without the use of formal measures such as those outlined previously. Simmons-Mackie and Damico (1996) developed the Communicative Profiling System (CPS), a form of **authentic assessment** based on ethnographic and conversational analysis research methods. The CPS incorporates five basic

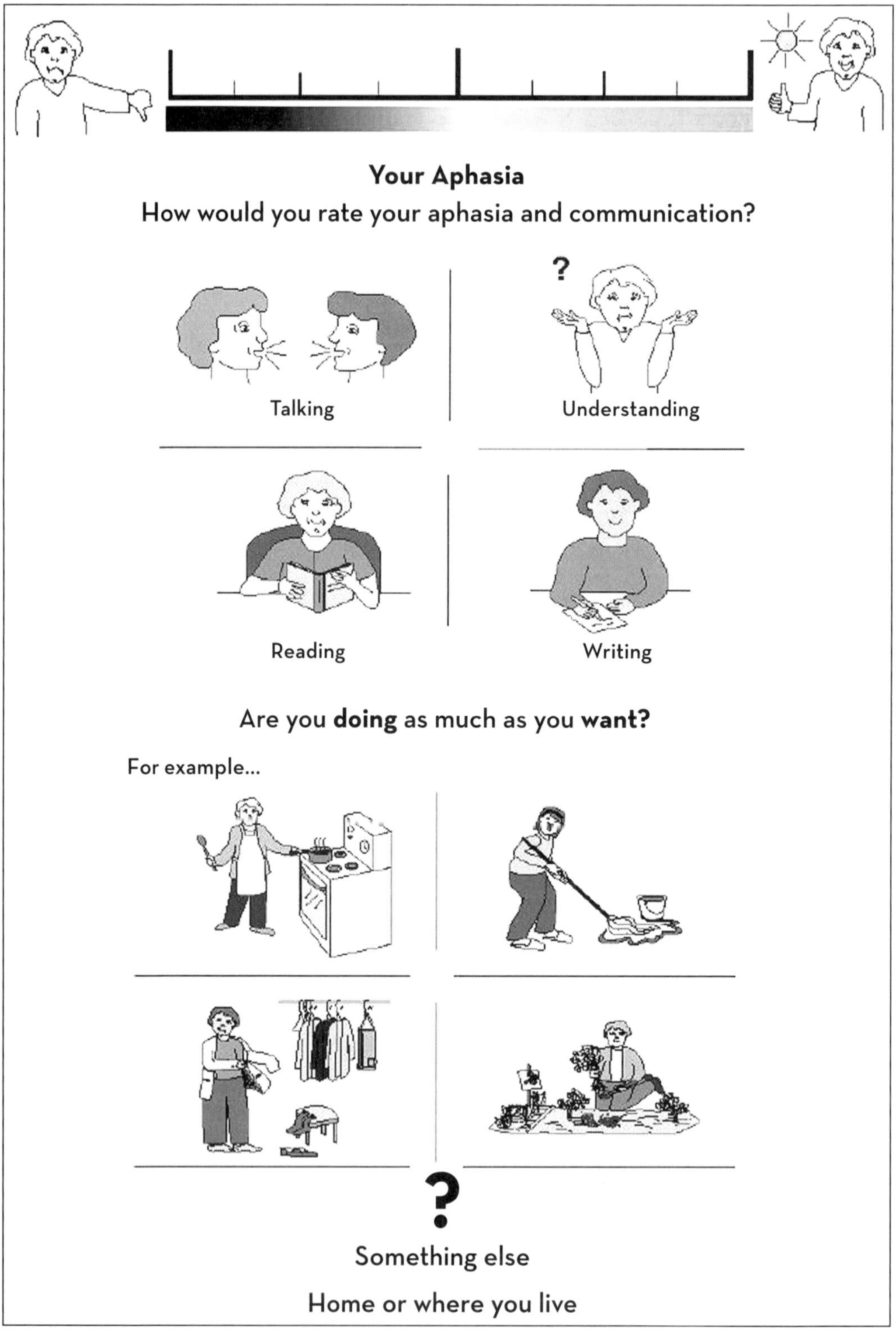

Figure 8-1. Examples of the rating scale and items from the *Assessment for Living With Aphasia*. Note. From *Assessment for Living With Aphasia*, by A. Kagan, N. Simmons-MacKie, J. C. Victor, A. Carling-Rowland, J. Hoch, M. Huijbregts, D. Streiner, and A. Mok, 2010, Aphasia Institute, Toronto, Ontario, Canada. Copyright 2010 by the Aphasia Institute. Reprinted with permission.

assessment principles: (1) Assessment addresses communication in real-life situations, (2) assessment considers the contexts in which communication takes place, (3) systematic data collection procedures are employed, (4) data are subjected to systematic qualitative analyses, and (5) conclusions are developed specifically for planning intervention.

Each of the four phases of the CPS involves data collection and analysis. In Phase One, the clinician develops a broad perspective of the patient's communication behaviors by interviewing individuals who communicate with the patient. The ethnographic interview is open-ended and informant driven (Simmons-Mackie & Damico, 2001). This is an important difference from the self-reported measures described earlier in this chapter, most of which involve a finite list of items that are administered to all respondents, regardless of their responses. Asking open-ended questions and allowing the patient's or family member's responses to direct the subsequent questions help the clinician identify the behaviors, contexts, and interactants that will be incorporated in the next phases of assessment. The second phase of the CPS involves direct observation of communicative interactions. Simmons-Mackie and Damico suggested that the clinician engage in participant-observation rather than attempting to contrive situations that mimic real-life contexts. Also included in Phase Two is collection of anecdotal reports of specific communicative interactions (e.g., the patient's spouse may describe the patient's attempt to order at a restaurant). The clinician considers the information gained in Phases One and Two to identify communicative patterns that warrant closer assessment.

Phase Three involves collecting and analyzing videotaped samples of communication in authentic contexts selected based on the communicative behaviors, contexts, and interactants deemed most relevant during earlier CPS phases. Further examination of the information obtained in Phases One through Three allows the clinician to explore more fully the interactions between communication behavior and context (Phase Four) as a means of identifying the purposes specific communicative behaviors might serve, as well as noting the communication strategies the patient may select in different contexts. Through this assessment process, the clinician will likely have obtained information regarding the ICF constructs of activity and participation, as well as environmental factors. The information obtained during initial data gathering will inform treatment planning, as well as serve as a baseline against which the effectiveness of treatment can be judged. Data collection should be ongoing, however, in recognition that communication behaviors and contexts are not static (Simmons-Mackie & Damico, 2001). Individuals learn new compensatory strategies, take on new responsibilities and roles, gain or lose communication partners, suffer medical setbacks, or experience any of the nearly limitless ways life situations can change. Dynamic, patient-driven, authentic assessment helps the clinician keep abreast of these changes and modify management strategies accordingly.

The authentic assessment process described by the CPS may be particularly useful when standardized tools are deemed inappropriate, inadequate, or both for addressing a specific patient's concerns. For example, a young adult experiencing a stroke, a patient who is deaf or multilingual, or a patient who has family members who also exhibit communication impairments will each likely demonstrate unique needs that may not be addressed by tools designed for more typical patient groups. The CPS provides a system for identifying and gaining an understanding of unique contexts and interactants that impact the patient's communication function, life participation, and quality of life. Nonetheless, given both the training needed to use the CPS effectively and the time required to implement it appropriately, the CPS should not be undertaken casually. Clinicians may incorporate principles of authentic assessment (e.g., patient-driven interviewing, direct observation of communication in context) as they seek to understand the impact of a patient's language or cognitive impairments on functional communication, participation, and quality of life.

Summary

This chapter concludes the discussion of assessment of neurogenic language and cognitive disorders. The assessment strategies described will help clinicians identify the impairments contributing to the communication and cognitive limitations experienced by patients, as well as the impact of these limitations on their function, life participation, and overall quality of life. Only when information about all of these factors is obtained can a complete diagnosis be determined, a reliable prognosis established, and an effective treatment program planned. Furthermore, the assessment process does not end here. As previously stated in Chapter 4, continued assessment throughout the treatment process is critical both to ensuring that treatment is effective and to monitoring the patient for signs of disease progression or new disease onset. The methods described in Chapters 4 through 8 are appropriate for initial evaluation, as well as for ongoing assessment and evaluation of treatment outcomes. The remaining chapters will focus on developing and evaluating treatment strategies that address the impairments, activity limitations, and participation restrictions identified in the assessment process.

Discussion Questions

1. What type of outcome measures do you think patients and their families would find most meaningful?
2. What is the value of combining measures addressing underlying impairment, functional communication, participation, and quality of life?
3. Are disease-specific measures of function, participation, and quality of life needed? Why or why not?
4. How could the presence of a communication or cognitive impairment influence the administration, scoring, and interpretation of measures of participation and/or quality of life?

Remediation of Body Structure and Function: Behavioral Approaches for Linguistic Disorders

chapter 9

Learning Objectives

After reading this chapter, you should be able to:

- Compare and contrast stimulation and cognitive neuropsychological approaches to treating language impairments at the ICF level of body structure and function
- Describe specific behavioral treatment procedures for addressing phonological, orthographic, lexical–semantic, morphosyntactic, or pragmatic impairments
- Discuss the strengths and weaknesses of utilizing commercially available workbooks and computer software programs when treating neurogenic language disorders
- Discuss linguistic treatment planning issues pertaining to the generalization and transfer of treatment effects

Key Terms

- barrier games
- coarse coding
- cognitive neuropsychological treatments
- constraint-induced aphasia therapy
- conversational script training
- cueing hierarchy
- mapping therapy
- Melodic Intonation Therapy
- Multiple Oral Rereading
- reauditorization
- repetitive transcranial magnetic stimulation
- Response Elaboration Training
- Semantic Feature Analysis
- stimulation treatments
- transcranial direct current stimulation
- Treatment of Underlying Forms
- Voluntary Control of Involuntary Utterances

Introduction

Clinicians face many challenges when planning and providing treatment for the linguistic impairments of patients with neurogenic language and cognitive disorders. First, clinicians must often prove to those making the referrals and those funding the therapy that linguistic treatments do indeed work. Although a significant and growing research literature supports linguistic treatment efficacy (e.g., Basso et al., 2011; M. Brady, Kelly, Godwin, & Enderby, 2012; Cicerone et al., 2011), speech-language pathology services continue to be declined or restricted by many insurers (Code, 2012; Code & Petheram, 2011; Katz et al., 2000). Inadequate provision of communicative therapy services is perhaps most pervasive with respect to the dementia patient population. As several investigators have noted, when clinicians do receive referrals for dementia patients, it is typically for dysphagia assessment and treatment, as health-care providers often (a) view behavioral intervention for these patients as inappropriate given the progressive nature of dementia, or (b) are unaware that intervention can produce significant improvements in these patients' abilities (Cleary et al., 2003; Hopper, Bayles, Harris, & Holland, 2001; Mahendra & Arkin, 2003). Accordingly, it is imperative that clinicians keep abreast of the empirical findings that support the provision of linguistic treatments for neurogenic disorders, and have on hand a list of research citations that can be forwarded to referral sources or funding agencies when advocating for treatment services.

A second challenge clinicians face is selecting from the plethora of treatment approaches the technique or techniques that will be most appropriate for each individual patient. This selection will be facilitated in part by a comprehensive evaluation that provides data pertaining to patients' linguistic strengths and weaknesses, as well as their daily communicative needs (see Chapters 4–8). Having a critical understanding of the variety of therapies currently available also is essential to selecting and providing the most suitable and efficient treatment for a given patient, particularly when the clinician's initial treatment choice proves ineffective.

To help resolve these challenges, we review in this chapter a variety of treatment procedures that have been developed to remediate neurogenic language disorders at the ICF level of body structure and function. Most of the behavioral treatments reviewed in this chapter were developed for language disorders associated with aphasia, as aphasia has been studied and clinically managed for much longer than language symptoms associated with right hemisphere brain damage (RHD), traumatic brain injury (TBI), or dementia. Over the last two decades or so, however, researchers and clinicians have begun to identify language interventions that can be effective with a variety of patient populations, or that are more specific to the language needs of patients with RHD, TBI, or dementia.

Two general treatment approaches encompass the majority of the behavioral procedures currently available for remediating the linguistic impairments of patients with neurogenic language and cognitive disorders: the linguistic stimulation approach and the cognitive neuropsychological approach. The **stimulation approach** is the most widely used linguistic treatment approach in the United States, and, as Coelho, Sinotte, and Duffy (2008) conjectured, "may be thought to encompass all approaches to aphasia rehabilitation" (p. 403). Basically, **stimulation treatments** emphasize understanding what stimulus factors may impede or enhance patients' current linguistic abilities, and then expose patients to stimulus and task hierarchies that will "stimulate" functioning of compromised language functions and modalities. In contrast, in **cognitive neuropsychological treatments**, models of normal and/or disordered language are used to motivate treatment targets and procedures (Whitworth et al., 2005; see also Chapter 1). Following a comprehensive assessment designed to delineate which specific linguistic processes (e.g., phoneme-to-grapheme conversion, phonological output lexicon) have been compromised (for further description of cognitive neuropsychological assessment procedures, see Chapter 6), the focus of cognitive neuropsychological treatments is to improve the disrupted processes or to capitalize on more intact processes, and then to evaluate how therapy effected change in trained (as well as untrained) linguistic stimuli, functions, and modalities. It is important to note that although the therapy procedures used when adhering to a cognitive neuropsychological treatment approach are often similar to those developed out of the stimulation approach, the rationale for these procedures is not. This chapter will review stimulation and cognitive neuropsychological treatments that have been developed to address linguistic impairments at the International Classification of Functioning, Disability, and Health (ICF; WHO 2001) level of body structure and function.

> ### Treatment Selection and Justification: Going Beyond "Because It Works!"
>
> How important is it to understand the theoretical framework behind a treatment? If a treatment works, why not just use it? There are at least two good reasons for clinicians to understand the philosophy guiding a given intervention strategy. The first reason is that clinicians should be able to explain to patients, their families, or both the purpose of a treatment activity. Patients who understand how the treatment is intended to help them will be more motivated to participate in treatment and devote energy to the tasks and strategies. Furthermore, caregivers are more likely to follow through with carryover activities if they understand their purpose. The second reason clinicians should understand the theory driving the intervention strategy is to provide the basis on which the therapy tasks can be modified to meet the needs of individual patients. To illustrate this concept, consider a treatment activity during which the patient is attempting to name pictures of common nouns. In a stimulation-based treatment (described later in this chapter), the clinician provides various semantic, phonologic, or other cues based on which cues elicit the appropriate response. Thus, within this framework, the clinician modifies the intervention task based on how the patient responds to various cues. In contrast, in the cognitive neuropsychologically based treatment of semantic feature analysis (also described later in this chapter), "cues" are limited to semantic features. Thus, although the clinician might modify which semantic features are targeted, all identified features would be reviewed even if some features were not particularly helpful to the patient in generating the target name. Although these two treatment strategies may look very similar to a naïve observer, the informed clinician will understand how their purposes differ, as well as how each can be modified to meet the needs of individual patients.

Phonological and Orthographic Treatments

As discussed in Chapter 6, assessment and consequently treatment of phonological and orthographic processes are most common when dealing with patients with aphasia. In contrast, patients with other types of neurogenic disorders do not frequently exhibit impairments at this language-processing level, and when such impairments are present, they are typically not a rehabilitation priority. Accordingly, most treatment procedures reviewed in this section were developed for, and thus are most suitable for, patients with aphasia.

Phonological Treatments

Although deficits of segmental and suprasegmental aspects of phonology are possible in patients with neurogenic language and cognitive disorders, there are currently limited treatment options available for remediating these types of language impairments. That is, most research to date has focused on qualifying and quantifying phonological impairments, rather than developing and validating treatment procedures. Accordingly, many of the therapy approaches and activities described require further empirical investigation to establish the validity and reliability of their effects.

Treatment of Segmental Impairments

Difficulties with discriminating or perceiving segmental aspects of phonology have been hypothesized to underlie the spoken and written word comprehension deficits of many patients with aphasia. Despite the possible prevalence of impairments at this level of language processing (Alexander & Hillis, 2008), only a few treatment approaches have been described or evaluated in the research literature.

One approach to remediating phonological decoding problems involves practicing speech discrimination tasks. For example, in a case study by J. Morris, Franklin, Ellis, Turner, and Bailey (1996), a patient with global aphasia and significant speech perception problems was provided a set of treatment activities designed to improve his discrimination of auditory speech stimuli. Treatment tasks included the following: (a) phoneme–grapheme matching—choosing which of three letters matched a spoken stimulus; (b) phoneme discrimination—deciding if a pair of spoken syllables was the same or different; (c) auditory word–picture matching—choosing which of three pictures matched a spoken word; (d) written word–auditory word matching—selecting which of three written words matched a spoken word, (e) correct/incorrect judgment—deciding if a spoken word matched a written word or picture; and (f) nonword syllable same-or-different judgment—deciding if pairs of spoken consonant-vowel syllables were the same or different. Treatment stimuli were selected so that initially the patient practiced discriminating spoken stimuli that differed significantly, with respect to phoneme characteristics such as the distinctive features of voice, place, and manner of articulation (e.g., "cot" vs. "lock"). As he progressed, the stimuli more closely approximated each other (e.g., "cot" vs. "pot"). Following 12 therapy sessions, the patient's phoneme discrimination and repetition of untrained stimuli significantly improved; positive but nonsignificant changes on auditory lexical decision and synonym judgment tasks also were observed.

Corsten and colleagues (2007) also examined the effects of speech discrimination treatment, but they utilized a computerized protocol. Their patient with phonological difficulties practiced twice daily (a total of 60 sessions across 6 weeks) discrimination tasks (i.e., determining if two auditory stimuli were the same or different), identification tasks (i.e., identifying an auditory target among four written choices), and reproduction tasks (i.e., repeating or reading aloud an auditory target when shown four written choices). As the patient improved, training tasks were made more difficult by increasing the number of targets (e.g., identifying two vs. one auditory target) and manipulating linguistic variables (e.g., increasing the phonological similarity of target and distracter items; placing the phonetic contrast at the beginning vs. end of items). Post-treatment, the patient demonstrated significant improvements in identifying and repeating words and pseudowords, reproducing words, and making rhyme judgments. Few of these improvements, however, were maintained three months post-treatment.

In another case study, the commercially available *Auditory Discrimination in Depth* (ADD; Lindamood & Lindamood, 1975), currently referred to as the *Lindamood Phoneme Sequencing Program for Reading, Spelling, and Speech* (LiPS; Lindamood & Lindamood, 2011), was used to improve the phonological awareness, reading, and spelling abilities of a patient with mild, acquired alexia and agraphia (T. Conway et al., 1998). As shown in Table 9-1, initial ADD treatment sessions focus on increasing patients' awareness of how phonemes are produced. Next, treatment targets patients' ability to break down and, consequently, read and spell short nonword syllables into their component speech sounds. The final stages of the ADD program involve increasing the complexity and length of the spoken stimuli. Following intensive daily treatment (i.e., 2–4 hours per day for a total of over 100 hours), Conway and colleagues' patient demonstrated improvements in reading aloud and spelling nonwords and regularly spelled words, in word and passage reading comprehension, and in reading rate. More recently, similar positive outcomes have been reported when modified versions of the ADD program (Kendall, Conway, Rosenbek, & Gonzalez Rothi, 2003; Kendall et al., 2006) or different commercially available programs like the *Wilson Reading System* (B. Wilson, 1996) have been used to target phonological awareness in patients with aphasia (Yampolsky & Waters, 2002).

Collectively, there is a growing literature documenting that auditory discrimination and, more broadly, phonological awareness treatments may remediate problems discriminating or perceiving segmental aspects of phonology (and, in some cases, production problems as well) in patients with aphasia (Conway et al., 1998; Franklin, Buerk, & Howard, 2002; Kendall et al., 2003, 2006, 2008; Waldron, Whitworth, & Howard, 2011), as well as individuals with pure word deafness (Slevc et al., 2011; Tessier, Weill-Chounlamountry, Michelot, & Pradat-Diehl, 2007). Because variable degrees of success on training tasks as well as generalization (to untrained stimuli and/or tasks) and maintenance of treatment effects have been reported (e.g., Kendall et al., 2006, or Waldron et al., 2011, vs. Kendall et al., 2003, or Franklin et al., 2002), future research will need to identify which participant and/or training protocol characteristics are influencing the outcomes of these phonological treatments.

Because problems producing segmental aspects of phonology are often attributed, at least in part, to motor planning (i.e., apraxia of speech) or production (i.e., dysarthria)

TABLE 9-1
Stages of the *Auditory Discrimination in Depth* (ADD) Program
(Lindamood & Lindamood, 1975)

STAGE	PURPOSE AND DESCRIPTION
Oral awareness training	Increase awareness of how individual phonemes are produced by providing visual cues (e.g., use of a mirror during phoneme production, drawings of articulators' positions) and verbal cues (e.g., provide names for particular articulator movements and voicing, such as "noisy lip-popper" for the phoneme /b/). Patients also are instructed to attend to tactile and kinesthetic feedback when producing individual phonemes (e.g., feel how and where the tongue touches the roof of the mouth when producing the /t/sound).
Simple nonword training	Improve the ability to parse simple nonword syllables into individual phonemes by using visual cues and the oral awareness skills trained in the first treatment stage. Patients must determine how many phonemes are in a target stimulus, the order of these phonemes, and, over time, similarities and differences between two target stimuli. At this stage, the ability to read and spell nonword syllables also is trained. Initially, patients point to drawings of articulators' positions to indicate the phonemic composition of target stimuli. As treatment progresses, the drawings are replaced by colored blocks (e.g., after hearing /ipi/, the patient points to a green block, a red block, and then another green block), letter tiles, and handwritten letters.
Complex nonword–word training	Train parsing, reading, and spelling of longer nonword and word monosyllabic stimuli using the methods described for Simple Nonword Training. Training of some common grapheme-to-phoneme conversion rules also is introduced (e.g., "qu" = /kw/).
Multisyllable nonword–word training	Train parsing, reading, and spelling of longer nonword and word multisyllabic stimuli using the methods described for Simple Nonword Training. Passage reading and training of common affixes also are introduced.

deficits, treatments for these output difficulties typically focus on motor speech skills and follow or occur concurrently with language treatments that ensure that patients have a sufficient linguistic base on which they can practice motor speech skills (see included DVD: Patient 6a); however, it should be noted that some of the phonological treatment tasks described above have also been used to target output problems (e.g., Franklin et al., 2002; Kendall et al., 2008). When treating patients with neurogenic language and cognitive disorders who have concomitant apraxia, dysarthria, or both, clinicians should consult textbooks, such as that of Freed (2012) or Duffy (2013), for ideas regarding motor speech therapy approaches and activities.

Treatment of Suprasegmental Impairments

For a limited number of patients with RHD or TBI, treatment of suprasegmental phonology skills (i.e., production and comprehension of prosody) may be necessary. We emphasize that improving suprasegmental processing will only infrequently be an appropriate treatment goal because in most patients (a) other deficits underlie their apparent difficulties with this aspect of language (e.g., dysarthria may cause impaired production of prosody or stress, attention deficits may limit suprasegmental comprehension; Bruck et al., 2011; Rodriguez, 2009) (see included DVD: Patient 9c), and consequently treatment should be directed toward these other deficits, and/or (b) treating other linguistic and cognitive deficits, even those unrelated to their suprasegmental difficulties, will often have a greater impact on their recovery and return to daily activities and communicative interactions. Additionally, although several treatment procedures are briefly described below, few of these have been subjected to empirical study, and thus their efficacy has yet to be confirmed (Lehman Blake, 2007; Wymer, Lindman, & Booksh, 2002).

If comprehension of suprasegmental aspects of language is deemed to affect significantly a given patient's daily communication interactions and thus is considered a suitable treatment target, clinicians might exploit one or more of the following tasks, depending on the exact nature of the patient's impairment:

- Present sentence stimuli that vary in terms of stress and intonational cues and have the patient explain or identify the correct interpretation of the stimuli or the correct interaction context for the prosodic cues. For example, the patient might be asked to contrast the meanings of "**You** went where?" versus "You went **where**?" in which the bold font indicates the most stressed word in the question.
- Present pairs of stimuli, such as short phrases or sentences, that slightly to substantially differ in terms of durational, intensity, and/or fundamental frequency cues and have the patient discriminate whether the two stimuli are the same or different and, if different, explain how they are different.
- Present a pictured scene and a spoken sentence and ask the patient to identify the mood or attitude being communicated.
- Present a short story and have the patient determine if there was a discrepancy between the linguistic content of any sentences in the story and the stress and/or intonation with which the sentences were spoken.

For the above or other prosody comprehension tasks, clinicians should consider using prerecorded stimuli to ensure that stimulus presentation is reliable across different sessions or within a session when the patient requests a repetition. Furthermore, recorded stimuli allow the clinician to pilot the stimuli on adults with no brain damage to ensure that the target prosody cues are apparent (i.e., listeners without brain damage should be able to discriminate or explain the prosodic cues).

In terms of prosody production, our clinical experiences indicate that only patients who rely on their speech as a source of income (e.g., radio announcer, actor) are typically interested in working on this aspect of language. In these cases, clinicians might consider treatment procedures such as contrastive stress exercises, which were developed for dysarthria (e.g., Duffy, 2013) (see Table 9-2). Alternate therapy activities include the following: (a) Provide patients with a set of spoken or written linguistic stimuli (e.g., word, phrase, complete sentence), and require them to say each stimulus with

TABLE 9-2
Contrastive Stress Procedures for Treating Prosody Production

STEPS	EXAMPLE
1. Present the patient with a sentence stimulus.	CLINICIAN: Dylan and Dennis played tennis yesterday.
2. Ask the patient a series of questions about the sentence and require the patient to answer by restating the sentence with stress or emphasis on the appropriate word or words.	CLINICIAN: When did Dylan and Dennis play tennis? PATIENT: Dylan and Dennis played tennis **yesterday**. CLINICIAN: What did Dylan and Dennis play yesterday? PATIENT: Dylan and Dennis played **tennis** yesterday.
3. Provide the patient with feedback regarding the adequacy of his or her response. Cues to elicit the appropriate response include: a. Describe ways in which speech rate or vocal loudness or pitch can be used to indicate stress or emphasis. b. Provide the sentence stimulus in both spoken and written formats to reduce memory demands, and have the patient identify the word or words to be stressed on the written stimulus before attempting a verbal production. c. Audio- or videotape the patient's responses so that the patient can make off-line judgments regarding the adequacy of his or her responses. d. Utilize software such as Visipitch or SpeechViewer or equipment such as a sound level meter to provide visual feedback concerning the adequacy of the patient's responses.	

Note. Words in bold font are those that should be emphasized or stressed by the patient.

a prescribed linguistic (e.g., declarative sentence vs. question intonation) or emotional (e.g., nervous vs. angry) prosody; (b) show patients pictured scenes and have them generate a sentence that one of the characters in the scene might be saying with linguistic and/or emotional prosody that is appropriate to the picture's context; and (c) require patients to read short scenarios and then read aloud or generate a final quotation for one of the story characters with appropriate linguistic and/or emotional prosody.

There is some empirical support for the use of these activities. For example, Stringer (1996) provided two months of "affective communication treatment" to a patient with prosodic production problems subsequent to a TBI. The treatment included providing visual feedback from a computerized pitch analysis system, as well as modeling and generating different emotional intonations and facial expressions. Improvements were observed and maintained for at least two months following treatment termination. More recently, Rosenbek and colleagues (Leon et al., 2005; Rosenbek et al., 2006) examined the effects of two treatment approaches: One treatment involved imitating utterances with different types of emotional prosody, whereas the other, referred to as a "cognitive-linguistic treatment," involved learning the vocal characteristics of different types of emotional prosody by matching descriptors of the target prosody to cards with the written label and picture of the emotional expression. Patients responded to both treatment approaches, with some generalization to the production of untreated sentences but not of untreated emotional prosodies. Given the small number of patients who have participated in these treatment studies and other methodological concerns (e.g., inadequate description of the nature of the participants' prosodic problems), conclusions regarding the effectiveness of these treatment procedures await the completion of further research.

Orthographic Treatments

Treatments that target orthographic processing are designed to improve reading by enhancing letter recognition, grapheme-to-phoneme conversion, or both. They also may be used to improve spelling by training letter production, phoneme-to-grapheme conversion, or both. Because many of the following treatments for orthographic difficulties were designed for and evaluated on patients with relatively pure alexias or agraphias, further exploration of whether these programs are equally effective for patients demonstrating a broader spectrum of linguistic and cognitive symptoms is still needed.

Orthographic Treatments for Reading Problems

Several approaches have been used to remediate problems recognizing or decoding orthographic symbols. When problems recognizing individual letters appear to underlie patients' reading difficulties (e.g., patients can orally spell words but not read written versions of these words), a tactile-kinesthetic treatment may be utilized (Greenwald & Gonzalez-Rothi, 1998; E. Kim et al., 2011; Lott, Carney, Glezer, & Friedman, 2010; Lott & Friedman, 1999; Sage, Hesketh, & Lambon Ralph, 2005). The premise of this therapy is that although some patients may have limited access to orthographic information via the visual modality, this access can be facilitated through other modalities like touch or movement (see included DVD: Patient 11b). The initial focus of treatment is naming of individual letters. If patients are unable to name the letter shown to them on a computer screen or index card, they are required to trace or copy the letter and then asked to name it. The tracing or copying process elicits kinesthetic stimulation, and if this is done on the patient's hand, then tactile stimulation also is achieved. Once patients' letter recognition has improved, word- and subsequently sentence-level stimuli are introduced. Positive outcomes in terms of improved letter recognition, as well as word-reading accuracy and/or rate have been reported, even when patients have linguistic deficits beyond the orthographic level (e.g., Greenwald & Gonzalez-Rothi, 1998). Kim et al. (2011), however, recently presented a case in which the tactile-kinesthetic treatment approach was associated with only modest gains, which could not be maintained without exhaustive practice. Further analysis of their patient's symptoms led them to conclude that this treatment approach may be ineffective if patients have a lesion affecting connections between brain regions that support tactile/kinesthetic information processing and those that support letter naming.

Other treatments address reading problems stemming from the inability to decode individual letters and letter combinations into their corresponding phonemic representations (i.e., grapheme-to-phoneme conversion deficits) (Beeson, Rising, Kim, & Rapcsak, 2010; Greenwald, 2004; Luzzatti, Colombo, Frustaci, & Vitolo, 2000). In one approach, patients are taught to associate a keyword with each grapheme (de Partz, 1986); for example, the word "baby" might be paired with the letter "b." Not only should the keywords be personally relevant to the patient (e.g., a spouse's name serves as a keyword for a certain grapheme), but they also should be words that the patient can consistently retrieve and say (see included DVD: Patient 11c, 11d). During initial treatment sessions, patients are shown a letter and asked to provide the keyword for that letter; once they say the keyword, they are then asked to say just the first phoneme that corresponds to the sound of the target letter. As patients progress, they are encouraged to still think of the keyword but only say the sound. In the final stages, patients practice reading aloud, first nonwords (so that they don't use a whole-word reading strategy during therapy) and then real words using this keyword technique for each letter in the stimulus. Additionally, patients are explicitly taught at least a small number of grapheme-to-phoneme conversion rules (e.g., a "c" followed by an "a," "o," or "u" is pronounced /k/; in remaining contexts it is pronounced /s/). Although the findings from several studies indicate that patients can learn which phonemes go with which graphemes using this treatment approach (Beeson et al., 2010; de Partz, 1986; Hillis, 1993; Mitchum & Berndt, 1991), a few researchers found that their patients had difficulty learning how to blend phonemes once treatment progressed to the word level (e.g., Mitchum & Berndt, 1991). Accordingly, further research is needed to delineate which patient profiles are most suitable for this treatment approach, or to identify training steps that might specifically address blending difficulties.

Orthographic Treatments for Spelling Problems

A limited number of spelling treatments have been developed to address problems at the orthographic level. Many of these treatments are similar to those described in the previous section on orthographic treatments for reading problems. For example, the keyword approach has been successfully used to remediate phoneme-to-grapheme conversion problems in several patients (Beeson et al., 2010; Carlomagno, Iavarone, & Colombo, 1994; Greenwald, 2004; Hillis & Caramazza, 1994). In this treatment, keywords that the patients can spell are linked to target graphemes (e.g., "Robert" for the letter "r"). Patients are then taught how to use the initial sounds of their keywords to write single graphemes and, as they progress, to use these keywords covertly to help them sound out and spell nonwords and eventually real words. Specific phoneme-to-grapheme conversion rules also may be explicitly taught by first explaining the rule to patients and then having them practice using the rule during a variety of writing tasks, such as writing to dictation and completing written sentence closure tasks (de Partz, Seron, & Van der Linden, 1992). Most frequently, these spelling treatments produce improvements on trained nonwords and words, as well as untrained regularly spelled words.

Because irregularly spelled words violate common phoneme-to-grapheme correspondences and conversion rules, improved spelling of these words would not be expected following treatments that focus on phoneme-to-grapheme conversion. Instead, lexical–semantic treatment approaches are more appropriate when patients solely or primarily have problems spelling these types of words (for information on lexical–semantic treatments, see the following section of this chapter). Alternately, Beeson and colleagues (2010) described a two-stage treatment protocol in which patients first completed keyword training to address phoneme-to-grapheme conversion problems, and then were provided an "interactive treatment," which trained patients to self-detect and correct their spelling errors with the assistance of an electronic spelling aid. Following this combined approach, the two patients of Beeson et al. demonstrated improved spelling of both trained and untrained words and nonwords, including irregularly spelled words when writing with or without the electronic spelling aid.

For some patients, spelling problems stem from deficits of peripheral processes (Beeson & Rapcsak, 2002, 2010). These patients can often spell aloud nonwords and words, but display difficulty when required to write spontaneously and, in some cases, copy written stimuli. More specifically, peripheral deficits include problems recalling the visual and/or physical characteristics of individual letters (i.e., allographic conversion deficit), completing the visuomotor plan and requirements for writing letters (e.g., apraxia, hemiparesis, visuoperceptual deficit), and attending to the writing process (i.e., visual neglect). For patients with allographic conversion impairments, two treatment approaches have been suggested. One involves teaching compensatory strategies—such as using an alphabet card when handwriting as a reminder of letter shapes (Ramage, Beeson, & Rapcsak, 1998)—or typing on a typewriter or computer (Black, Behrmann, Bass, & Hacker, 1989). The second approach capitalizes on these patients' typically preserved oral spelling abilities by requiring them to self-dictate words before they write them. That is, patients dictate to themselves one letter at a time to help them write out words, checking after each letter for mistakes. Although this technique proved effective in two case studies (Pound, 1996; Ramage et al., 1998), less successful results were reported by Lesser (1990), indicating that further investigations are needed to specify which patients will benefit from this self-dictation procedure.

Several treatment strategies may be appropriate when motor, visuoconstruction, or attention problems underlie writing difficulties. For example, Beeson and Rapcsak (2002, 2010) recommended intensive immediate and delayed copying tasks to help restore and automate motor plans in patients with apraxic deficits. Empirical support for this recommendation is lacking, however, given that currently there are no published studies on treating apraxic writing problems. Treatments for other motor- and attention-based writing difficulties, however, have been described in the research literature. As shown in Table 9-3, all of these are primarily compensatory in nature and require further investigation to substantiate their effectiveness.

Lexical-Semantic Treatments

Of the various linguistic symptoms associated with neurogenic language and cognitive disorders, lexical–semantic processing deficits have without question been the focus of the greatest number of treatment studies. Although these deficits are possible following the onset of any type of neurogenic language or cognitive disorder (e.g., aphasia, dementia, cognitive-communicative disorders associated with TBI or RHD), the majority of procedures described below were designed for and evaluated on patients with aphasia. Therefore, when used with other patient populations, these treatments may need to be modified to circumvent or address a given patient's specific symptom profile (e.g., concomitant neglect or memory deficits). Furthermore, empirical investigations are still needed to examine the appropriateness and, consequently, effectiveness of these treatments for lexical–semantic problems associated with RHD, TBI, or dementia.

The Linguistic Stimulation Approach to Treating Lexical-Semantic Deficits

Many traditional lexical–semantic treatments are based on a stimulation therapy model and focus on identifying, providing, and ultimately fading cues to facilitate patients' lexical–semantic comprehension or production abilities. Additionally, therapy stimuli and activities in these traditional treatments usually are ordered such that those that are more difficult for patients are introduced later in the treatment process. Specific cues, stimuli, and activities should be selected on the basis of factors such as semantic category, stimulus length, or part of speech found to influence the patient's lexical–semantic abilities during the linguistic assessment (for a list of possible influential factors, see Table 6-4). Below we review some specific stimulation treatments that have been used successfully to target the spoken and/or written lexical–semantic processing abilities of patients with aphasia.

Stimulation Treatment for Lexical-Semantic Comprehension Deficits

One basic form of stimulation treatment has been traditionally used to remediate lexical–semantic comprehension deficits. This standard approach involves distinguishing one or more modalities through which a patient can access lexical–semantic information and then presenting treatment stimuli via these modalities to prime or "deblock" the impaired modality (Coelho et al., 2008; S. Small, 2009; Weigl, 1981). For example, if a patient has difficulty understanding spoken language, initial treatment activities

TABLE 9-3
Compensatory Strategies for Addressing Peripheral Writing Difficulties

COMPENSATORY STRATEGY	TARGET DEFICIT	AUTHOR(S)
Lined paper	Letter size and spacing problems due to micrographia, letter/word spacing problems and upward slant due to visual neglect	R. Oliveira, Gurd, Nixon, Marshall, & Passingham (1997); Tompkins (1995)
Self- or clinician-provided verbal cues (e.g., "write big," "look left")	Micrographia, visual neglect	Farley, Derosa, Koshland, Fox, & Van Gemmert (2006) R. Oliveira et al. (1997); Tompkins (1995)
Writing prosthesis (e.g., large-grip pen, forearm skateboard)	Dominant hand/arm hemiparesis	J. Brown, Leader, & Blum (1983); Leischner (1996) Papathanassiou, Filipovic, Whurr, & Jahnashahi (2003) Whurr & Lorch (1991)
Typewriter or computer keyboard	Allographic conversion deficit, apraxia	Beeson & Rapscak (2002, 2010) Black et al. (1989)

might involve presenting written, gestural, *and* spoken forms of the target stimuli and having the patient select the correct pictures or objects that correspond to the target. As the patient progresses on this task, the written and gestural cues could be faded so that eventually the patient is completing a spoken-word-to-picture matching task. The final stages of this treatment would focus on gradually increasing the complexity of the stimuli (e.g., decrease vocabulary familiarity, increase stimulus length to phrases or sentences, introduce various parts of speech) and the task demands (e.g., complete the task after a delay to increase memory demands, complete the task in a noisy environment to increase attention demands, increase the number and similarity of distracter items). Table 9-4 lists other therapy activities that might be used in stimulation treatments for lexical–semantic comprehension problems. Note that most of these activities can easily be adapted to target lexical–semantic production as well.

Stimulation treatment has been used successfully, even with patients who have severe comprehension deficits. For instance, Ulatowska and Richardson (1974) designed a series of deblocking activities that progressed from reading comprehension tasks (e.g., arranging written words into phrases) to auditory comprehension tasks (e.g., matching spoken phrases to the written phrases used in previous activities) and found that following this treatment, their patient with Wernicke's aphasia showed substantial improvements in his written and spoken comprehension skills. Similarly, Helm-Estabrooks and Albert (2004) have described a treatment program called Treatment for Wernicke's Aphasia (TWA), which is designed to improve auditory comprehension by capitalizing on patients' more intact reading and repetition skills. According to Helm-Estabrooks and Albert, TWA is most appropriate for patients with relatively preserved

TABLE 9-4
Therapy Activities for Addressing Lexical–Semantic Comprehension Deficits

ACTIVITY	EXAMPLES
Pointing tasks	• Point to the picture or object that represents the spoken, written, and/or gestured word stimulus. • Point to the written word that represents the spoken, written, and/or gestured word stimulus. • Point to the picture, object, or written word that represents the spoken and/or written definition (e.g., "Point to the color of bananas"). • Point to the picture, object, or written word that completes a spoken and/or written phrase or sentence (e.g., "The housekeeper _____ the floor"). • Point to the pictured scene that represents the spoken and/or written description.
Following directions	• Point to pictures or objects in the sequence specified by a spoken and/or written command (e.g., "Point to the girl in the pants and then to the boy in the hat"). • Manipulate an object or set of objects in the manner and sequence specified by a spoken and/or written command (e.g., "Sign your name and then fold the paper in half").
Answering questions	• Answer spoken and/or written yes/no questions about general information (e.g., "Is Canada south of the United States?"). • Answer spoken and/or written yes/no questions about pictured scenes or spoken and/or written stories or scenarios. • Answer spoken and/or written multiple-choice questions* about pictured scenes or spoken and/or written stories or scenarios.
Sentence verification	• Determine if a spoken and/or written sentence makes sense (e.g., "The dairy farmer kept the cows in the garage").

*Clinicians must keep in mind the increased memory demands involved in answering multiple-choice questions, particularly those presented verbally, compared to the other activities listed above.

reading comprehension, at least at the single-word level on an aphasia test. Steps of this treatment program include:

1. Patients complete written-word-to-picture matching tasks to enhance their reading comprehension skills.
2. Auditory comprehension is stimulated through a process called **reauditorization**, whereby patients are required first to read aloud the items trained in the reading comprehension step, and then to repeat aloud these items when provided with a spoken model and a picture stimulus. Patients are often better able to understand a word if they can say the word.
3. Patients complete spoken-word-to-picture matching tasks.

Although no formal evaluation of TWA has yet been completed, the authors summarized a successful case and additionally provided sufficient description of procedural details so that their program could be easily applied in future clinical practice or research endeavors.

In summary, the stimulation approach to treating lexical–semantic comprehension deficits is widely used clinically. Because of an inordinate research focus on treatments for lexical–semantic production versus comprehension problems, however, minimal empirical support for this treatment technique has accumulated thus far (Basso et al., 2011; Hough, 1993; Laska et al., 2011; R. Marshall & Neuburger, 1984; Ulatowska & Richardson, 1974). Additionally, Basso et al. (2011) suggested that the lack of research may reflect, at least in part, that comprehension at the word level typically recovers quickly and spontaneously compared with other linguistic deficits, and thus there has been less need to develop treatments for this type of linguistic problem. Nonetheless, patients with severe aphasia may still present with enduring word-level comprehension problems. Although the studies that have been completed have consistently reported that patients acquired comprehension of trained items following stimulation treatment, generalization effects to untrained items and modalities were variable. Accordingly, more research is necessary to determine the validity of these commonly used therapy procedures, particularly in terms of whether or not treatments evoke improvements in patients' understanding during their daily communication interactions and activities.

Stimulation Treatment for Lexical–Semantic Production Deficits

Numerous stimulation treatments described in the literature aim to remediate spoken or written lexical–semantic production problems. For instance, intensive practice at speech perception tasks (i.e., determining if a target spoken word matches a picture) has been found to improve spoken naming in patients with moderate, nonfluent aphasia and concomitant apraxia of speech (Fridriksson et al., 2009); this treatment resembles the deblocking approach described above with respect to stimulation treatments for lexical–semantic comprehension deficits. The most basic of stimulation treatments for lexical–semantic production deficits requires patients to practice intensively repeating or copying a set of target items so that eventually they can produce these items without a verbal or written model (see included DVD: Patient 6a). Indeed, intensive spoken and/ or written repetition of words, phrases, or both, has been found to produce positive outcomes, even in patients with severe language deficits, although additional research is needed to examine maintenance and generalization of these treatment effects (Boo & Rose, 2011; Kempler & Goral, 2011; Kumar & Humphreys, 2008; Nobis-Bosch, Springer, Radermacher, & Huber, 2011; Small, 2009).

As an example, the Copy and Recall Treatment (CART) program developed by Beeson and colleagues (Beeson, 1999; Beeson, Rising, et al., 2003) consists of having patients practice repeatedly copying written words (that are presented in concert with their pictured representations), followed by written picture naming (i.e., only the pictures are presented) (see included DVD: Patient 11a, 11b). These researchers have found that patients with severe writing deficits have been able to acquire and maintain production of trained vocabulary when this simple treatment was provided in either one-on-one therapy sessions and/or as a homework program (Beeson, 1999; Beeson, Rising, et al., 2003; E. Kim et al., 2011). Beeson, Rising, et al. (2003) noted that patients who fail to complete their assigned writing homework consistently and accurately, and who have significant concomitant semantic and cognitive impairments, are less likely to benefit from CART. More recently, CART has been paired with spoken repetition of target words to target both written and spoken naming (Ball, Riesthal, Breeding, & Mendozza, 2011; Beeson & Egnor, 2006; de Riesthal, 2007). To facilitate at-home spoken repetition practice, patients were given either video clips of someone saying the target words (Ball et al., 2011) or a device that provided the auditory model of target words (Beeson & Egnor, 2006; de Riesthal, 2007). The findings from these studies indicate that patients with severe aphasia consistently show improvements in writing trained stimuli, but those with coexisting apraxia of speech are less likely to show gains in their spoken naming, even with the inclusion of the device or video clips for home practice.

Perhaps one of the most frequently used stimulation techniques entails developing and applying a **cueing hierarchy** to facilitate patients' lexical–semantic production abilities. The first step to cueing treatments involves determining what cues facilitate the individual patient's word retrieval skills (see Table 9-5 for a list of possible cues). These cues are then arranged into a hierarchy. Cues at the top of the hierarchy are those that provide the least amount of external support, and thus are expected to help the patient the least. In contrast, cues falling at the bottom of the hierarchy are those that provide greater amounts of external support, and thus are expected to help the patient the most. Although the relative strength of the cues shown in Table 9-5 can vary across individual patients, initial phoneme and semantic cues, such as sentence completion, are frequently the most potent (Edwards & Tucker, 2006). It should also be noted that in some cueing hierarchies, especially those used in concert with errorless learning or vanishing-cues training protocols (training approaches that attempt to minimize patients giving inaccurate responses; see also Chapter 10 for a description of these training approaches), cues at the top of the hierarchy provide maximal support, whereas those at the bottom provide nominal support (Edwards & Tucker, 2006; Floel et al., 2011; Raymer et al., 2012).

Studies by Marshall, Freed, and colleagues (Freed, Celery, & Marshall, 2004; R. Marshall, Karow, Freed, & Babcock, 2002; Olsen et al., 2012) have shown that personalized cues also may be particularly potent for patients with aphasia. Personalized cues are ones that patients with aphasia create on their own to help them retrieve specific words. For example, a patient might come up with the cue "birthday" to help him retrieve the target word, "chocolate," because he always has chocolate cake for his birthday. Importantly, Marshall, Freed, and colleagues have found that compared to phonological cues, personalized cues can result in greater and more enduring word retrieval improvements. These researchers have also reported some evidence of improved word retrieval during more natural communication settings following training with personalized cues. Data from one participant with aphasia, however, suggested that personalized cues may not be beneficial for patients with word retrieval difficulties due to early dementia (Olsen et al., 2012): This patient demonstrated little improvement in response to this cueing approach and, shortly after her participation in the study, was unfortunately diagnosed with probable Alzheimer's disease.

Once a cueing hierarchy has been created, it is used to facilitate the patient's lexical–semantic production abilities while completing word retrieval tasks. That is,

TABLE 9-5
Cues That May Be Used to Facilitate Spoken and/or Lexical–Semantic Production

CUE TYPE	CUE EXAMPLE FOR THE TARGET
Semantically based	
Superordinate	"It's an *animal*."
Coordinate	"It's like a *cow*."
Associate	"It eats *hay*."
Function	"You can *ride* it."
Attribute	"It has a *mane*."
Phrase or sentence completion	"The jockey fell off of the ___."
Definition or description	"This is an animal that you can find on a farm or a ranch. You can ride or race them. You can see them at a rodeo...."
Antonym	N/A
Phonologically based	
Initial phoneme or syllable	"It's a /h/..."
Number of syllables	"It has one syllable."
Real word or nonword rhyme	"It rhymes with *course*." "It rhymes with *gorce*."
Repetition	"It's a horse. Say *horse*."
Unison speech or singing	"It's a horse. Now say that word with me—*horse*."
Orthographically based	
Initial grapheme	"It starts with an *h*."
Number of letters	"It has five letters."
Word shape	⌐▔▔▔▔▔▔▔⌐
Letter anagrams	o s h e r
Copying	"It's this word. Copy this word."
Reading aloud	"Here's the word. Read it aloud."
Others	
Sound effects	"neigh," "clip-clop"
Tactile	N/A
Pantomime or iconic gesture	Pretend to hold the reins and ride a horse.
Drawing	Clinician and/or patient draw a picture of a horse and then the patient tries to name it while drawing it.
Time delay	"Wait 5 seconds before telling me what this is."

Note. N/A = not applicable.

the patient cannot correctly complete an item, the clinician provides the first cue at the top of the hierarchy; if, following that cue, the patient still cannot complete the item correctly, the next cue is provided, with the clinician continuing to provide prompts until the patient is able to complete the target item correctly. Once the patient has provided a correct response, the patient can be required to work back up through the hierarchy to provide additional practice of the erred item, or, alternately, a new target item may be introduced. Figure 9-1 provides an example of a cueing hierarchy that might be used to target written naming.

Numerous studies have documented that cueing hierarchies or, more broadly, treatments that involve cueing combinations (e.g., semantic plus gestural cues) can improve the spoken (Boo & Rose, 2011; Cameron, Wambaugh, Wright, & Nessler, 2006; Edwards & Tucker, 2006; Ferguson, Evans, & Raymer, 2012; Floel et al., 2011; Raymer et al., 2012; Rose & Sussmilch, 2008) and/or written (Ball et al., 2011; Beeson, 1999; Marshall et al., 2012; L. Murray & Karcher, 2000) lexical retrieval abilities of patients with aphasia. Patients with progressive language disorders also benefit from cueing treatments (Dressel et al., 2010; Jokel & Anderson, 2012). Further, cueing hierarchies have proven effective not only in improving retrieval of several parts of speech (e.g., nouns, verbs), but also when implemented via direct therapy, computer-based treatments (e.g., word prediction software), homework activities, or some combination of these therapy formats. Although cueing treatments invariably lead to acquisition of trained items,

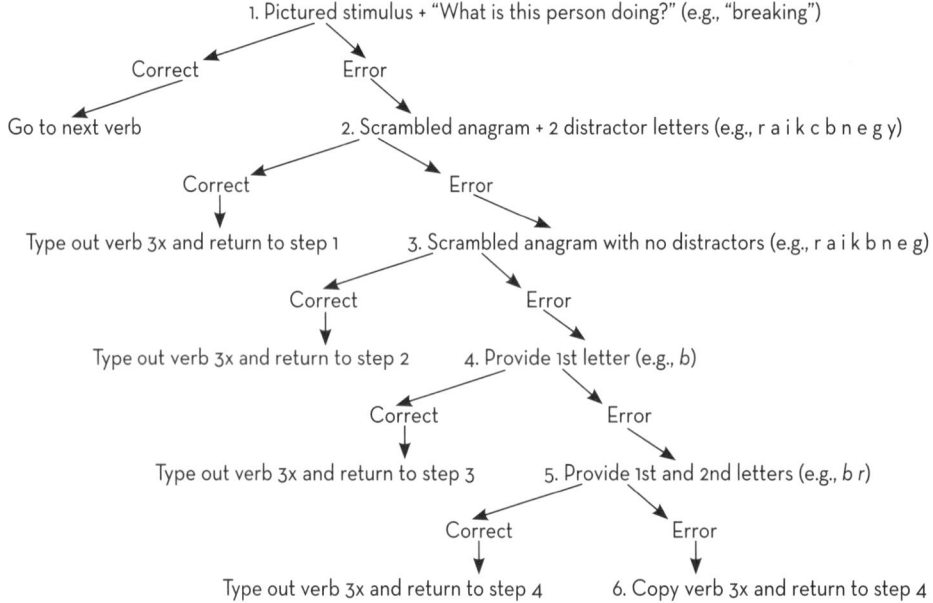

Figure 9-1. Example of a cueing hierarchy for training written naming of verbs. *Note.* Adapted from "A Treatment for Written Verb Retrieval and Sentence Construction Skills," by L. Murray and L. Karcher, 2000, *Aphasiology, 14,* pp. 585–602. Copyright 2000 by Taylor & Francis, Ltd., http://www.informaworld.com. Adapted with permission.

generalization to untrained items and/or language modalities and maintenance of treatment effects will depend on one or more of the following (DeDe et al., 2003; Ferguson et al., 2012; Floel et al., 2011; J. Marshall et al., 2012; Rayner et al., 2012): (a) the nature (e.g., semantic/conceptual vs. phonological access) and severity of the patients' lexical–semantic deficit and other language impairments, (b) whether or not the patients have concomitant cognitive or motoric problems (e.g., generalization of a writing treatment to verbal skills would be unlikely in a patient with concomitant apraxia of speech), (c) whether or not patients continue to practice or use the trained vocabulary, and (d) whether or not patients learn to generate these cues independently (i.e., acquire a word retrieval strategy).

A few stimulation programs have been developed for specific patient populations. For example, **Voluntary Control of Involuntary Utterances** (**VCIU**; Helm-Estabrooks & Albert, 2004) was designed to stimulate propositional (i.e., voluntary) verbal output in patients whose current spoken language abilities are restricted to involuntary production of a small set of real words (e.g., stereotypical utterances such as "That's good"). Basic steps to the VCIU program include the following:

1. Make a list of all real words the patient has been reported to produce spontaneously.
2. Write one of these words on a card and require the patient to read it aloud. If the patient correctly reads the word aloud, it becomes a target stimulus for homework and future therapy sessions. If the patient is unable to read the word aloud, it is discarded and the next word on the patient's list is written on a card. This step is repeated until the clinician has attempted to elicit reading aloud of all words on the patient's list.
3. Pictures of the words that the patient was able to read aloud are then presented, and the patient is required to name these pictures. If the patient is unable to complete confrontation naming of an item, he/she is shown the written word and asked to read it aloud. Note that if the patient produces an incorrect, real word while attempting to read aloud or name target stimuli, that incorrect word should be added to the patient's list, and thus should itself be evaluated to determine if it too may become a target stimulus.

Only one study to date has evaluated the effects of VCIU. In 1980, Helm and Barresi provided three to six months of VCIU to three patients with severely nonfluent output and mild to moderately impaired auditory comprehension abilities. Following treatment, all patients had acquired a spoken vocabulary of at least 250 words and showed improved scores on responsive naming, confrontation naming, and animal naming tests. Little change, however, was observed in their performance of oral reading tests. Whereas these findings and the anecdotal case reported by Helm-Estabrooks and Albert (2004) indicate encouraging outcomes, further studies with appropriate research design controls (e.g., larger sample size, assurance that all patients are beyond the spontaneous recovery period, inclusion of a control measure) remain needed to validate VCIU treatment effects.

Another stimulation program created for a specific patient group is **Response Elaboration Training** (**RET**; Kearns, 1985; Kearns & Scher, 1989). RET is designed to affect positively utterance length and information content in the verbal output of patients with nonfluent aphasia. It is considered a "loose training" program that involves incidental learning, reinforcement of patient-initiated output, and emphasis on utterance content (including lexical–semantic accuracy) versus form. A typical RET session includes the following:

1. The patient is asked to comment on a picture scene, making sure to discourage naming or concrete description.
2. The clinician models and reinforces the patient's initial utterance. For example, if the patient says "Man gun bad" in response to a newspaper picture of a war scene, the clinician might model "I agree, the soldier with the gun looks very mean or angry."
3. The clinician utilizes *wh-* questions to elicit further responses and to encourage the patient to elaborate on earlier responses. For example, the clinician asks, "Why do you think the soldier is angry?" and the patient responds, "Guy."
4. The clinician provides a model that combines the patient's previous responses. For example, the clinician responds, "I see, the soldier with the gun is mad at the prisoner."
5. The patient is asked to repeat the clinician's model. For example, the clinician says, "Now you try to say this whole sentence… 'The soldier with the gun is mad at the prisoner.'"
6. The clinician reinforces the patient's response and models the sentence again. For instance, the clinician states, "Great job. The soldier with the gun is mad at the prisoner."

Note that at no time does the clinician directly correct the patient's spontaneous utterances, but rather only provides indirect feedback via conversational modeling.

Several studies have shown that RET, by itself or in concert with other verbal output treatments, is an effective means by which to increase the informational content of patients with nonfluent aphasia and mild to moderate apraxia of speech (Gaddie, Kearns, & Yedor, 1991; Kearns, 1985; Kearns & Scher, 1989; Kempler & Goral, 2011; L. Murray, Timberlake, & Eberle, 2007), as well as those with nonfluent aphasia and severe apraxia of speech (Wambaugh & Martinez, 2000; Wambaugh, Martinez, & Alegre, 2001). That is, following treatment, patients have been found to display one or more of the following: (a) an increased number and variety of content words (e.g., nouns, verbs), (b) longer utterances, and (c) improvements in productive syntax (e.g., more grammatically complete utterances). Additionally, patients have been reported to show similar degrees of improvement with novel stimuli, conversational partners, and communicative settings and are able to maintain these gains over time. R. Marshall (2001) also presented a case in which a patient with Wernicke's aphasia successfully responded to this treatment approach, although clearly further research investigating the appropriateness of RET for patients representing a variety of language profiles is still needed.

To Modify or Not to Modify... That Is the Question

Programmatic intervention strategies such as RET, Melodic Intonation Therapy (see below), and SFA are often appealing to clinicians, particularly those new to managing neurogenic language and cognitive disorders, because procedures for these treatments are usually clearly described. Clinicians may wonder, however, whether it is appropriate to deviate from the treatment protocols specified in these programs. Several issues are relevant when considering this question. First, arguably the most important advantage of detailed treatment protocols is that they allow other clinicians and researchers to replicate the methods implemented by the original researchers. Careful review of groups of studies examining the same program, nevertheless, often reveal that program modifications are made to address the needs of the patients described in each study (e.g., Beeson, 1998, vs. Mayer & Murray, 2002). Second, it is common for the literature to include reports of treatment outcomes for only a small number of patients, perhaps none of whom exhibit precisely the same clinical presentation or activity and participation needs as the patient for whom the clinician is considering implementing the treatment. Thus, there are likely to be occasions when clinicians find it necessary to modify treatment procedures. Clinicians are encouraged, however, to be mindful of the theoretical framework driving the treatment program, and to develop modifications accordingly.

Melodic Intonation Therapy (**MIT**; Helm-Estabrooks & Albert, 2004; Sparks, 2001) is a stimulation treatment developed to alleviate the spoken language problems of patients with severe nonfluent aphasia. The impetus for its design was the clinical observation that patients with aphasia who have severely restricted verbal output often are able to retrieve and produce words correctly while singing. Accordingly, Albert, Sparks, and Helm (1988) created the structured, hierarchical MIT program in which patients move from initially producing words and phrases in an intoned and rhythmic manner (like singing) to eventually saying these words with natural prosody. The summary of MIT procedures listed in Table 9-6 provides an overview of the treatment program. More detailed descriptions of MIT can be found in Helm-Estabrooks and Albert (2004) or in the commercially available MIT kit (Helm-Estabrooks, Nicholas, & Morgan, 1989), which includes specific therapy instructions, picture stimuli, scoring sheets, and a DVD with a demonstration of all MIT levels.

Although most studies have primarily included participants with moderate to severe nonfluent aphasia, prior research indicates that MIT can improve production of trained words and phrases in patients representing a variety of aphasia profiles (F. Baker, 2000; Bonakdarpour, Eftekharzadeh, & Ashayeri, 2003; Goldfarb & Bader, 1979; Hough, 2010; Schlaug, Marchina, & Norton, 2008; Vines, Norton, & Schlaug, 2011; S. Wilson, Parsons, & Reutens, 2006). Generalization in terms of increased utterance lengths, higher informational content, and improved lexical retrieval on untrained speech tasks and stimuli is most likely, however, only in patients with nonfluent aphasia whose lesions

TABLE 9-6
Levels and Steps to Administering Melodic Intonation Therapy

LEVEL	STEP	DESCRIPTION
1	1. Humming	The clinician hums a tonal pattern for the target word or phrase while pointing to a picture or other cue related to the target. While the clinician hums the tonal pattern, he or she also taps the patient's left hand once for each syllable. No patient response is required at this level.
	2. Unison singing	The clinician and patient hum or intone the target word or phrase together while the clinician taps the patient's hand.
	3. Unison singing with fading	Same as previous step except halfway through the word or phrase, the clinician stops intoning.
	4. Immediate repetition	The patient repeats the clinician's model of the intoned and tapped word or phrase. During the patient's production, the clinician still taps the patient's hand.
	5. Response to a probe question	After the patient successfully repeats the intoned word or phrase, the clinician asks the patient an intoned question pertaining to the word or phrase (e.g., "What did you ask for?" for the target "Coffee, please"). The clinician may still tap the patient's hand when the patient answers the question with the intoned target.
2	1. Introduce the target	Same as Step 1 of Level 1.
	2. Unison with fading	Same as Step 3 of Level 1.
	3. Delayed repetition	The patient repeats the clinician's model of the intoned and tapped word or phrase after a delay of approximately 6 seconds. During the patient's production, the clinician still taps the patient's hand.
	4. Response to a probe question	Approximately 6 seconds after the patient successfully completes Step 3, the clinician intones a probe question to elicit another production of the intoned target by the patient.
3	1. Delayed repetition	Same as Step 3 of Level 2.
	2. Introduce sprechgesang	The clinician models the target word or phrase in sprechgesang (speaking with accentuated rhythm and stress, but normal intonation or pitch) and taps the patient's hand. No patient response is required at this level.
	3. Sprechgesang with fading	Like Step 2 of Level 2, except sprechgesang rather than intoning is used.
	4. Delayed spoken repetition	The patient repeats with normal speech prosody the clinician's spoken model of the target word or phrase after a delay of approximately 6 seconds. No hand-tapping cue is provided.
	5. Response to a probe question	Like Step 4 of Level 2, except both the clinician's question and the patient's response should be produced with normal speech prosody.

Note. From *Manual of Aphasia and Aphasia Therapy* (3rd ed.), by N. Helm-Estabrooks, M. Albert, and M. Nicholas, in press, Austin, TX: PRO-ED. Copyright 2014 by PRO-ED. Adapted with permission.

spare the temporal lobe, and who relatedly have relatively good auditory comprehension (Bonakdarpour et al., 2003; Naeser & Helm-Estabrooks, 1985; Sparks, Helm, & Albert, 1974; Vines et al., 2011). MIT has been shown effective when (a) caregivers were trained to administer the treatment protocol (Goldfarb & Bader, 1979), (b) it was adapted for other languages (Bonakdarpour et al., 2003; Popovici, Mihailescu, & Voinescu, 1992), (c) it was modified for patients who did not benefit from the more traditional MIT format (F. Baker, 2000; Hough, 2010), (d) it was provided in concert with non-invasive brain stimulation (i.e., transcranial direct current stimulation; Vines et al., 2011), and (e) it was used in the acute-care setting (Conklyn, Novak, Boissy, Bethoux, & Chemali, 2012). The melodic and rhythmic aspects of MIT appear to be particularly important in terms of producing improvements in verbal output: When compared to intervention protocols that are similar to MIT except they lack intoning and/or tapping steps (see Table 9-6), MIT treatment outcomes are superior in terms of the amount and maintenance of progress (Schlaug et al., 2008; Wilson et al., 2006). Despite numerous prior studies documenting the positive effects of MIT, recent critical and systematic reviews of MIT have highlighted the need for further research, particularly in terms of delineating MIT candidacy requirements, specifying the neural and behavioral mechanisms driving MIT outcomes, and determining the effects of MIT on the ICF levels of activity and participation (Hurkmans et al., 2012; van der Meulen, van de Sandt-Koenderman, & Ribbers, 2012).

We Want MIT—It Worked for Gabby Giffords, Right?

One of the more recent rounds of speech-language pathology in the mainstream press involved the case of former congresswoman Gabrielle (Gabby) Giffords. She was shot in the head when meeting with constituents in Tucson in January 2011. When clips of her early rehabilitation were aired on television, the general public observed how music, more specifically melodic intonation therapy (MIT), could be used to aid in the recovery of language abilities. Almost immediately after the media began covering Gabby's rehabilitation and progress, we began receiving requests from patients and families dealing with aphasia or other neurogenic language and cognitive disorders to receive MIT or to ask why they hadn't received MIT when they were receiving services.

Although indeed Gabby did receive MIT initially, Dr. Helm-Estabrooks, who played an integral role in her aphasia treatment program, noted that MIT was only used initially while Gabby was an inpatient (Murray Law, 2012). Instead, much of her post-acute language intervention has focused on activities that address her agrammatism and reduced utterance length.

Accordingly, we were sure to point out to those making inquiries about MIT that, as with any treatment, it is not necessarily appropriate for all types and severities of aphasia or for all types of neurogenic language or cognitive disorders. Likewise, we noted that Gabby's remarkable recovery could not be solely attributed to MIT, even though the media's coverage of her case might have suggested that was the case.

Finally, conversational coaching or **conversational script training** might be considered a lexical–semantic stimulation approach as it primarily focuses on improving output content at the discourse level (Cherney & Halper, 2008; Cherney, Halper, Holland, & Cole, 2008a; Holland, 1991). This treatment begins with the patient and clinician developing a script that can be used by the patient in one or more social settings outside of therapy. Scripts may consist of conversational or monologue discourse. For example, if a patient has an upcoming family reunion to attend, he might want to develop a script that will allow him to update his relatives on what he has been doing at work and how his wife and children are doing; such a script would also be helpful when visiting with friends. Once the clinician and patient have created the script, the patient practices communicating it with the clinician. The practice sessions can be videotaped so that the clinician and patient can identify what was and was not shared successfully, and when information was not successfully shared, what strategies might be used to facilitate communication success (e.g., rather than struggling to say the name of the company at which he works, he should refer to his smartphone where it is listed under his contacts). The next steps involve practice at conveying the script with familiar and unfamiliar conversational partners, again with feedback to identify positive and negative communication behaviors. In more recent versions of this treatment, patients practice their scripts with a virtual clinician as part of a software program (e.g., Lee, Kaye, & Cherney, 2009) or in response to conversations videotaped in real-life settings (e.g., ordering at a restaurant) with amateur actors (Bilda, 2011). In these newer script training protocols, patients move from maximal to minimal cueing practice levels.

Data accrued from several recent studies indicate that patients with a variety of types and severities of chronic aphasia respond positively to conversational script training (Bilda, 2011; Cherney & Halper, 2008; Cherney, Halper, et al., 2008a; Lee et al., 2009; Manheim, Halper, & Cherney, 2009; Youmans, Holland, Munoz, & Bourgeois, 2005). That is, they show not only improved production of the treated scripts (e.g., faster speech rate, fewer word retrieval errors) but also generalization to untreated language behaviors, such as the more accurate production of untrained scripts, general language gains on aphasia batteries, and more positive perceptions of the patients' communication abilities as rated by the patients themselves as well as by their caregivers. Larger and more enduring improvements have been reported following more intense conversational script training (Bilda, 2011; Lee et al., 2009).

Cognitive Neuropsychological Approaches to Treating Lexical–Semantic Deficits

Another approach to treating lexical–semantic deficits has been to utilize therapies based on cognitive neuropsychological models of language processing (see Chapter 1). Two general categories of model-based treatments have thus far been developed and evaluated: semantic-based treatments, which aim to remediate problems related to the integrity of or access to semantic or conceptual representations, and phonological-based treatments, which focus on deficits related to breakdowns within or in accessing phonological representations. Both of these approaches are described below in terms of specific therapy activities and current empirical support.

Semantic Treatment Approaches

Several treatments for spoken or written word processing difficulties have been developed to strengthen semantic representations, access to or from semantic representations, or both. Semantic-level treatments should theoretically evoke improvements in *both* comprehension and production (B. Rapp & Caramazza, 1998). That is, according to many cognitive neuropsychological models of language, only one set of semantic representations is proposed to support comprehension and production of both spoken and written language. Thus, strengthening semantic representations, the organization of these representations, or both should positively affect both comprehension and production abilities. Specific tasks that are frequently used to target semantic processing skills include:

- Sorting or matching picture or word cards by semantic categories or associations
- Spoken- or written-word-to-picture matching tasks in which distracter items are semantically related to the target items (e.g., for the target "hamburger," distracters might include "hot dog," "sandwich," and "ketchup")
- Spoken or written naming tasks in which one or more semantic cues such as the superordinate category, function, attributes, or semantic associates of the target item are provided to elicit the correct response (for a list of semantic cues, see Table 9-5)
- Spoken or written phrase or sentence completion tasks
- Answering spoken or written semantically based questions about the target items (e.g., for the target "hamburger," questions might be, "Do you eat hamburgers for breakfast?" or "Do you boil hamburgers?")
- Matching pictures or written words to spoken definitions
- Completing odd-one-out tasks in which the picture or written word that does not belong with the other pictures or words must be identified
- Generating, comparing, and/or contrasting attributes for the target items

Semantic Treatments for Comprehension Problems. Few studies have examined whether these types of semantic tasks can help address auditory comprehension problems related to lexical–semantic processing deficits. Furthermore, the investigations that have been completed thus far have produced mixed results. For example, B. Jacobs and Thompson (1992) provided a series of semantic comprehension tasks to a patient with global aphasia and found only minimal improvements in his ability to identify spoken words and sort pictures of items from trained semantic categories; their patient also displayed little generalization to untrained comprehension or production tasks. In contrast, other studies reported remarkable improvements in auditory comprehension when similar semantic-based tasks were used with patients with aphasia or semantic dementia (Behrmann & Lieberthal, 1989; C. Davis, Harrington, & Baynes, 2006; Grayson,

Hilton, & Franklin, 1997; Jokel & Anderson, 2012). The patients in these investigations, however, appeared to have less severe and/or more circumscribed deficits compared to those of Jacobs and Thompson's (1992) patient. Therefore, further research is needed to resolve these inconsistent findings pertaining to the effects of semantic treatments on auditory lexical–semantic comprehension deficits.

In terms of reading comprehension, a few semantic-based treatment approaches have been developed to increase patients' reliance on whole-word reading, which is also referred to as the "lexical–semantic route for reading comprehension" (Beeson & Henry, 2008; Friedman & Lott, 2000; Rothi & Moss, 1992). In one treatment, patients, particularly those who solely rely on a slow and thus inefficient letter-by-letter reading strategy, are briefly (e.g., 50 milliseconds) shown a written word, typically on a computer screen, and then asked to do one or more of the following: (a) read the word aloud, (b) determine if the word belongs to a target semantic category, (c) decide if the stimulus was a real or made-up word, or (d) determine if the word was part of an orally presented sentence. Improvements such as increased reading rates, improved recognition of trained words, and improved oral reading of trained and untrained words have been reported. Because less-positive outcomes also have been reported (e.g., Maher, Clayton, Barrett, Schober-Peterson, & Rothi, 1998), further research is necessary to identify which patients are most likely to benefit from this type of reading treatment.

Multiple Oral Rereading (**MOR**; Beeson, 1998; Beeson & Insalaco, 1998) is another treatment designed to increase use of whole-word reading in patients who rely on letter-by-letter reading. In MOR, patients read aloud repeatedly a preselected text to increase their reading rate. It is hypothesized that because repeated readings will allow increased familiarity with the content and syntactic structure of the text, patients will be able to shift over time to the more efficient whole-word reading strategy. Although patients have achieved faster text-reading rates following MOR (Beeson, 1998; Beeson & Insalaco, 1998), whether or not their reading comprehension was enhanced was not examined.

Accordingly, Mayer and Murray (2002) developed a modified version of MOR to encourage text comprehension by having their patient answer a set of questions following each reading aloud of target passages. Despite the addition of these comprehension questions, their patient demonstrated improvements only in reading rate. These researchers identified several factors that may have limited their ability to identify or elicit comprehension improvements, including the low intensity of their treatment schedule and the use of inordinately difficult reading probe passages (i.e., probes were at a Grade 15 level, whereas treatment passages were near a Grade 9 level). Therefore, although MOR has consistently been found to improve reading rate in patients with a variety of symptom profiles, further investigations are needed to delineate the effects of this treatment on reading comprehension and to determine whether or not MOR is any more effective than simply practicing reading on a regular basis.

Semantic Treatments for Production Problems

In contrast to the limited database pertaining to the effects of semantic treatments on spoken or written lexical–semantic comprehension, numerous studies have examined whether these treatments can ameliorate lexical–semantic produc[tion, particu]larly spoken naming impairments (C. Davis et al., 2006; de Jong-H[agelstein;] Doesborgh et al., 2004; Ennis, 2001; Wambaugh, 2003; Wambau[gh] & Kalinyak-Fliszar, 2002). In these investigations, patients were p[rovided] of the previously described semantic-based therapy activities, such [as sorting] into semantic categories, answering semantic judgment questions, or completing naming tasks with the provision of semantic prompts (e.g., superordinate or attribute cue; see also Table 9-5). Collectively, the results of these studies indicate that semantic treatments can evoke positive gains in the spoken word retrieval of patients with aphasia, regardless of what processing deficits (i.e., semantic, phonological, or both) underlie their naming impairments. There is some emerging evidence that semantic treatments can also facilitate naming abilities in patients with progressive disorders such as semantic dementia, albeit to a lesser extent than that observed in patients with aphasia due to static lesions (Bier et al., 2009; Henry, Beeson, & Rapcsak, 2008; Jokel & Anderson, 2012). Whereas initial research suggested that semantic therapies are superior to phonological therapies in terms of the durability of treatment effects on spoken naming abilities (Nickels & Best, 1996), more recent data do not support this contention (de Jong-Hagelstein et al., 2011; Doesborgh et al., 2004; Wambaugh, 2003).

One specific semantic treatment that has been the subject of a growing number of studies is **Semantic Feature Analysis** (SFA; Boyle, 2001, 2004, 2010; Coelho, McHugh, & Boyle, 2000). In SFA, which can be used in both individual and group therapy settings (e.g., Antonucci, 2009; Falconer & Antonucci, 2012), a chart such as that shown in Figure 9-2 is typically used to help patients generate words that are semantically related to the target item. More specifically, patients are shown a picture and asked to name that

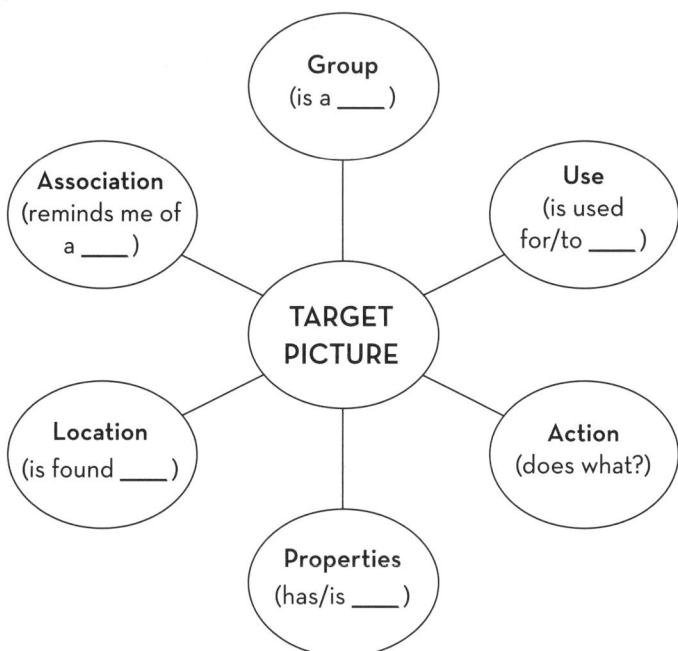

Figure 9-2. Example of a chart that may be used during Semantic Feature Analysis treatment.

...re. Regardless of their response accuracy, they are asked to come up with words that will fill each bubble on the chart, and these words in turn are written onto the chart either by the clinician or the patients themselves. If patients have difficulty generating these semantic features, the clinician provides cues regarding possible features, and if those don't assist the patients, supplies the features and adds them to the chart. Once the chart has been completed, patients are again asked to name the target item; if they still are unable to name the item, the clinician models the appropriate label. The goal of SFA is to activate the semantic network (via elicitation of semantic features) to which the target item belongs, and this activation in turn should facilitate access to, and thus production of, the target item. Additionally, it is hoped that patients will begin to generate independently semantic features to self-cue themselves in communicative activities outside of the therapy room.

With SFA, patients with a variety of aphasia types and severities (Antonucci, 2009; Boyle, 2001, 2004; Conley & Coelho, 2003; Falconer & Antonucci, 2012; Rider, Wright, Marshall, & Page, 2008), as well as those with naming difficulties subsequent to TBI (Coelho et al., 2000; Falconer & Antonucci, 2012; Massaro & Tompkins, 1992), have shown improved spoken naming of trained and, in some cases, untrained nouns with good maintenance of these improvements. SFA has also been used to target verb retrieval and has been similarly found to improve naming of trained verbs (that was maintained by most patients), but with little change in untrained verbs (Boo & Rose, 2011; Wambaugh & Ferguson, 2007). Some generalization to discourse, particularly in terms of increased informativeness and communicative efficiency, has been reported when SFA has been used to train noun or verb retrieval (Antonucci, 2009; Boyle, 2004; Coelho et al., 2000; Falconer & Antonucci, 2012; Wambaugh & Ferguson, 2007). Comparable positive outcomes have been observed when a semantic specification treatment similar to SFA was applied to improve written naming in a patient with semantic-level deficits (Hillis, 1991). That is, this patient demonstrated improved written naming of trained items, and generalization to written naming of untrained exemplars of trained categories and to spoken naming and auditory comprehension of trained and untrained exemplars of trained categories. Because varying degrees of improvement and generalization were reported in previous SFA studies, further investigations are needed to identify which patient (e.g., aphasia severity, aphasia type, etiology) and procedural factors (e.g., treatment length, individual vs. group format, nouns vs. verbs) are most influential on SFA outcomes.

A treatment similar to SFA has been developed by Edmonds and colleagues to address verb retrieval skills (Edmonds & Babb, 2011; Edmonds, Nadeau, & Kiran, 2009). Verb Network Strengthening Treatment (VNeST), like SFA, requires patients to generate words that are related to the target stimulus. In VNeST the target stimulus is a verb and patients are asked to name three to four pairs of agents (the action doer) and patients (the action receiver) for each target word (see Figure 9-3 for an example). Patients are asked to try to make one of these word pairs personal, and across sessions, the pairs they generate for a given verb are allowed to vary. If patients have difficulty generating these word pairs, they are given word cards (which include foils) from which they must

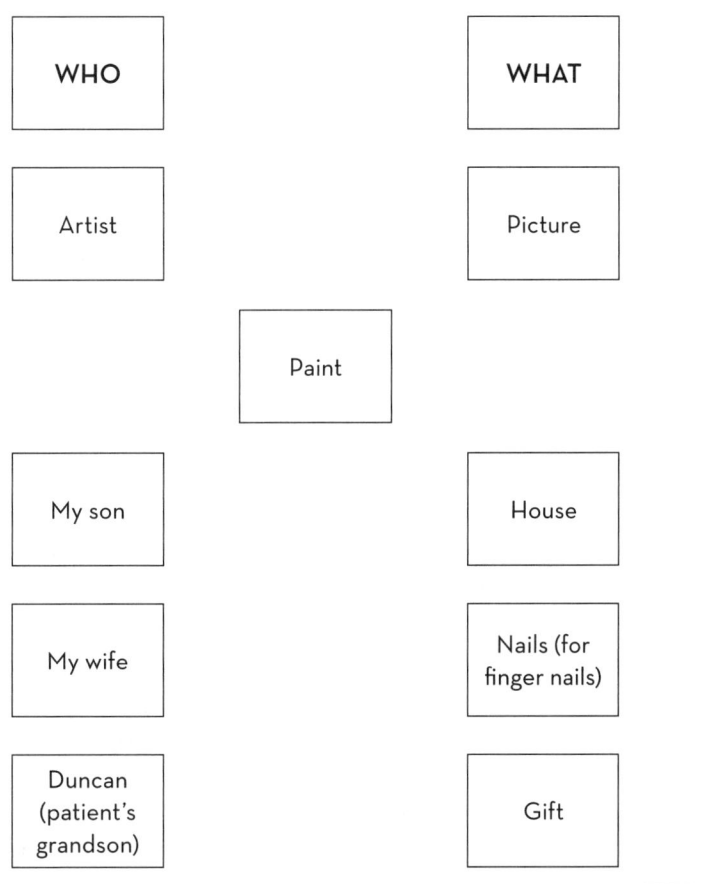

Figure 9-3. Example of word cards for training a target verb via Verb Network Strengthening Treatment. *Note.* The target verb is "paint" and the "WHO" and "WHAT" cards serve to indicate that the patient must generate agent and patient pairs, respectively.

select appropriate agents and patients. Next, patients read aloud the agent-verb-patient combinations that have been generated and answer a *wh-* question (*where, when, why*) regarding one combination. For instance, the patient might be asked, "Why was your wife measuring windows?" for the target verb and word pairs shown in Figure 9-3. The goal of VNeST is to facilitate access to verbs and words related to them, which in turn should facilitate production of these words in connected language contexts (i.e., sentence and discourse levels).

Edmonds and colleagues (2009; Edmonds & Babb, 2011) have found that patients with moderate or moderate-to-severe fluent or nonfluent aphasia benefit from VNeST. Treated patients have demonstrated improvements on several or all of the following: (a) naming of verbs and nouns, (b) retrieval of content words when producing sentences for the trained verbs as well as untrained verbs that were semantically related to the trained verbs (e.g., if "measure" was trained, improvements in production of a sentence for the verb "weigh" was observed), and (c) production of complete utterances (i.e., contain both subjects and verbs) and informative content in discourse samples. As might be expected, patients with more severe aphasia required a longer treatment period and showed more modest gains. Importantly, a protocol similar to VNeST was associated with similar improvements in a case study presented by Webster and Gordon (2009).

Kiran and colleagues (Kiran, 2008; Kiran & Johnson, 2008; Kiran, Sandberg, & Sebastian, 2011; Kiran & Thompson, 2003) have explored how to maximize the generalization effects of semantic treatments aimed at improving noun retrieval. These researchers have proposed that generalization may be enhanced by attending to the complexity of the trained stimuli. That is, given that training more "complex" syntactic structures (e.g., Thompson & Shapiro, 2007) and phonological forms (e.g., Gierut, 2007) has been shown to evoke improvements in untrained, simpler syntactic structures and phonological forms, respectively, Kiran and colleagues have investigated whether training atypical (i.e., more complex) category exemplars results in improved naming of untrained, typical (i.e., less complex) category exemplars. For example, in their initial study, Kiran and Thompson (2003) provided four patients with moderately severe aphasia a semantic-based naming treatment that involved both comprehension and production activities (e.g., picture sorting, semantic judgment questions). They found that when atypical items of a target category were trained, generalization to untrained typical and intermediate exemplars of that treated category occurred. In contrast, minimal generalization was observed when typical items were trained. In their more recent investigations, a similar pattern of treatment effects (i.e., training atypical generalizes to typical but not vice versa) has been observed on confrontation naming, as well as verbal fluency or generative naming tasks for most of their participants (Kiran, 2008; Kiran & Johnson, 2008; Kiran et al., 2011).

The majority of participants involved in the work of Kiran and colleagues have had mild to moderate language impairments; Mayer, Murray, and Karcher (2004) attempted to elicit these complexity effects in three patients with severe to profound aphasia. In contrast to Kiran and Thompson, Mayer et al. found only item-specific training effects with no generalization to untrained exemplars, regardless of whether atypical or typical exemplars were treated. It is important to note, however, that Mayer and colleagues utilized a more traditional cueing hierarchy treatment because the semantic judgment questions used by Kiran and Thompson were beyond the comprehension capabilities of Mayer and colleagues' patients. Accordingly, further research is needed to determine if (a) training complex stimuli evokes generalization in only certain patient populations or (b) the combination of a semantic-based treatment *and* training complex stimuli is necessary to evoke generalization.

Should Clinicians Focus on Only One Treatment Strategy?

Describing intervention strategies individually can be misleading because of the potential implication that there is a single treatment that is "best" for each patient. Instead, clinical experience shows us that most patients with neurogenic language and cognitive disorders exhibit impairments of many linguistic processes that are most effectively addressed with different intervention strategies. Consider Helen, a 45-year-old woman who had experienced a stroke resulting in moderate anomia, alexia, and agraphia. During assessment, it was revealed that Helen exhibited impairments in both semantic and phonological domains. Further, she displayed mild right-sided inattention. Helen's goal was to return to her former position as a volunteer receptionist for a local nonprofit agency. Treatment therefore emphasized the skills pertinent to this position (e.g., answering the telephone, writing down phone numbers). Because Helen's word finding was facilitated by visual and/or kinesthetic cueing (i.e., writing the word with a pencil or spelling the word in the air), treatment initially targeted developing this compensatory strategy as a means of facilitating verbal expression, as well as addressing some of the skills relevant to her vocational goals. Unfortunately, it soon became apparent that Helen also experienced difficulty with grapheme-to-phoneme conversion. Thus, even while the physical act of attempting to write the word facilitated her verbal expression, her written production of the target word was often spelled incorrectly. Moreover, her attempts to read back what she had written were limited by her right-sided inattention. Ultimately, Helen devised separate strategies for spoken and written expression. To facilitate accurate recording of telephone messages, Helen asked speakers to spell names letter by letter, which she would then read back letter by letter. She used a similar strategy for phone numbers.

Phonological Treatment Approaches

Phonological Treatments for Comprehension Problems. Phonological treatments are designed to strengthen the integrity of or facilitate access to phonological representations. When comprehension is being trained, spoken-word-to-picture or object matching and/or spoken-word-to-written word matching might be used. To stress phonological processing skills, distracter items for these tasks should be phonologically related to the target stimuli. For example, for the target "phone," distracter items might be "cone," "fawn," and "fin." Additional tasks include answering phonological judgment questions (e.g., for the target "phone," "Does this word rhyme with *moan*?" "Does this word have one syllable?"), or completing phonemic perception and discrimination tasks (see the "Treatment of Segmental Impairments" section at the outset of this chapter). Although these treatment activities are commonly used in daily clinical practice, there is a dearth of research regarding their potential effects on patients' lexical–semantic comprehension abilities. When these tasks have been used in formal investigations, they were typically administered in concert with or subsequent to semantically based comprehension activities (e.g., Ennis, 2001; de Jong-Hagelstein et al., 2011). Accordingly, the effects of phonological tasks by themselves on lexical–semantic comprehension, including to what extent they can evoke generalization to untrained stimuli and activities, remains to be proven.

Phonological Treatments for Expression Problems. In contrast to the above description of comprehension treatments, many researchers have used phonologically based treatments to remediate lexical–semantic production in patients with aphasia. When production is being trained, one or more of the following tasks might be utilized: (a) repeating, (b) reading aloud, (c) making phonological judgments or identifications, and (d) naming following or in concert with the provision of one or a hierarchy of phonologically based cues (see Table 9-5) (see included DVD: Patient 6a, 6b). Extensive research indicates that phonological treatments can facilitate spoken word retrieval in patients whose naming deficits have been traced to problems at primarily phonological output levels (Kendall et al., 2008; Murray & Kim, 2004; Tuomiranta, Rautakoski, Rinne, Martin, & Laine, 2012; Waldron et al., 2011), those with predominately semantic-level problems (Raymer, Thompson, Jacobs, & Le Grand, 1993; Wambaugh, 2003), and those with semantic and phonological problems (de Jong-Hagelstein et al., 2011; Doesborgh et al., 2004). Inconsistent findings, however, have been reported concerning whether phonological treatment effects are maintained over time (e.g., Nickels & Best, 1996, vs. Tuomiranta et al., 2012) or generalize to untrained items and modalities (e.g., Waldron et al., 2011, vs. Vitali et al., 2010). Factors that may influence the degree and persistence of improvements following phonological treatment include the part of speech being trained (e.g., noun vs. verb; Wambaugh et al., 2002), the degree to which patients actively participate in choosing or self-generating the cue (DeDe et al., 2003; Vitali et al., 2010), lesion size (Vitali et al., 2007), and presence and severity of concomitant cognitive and/or motor speech deficits (Tuomiranta et al., 2012; Waldron et al., 2011).

Combined Semantic and Phonological Treatment Approaches

A review of the effects of semantic- versus phonological-based treatments indicates that there does not appear to be a direct relationship between type of lexical–semantic deficit (i.e., semantic level vs. phonological level vs. both) and the most effective or efficient treatment approach. That is, investigators have found that patients with phonological-level deficits are not the only ones to benefit from phonological-based treatment, just as patients with semantic-level deficits are not the only ones to benefit from semantic-based treatment (e.g., de Jong-Hagelstein et al., 2011; Doesborgh et al., 2004). Accordingly, for many patients a therapy program that combines semantic and phonological protocols will be most efficient.

Oral Reading for Language in Aphasia (ORLA) exemplifies a treatment designed to strengthen both phonological and semantic reading routes (Cherney, 2004, 2010a, 2010b). Steps to the ORLA protocol are as follows:

1. The clinician reads aloud while pointing to each word, as the patient follows along by reading silently.
2. The same procedures are followed as in step 1, except the patient should also point to each word.
3. The clinician and patient read aloud together (i.e., choral reading) while both point to each word.

4. The patient has to point to the one word read aloud by the clinician for each line or sentence within the trained text.
5. The clinician has to point to the one word read aloud by the patient for each line or sentence within the trained text.
6. The clinician and patient again read aloud together.

ORLA has four levels through which patients progress. For the first level, trained text is at a first-grade reading level (i.e., 3–5-word sentences with simple syntax); for the final level, the paragraph-length text is at a sixth-grade reading level (4–6 sentences in length for a total of 50–100 words).

Treatment outcomes following ORLA provided via a clinician or computer have included improvements in not only reading comprehension but also spoken language, writing, and auditory comprehension and, therefore, overall aphasia severity (Cherney, 2004, 2010a, 2010b). How well these gains are maintained, however, has not yet been examined. Additionally, although patients with a variety of aphasia types and severities have responded positively to ORLA, some patients show minimal change. Therefore, further research is needed to identify patient characteristics (e.g., lesion location, demographic variables) that may assist in determining for whom ORLA may be most appropriate.

Brain Stimulation Approaches to Treating Lexical–Semantic Deficits

Recently researchers have begun to explore the potential of non-invasive electrophysiological techniques to address lexical–semantic deficits in individuals with neurogenic language and cognitive disorders. The two techniques that have been used thus far are **transcranial direct current stimulation (tDCS)** and **repetitive transcranial magnetic stimulation (rTMS)**. Briefly, in tDCS, a continuous, weak, direct current is applied to the scalp to increase (via anodal polarization) or decrease (via cathodal polarization) the firing rates of neurons (Chrysikou & Hamilton, 2011; Nitsche & Paulus, 2011; Vines et al., 2011). In rTMS, an electrical current, which like in tDCS can be used to excite or inhibit neural tissue activity, is created via magnetic pulses (Chrysikou & Hamilton, 2011; Rossi, Hallett, Rossini, Pascual-Leone, & the Safety of TMS Consensus Group, 2009). As might be expected, given that cortical activity levels respond to this type of electrical stimulation, regional blood flow changes have been identified, even after the stimulation has been turned off (Zheng, Alsop, & Schlaug, 2011). For a detailed review of tDCS and rTMS procedures and applications, see Chrysikou and Hamilton (2011).

Initial research indicates that when used by themselves or in concert with one of the other lexical–semantic stimulation or cognitive neuropsychological approaches described above, tDCS (Floel et al., 2011; Fridriksson, Richardson, Baker, & Rorden, 2011; Monti, Cogiamanian, Marceglia, Ferrucci, & Mameli, 2008; Nitsche & Paulus, 2011; Vines et al., 2011) and rTMS (Kakuda, Abo, Kaito, Watanabe, & Senoo, 2010; P. Martin et al., 2009; Medina et al., 2012; Naeser et al., 2005, 2010; Szaflarski et al., 2011) can evoke positive changes in the lexical–semantic retrieval abilities of individuals with chronic aphasia; further, these changes are well maintained following discontinuation of the stimulation. Across these studies, the vast majority of patients have presented with nonfluent aphasia, and treatment outcomes have primarily focused on naming abilities (e.g., verbal fluency, confrontation naming). A limited number of investigators, however, have examined whether language benefits might extend beyond naming and have documented spoken discourse improvements in terms of the quantity and quality of the output (e.g., increased number of closed class words, larger number of nouns used; increased utterance length), gains in spoken language comprehension, or both (Barwood et al., 2011; R. Hamilton et al., 2010; Medina et al., 2012; Naeser et al., 2010; You, Dae-Yul, Chun, Jung, & Park, 2011). In contrast, productive syntax abilities appear less responsive to stimulation procedures. Initial findings also suggest that the naming abilities of patients in the more acute phases of aphasia recovery (e.g., first few months post-onset; Weiduschat et al., 2011; You et al., 2011) or with fluent aphasia profiles (Fridriksson et al., 2011) will benefit from these stimulation techniques.

It is important to point out that not all aphasic patients respond to tDCS or rTMS, with some patients showing limited changes in their language abilities (P. Martin et al., 2009; Szaflarski et al., 2011). Further, some patients will have concomitant symptoms that will disqualify them from these stimulation techniques. For example, rTMS is not recommended for patients with a history of seizures. Additionally, both stimulation techniques require MRIs to determine the appropriate site of neural stimulation so patients who do not meet the inclusionary criteria for MRIs (e.g., have metal implants) will also not qualify for tDCS or rTMS.

Collectively, the findings from tDCS and rTMS studies thus far are quite encouraging. Overall, however, many of the treatment investigations have had relatively weak study designs (e.g., case reports, no control or sham group), indicating a need to verify their results. Likewise, the benefit these stimulation techniques might hold for a broad range of language impairments (e.g., morphosyntactic comprehension) and patient profiles (e.g., dementia, TBI, RHD) needs to be explored. Finally, further research is required to determine the stimulation protocol most likely to maximize language outcomes (e.g., ideal stimulation sites; stimulation to excite or inhibit neural activity; number, length, and frequency of stimulation sessions).

Morphosyntactic Treatments

Whereas substantial research has aimed at qualifying and quantifying the morphosyntactic processing deficits associated with aphasia (e.g., Bastiaanse & Edwards, 2001; Goodglass, 1993), a more limited literature has examined treatments for these deficits. Because there is a dearth of research pertaining to the integrity of morphosyntactic processing following TBI, RHD, or the onset of dementia, as well as treatments for these possible deficits, our discussion will focus on morphosyntactic procedures developed for patients with aphasia; whether these procedures can or should be used with other neurogenic patient populations remains to be proven.

The Linguistic Stimulation Approach to Treating Morphosyntactic Deficits

Stimulation treatments for morphosyntactic deficits often involve determining a hierarchy of difficulty for comprehending and producing morphosyntactic structures, and then, in treatment, progressing through that hierarchy from the easiest to the most complex structures. Morphosyntactic production deficits are typically remediated by having patients practice producing sentences that include the target morphosyntactic structure(s). Morphosyntactic comprehension deficits may be addressed through activities that require patients to identify the target morphosyntactic structures, such as pointing to the picture that corresponds to the target sentence or manipulating objects so as to act out the target sentence.

Although stimulation activities to target morphosyntactic production or comprehension are frequently described in textbooks and therapy workbooks (e.g., Coelho et al., 2008), empirical investigation of the efficacy of these tasks has almost exclusively focused on production treatments (Kempler & Goral, 2011; McCall, Virata, Linebarger, & Berndt, 2009; L. Murray & Karcher, 2000; Webster & Gordon, 2009). For example, one of the more popular morphosyntactic stimulation approaches described in the research literature is the *Helm Elicited Program for Syntax Stimulation* (HELPSS; Helm-Estabrooks, 1981; Helm-Estabrooks & Albert, 1991). Based on earlier research by Gleason, Goodglass, Green, Ackerman, and Hyde (1975), the HELPSS trains production of the hierarchy of sentence constructions shown in Table 9-7. Each sentence construction is practiced at two levels: Level A, which elicits delayed imitation, and Level B, which elicits a spontaneous response via story completion cues. At both Level A and Level B, the patient is read a short story and shown a picture depicting that story. For example, to elicit the Direct and Indirect Object sentence "They give Pat a cake" at Level A, the clinician would read the following: "It's Pat's birthday. Her friends want to celebrate, so they give Pat a cake. What do they do?" (Helm-Estabrooks & Albert, 1991, p. 226). To elicit that same sentence at Level B, the clinician would read, "It's Pat's birthday and her friends want to celebrate, so what do they do?" (Helm-Estabrooks & Albert, 1991, p. 226). Treatment proceeds by first training at Level A the simplest sentence construction that the patient has difficulty producing. Once the patient completes Level A probes for that sentence construction with 90% accuracy, Level B probes for that sentence construction are introduced. When the patient can complete Level B probes with 90% accuracy, Level A probes for the next most difficult sentence construction in the hierarchy are trained. Treatment continues until the patient has progressed through the hierarchy of sentence types.

In 2000, Helm-Estabrooks and Nicholas published a revised version of the HELPSS, referred to as the *Sentence Production Program for Aphasia* (SPPA). Differences between the HELPSS and the SPPA include the following: (a) The SPPA targets only eight

TABLE 9-7
Hierarchies of Syntactic Constructions for the *Helm Elicited Program for Syntax Stimulation* (HELPSS) and the *Sentence Production Program for Aphasia* (SPPA)

SENTENCE CONSTRUCTION TYPE (from easiest to most complex)	EXAMPLES
Imperative intransitive	"Lie down." "Wake up."
Imperative transitive	"Wash the dishes." "Drink your milk."
Wh- interrogative	"What are you writing?" "Where are my shoes?"
***Wh-* interrogative: *what* and *who* (SPPA only)**	"Who is coming?" "What are you watching?"
***Wh-* interrogative: *where* and *when* (SPPA only)**	"Where is the hospital?" "When are we landing?"
Declarative transitive	"She cleans teeth." "He teaches school."
Declarative intransitive	"She skates." "He swims."
Comparative	"They are funnier." "She is taller."
Passive	"The suitcases were lost." "The car was towed."
Yes/No questions	"Did you buy the paper?" "Is it sad?"
Direct and indirect object	"They give Pat a cake." "He reads his grandchild a story."
Embedded sentences	"She wanted him to be healthy." "She wanted him to be rich."
Future	"He will hike." "He will sleep."

Note. Only those sentence constructions in bold font are trained as part of the SPPA (Helm-Estabrooks & Nicholas, 2000). The HELPSS (Helm-Estabrooks, 1981) trains those in bold and regular font, unless otherwise noted.

sentence constructions (see Table 9-7) by excluding the HELPSS sentence constructions that are viewed as less applicable in daily communication interactions and that are particularly challenging for patients with aphasia, such as passives and embedded clauses; (b) the SPPA includes a similar number of exemplars for each sentence construction; and (c) the SPPA stimuli revolve around a restricted set of characters who represent a range of ages and ethnicities.

There is some empirical support for using the HELPSS to improve the morphosyntactic production abilities of patients with aphasia, at least those with nonfluent language profiles. For example, researchers have reported that patients with chronic Broca's aphasia demonstrate increased phrase length and sentence grammaticality in their spoken discourse following the HELPSS (Fink et al., 1995; Helm-Estabrooks, Fitzpatrick, & Barresi, 1981; Helm-Estabrooks & Ramsberger, 1986b; Murray & Ray, 2001). These improvements have even been reported when the HELPSS was provided over the telephone to patients who were unable to attend clinic sessions (Helm-Estabrooks & Ramsberger, 1986a). Generalization of treatment effects, however, has most frequently been limited to untrained exemplars of trained sentence constructions, rather than extending to untrained sentence constructions (e.g., Doyle, Goldstein, & Bourgeois, 1987;

Fink et al., 1995). Currently, there are no published studies evaluating the efficacy of the SPPA. Likewise, researchers have yet to explore whether or not the HELPSS or the SPPA are appropriate for patients with fluent language profiles or for written morphosyntactic deficits. Finally, given that most research has focused on stimulation treatments for morphosyntactic production impairments, the development and examination of stimulation activities that target morphosyntactic comprehension abilities are still needed.

Linguistic Theory Motivated Approaches to Treating Morphosyntactic Deficits

In contrast to stimulation morphosyntactic treatments, which tend to target sentence structures on the basis of overt impairment rather than theory, other treatment procedures have been developed to reflect linguistic models of morphosyntactic processing in adults with or without aphasia. In particular, two theoretically motivated approaches, **mapping therapy** and **Treatment of Underlying Forms**, have been created to treat deficits of grammatical production, comprehension, or both, and to date have proven effective for at least some patients with aphasia.

Mapping Therapy

The theoretical impetus of mapping therapy is M. Garrett's (1988) model of sentence production. According to Garrett, there are two levels of representation that contribute to the final production or comprehension of a sentence: (a) the Functional, or semantic, level, at which words are assigned a thematic role (e.g., agent, or who is doing the action), and (b) the Positional level, at which words and morphemes are arranged into syntactic frames and assigned phonological forms. Advocates of mapping therapy propose that patients with agrammatism experience problems "mapping relations between the abstract functional level and surface syntax at the positional level" (Rochon & Reichman, 2003, p. 203). These difficulties in turn result in problems processing sentences like those shown below. Sentence 1 is noncanonical (i.e., the second vs. first noun is the agent or action "doer"), and sentence 2 is reversible (i.e., either noun could feasibly serve as the agent). Most difficult would be noncanonical, reversible sentences like that shown in sentence 3 below.

1. **Passive sentence with noncanonical order:** The guitar was played by Dylan.
2. **Reversible sentence:** Dylan was chasing the dog.
3. **Noncanonical, reversible sentence:** Dylan was chased by the dog.

The overall goal of mapping therapy, therefore, is to improve patients' ability to map or understand the connection between the Positional and Functional levels of sentences such as those exemplified above (i.e., noncanonical and/or reversible), which in turn is expected to alleviate their grammatical comprehension and/or production impairments (Harris, Olson, & Humphreys, 2012; Rochon, Laird, Bose, & Scofield, 2005; Rochon & Reichman, 2003, 2004; M. Schwartz, Saffran, Fink, Myers, & Martin, 1994). Although there has been some divergence in the activities and language behaviors targeted during treatment (e.g., target sentence structure, comprehension vs. production), most mapping therapies have utilized a sentence query procedure to increase patients' awareness of the relationship between words' thematic roles and their location within a sentence. For example, steps for a mapping therapy session might include the following:

1. Present a pictured scene and/or a spoken or written model of the target sentence structure (e.g., "The nurse was greeted by the doctor"), and ask the patient to identify the action (i.e., verb) by manipulating objects to demonstrate the action and/or underlining or saying the appropriate word in the sentence stimulus.
2. Next, require the patient to identify who was doing the action (i.e., agent) by pointing to the correct object/figure and/or underlining or saying the appropriate word in the sentence stimulus.
3. Instruct the patient to identify whom the action was done to (i.e., theme) by pointing to the correct object/figure and/or underlining or saying the appropriate word in the sentence stimulus.
4. If sentence production is being targeted, the final step would be to have the patient produce the correct sentence structure in response to the picture stimulus.

The results of several treatment studies indicate that mapping therapy can positively affect the sentence processing abilities of patients with nonfluent (Byng, 1988; Harris et al., 2012; Rochon et al., 2005; M. Schwartz et al., 1994; Wierenga et al., 2006) or mixed aphasia profiles (Rochon & Reichman, 2003, 2004), keeping in mind that not all patients like or respond to mapping therapy activities (e.g., Webster & Gordon, 2009). That is, patients have been found to improve on trained sentence structures (i.e., primarily passives and/or object clefts) with generalization to untrained exemplars of the trained structures. Further, when sentence comprehension abilities have been trained, some generalization to production at the sentence or discourse level has been observed (Byng, 1988; Rochon & Reichman, 2004; M. Schwartz et al., 1994). In addition to addressing sentence processing deficits, Harris and colleagues (2012) demonstrated that their mapping therapy protocol resulted in improved production of both regular and irregular past tense verbs, with generalization to untrained regular verbs, as well as untrained irregular verbs that shared characteristics with the trained irregular verbs (e.g., if "led" for "lead" was treated, other irregular past tense verbs formed in the similar manner improved, like "fed" for "feed"). In contrast, studies have not yet consistently demonstrated that sentence production training improves sentence comprehension or that either sentence production or comprehension training generalizes to untrained sentence structures (Harris et al., 2012; Rochon & Reichman, 2003; Rochon et al., 2005; Wierenga et al., 2006).

Treatment of Underlying Forms (TUF)
TUF, previously referred to as Linguistic Specific Treatment, is based on Chomsky's government binding theory (for a review, see Shapiro, 1997) and the proposition that

patients with agrammatism have difficulty processing grammatically complex sentences in which there has been phrase movement (e.g., passives, sentences with embedding) (K. Ballard & Thompson, 1999; Thompson, 2008; Thompson & Shapiro, 2005, 2007). An additional tenet of TUF is that targeting syntactically complex sentence types, in particular those with noncanonical order (i.e., phrase movement), should effect generalization to syntactically related, but less complex sentence types; this tenet has been referred to as the Complexity Account of Treatment Efficacy, or CATE. For example, treating sentences with *wh-* movement (such as that shown in sentence 1 below) should result in improved processing of other less complex *wh-*movement sentence forms (such as that shown in sentence 2 below), but evoke no change in processing sentences with other, unrelated forms of movement (such as that shown in sentence 3 below).

1. More complex *wh-*movement structure: [IPI know [CPwho$i$ [IPDylan kissed *trace$i$*]]]
2. Less complex *wh-*movement structure: [$_{CP}$Who$i$ has [$_{IP}$Dylan kissed *trace$i$*]]
3. Unrelated, noun phrase movement structure: [$_{IP}$The girl$i$ was kissed *trace$i$* by Dylan]

The overall goal of TUF, therefore, is to remediate patients' ability to process phrase movement by increasing their awareness and understanding of verbs, verb argument structure, and how certain sentence constituents move to form noncanonical sentence types, and by requiring them to practice producing noncanonical sentence types. Thus, some components of TUF are similar to those described above for mapping therapy (e.g., identifying the agent and theme in a target sentence). Specific TUF steps include the following:

1. Provide a spoken model of the target sentence structure (e.g., "I know who the girl splashed"), and require the patient to produce a similar sentence with the same sentence form that corresponds to a picture stimulus (e.g., "I know who the boy splashed").
2. Regardless of the patient's accuracy in step 1, present a set of written word/phrase cards that make up the canonical (i.e., active form) sentence (e.g., "The boy splashed the girl"), and have the patient identify the verb, the agent (e.g., "the boy"), and the theme (e.g., "the girl").
3. Provide the additional written word/phrase cards necessary to complete the target sentence structure, and model how to arrange all the cards to form the target sentence structure (e.g., "I know who the boy splashed"). Require the patient to read this target sentence aloud and then identify which words within it represent the verb, agent, and theme.
4. Shuffle the word/phrase cards, and then have the patient form and read aloud the target sentence structure.
5. Remove the word/phrase cards, and have the patient provide the target sentence structure.

A software version of the TUF protocol, Sentactics, has been developed (Thompson, Choy, Holland, & Cole, 2010). Such software might aid clinicians who lack familiarity with the linguistic theory and structures inherent to TUF, as well as offer a convenient mechanism for TUF home practice. Initial data indicated that patients who receive TUF via Sentactics demonstrate a similar improvement pattern as that described below and achieved by patients receiving clinician-delivered TUF.

Several investigations have been conducted to determine the effects of TUF on the grammatical production abilities of patients with Broca's or agrammatic aphasia profiles (K. Ballard & Thompson, 1999; B. Jacobs, 2001; B. Jacobs & Thompson, 2000; L. Murray et al., 2007; Stadie et al., 2008; Thompson, Ballard, & Shapiro, 1998; Thompson, Shapiro, Kiran, & Sobecks, 2003). Data from these studies indicate that TUF can evoke improvements in these patients' production of trained and linguistically related, untrained sentence structures. Modest generalization to untrained production tasks (i.e., narrative discourse) and output modalities (i.e., writing if speech was trained and the inverse pattern as well) also has been reported. Notably, less impressive findings were obtained when patients displayed one or more of the following: a fluent or mixed aphasia profile, concomitant cognitive deficits, or significant auditory comprehension deficits (Dickey & Yoo, 2010; L. Murray, Ballard, & Karcher, 2004): Although these patients did acquire the trained complex sentence structures, they demonstrated minimal or erratic generalization effects. These results suggest that patients with more isolated grammatical difficulties may be the best candidates for TUF.

The above review indicates that morphosyntactic treatments that are motivated by linguistic theory can be effective in improving the deficits of sentence comprehension, production, or both that are associated with chronic aphasia. With few exceptions (e.g., L. Murray et al., 2004; Rochon & Reichman, 2004), however, the effects of these treatments have been explored with only patients who have Broca's or nonfluent aphasia. Consequently, future research should determine if these treatments are equally effective for patients with other language profiles, identify what treatment adaptations may be necessary when working with these patients, or both. Likewise, the vast majority of prior studies have focused on treating morphosyntactic production deficits. Although a few protocols for addressing morphosyntactic comprehension deficits have been described and evaluated (e.g., Kiran et al., 2012; M. Schwartz et al., 1994), further examination of these treatments is clearly needed.

What to Do When You're Monolingual, but Your Client Is Bilingual or Multilingual?

Given that individuals who speak more than one language are one of the fastest growing segments of the U.S. population and that over half of the world's population is bilingual, it is quite likely that monolingual clinicians will at some point in their career be faced with providing services to patients who use a number of languages (Centeno, 2009; D'Souza, Kay-Raining Bird, & Deacon, 2012). In terms of providing language intervention to such clients, some key questions monolingual clinicians might have include the following:

(a) Should treatment target one or all of the client's languages?
(b) If just one language is treated, which one should be selected?
(c) If just one language is treated, will the untreated language get better (i.e., cross-linguistic transfer)?
(d) What client variables should be considered when trying to answer questions (a) and (b)?

Aphasia researchers are attempting to find answers for such questions, with initial findings suggesting that improvements occur if either unilingual or multilingual treatment is provided or if either the patient's first or second language is treated (Faroqi-Shah, Frymark, Mullen, & Wang, 2010; Gitterman, Goral, & Obler, 2012; Kohnert, 2009). How to foster cross-linguistic transfer, however, has yet to be resolved, given that mixed results have been reported following unilingual as well as bilingual language treatment (e.g., Miertsch, Meisel, & Isel, 2009, vs. Meinzer, Obleser, Flaisch, Eulitz, & Rockstroh, 2007b). Similarly, given that a relatively small number of patients have been described in the bilingual and multilingual treatment literature thus far, with little consistency across studies in terms of patient (e.g., which languages the patient uses, type and severity of aphasia, aphasia chronicity) or treatment variables (e.g., focus on word retrieval vs. morphosyntax; number, length, and intensity of treatment sessions), client characteristics that might assist in driving unilingual and/or multilingual treatment decisions have yet to be identified. Unfortunately, there is a dearth of research to guide intervention decisions when working with multilingual patients who have language deficits subsequent to RHD, TBI, or the onset of a progressive disorder.

Treatments for Pragmatic and Discourse-Level Impairments

Although a rich literature describes the nature of pragmatic and discourse-level impairments common in several types of neurogenic language and cognitive disorders (see Chapter 2), and a number of tools are available to aid in identifying such impairments (see Chapter 6), comparatively fewer data exist to guide treating pragmatic or discourse-level impairments. Nonetheless, clinicians can refer to a number of theory-driven intervention approaches that have been described, as well as develop individualized interventions based on current theoretical models of pragmatics or discourse (E. Armstrong, 2012; E. Armstrong, Ferguson, & Simmons-Mackie, 2011; Sohlberg & Turkstra, 2011; Tompkins, 2012).

Pragmatic aspects of communication and discourse-level skills (e.g., conversational turn-taking) are highly context dependent and are further influenced by cultural norms and individual subjectivity (McGann & Werven, 1999). These features of pragmatic and discourse behaviors have several implications for planning treatment activities. First, clinicians should be mindful of subjectivity and cultural variations when selecting treatment goals, stimuli, and activities. For example, cultures can vary in terms of which discourse genres are more highly valued, encountered, or both, and thus the patient's culture must be considered when choosing what genre will be targeted in treatment. Likewise, pragmatic conventions of some cultures are particularly sensitive to age or class differences between communication participants, whereas other cultures may be more or less accepting of irony or sarcasm as acceptable communication styles. The nature of prosodic markings also differs across cultures and dialects. Accordingly, if the clinician does not share the culture, dialect, or both of the patient, or if the clinician has idiosyncratic pragmatic behaviors, it may be helpful to utilize standardized treatment materials appropriate to the patient. Recorded stimuli (e.g., Tompkins, 1995) and standardized scenarios (e.g., Bayles & Tomoeda, 1993; Nicholas & Brookshire, 1993) may be used, or if such materials are inappropriate, the clinician may choose to invite other individuals whose communication behaviors share the same pragmatic or discourse conventions as the patient's to participate in treatment activities (e.g., Wiseman-Hakes, Stewart, Wasserman, & Schuller, 1998).

Second, because pragmatic and discourse-level aspects of both language comprehension and production are highly influenced by context, clinicians may find it difficult to address these skills in relatively context-free activities or environments, such as stimulus-response drills or in individual sessions in the speech-language therapists' office, respectively (Cherney & Halper, 2000; Sohlberg & Turkstra, 2011). Relatedly, discourse treatments by necessity incorporate extended text, messages, and/or exchanges and emphasize the construction and/or integration of meaning beyond the sentence level. Accordingly, clinicians will find that group treatment and activities such as role-playing or perspective taking, all of which incorporate rich contextual cues and require discourse comprehension and production, are particularly useful (Elman, 2007; A. Holland & Hinckley, 2002; Sohlberg & Turkstra, 2011). In fact, some texts incorporate treatment of pragmatics and discourse into the discussion of treatment at the ICF levels of activity and participation (see Chapter 12), particularly when addressing these aspects of communication for patients with aphasia (e.g., A. Holland & Hinckley, 2002; Wright & Newhoff, 2005).

Finally, it is helpful to remember that many pragmatic and discourse-level conventions are learned implicitly, that is, without conscious awareness. Although many adults experienced direct instruction in phonics, reading, writing, and grammar, it is unlikely that they had school coursework on appropriate loudness levels, how to alter intonation to change sentence meaning, how close to stand to individuals when speaking (i.e., proxemics), how to know when it is their turn to add to a conversation, or other pragmatic or discourse behaviors. Thus, developing metalinguistic awareness of these aspects of communication may be the first step in addressing specific pragmatic or discourse skills (Sohlberg & Turkstra, 2011; Tompkins, 1995) (see included DVD: Patient 7). Clinicians should also consider that given the automatic nature of many pragmatic processes, metalinguistic tasks, like those used to evaluate and remediate pragmatic problems, may mask underlying pragmatic competence. For further discussion of these issues and the implication for assessment and treatment, see Tompkins (1995, 2012) and Lehman Blake (2007).

The following sections of this chapter discuss strategies for addressing various aspects of pragmatic and discourse-level abilities. Although the discussion is organized with respect to specific pragmatic and discourse skills, many skill areas overlap; consequently, several treatment strategies are appropriate for addressing a variety of pragmatic and discourse symptoms. Because disruptions in pragmatic behaviors are most apparent in individuals with RHD and TBI, clinicians also may wish to consult the more detailed discussions of pragmatic treatment included in texts that exclusively focus on these populations (e.g., Myers, 1999; Sohlberg & Turkstra, 2011; Tompkins, 1995).

Figurative Language and Alternative Meanings Treatments

Many linguistic messages are ambiguous or have two or more alternative interpretations, depending on the communicative context. Lexical–semantic ambiguity results when single words have more than one meaning. For example, the homograph "block" can be used to denote a child's toy, a city division, an obstacle, or a strategic movement in the game of football or volleyball. Similarly, the homophones "hair" and "hare" have different meanings. Linguistic ambiguity may be most apparent in the case of figurative language, which includes metaphors (e.g., "He's a snake"), similes (e.g., "He's as happy as a clam"), and idioms (e.g., "She has her hands full"). When linguistic ambiguity is present, the task for the listener is to generate word features and plausible meanings (sometimes referred to as **coarse coding**) and then determine which is most appropriate to the communicative context (which involves suppressing incompatible word features and meanings), keeping in mind that the communicative context includes information pertaining to (a) the current physical environment (e.g., location of current communicative interaction, number of communicative partners, time of day), (b) the social and cognitive environment (e.g., social status of communicative partners, amount of knowledge shared among the communicative partners, emotional status of communicative partners), and (c) the verbal and nonverbal environment (e.g., colloquial vs. formal vocabulary, body language and/or facial expressions of communicative partners).

An essential first step to remediating difficulties with figurative language and other forms of alternate meanings is to ensure appropriate awareness of linguistic ambiguity. The clinician can identify examples of homographs, idioms, and metaphors to prompt discussion of alternative interpretations, including consideration of the contexts in which each meaning is most likely to apply. Many patients, however, who show apparent figurative language deficits in structured clinical tasks with such metalinguistic demands often demonstrate greater competence when figurative language is used in conversation (Myers, 1999; Tompkins, Klepousniotoou, & Gibbs Scott, 2011). For these patients, targeting awareness of lexical ambiguity may not be necessary. Instead, if it is clear the patient understands the concept of ambiguity, the clinician can devise scenarios and have the patient determine the most appropriate interpretation of messages within a given context. If necessary, the clinician can assist the patient in identifying the most important contextual features to assist in determining the meaning of ambiguous messages (Ferre, Ska, Lajoie, Bleau, & Joanette, 2011; Lehman Blake, 2007; Penn, Jones, & Joffe, 1997; Tompkins, 1995). Myers (1999) also described a variety of activities for targeting activation of alternative meanings (e.g., developing semantic associations for homographs: stand/sit, stand/platform), as well as suppression of inappropriate interpretations (e.g., selecting the appropriate interpretation when several possible alternatives have been identified).

Approaches for Figurative Language Comprehension Problems

Only recently has there been any empirical evaluation of interventions designed to enhance figurative language comprehension abilities. Tompkins (2012) and Tompkins, Blake, Wambaugh, and Meigh (2011) have developed Contextual Constraint Treatment, which has one version to address coarse coding (CC) problems and one version to target suppression (SUPP) issues (see Chapter 2 for a review of sources of RHD language symptoms). The treatment can be used to target response accuracy as well as speed, the latter of which is typically more problematic for patients who have difficulties with CC, SUPP, or both. The intervention protocol involves listening to cues that "prestimulate the target concept" (Tompkins, Blake, et al., 2011, p. 794): For the CC version, the target is the distant semantic feature, and for the SUPP version, the target is the contextually biased interpretation. The following hierarchy of pre-stimulation cues was developed: (a) the *strong-constraint context*, in which two cueing sentences are provided, the first of which offers a strong bias and the second of which offers a moderate bias for the target concept; (b) the *moderate-constraint context*, in which only one sentence with moderate bias is presented; and (c) the *minimal-to-none condition* (for the CC version only), in which no pre-stimulation cue is provided (Tompkins, 2012; Tompkins, Blake, et al., 2011). Patients must meet accuracy and response time criteria to move from the strong- to moderate- to no-constraint condition. In the CC version, after listening to the cues, patients hear a probe stimulus (a semantically neutral sentence followed by a target word) and must decide if the target word is a real or made-up word (i.e., a lexical decision task). In the SUPP version, after the cues, patients hear a probe stimulus (a sentence with an ambiguous final noun followed by a target word) and must decide if the target word fits with the meaning of the probe sentence. Stimulus examples are provided in Figure 9-4.

Initial data from four patients with RHD indicate that Contextual Constraint Treatment holds promise (Tompkins, 2012; Tompkins, Blake, et al., 2011). With treatment, all participants achieved a higher percentage of accurate responses that fulfilled pre-specified response time criteria. Importantly, maintenance and generalization (to untrained items, as well as comprehension of implied information at the discourse level) of treatment effects were observed, although data pertaining to maintenance and generalization are available for only a few participants thus far.

Example stimuli for the Coarse Coding version of the Contextual Constraint Treatment

    Strong Constraint Cues
        The pilot checked the gauges. He landed on the runway.

    Probe Stimulus
        There was an airplane—*captain*

    Task: Patient listens to the constraint cues and probe stimulus and must decide as quickly and accurately as possible if the target word (italicized) is real or made up.

Example stimuli for the Suppression version of the Contextual Constraint Treatment

    Strong Constraint Cues
        The girl bought a balloon. The balloon was filled with helium.

    Probe Stimulus
        She watched as it rose—*daisy*

    Task: Patient listens to the constraint cues and probe stimulus and must decide as quickly and accurately as possible if the target word (italicized) is related to the meaning of the directly preceding probe stimulus sentence.

Figure 9-4. Example stimuli from the Contextual Constraint Treatment of Tompkins and colleagues (Tompkins, Blake, Wambaugh, & Meigh, 2011; Tompkins, Scharp, Meigh, Blake, & Wambaugh 2012). Stimuli were taken from Tompkins, Blake, et al. (2011).

A protocol for targeting metaphor comprehension has also been recently developed (Lundgren, Brownell, Cayer-Meade, Milione, & Kearns, 2011). The Metaphor Training Program (MTP) focuses on highlighting possible semantic associations for each component of the metaphor and then on selecting which of those associations are most appropriate for the given metaphor. As illustrated in Figure 9-5, a graphic display, or bubble map, is used to highlight the components of the metaphor (which are located in the main circles), associations for each metaphor component (which are located in outer circles), and links between main and outer circles (lines connecting the circles). Specific MTP steps include the following:

1. For each component of the metaphor (e.g., "game" and "nightmare" for the metaphor "the game is a nightmare"), patients answer yes/no questions regarding possible connotative meanings (e.g., Is "nightmare" typically considered "peaceful?"; Is it typically considered "tense?").
2. For each component of the metaphor, patients answer yes/no questions regarding possible concrete associations (e.g., Is "nightmare" typically associated with "bed?"; Is it typically associated with "sun?").
3. Using a separate bubble map for each metaphor component, patients generate typical associations.
4. Using a double bubble map (like that shown in Figure 9-5), patients generate associations for one metaphor component and then answer yes/no questions

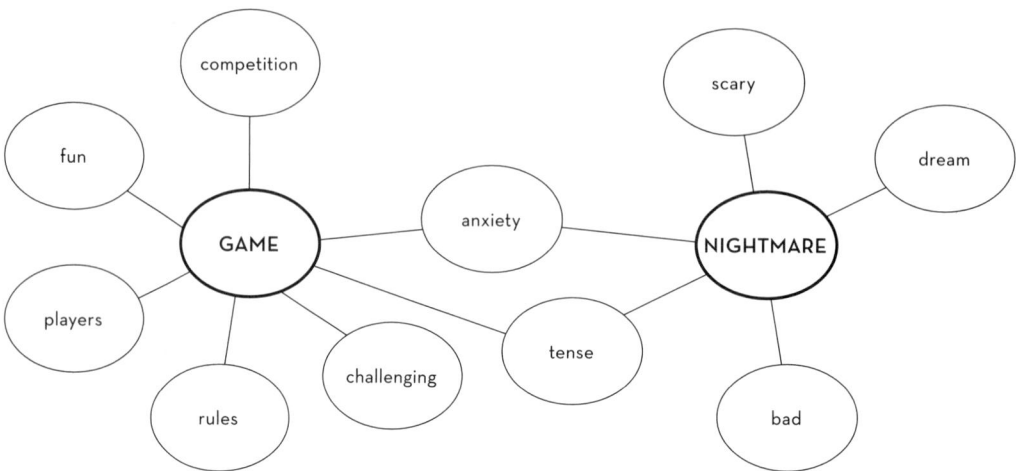

Figure 9-5. An example bubble map from the Metaphor Training Program (Lundgren et al., 2011) for the target metaphor "The game is a nightmare."

regarding whether these associations would also be appropriate for the other metaphor component.
5. Patients identify the correct metaphor interpretation from a choice of three (i.e., correct, literal interpretation, interpretation from a somewhat similar metaphor).

Only a limited number of RHD patients (i.e., $n = 5$) have completed MTP thus far, but with training, all patients displayed significant improvements in providing oral interpretation of metaphors; the majority also maintained their improvements at the three-month follow-up. Given that different degrees of improvement were observed among the patients, additional research is needed to explore influential participant variables (e.g., presence and severity of concomitant deficits) and to establish the reliability of these initial treatment outcome data.

Approaches for Figurative Language Expression Problems

Although patients with neurogenic language or cognitive disorders may exhibit reduced use of figurative language, this characteristic may interfere minimally with communication because explicit language is generally easily understood by communication partners. However, if it is deemed appropriate, clinicians may target production by devising scenarios in which the use of idioms, metaphors, and other forms of figurative language is appropriate. Treatment might begin with forced choice, in which the patient identifies the expression that best matches a presented context. For example, presented with an illustration of a man with money overflowing from his wallet, the patient selects the most appropriate metaphor from the choices, "He's loaded," "He's a gas," or "He's cold-hearted." Eventually, the patient is responsible for generating independently appropriate metaphors/idioms for pictured, written, or live-action stimuli and scenarios.

Training alternative meanings also may be necessary to help patients apply newly acquired language skills or strategies to a variety of communicative settings. For example, Robson and colleagues found that although their patients with severe aphasia and jargon were able to acquire a small written vocabulary via a writing treatment program, few of these patients used their written vocabulary during daily communicative activities (Robson, Marshall, Chiat, & Pring, 2001; Robson, Pring, Marshall, Morrison, & Chiat, 1998). Therefore, these researchers added a "message therapy" to their writing treatment protocol that included (a) tasks to show explicitly how patients could use their "new" words to represent more complex messages (e.g., "shoe" might be used not only to label the object but also to ask for help finding one's shoes, to indicate that one wants to go for a walk, to indicate that one's feet are cold, etc.) and (b) tasks to practice communicating these more complex messages to their daily communicative partners. Following the inclusion of these tasks that directly targeted the communicative uses (or alternative meanings) of trained written vocabulary, Robson et al. found remarkable improvements in the functional communication abilities of their patients with severe aphasia.

Topic Coherence and Cohesion

Topic coherence and cohesion skills are vital to effective discourse production. Because these skills rely on lexical–semantic and grammatical markers, it may be helpful to target deficits in lexical–semantics, morphosyntax, or both prior to or concurrently with discourse targets. Many patients with discourse deficits will benefit from treatment activities that facilitate awareness of their coherence and cohesion errors (e.g., abrupt topic shift, inappropriate use of ellipsis or vague reference), as well as their understanding of strategies to enhance their coherence (e.g., use of disjunctive markers), cohesion (e.g., use of synonyms instead of exact repetition), or both. Barrier games and practice with discourse genres such as storytelling and conversation (see also Chapter 12) may provide a context for not only error detection, but also discourse production practice and self-monitoring (C. Busch, Brookshire, & Nicholas, 1988; Tompkins, 1995; R. Wilkinson, 2010).

Because **barrier games** are particularly helpful for addressing a variety of pragmatic and discourse goals (Ferre et al., 2011), it is appropriate to provide a more detailed description of how to set up this type of activity. The basic premise of a barrier activity is to place a solid barrier (e.g., a game board or a large book standing on its side) between the patient and the clinician or other communication partner so as to create a more "natural" communication context. For example, the barrier can create the communicative need for communication partners to establish a conversational topic, provide accurate and specific referents, and so forth. Typically, similar sets of treatment stimuli or materials are placed on the patient's and the clinician's sides of the barrier, and activities such as describing a specific stimulus (e.g., a specific person in a group photograph), giving instructions (e.g., "First, put the family reunion photo above the summer vacation photo. Second, put the graduation photo below the summer vacation photo"), or asking questions about the materials (e.g., "Do you have a picture of a short woman wearing a black hat?") are completed. Because each communication partner cannot see, or, more ideally, does not know, what materials the other communication partner has access to, successful communicative exchanges during barrier activities will require each partner not only to utilize specific and efficient language output, but also to pay close attention to the other partner's verbal output, as many nonverbal cues have been eliminated. Examples of the numerous discourse and pragmatic behaviors that can be practiced via barrier games include production and/or comprehension of indirect requests, reduction of tangential comments, and use of specific vocabulary or referents (vs. nonspecific pronouns or content words).

Two aspects of topic coherence that are easily targeted in barrier games or other discourse activities are topic management skills such as topic initiation and maintenance. Early treatment activities may be relatively didactic, with the clinician asking patients to simply identify the topic and/or main idea of a spoken or written discourse sample such as a brief story or narrative. Initially, the clinician may also choose to alert the patient to coherence breakdowns in an online manner. As the discourse sequences become longer or as the patient gains skill in aspects of topic management, however, video and other recordings, including dictation or written discourse, may facilitate development of online self-evaluation skills (Ferre et al., 2011). Subsequent treatment activities may be elaborated to include sequential or concurrent stimuli for which patients must identify when new information is available, as well as when content is repeated (Tompkins, 1995). Finally, patients can practice identifying or utilizing discourse markers that indicate when new information is consistent with (e.g., "In addition..."), related to (e.g., "Similarly..."), or inconsistent with/unrelated to (e.g., "In contrast...") the previous or current content or topic (Wiseman-Hakes et al., 1998).

To address reading comprehension deficits at the discourse level, clinicians might utilize or adapt one of the techniques used in the education literature (e.g., Penn et al., 1997; Winograd & Hare, 1988). For example, patients who have difficulty identifying relevant information or integrating information across a text could be taught to complete the following steps when reading: (a) preview headings and subheadings to identify the main ideas, (b) write down questions about those main ideas, (c) read the text so that those questions can be answered, (d) paraphrase or summarize what has been read, and (e) review the text again to ensure understanding of the text and that questions were answered correctly.

Treatment of topic cohesion entails more sophisticated metalinguistics than are necessary for activities targeting topic maintenance or coherence. Effective topic cohesion requires speakers to be aware of not only the information that has been communicated, but also the specific lexical and morphosyntactic structures used to communicate the information. For example, effective use of pronouns (e.g., *it, those, his*) requires that the appropriate referents have been specified earlier in the discourse (e.g., referent and pronoun agree in number and gender). Likewise, an elliptical statement such as "They did." is appropriate only following a syntactically elaborated preface such as "I thought Sarah and Lucy said they'd meet us here." Although topic cohesion may be a more subtle skill than topic coherence, many of the treatment strategies discussed with respect to coherence also are appropriate for cohesion. For example, given a context-rich stimulus, the clinician can prompt the patient first to identify the topic and then to formulate one or two sentences summarizing the main ideas. As the patient elaborates the discourse sequence, specific cohesion strategies (e.g., pronouns, synonymy, ellipsis) can be targeted.

As will be elaborated on in Chapter 12, involving patients' daily communication partners in coherence and cohesion treatment activities may be a particularly efficient approach to discourse intervention. That is, the discourse skills of just one or both members of the patient–partner communication dyad can be targeted (Simmons-Mackie, Kearns, & Potechin, 2005; R. Wilkinson, Bryan, Lock, & Sage, 2010; R. Wilkinson, Lock, Bryan, & Sage, 2011). For example, R. Wilkinson and colleagues (2011) trained both a wife with aphasia and her husband, with the goal of improving the topic initiation skills of the wife. Prior to training, the wife with aphasia often abruptly changed topics, resulting in her husband not understanding the new topic and in turn leading to a conversational breakdown. Training first involved general education regarding topic initiation and its role in conversation, followed by discussion of the pattern of topic initiations observed when the couple conversed. Next, strategies were reviewed and practiced that would result in more collaborative and gradual topic initiations or shifts in the couple's conversations (e.g., the wife using a phrase like "by the way" to indicate a new topic; the husband providing more time if he noted that his wife was attempting to initiate a new topic). Following treatment, successful topic initiations were observed with a concomitant decrease in conversational breakdowns. The researchers also observed the wife with aphasia successfully shifting topics when conversing with a close friend in a sample collected close to two years following her training.

Inferencing

"Inferencing," or "gleaning information that is not specifically provided" (Tompkins, 1995, p. 254), is a communicative skill frequently enlisted in discourse. Treating inferencing involves first helping the patient become aware of implied meanings. This process is very similar to what was described in earlier sections addressing awareness of ambiguity. Specifically, using picture description or story retelling, the patient, with or without assistance from the clinician, can identify stated or explicit information. The clinician can then propose additional implied meanings or information, discussing the cues that led to each inference (Ferre et al., 2011; Penn et al., 1997). A number of activities can provide patients with practice identifying cues leading to inference, including describing relationships among stimuli (e.g., categorizing), speculating about characters' motives, and identifying incongruities and absurdities. Ultimately, patients can be asked to draw inferences from larger discourse texts and to develop text from which listeners or readers must draw inferences.

Conversational Skills

Effective conversations not only are characterized by coherence and cohesion, and may include the use of implied meanings, but also depend on appropriate use and comprehension of prosodic and nonverbal cues and figurative language, as well as adherence to social convention. Thus, treatment targeting conversational skills may incorporate the activities addressing these related abilities that are discussed in other sections of this chapter. In addition to these skills, turn taking is a key conversational skill.

To increase patients' awareness of turn-taking behaviors, the clinician may first describe verbal and nonverbal behaviors that signal the beginning or end of a conversational turn (e.g., significant pause, direct questions, eye contact) (Tompkins, 1995; Wiseman-Hakes et al., 1998). The clinician and patient can then review audio or video recordings of conversations, identifying where specific turn-taking cues were used and whether or not the cues were effective. Similar activities can be used to address other aspects of turn taking, such as length of turn, signaling the desire to have a turn, and inappropriate interrupting (Snow & Douglas, 2000). As suggested previously for treating pragmatic targets, conversational skills may be effectively addressed during group treatment, affording patients an opportunity to evaluate and provide feedback about other participants' conversational skills, while at the same time practicing their own. Reviewing videotapes or transcripts of the patient's conversations, including those occurring during group treatment, may also be helpful.

It also is important to keep in mind that as patients progress in the treatments previously described to target specific phonological, lexical–semantic, or morphosyntactic deficits, practice of trained behaviors at a conversational level should also be included. That is, many previously reviewed treatments primarily focus on training production or comprehension of language targets at the word or sentence level, with the assumption that if patients become competent at word or sentence levels, their ability to apply trained behaviors to discourse and conversation should also improve. Research, however, indicates that meaningful improvements at the discourse and conversational levels are more likely when treatment specifically includes activities at these language levels (M. Brady et al., 2012; L. Murray et al., 2007; Peach & Wong, 2004).

Social Conventions Treatments

Patients with TBI and certain forms of dementia (e.g., behavioral variant of frontotemporal lobar degeneration) are particularly prone to deficits in the social aspects of communication (see Chapter 2), although these deficits may also be observed in patients with RHD or other types of dementia (e.g., Alzheimer's disease), and less frequently in those with aphasia. Social communication incorporates behaviors related to prosody, nonverbal communication, as well as discourse and many cognitive (e.g., inhibition) skills. Thus, in addition to the techniques described below, strategies already described in this chapter, as well as some of those reviewed in Chapters 10 and 12, may be suitable for addressing social skills.

A key social skill influencing the effectiveness of communication is sensitivity to the listener and to the environment (Tompkins, 1995). Typical communication exchanges, including what information is exchanged, in what detail, and with which words and grammatical structures, are strongly influenced by what each participant presupposes about the listeners, as well as by the communication context. As is true for many pragmatic behaviors, sensitivity to listener needs and contextual influences occurs relatively automatically. Patients with neurogenic language or cognitive disorders, however, may need to develop greater conscious awareness of these issues, as well as explicit knowledge of how communication behaviors must be modified once listener or environmental cues are identified (Ferre et al., 2011). The clinician may devise scenarios in which the patient must anticipate a listener's prior knowledge about a potential conversation topic (e.g., talking to a spouse about work, talking to a vocational rehabilitation agent regarding accommodation needs). The clinician and patient may then discuss or role-play communication interactions related to the different scenarios. Video recordings or transcripts of simulated or real interactions, as well as participation in group treatment sessions, may assist the patient in identifying mismatches in communication style and listener needs/environmental context.

For some patients, emotion perception deficits may negatively affect their sensitivity to their communication partners (McDonald, 2012; McDonald & Flanagan, 2004). Accordingly, for these patients, intervention might focus on one or several skills related to emotion perception, such as discriminating and then interpreting changes in facial features and expressions, body posture and gestures, and prosody associated with nonverbal emotion expression (McDonald et al., 2009; Radice-Neumann, Zupan, Tomita, & Willer, 2009). Other activities might involve identifying emotional states related to scenarios that frequently occur in patients' everyday activities (e.g., a patient who was a car salesman being able to list emotions and identify verbal and nonverbal behaviors indicative of those emotions that potential car buyers might display when at his dealership), or comparing and contrasting similar emotions (e.g., relief and happiness) or dissimilar emotions (e.g., excitement vs. boredom). Hierarchies of stimulus and task difficulty can be developed for each patient. For example, easier target emotions might be those that occur frequently or have obvious nonverbal correlates, whereas easier tasks might involve providing response choices for patients or having target emotions depicted in a static state (e.g., line drawing, photograph). Although emotion perception treatment studies are lacking, the initial findings of Radice-Neumann and colleagues (2009) indicate that activities similar to those described above may evoke improvements in emotion processing in individuals with TBI.

Communication: A Focus of Study and Service in Disciplines Other Than Speech-Language Pathology

The nature of communication exchanges among normal adults is in itself an entire field of study. University communication departments typically offer courses in topics such as organizational communication, small-group communication, interpersonal communication, and nonverbal communication, recognizing that each of these communication contexts has unique characteristics and influences. Clinicians are encouraged to explore the wealth of information available regarding normal adult communication to assist in both assessment and remediation of higher-level communication deficits.

Another aspect of social communication that may be targeted for intervention is humor (Parenté & Herrmann, 2010). "Sense of humor" is a highly personal characteristic and varies considerably, even among individuals without neurogenic language and cognitive disorders. Tompkins (1995) argued that distressing changes in sense of humor accompanying neurogenic language and cognitive disorders likely reflect difficulties in one or more of the following: interpreting nonverbal cues, making inferences, or comprehending intentional use of alternate meanings of words and phrases. The treatment activities for addressing each of these skills suggested earlier in this chapter can easily be modified to incorporate stimuli with humorous content, such as riddles that use plays on words, or comic strips depicting characters using facial expressions.

The social conventions of compliments, politeness, criticism, social confrontation, topic selection, and questions/answers are also appropriate targets for pragmatic treatment. In a study examining the benefit of group social skills treatment for patients with TBI, Braunling-McMorrow, Lloyd, and Fralish (1986) described a variation of the "Sorry" board game in which the standard game cards were replaced with cards describing social situations, along with a prompt to elicit appropriate communicative responses to the scenario. During the game, each patient developed a response to the prompt on the card drawn during his or her turn. If the response was judged by the clinician to be appropriate, the patient moved a game piece forward on the board. Feedback was provided following inappropriate responses. The authors reported that their patients with TBI demonstrated increased frequency of appropriate social responses both during the treatment activity and on generalization measures obtained outside of treatment. Although not specifically described in the study, this game could easily be modified so that group participants are responsible for judging the appropriateness of a response, providing feedback about how to improve the response, or both.

Social skills intervention groups, in which patients partake in discussions about appropriate and inappropriate social and conversational behaviors (e.g., how to start and keep conversations going, social boundaries, how to deal with disagreements), role-playing scenarios, and problem-solving activities (e.g., generating solutions and strategies for inappropriate behaviors), have also proven effective for addressing a variety of social convention and discourse-level deficits. For a detailed example of the curriculum often used in these intervention groups, see Hawley and Newman (2010), who reviewed the content, procedures, and theoretical rationale of their Group Interactive Structure Treatment (GIST) protocol. Importantly, a number of recent studies have examined the effects of social skills group training for patients with TBI who are in the chronic stages (Braden et al., 2010; Dahlberg et al., 2007; McDonald et al., 2008) or more acute stages (Appleton et al., 2011) of recovery. Across these studies, intervention lasted at least 12 weeks, with sessions ranging in length from 1.5 to 3 hours. In these studies, intervention resulted in improvements in specific social and discourse behaviors, although changes in self- and caregiver reports of daily social activities and participation were less substantial; furthermore, in several of these studies, gains were maintained three to six months post-treatment (Appleton et al., 2011; Braden et al., 2010; Dahlberg et al., 2007).

In summary, although a variety of treatment activity options are available, particularly to the creative clinician, to address the pragmatic and discourse-level impairments of patients with neurogenic language or cognitive disorders, empirical verification of the effectiveness of many of these activities is still lacking (Ferre et al., 2011; Koul & Van Sickle, 2010; Lehman Blake, 2007; Sohlberg & Turkstra, 2011). A few areas in need of further research include determining which patient populations respond best to which treatment approach (e.g., TBI vs. RHD, patients with poor vs. good awareness of deficits, mild vs. severe linguistic and/or cognitive impairments); examining whether treatment effects are maintained following treatment termination; documenting which treatment protocols result in generalization to untrained stimuli, tasks, and contexts; and utilizing more rigorous study designs when examining novel, as well as existing, interventions.

Use of Commercially Available Workbooks and Computer Software and Applications

To allow quick identification of treatment stimuli and activities, numerous commercially available workbooks and computer software programs and applications have been developed. As shown in Table 9-8, some workbooks and software programs provide activities for a broad range of both linguistic and cognitive deficits (e.g., *Workbook of Activities for Language and Cognition–5: Neurological Rehab;* Arnold, 2003), whereas others focus on a narrower range of language impairments (e.g., *Idioms Workbook–Second Edition*; Auslin, 2003) or neurogenic patient populations (e.g., *Workbook of Activities for Language and Cognition: Aphasia Rehab (Spanish)*; Tomlin, 2007). The functionality of these workbook and software program tasks also varies, from contrived (e.g., making a list of words that start with a given letter to target written word retrieval) to more applied and realistic activities (e.g., identifying important information on medicine prescriptions to target reading comprehension). Given the abundance of material choices and the range in quality of these materials, clinicians should carefully consider the following advantages and disadvantages associated with workbook or computerized activities. Such advantages and disadvantages should also be considered when selecting applications for smartphones or computer tablets (as discussed in Chapter 12).

There are a number of possible incentives to using commercially available workbooks, computer software programs, or both in linguistic treatments. For example, these published products may improve the cost effectiveness of treatment by increasing the amount of time patients are involved in treatment tasks, without increasing the amount of direct clinician contact time necessary (Katz & Wertz, 1997; van de Sandt-

TABLE 9-8
Examples of Workbooks and Software Programs for Treating Linguistic Disorders

	PRIMARY TARGET AREA(S)	AUTHOR(S)
Workbooks		
Behavior: Functional Rehabilitation Activity Manual	Pragmatics	Messenger & Ziarnek (2004)
Focus on Function–Second Edition	Various linguistic abilities	E. Klein & Hahn (2007)
Functional Vocabulary for Adolescents and Adults	Lexical-semantic production and comprehension	Plass (2005)
Improving First Impressions: A Step-by-Step Social Skills Program	Pragmatics and discourse-level skills	McDonald et al. (2009)
Narrative Story Cards	Narrative discourse skills	Helm-Estabrooks & Nicholas (2003)
The Idioms Workbook–Second Edition	Idiom comprehension	Auslin (2003)
Workbook of Activities for Language and Cognition–5: Neuro Rehab	Various cognitive and linguistic skills	Arnold (2003)
Workbook of Activities for Language and Cognition–1: Aphasia Rehab (Spanish)	Reading and writing (single-word through paragraph/page level)	Tomlin (2007)
Software		
Aphasia Tutor	Various linguistic skills	Bungalow Software (2004)
Language Activity Resource Kit–Second Edition (CD-ROM)	Various linguistic skills	Matesich & Dressler (2006)
MossTalk Words	Lexical-semantic retrieval	Fink et al. (2002)
No-Glamour Sentence Structure Interactive Software	Syntax production and comprehension	Gustafson (2006)
Parrot Software	Various cognitive and linguistic skills	Parrot Software (1982–2003)
Rosetta Stone Language Learning Programs	Various linguistic skills	Fairfield Language Technologies (2001)
SentenceShaper 2	Syntax and connected speech production	Psycholinguistic Technologies (2012)
Spotlight on Social Skills Adolescent Interactive Software	Pragmatic and discourse skills	P. Johnson & LoGiudice (2011)

Koenderman, 2011; Varley, 2011; Wertz & Katz, 2004). Relatedly, they serve to provide additional at-home practice opportunities, and in some cases, such at-home practice may also serve as some respite for caregivers if patients can independently utilize the workbook or software activities. For software programs, computer use is now pervasive across all age groups, and thus the vast majority of patients will have computer access and may even prefer home computer practice versus paper-and-pencil tasks. Finally, and most importantly, a growing number of studies have reported positive and enduring improvements in a number of linguistic abilities, such as written and spoken lexical retrieval, syntax production and comprehension, and reading, when computer-assisted therapy programs have been utilized, particularly when close supervision of a clinician was available (Aftonomos, Appelbaum, & Steele, 1999; Cherney, 2010a, 2010b; Cherney, Halper, et al., 2008; Crerar, Ellis, & Dean, 1996; Fink, Brecher, Schwartz, & Robey, 2002; Katz & Wertz, 1997; McCall et al., 2009; Thompson et al., 2010). However, it is important to keep in mind that the software used in these studies (e.g., AphasiaScripts, ORLA, Sentactics) is not always widely available to clinicians (i.e., not distributed by the larger publishers of rehabilitation tests or materials).

Unfortunately, several problems also have emerged as clinicians have begun to exploit these treatment materials (Katz, 2000; van de Sandt-Koenderman, 2011; Wertz & Katz, 2004). First, many workbooks—and, to a lesser extent, software programs—consist of repetitive drills that lack the flexibility to adjust the stimuli, task procedures, or both to meet the needs of individual patients. For example, the target words in the word retrieval activities of workbooks or software programs may lack personal relevance to the patient; in turn, the patient may be less motivated to practice such words, have few opportunities to use such words in his daily communicative interactions, or both. Second, obtaining financial support to purchase computers or software is difficult. Nonetheless, many companies (e.g., Parrot Software) offer monthly subscriptions to software programs or packages, which may be more affordable to patients if they must pay out-of-pocket. Third, many workbooks and software programs lack construct validity in that there is no research to support that the linguistic processes they purport to address are actually being addressed. Fourth, these types of published materials are limited in terms of what areas of language can be targeted. For example, because most of these materials focus on basic language abilities and have limited application to nonverbal communication (e.g., facial expressions, gestures, contextual cues) or spoken language skills (beyond naming or isolated sentences), they are often inadequate for addressing the social communication or high-level language difficulties that are common among patients with neurogenic language and cognitive disorders; they are also often not challenging enough for patients with mildly impaired language abilities. Fifth, extensive time practicing workbook or software activities may lead to social isolation, which is already problematic in many patients with neurogenic language and cognitive disorders. Finally, within the research literature examining the effectiveness of computerized programs, not all patients respond positively, and/or often there is minimal generalization to untrained stimuli or tasks, including daily activities (e.g., Albright & Purves, 2008; Cherney, 2010a; Fink et al., 2002; Katz & Wertz, 1997; Nobis-Bosch et al., 2011). There is also a deficiency of formal, well-designed studies evaluating the use of workbook activities in treatment.

The above review indicates that workbooks and computer software can foster improvements in the linguistic abilities of at least some patients with neurogenic language and cognitive disorders if clinicians take an active role in evaluating the appropriateness of the workbook or software activities for each individual patient and regularly monitor patients' progress with these activities. Because of limitations such as suspect validity and restricted usefulness for targeting certain linguistic abilities (e.g., prosody production), most researchers concur that currently, the use of workbooks, computer software, or both should, at most, be considered "a component in an organized treatment program versus being improperly viewed as treatment itself" (Matthews, Harley, & Malec, 1992, p. 122) and recommend further research to determine which patients are most likely to benefit from these treatment activities.

Maintenance, Generalization, and Transfer of Learning

Regardless of which linguistic ability is being targeted, or which treatment approach is being used, clinicians must incorporate treatment procedures to ensure that patients will carry over and transfer trained behaviors and strategies to daily activities and environments. Without conscious efforts to target maintenance and generalization, patients might display unstable, task-specific improvements: Although task-specific improvements may still be a positive outcome if they are maintained, they are not as positive an outcome as those that transfer to untrained contexts. Research indicates that considering the following factors when selecting treatment stimuli, activities, and approaches will help ensure maximal maintenance and generalization of treatment effects (Basso et al., 2011; Golisz, 1998; Lloyd & Cuvo, 1994; S. Small, 2009; Wressle et al., 2002).

First, treatments that incorporate a variety of tasks, contexts, and stimuli produce greater success and generalization. For example, several pictures (e.g., photograph, line drawing, cartoon) of a word being trained as part of a word retrieval treatment should be used; likewise, text written in different font styles, colors, and sizes might be used during a reading treatment program. Training sessions might alternate between the therapy room, the patient's hospital room, and the clinic waiting room to vary the environmental context. These types of manipulations overtly teach the patient that the strategy or behavior being taught applies for general use and multiple contexts. Clinicians should keep in mind that this variability tends to reduce the rate of knowledge or skill acquisition, and thus should counsel patients and caregivers accordingly, emphasizing the long-term benefits (i.e., increased generalization) of such a treatment approach.

Second, training should include functional and personally relevant stimuli and strategies or, relatedly, should target linguistic or cognitive goals and functions that correspond to patients' daily needs and activities (see included DVD: Patient 8m). Patients will find it easier to relate these types of stimuli and behaviors to their existing knowledge and experience base, be motivated to practice and utilize the skills being trained, and consequently be more likely to apply trained skills within their daily environments. Caregivers also will be more likely to reinforce patients' use of trained skills if they too can see the functional benefits of such skills.

A final factor to consider when planning treatments that will ensure or maximize the probability of maintenance and generalization is the amount of practice or training provided (E. Baker, 2012; Cherney, Patterson, et al., 2008; S. Small, 2009; Varley,

2011). With few exceptions, those treatment approaches previously described in this chapter that facilitated improvement to untrained stimuli, skills, or contexts and produced enduring positive outcomes provided patients with intensive and/or extensive practice. For example, treatment intensity is a fundamental principle of **constraint-induced aphasia therapy (CIAT)**, a protocol that incorporates several stimulation-based procedures (e.g., cueing hierarchies) described earlier in this chapter to foster recovery of spoken language production abilities (e.g., Kurland, Baldwin, & Tauer, 2010; Kurland, Pulvermuller, Silva, Burke, & Andrianopoulos, 2012; Maher et al., 2006; Meinzer, Streiftau, & Rockstroh, 2007). That is, in CIAT, patients minimally partake in three-hour therapy sessions for at least five days a week for two weeks. Although another principle of CIAT is the constraint of modalities other than spoken language, the intensive therapy schedule appears to be a particularly influential component of this treatment (Barthel, Meinzer, Djundja, & Rockstroh, 2008; Cherney, Patterson, et al., 2008; Szaflarski et al., 2008). Likewise, Bhogal, Teasell, and Speechley (2003) examined the aphasia treatment literature and observed that study participants who received approximately nine hours of treatment per week for at least 11 weeks were most likely to demonstrate significant treatment effects; in contrast, study participants who received two hours or less of treatment per week were unlikely to achieve significant treatment effects, even when treatment was offered over a longer span of weeks (i.e., more than 20 weeks). This finding has been recently confirmed by M. Brady et al. (2012), who completed a systematic review of aphasia intervention studies, and Basso and colleagues (2011), who examined treatments for language and related disorders due to vascular disorders: Studies with positive treatment effects included more treatment time than those reporting no positive effect. Researchers have noted, however, that there remains a need to identify optimal intensity recommendations for specific interventions, including how intervention intensity might need to be modified based on consideration of patient-, clinician-, disorder- and service-related variables (E. Baker, 2012; Cherney, 2012).

Currently, in most health-care settings, funding or approval of direct treatment is typically restricted (for further discussion of funding issues, see Chapter 13). Clinicians can still ensure sufficient opportunities for practice by developing detailed homework programs, training families or other caregivers to administer the treatment protocol, or both (e.g., Nobis-Bosch et al., 2011). Furthermore, given the importance of evidence-based practice in today's health-care system, clinicians should draw the attention of funding agencies to the growing empirical literature documenting the need for intensive and extensive treatment and thus advocate for patients with neurogenic language and cognitive disorders at risk of receiving inadequate access to language intervention (Code, 2012; Code & Petheram, 2011).

Summary

Numerous treatment approaches and procedures have been developed to facilitate the linguistic recovery of patients with neurogenic language and cognitive disorders, or in the case of progressive disorders, slow the rate of deterioration in linguistic abilities. As reviewed in this chapter, however, few treatments have been sufficiently investigated with respect to which patient populations might benefit from the approach (e.g., those with aphasia vs. TBI, those with acute vs. chronic deficits), how well treatment effects are maintained over time, and whether treatment effects generalize to real-world contexts and thus are truly compatible with patients' activity and participation needs. Furthermore, despite the number of therapy options currently available, there remains a desperate need to develop and critically examine treatments for certain symptoms (e.g., severe auditory comprehension deficits, impaired inferencing) and, relatedly, certain patient populations (e.g., patients with RHD, patients with Wernicke's aphasia). Finally, the benefits of combining two or more of the linguistic treatments described in this chapter or of coalescing therapy procedures mentioned in this chapter with those described in Chapters 10, 11, or 12 have yet to be systematically explored. Despite these research needs, clinicians should be assured that sufficient empirical support has accumulated to justify providing language treatment services to patients with neurogenic language and cognitive disorders (Basso et al., 2011; Berthier, 2005; M. Brady et al., 2012; Cicerone et al., 2011). By keeping abreast of research developments, clinicians will be able to not only advocate effectively for treatment services for their patients, but also select and provide treatment procedures that are most suitable for each individual patient.

Discussion Questions

1. Compare and contrast a stimulation treatment with a cognitive neuropsychological treatment for addressing syntactic comprehension problems.
2. What types of patients are most likely to need and/or benefit from treatments to enhance prosody production? Develop a treatment protocol for one of these patients.
3. Which treatment for morphosyntactic production problems might be most appropriate for a patient with severe Wernicke's aphasia? A patient with mild Broca's aphasia?
4. Identify a computer software program that might be appropriate for training written word retrieval at the sentence and discourse levels. Evaluate the program in terms of the following:
   (a) Which patients would most likely benefit from its use (e.g., aphasia type or severity, presence of hemiparesis, static vs. progressive disorder)
   (b) Its construct validity
   (c) Its ecological validity and, relatedly, whether generalization to untrained daily writing activities would be expected
   (d) Cost
5. Develop a treatment activity that would be appropriate for addressing the inferencing problems that a patient with right hemisphere brain damage encounters when reading.

Remediation of Body Structure and Function: Behavioral Approaches for Cognitive Disorders

chapter 10

Learning Objectives

After reading this chapter, you should be able to:

- Describe specific behavioral treatment procedures for addressing attention, memory, or executive function impairments
- Describe cognitive approaches for addressing neurogenic language disorders
- Discuss the strengths and weaknesses of utilizing commercially available workbooks and computer software programs when treating cognitive disorders in patients with neurogenic language and cognitive disorders
- Discuss cognitive treatment planning issues pertaining to the generalization and transfer of treatment effects

Key Terms

- backward chaining
- effortful or errorful learning
- errorless learning
- Goal Management Training
- limb activation
- metacognitive training
- mnemonic strategies
- prism lenses
- spaced retrieval
- strategic learning techniques
- verbal mediation

Introduction

The previous chapter reviewed numerous approaches that have been developed to address *linguistic problems* in patients with neurogenic language and cognitive disorders. This chapter will review a variety of treatment procedures that have been developed to remediate these patients' *impairments of cognition* at the ICF (International Classification of Functioning, Disability, and Health; WHO, 2001) level of body structure and function. Although so far most cognitive treatment research has involved patients with right hemisphere brain damage (RHD), traumatic brain injury (TBI), or dementia, some initial investigations have also focused on developing cognitive interventions for patients with aphasia. This chapter summarizes behavioral therapies aimed at facilitating recovery of cognitive impairments in a variety of patient populations.

Generally, two treatment approaches have been exploited to remediate cognitive impairments associated with neurogenic language and cognitive disorders: behavioral or cognitive rehabilitation and pharmacotherapy (see Chapter 11). In terms of cognitive rehabilitation, most programs, particularly those that were first developed, are similar to stimulation language therapies. For example, these programs provide extensive practice at responding to stimuli and activities that gradually increase in complexity in order to facilitate functioning or restoration of the impaired cognitive process or processes. Unfortunately, few of these traditional therapies have produced remarkable generalization to untrained stimuli and daily activities. More recently developed programs, however, extend beyond stimulating the impaired cognitive function and additionally incorporate training compensatory strategies (sometimes referred to as **metacognitive training**), practicing with stimuli and tasks that are encountered in the patients' daily routines, or both. This chapter provides examples of these varied forms of cognitive rehabilitation that have been used to address the concomitant attention, memory, and executive function impairments of patients representing a variety of neurogenic language and cognitive disorders.

Attention Treatments

Given that attention impairments are perhaps the most frequently occurring symptom following the onset of brain damage or disease, regardless of severity, and that they can have dire consequences on rehabilitation and functional outcomes, it is not surprising that numerous treatment protocols have been developed to address this pervasive cognitive problem. Whereas one group of attention interventions aims to remediate neglect, other interventions were designed to address deficits in other aspects of attention (e.g., sustained attention, divided attention). Each of these types of attention intervention is described below.

Treatment of Neglect

Currently, several therapy approaches have been developed to address the attentional problem of neglect. These interventions vary from environmental modifications to attempting to remediate cognitive deficits contributing to neglect. Whereas there is some evidence to indicate that provision of one or several of these neglect treatments may result in greater neglect recovery than when a general cognitive retraining program is used (Kortte & Hillis, 2009, 2011; Paolucci et al., 1996), only a few neglect treatments have yet proven effective in producing gains that persist beyond treatment termination or that generalize to daily living activities (Proto, Pella, Hill, & Gouvier, 2009; Zoccolotti et al., 2011). Accordingly, unless otherwise stated, clinicians should primarily expect task-specific gains when applying one or more of the neglect treatments described in this chapter.

Environmental and Task Modifications

Environmental and task modifications such as drawing a red line down the neglected side of a page to assist reading, placing a brightly colored bracelet or sweatband on the patient's neglected wrist to encourage visual attention to that side of the body, or putting brightly colored clothes or a flashing light on the neglected side of a clothes closet can help reduce the negative consequences of neglect, particularly in patients who have little awareness of their neglect (see Chapter 12 for further examples of environmental modifications). Additionally, the following are examples of devices and procedures that provide patients with the impression that their environment has been shifted toward their neglected side. These devices and procedures thus can reduce the effects of neglect, at least in some patients, while (or immediately after) they utilize the device or receive the stimulation:

- *Monocular eye patching:* The lens of the non-neglected side is blocked or shaded on a pair of glasses (Walker, Young, & Lincoln, 1996). This technique is not recommended, given that in some patients eye patching has been shown to aggravate rather than alleviate neglect, and there is no evidence for whether the effects on neglect are stable or transfer to daily functioning (Barrett, Crucian, Beversdorf, & Heilman, 2001; Zoccolotti et al., 2011).
- *Hemispatial patching or sunglasses:* The non-neglected hemifield of each lens is shaded or completely occluded to force the patient to attend to the neglected visual field (Beis, Andre, Baumgarten, & Challier, 1999; Tsang, Sze, & Fong, 2009). With extensive exposure to this device, improvements in neglect have been reported, even when the patient is not wearing the sunglasses (Beis et al., 1999).
- **Prism lenses:** The patient wears specially designed glasses that optically displace visual targets rightward (e.g., 15 degrees), and that after wearing cause a natural adjustment of the eyes to shift visual focus toward the neglected side (Frassinetti, Angeli, Menghello, Avanzi, & Ladavas, 2002; Shiraishi et al., 2008; Watanabe & Arnimoto, 2010). Enduring improvements to untrained and functional tasks (e.g., wheelchair navigation, posture stability) are most likely if patients practice tasks such as pointing, searching, playing darts, and scanning while wearing the glasses, and receive such training over a long period of time (e.g., 5–6 weeks).
- *Other stimulation techniques:* Other forms of stimulation involve excitment of vestibular organs on the neglected side via ear irrigation (Adair, Adair, Na, Schwartz, & Heilman, 2003; Rode et al., 2002), optokinetic or visual motion stimulation (e.g., stimuli are shown on a computer or video monitor moving from the neglected to the non-neglected side; Kerkhoff et al., 2012; Schroder, Wist, & Homberg, 2008; Thimm et al., 2009), or vibrotactile or electrical somatosensory stimulation of the neck or hand (Karnath, 1994; Polanowska, Seniów, Paprot, Le niak, & Członkowska, 2009; Schroder et al., 2008). Again, maintenance of treatment effects and generalization to untrained and more functional daily tasks is most likely when patients receive extended exposure to the stimulation (e.g., Schroder et al., 2008).

To reiterate, neglect improvement dissipates after these devices or forms of stimulation are removed, unless the patients have had intensive and prolonged exposure to the device or stimulation and practice tasks that involve scanning and attending to the full visual field while wearing the device or receiving the stimulation (e.g., Kerkhoff et al., 2012; Watanabe & Arnimoto, 2010). Generalization should not necessarily be expected, given that the above devices or stimulation, by themselves, do not necessarily attempt to reduce the underlying impairment contributing to the patient's neglect, but rather focus on changing variables in the environment, modifying task demands, or altering visual or vestibular input. Furthermore, not all patients experience neglect dissipation when exposed to these adaptations (e.g., Shiraishi et al., 2008). Accordingly, environmental modifications will likely be most appropriate when (a) the patient is willing to wear the device or receive the stimulation over extended periods and shows some immediate effects, and/or (b) other cognitive or linguistic impairments are being treated and such devices/stimulation reduce the probability that neglect will interfere with the patient's performance of therapy activities.

Attention Training or Retraining Treatments

Another approach to treating neglect focuses on remediating cognitive problems that contribute to neglect. For instance, because patients with neglect inadequately move their eyes, head, or body to attend to stimuli or activities on their neglected side, treatment aims to increase their active attention to the neglected side. In therapy, patients practice activities in which they demonstrate neglect, and during the practice clinicians provide one or several cues to encourage patients to attend to their neglected side. These cues might be verbal, such as "Don't forget to look all the way to left side of the page"; visual, such as flashing a light on the neglected side or placing a visual "anchor" such as a red line on the neglected side; auditory, such as presenting a tone burst on the neglected side; or tactile, such as tapping the neglected hand. Over time, clinician cueing should be faded as patients' performances improve. Most frequently, clinicians require patients to practice repetitively visual scanning, figure copying, and cancellation tasks similar to those used to diagnose neglect (see Chapter 7). These might be completed with real objects or paper and pencil, or as computerized activities.

Even though these tasks are popular and, with practice, patients can indeed improve their performance on them (or tasks that are similar to the practiced tasks), there is little empirical support for their use given that they fail to evoke generalization to more functional, real-world activities, particularly if patients have more severe cognitive deficits and/or have awareness issues (Kerkhoff et al., 2012; Kortte & Hillis, 2009, 2011; Manly, 2002; Proto et al., 2009; Zoccolotti et al., 2011). Accordingly, if this approach to neglect treatment is adopted, clinicians *must* incorporate functional activities such as dressing, writing emails, texting, or cooking, rather than contrived tasks such as line bisection or canceling out target letters or symbols.

Cueing Approaches

A related approach is to teach patients to cue themselves. This approach may result in generalization as long as patients are sufficiently aware of their neglect and the possible consequences of that neglect (Golisz, 1998; Kortte & Hillis, 2011; Manly, 2002;

Proto et al., 2009). For instance, Niemeier (1998; Niemeier, Cifu, & Kishore, 2001) has taught, in both inpatient and outpatient settings, a "lighthouse" imagery strategy to patients with neglect due to stroke or other forms of acquired brain damage (e.g., TBI, brain tumor). Patients were asked to imagine that their eyes were like the light in a lighthouse sweeping all the way from the left to the right. While completing a variety of tasks (e.g., computer activities, locating items in the room), patients were initially cued by their clinicians to use the strategy; family and other health-care team members also were educated about the strategy and encouraged to remind patients about its use. Over time, cues were faded as patients' performances improved and they began to apply the strategy independently. Following treatment, patients in Niemeier's 1998 study not only demonstrated significant improvements on tests of neglect and attention, but also performed these tests better than a group of patients who did not receive the imagery training. Additionally, the subjective reports of the family and caregivers suggested reductions in neglect when patients completed activities in settings outside of the rehabilitation facility. In the 2001 study, treated patients additionally achieved significant gains on functional tasks such as route finding, wheelchair negotiation, and problem-solving tasks.

Limb activation represents another effective technique that patients can learn as a self-cue or strategy to help alleviate neglect symptoms. This technique involves training patients to move some part of the neglected side of their body in the neglected hemispace while they complete daily activities that might be negatively affected by their neglect (Kortte & Hillis, 2011; Robertson, Hogg, & McMillan, 1998; Robertson, North, & Geggie, 1992). For example, a patient with left neglect might be trained to tap the fingers of his left hand on his left knee during reading tasks. This limb movement is proposed to decrease neglect symptoms by increasing activation within the neural areas of the damaged hemisphere, which contribute to attention. As in other cueing approaches, training proceeds with the clinician initially reminding patients to use limb activation while they complete therapy activities; as the patients' performances improve, clinician cueing is faded so that patients become responsible for remembering to utilize the strategy. For patients who have difficulty remembering to use the strategy, Robertson and colleagues (1992) created a small "neglect-alert device." The device has a handheld button that has to be pressed on a regular basis (e.g., once every five seconds) to avoid setting off a buzzer.

Several studies have shown that limb activation training with or without the use of this device can alleviate neglect symptoms, regardless of whether the movement of the neglected limb is part of the target activity (Luukkainen-Markkula, Tarkka, Pitkanen, Sivenius, & Hamalainen, 2009; Robertson et al., 1992; Samuel et al., 2000; B. Wilson, Watson, Baddeley, Emslie, & Evans, 2000). Not all patients, however, benefit from this technique, and obviously it is inappropriate for patients with dense hemiplegia (Kortte & Hillis, 2011; Manly, 2002). Furthermore, variable degrees of generalization and maintenance of treatment effects have been reported (e.g., Maddicks, Marzillier, & Parker, 2003, vs. Samuel et al., 2000), which may be, at least in part, related to procedural differences among previous investigations. For example, some studies examined upper limb activation, whereas others examined lower limb activation. Some studies included patients who were in the acute stages of recovery, whereas more chronic patients participated in other studies. Finally, some studies evaluated limb activation by itself, whereas others evaluated limb activation in combination with other neglect treatment procedures. Accordingly, further research is needed to help delineate when and to whom this treatment should be taught.

Interestingly, George, Mercer, Walker, and Manly (2008) examined whether giving instructions indicating a time limit versus giving instructions with no indication of a time limit would influence the cancellation task performances of patients with neglect. The premise for this task instruction manipulation was that neglect symptoms can be reduced by increasing overall alertness levels (akin to the "neglect-alert device" described above), and that, relatedly, time pressure is associated with higher subjective levels of arousal. The researchers found that patients' performances were more accurate and faster when they were told versus not told there was a time limit (even though there wasn't one). Therefore, giving oneself a time limit might serve as another cueing technique for neglect, although the intervention application of this approach has not yet been investigated.

A Little Zap Will Do Ya

Initial research is now under way to explore whether repetitive transcranial magnetic stimulation (rTMS) or transcranial direct current stimulation (tDCS) can reduce neglect (see Chapter 9 for a description of these procedures). Preliminary findings indicate that rTMS to the left parietal cortex (Song et al., 2009) or tDCS to the right posterior parietal cortex (Ko, Han, Park, Seo, & Kim, 2008) can improve scores on standard neglect tests. Investigators have also begun to explore whether these and other noninvasive stimulation approaches might remediate other cognitive deficits (e.g., episodic memory, working memory, sustained attention) (Cotelli, Manenti, Zanetti, & Miniussi, 2012; L. Murray, 2012c; Nitsche & Paulus, 2011; Utz, Dimova, Oppelander, & Kerkhoff, 2010). Additional research is necessary, however, before recommending that patients look into getting "zapped," as these studies typically involve small samples, have not examined maintenance or generalization of treatment effects, and have yet to evaluate the possibility of long-term exposure risks.

Review of the neglect treatment literature indicates that only a few treatments evoke remarkable maintenance of treatment effects, generalization to untrained everyday tasks, or both. More positive findings, however, are beginning to accrue when two or more of these treatments are used in concert (Kortte & Hillis, 2011; Polanowska, Seniów, Paprot, Leśniak, & Członkowska, 2009). For example, Schindler, Kerkhoff, Karnath, Keller, and Goldenberg (2002) found that compared to visual exploration/scanning activities by themselves, providing neck stimulation along with visual exploration/ scanning activities resulted in greater improvements in activities of daily living and untrained visual and tactile search tasks. Therefore, researchers should focus future efforts on evaluating the effects of other neglect treatment combinations, particularly in terms of carryover to untrained functional tasks. Finally, given that the above research has almost exclusively focused on visual neglect (although for an example of a protocol for auditory neglect, see Kerkhoff et al., 2012), there is an immediate need to determine if these treatments are effective at remediating neglect symptoms in other modalities.

Treatments for Other Attention Deficits

Like neglect, several treatment approaches have been developed to address attention deficits related to acquired brain damage and disease. Generally, these treatments focus either on stimulating impaired attention functions or on training strategies to help patients accommodate for their attention limitations. Each of these attention treatment approaches is briefly reviewed.

Attention Training or Retraining

Several protocols attempt to retrain directly one or more attention functions through a structured hierarchy of paper-and-pencil or computerized attention tasks (e.g., Galbiati et al., 2009; Sturm et al., 2004; Sturm, Willmes, Orgass, & Hartje, 1997). That is, patients are given intensive and repetitive practice at completing sets of tasks, which are organized not only in terms of general difficulty or complexity but also in terms of what specific attention function they target (e.g., sustained attention, attention switching, divided attention). As the patients progress on the simpler tasks that target less complex attention functions (e.g., sustained attention), new tasks that are more difficult and target the same attention function or a more complex attention function (e.g., selective attention) are introduced.

Sohlberg, Mateer, and colleagues have developed three structured programs, *Attention Process Training* (APT; Sohlberg & Mateer, 1986), *Attention Process Training–II* (APT-II; Sohlberg, Johnson, Paul, Raskin, & Mateer, 2001), and *Attention Process Training–III* (APT-III; Sohlberg & Mateer, 2010), that are good examples of attention retraining protocols. All programs consist of tasks that are graded in difficulty and target a number of attention functions in auditory and/or visual modalities (for examples, see Table 10-1). APT was designed for patients with TBI who have moderate to severe attention problems, and because APT-II contains more complex and demanding attention tasks, it is recommended for patients with mild attention problems. The newest APT-III comes on a USB drive (i.e., no software is installed onto the user's computer), which allows presenting the tasks on either a PC or Mac computer. Compared to APT and APT-II, APT-III offers more flexibility in terms of manipulating task parameters and thus is suitable for patients representing severe through quite mild attention symptoms.

Researchers have found that patients with TBI (Palmese & Raskin, 2000; N. Park, Proulx, & Towers, 1999; Pero, Incoccia, Caracciolo, Zoccolotti, & Formisano, 2006;

TABLE 10-1
Examples of Activities From the *Attention Process Training-III* (APT-III) Program (Sohlberg & Mateer, 2010)

ATTENTION DOMAIN	EXAMPLE ACTIVITY	PERFORMANCE MEASURES
Basic sustained attention	Respond to a target sound embedded in series of sounds (e.g., tone, car honking).	Accuracy, omissions, false positives, patient rating of task difficulty and his or her motivation
Executive control: Working memory	Listen to a number sequence and then respond with that sequence in the reverse order	Accuracy, order errors, patient rating of task difficulty and his or her motivation
Executive control: Selective attention	Respond when two consecutive numbers in a series of numbers are presented in descending order in the presence of background noise	Accuracy, omissions, false positives, patient rating of task difficulty and his or her motivation
Executive control: Suppression	Respond to the words "happy" and "sad" only when these words are spoken with the correct emotional prosody	Accuracy, omissions, false positives, patient rating of task difficulty and his or her motivation
Executive control: Alternating attention	Respond to a word (i.e., "adult" or "child") when the word matches the speaker's voice (i.e., adult vs. child voice), and then switching when prompted to respond if a word does not match the speaker's voice	Accuracy, switching errors, patient rating of task difficulty and his or her motivation

Sohlberg, McLaughlin, Pavese, Heidrick, & Posner, 2000), aphasia (Coelho, 2005; L. Murray, Keeton, & Karcher, 2006; Sinotte & Coelho, 2007), RHD (Barker-Collo et al., 2009; Boman, Lindstedt, Hemmingsson, & Bartfai, 2004), or mild cognitive impairment (Mayer, Murray, & Bishop, 2012) show improved performance of trained tasks after receiving APT or APT-II. Conflicting results, however, have emerged with respect to generalization to untrained attention tasks, measures of other cognitive abilities, or functional outcomes. For example, whereas Sohlberg, McLaughlin, Pavese, Heidrich, and Posner (2000) reported improvements in memory, learning, executive functioning, and functional independence following APT, N. Park and colleagues (1999) found minimal change in their patients' performance of a memory test after receiving APT. As APT-III is relatively new, no studies have yet been published documenting its effectiveness.

In an attempt to resolve these and other discrepancies in the attention retraining literature, particularly with respect to maintenance and generalization effects, several comprehensive review papers have been written (Cicerone et al., 2011; N. Park & Ingles, 2001; Sohlberg et al., 2003; Zoccolotti et al., 2011). Collectively, the authors of these reviews have concluded that optimal improvements are more likely if (a) the structured, attention retraining tasks are *combined* with strategy training (see below for a description of strategy training treatments), (b) intensive training is provided with an optimal session length of 60 minutes, (c) complex (e.g., divided attention) rather than simple attention functions (e.g., sustained attention) are trained, and (d) only tasks that target the specific needs and deficits of a given patient are utilized, rather than progressing through standard programs in their entirety.

Strategy Training

Researchers have also explored the utility of treatments in which patients are taught strategies to help manage or monitor their attention (Butler & Copeland, 2002; Catroppa & Anderson, 2006; Cicerone, 2002; Fasotti, Kovacs, Eling, & Brouwer, 2000; Winkens, Van Heugten, et al., 2009). Typically in these treatments, patients are trained to use their strategies (e.g., completing tasks or task steps in a serial manner vs. concurrently) while completing tasks like those found in the previously described attention retraining programs. In fact, in several of the studies cited in the above section on attention retraining, strategy training was incorporated into the intervention program (e.g., Boman et al., 2004; Galbiati et al., 2009; Mayer et al., 2012).

As an example of a strategy-training protocol, Cicerone (2002) gave four patients with TBI his "working attention" treatment, and compared their pre- and post-treatment test performances to those of four patients with TBI who had been referred for treatment but could not attend. Cicerone's treatment consisted of two components. For the first half of each therapy session, patients completed a working memory task under different attention conditions. For the working memory task, patients worked through a stack of playing cards by recalling the number on the card that was one, two, or three back from the card currently being viewed. In more complex divided attention conditions, patients completed this task while (a) sorting the cards according to suit, (b) completing a verbal fluency task, or (c) completing a secondary task similar to one of their daily activities (e.g., a patient who previously made a lot of conference calls shadowed audiotaped lectures while completing the working memory task). During the latter half of each session, patients were (a) counseled regarding their performance of treatment tasks; (b) assisted with identifying task and emotional variables that influenced their performance; and (c) taught strategies to aid their performance, including use of verbal mediation, rehearsal, self-pacing, task demands estimation, and positive self-statements. Patients also completed emphasis-change training, which involved practicing to shift attentional priority during the divided attention activities.

Cicerone (2002) reported that patients receiving his working attention treatment achieved better attention test scores and reported fewer attentional difficulties during daily tasks than those patients who could not attend treatment. Additionally, whereas all treated patients returned to work, none of the control group did so. Cicerone's findings, as well as those from other strategy-training treatment studies (e.g., Butler & Copeland, 2002; Galbiati et al., 2009), are encouraging and indicate a need to further explore strategy training to delineate which patients and what type of attention problems might be best served by this form of attention treatment.

Who Wants to Treat Attention Disorders—Anyone or Everyone?

As discussed in Chapters 4 and 7, disciplines other than speech-language pathology often address the attention impairments that may accompany neurogenic language and cognitive disorders. In particular, rehabilitative neuropsychologists may target various aspects of attention in their treatment. Occupational therapists often target neglect as a component of a treatment plan addressing bathing, grooming, feeding, and other activities of daily living. More recently, physical therapy has also begun to incorporate dual-task or divided attention methods into mobility interventions (for an example, see Evans, Greenfield, & Wilson, 2009). Accordingly, clinicians may find it helpful to collaborate with these other rehabilitation disciplines when developing attention treatment goals, designing specific intervention activities, or both to ensure that services aren't being duplicated across disciplines or, alternatively, that services are not overlooked because each therapist incorrectly assumed that another discipline would take responsibility.

Combined Approaches

Another approach to remediating attention that has produced positive outcomes involves incorporating aspects of attention retraining, strategy training, and functional attention tasks that resemble patients' everyday communicative and cognitive activities into treatment. For example, the attention treatment program developed by C. Wilson and Robertson (1992) evolved from the complaint of their patient with TBI of frequent attention slips while reading. Each day, the patient completed short homework sessions during which he read a novel and kept track of how long he read before experiencing an attention slip. Additionally, prior to reading, the patient completed relaxation exercises such as controlled breathing to help alleviate negative thoughts or emotions that might interrupt his concentration and reading. By the end of treatment, the patient had progressed from one and one-half minutes of reading without an attention slip in a quiet environment to five minutes of reading without an attention slip in the presence of distraction (i.e., talk radio programs). The patient also showed improvements in reading untrained text and reported that following treatment, he had resumed reading for pleasure.

Importantly, attention retraining programs have begun to acknowledge the importance of integrating into therapy more functional versus contrived tasks (e.g., scanning the financial section of a newspaper for a certain stock vs. scanning a worksheet to circle a certain abstract design). For example, in their APT-II and APT-III programs, Sohlberg and colleagues (Sohlberg et al., 2001; Sohlberg & Mateer, 2010) recommended identifying and utilizing daily activities that involve the same attention functions being targeted by APT-II or APT-III tasks in order to maximize generalization of retrained attention skills to patients' everyday functioning.

In summary, a growing literature indicates that cognitive rehabilitation can positively affect the attention abilities of patients with TBI (Cicerone et al., 2011; Zoccolotti et al., 2011). Those programs that incorporate strategy training and functional daily activities are more likely to encourage generalization to untrained, real-world stimuli, tasks, and environments than protocols that rely solely on retraining attention via structured and controlled, but artificial, exercises. To further our understanding of how best to remediate attention disorders, future studies should explore the effects of existing treatment protocols on a broader range of patient populations (e.g., RHD, dementia, aphasia), as only a limited set of studies has thus far examined application of the above treatment protocols with these patient populations. Additionally, research is needed to specify when we should be treating which attention functions (e.g., acute vs. chronic stages of recovery), whether certain attention functions or modalities or patient profiles respond better to certain therapy approaches, and how much training is necessary to optimize maintenance and generalization of treatment effects.

Memory Treatments

The types of treatment approaches developed to address memory impairments in patients with neurogenic language and cognitive disorders are very similar to those just reviewed for attention intervention. That is, some memory therapy approaches have been designed to train or stimulate overall memory functioning, whereas others focus on strategy training. Additionally, another approach to addressing memory problems incorporates procedures for training the recall of specific information or procedures (e.g., spaced retrieval).

General Memory Stimulation Approaches

Those programs that attempt to restore general memory abilities typically involve structured and repetitive drills such as digit or word span tasks or list-learning activities (Piras, Borella, Incoccia, & Carlesimo, 2011; Sohlberg & Mateer, 2001). During these activities, patients are presented with novel information and then asked to recall that information at a later time, following a filled or unfilled delay. By manipulating one or more of the variables listed in Table 10-2, clinicians can make memory activities more difficult or easier (Bayles & Kim, 2003). Given the abundance of workbooks and computer software programs that contain these types of tasks, this approach to treating memory continues to appear quite popular.

Numerous studies and evidence-based reviews, however, have indicated that even though these treatments may result in improved recall of trained stimuli, generalization to untrained stimuli and novel everyday contexts is unlikely unless such activities are paired with strategy training (Cornis-Pop et al., 2012; das Nair & Lincoln, 2008; Ehlardt

TABLE 10-2
Variables for Manipulating the Difficulty of Memory Activities

VARIABLE	POORER RECALL IF...
Amount of to-be-remembered information	More information
Type of to-be-remembered information:	
• Syntactic complexity	More complex syntax
• Emotional valence	Lower emotional content
• Self- vs. clinician-generated	Clinician-generated material or cues
• Modality	Dependent on other concomitant deficits (e.g., for certain aphasia and dementia patient populations, spoken language may be more difficult to remember than written language) and premorbid learning preferences (e.g., prior to his stroke, the patient was better at learning and recalling material presented visually vs. an auditory format)
• Similarity of encoding and retrieval conditions	Dissimilar encoding and retrieval conditions
• Encoding strategy	Shallow strategy (e.g., rote rehearsal vs. semantic elaboration)
• Type of recall task	Free recall (vs. recognition or cued recall)
• Time demands	Increased time pressure (vs. less time pressure or no time constraint)

et al., 2008; Fraas, 2006; L. Murray, 2012c; Piras et al., 2011). Nevertheless, in certain cases, retention of only trained material may still represent clinical success and have positive effects on patients' everyday functioning, particularly when the trained material is functional. For example, Arkin (1991, 1998) provided patients in the early and middle stages of Alzheimer's disease with audio- or videotaped narratives about their own autobiographical or factual information. After the narrative was presented, the patients completed a quiz about facts within the narrative (with the correct answers provided on the tape). Arkin found that these patients could learn and retain the material for periods as long as one month following their last supervised practice session. These improvements in recalling the trained information also resulted in more positive views of the patients' abilities, not only by the caregivers, but also by the patients themselves.

Strategy Training

Patients also might be trained to use internal **mnemonic strategies** to enhance memory encoding (temporary maintenance, as well as long-term storing) and retrieval. Examples of internal mnemonic strategies include the following: (a) *visual imagery*, which includes techniques such as self-imaging (i.e., patients imagine themselves interacting with or completing the to-be-remembered information or task, respectively) and the method of loci (i.e., patients imagine keywords in the to-be-recalled information linked to specific locations, such as along a familiar route or on their body); (b) *semantic elaboration*, in which, when presented with a to-be-recalled object, patients think about a number of the object's semantic features, such as its use, location, or composition; (c) *verbal organization*, in which patients create acronyms or paired associations to encode and recall information (d) *dual coding*, which involves verbalizing and visualizing to-be-recalled information; (e) *rote rehearsal* or repetition; and (f) *alphabet search*, in which patients go through the alphabet to see whether each letter might cue their recall of the target information. Relatedly, **strategic learning techniques** (e.g., the PQRST technique) might be taught that focus on identifying relevant versus irrelevant information, as well as the synthesis of information to determine the overall meaning or gist of the to-be-remembered information.

Within sessions, patients are first provided with a description and examples of the target mnemonic strategy or strategic learning technique. Next, they are instructed to utilize one or more of these strategies when presented with to-be-recalled information, and may also be cued to apply these strategies when attempting to recall the information. Extensive practice with applying these strategies in a variety of everyday contexts and with a variety of to-be-remembered information is required so that strategy use becomes independent (i.e., clinician cueing is faded over time) and relatively automatic. Training of these memory strategies has been conducted successfully in both individual and group settings (Radford, Lah, Thayer, Say, & Miller, 2012). For further description of the treatment steps involved in strategy training, see Chapter 12, as well as Sohlberg and Turkstra (2011).

Research indicates that although patients with a variety of forms of brain damage (e.g., stroke, TBI, infection, epilepsy) may improve their recall of trained material or tasks using internal strategies or strategic learning techniques, only those with relatively mild and stable (i.e., not progressive) impairments who are motivated to use such strategies or techniques demonstrate spontaneous, independent use of these strategies with untrained material or outside of therapy (Cicerone et al., 2011; Cook et al., 2011; Cotelli et al., 2012; Duval, Coyette, & Seron, 2008; Grilli & McFarland, 2011; O'Neil-Pirozzi et al., 2010; Piras et al., 2011; Radford et al., 2012; Thickpenny-Davis & Barker-Collo, 2007). Additionally, it is likely that strategies with language demands (e.g., rehearsal, semantic elaboration) will be inappropriate for patients with aphasia, and indeed these patients are often excluded from studies examining mnemonic techniques (e.g., Fraas, 2006; Thickpenny-Davis & Barker-Collo, 2007). Given that executive functions such as initiation, self-regulation, and problem solving help support autonomous use of internal mnemonic strategies and strategic learning techniques, and that many patients with memory disorders have concomitant executive functioning deficits, it is not surprising that only patients with mild and relatively isolated memory impairments are able to apply these strategies independently in real-life contexts (Cicerone et al., 2011; Kaschel et al., 2002; Radford et al., 2012).

Again, however, if only treatment-specific gains are wanted, training use of one or more of these strategies may be appropriate. For example, Oberg and Turkstra (1998) taught two adolescent patients with TBI an elaboration strategy that resulted in their acquisition of vocabulary needed for school. Although these patients continued to require clinician assistance to apply the strategy, they were able to learn and retain the trained material that they needed for their current school activities. In this case, even though generalization was not achieved, the domain-specific effects still resulted in functional gains for the patients.

Training or Instructional Approaches

Several training protocols have been developed to help patients with neurogenic language or cognitive disorders recall specific information, procedures, or both. The four training protocols reviewed in this section—PROMPT, spaced retrieval, chaining, and errorless learning—may be used by themselves, in combination with each other, or in concert with other treatment approaches to address memory or other cognitive-linguistic problems in a variety of patient populations.

PROMPT

Sohlberg, White, Evans, and Mateer (1992) developed PROMPT (Prospective Memory Process Training) to address problems with prospective memory, or the ability to recall and carry out future intentions (see Chapter 1 for a description of prospective memory). The goal of this program is to extend the amount of time a patient is able to remember to carry out specified tasks at specified times. Thus, PROMPT's focus is on the more complex, time-based prospective memory skills. In its most basic form, patients are instructed to complete a task after a set time interval. If patients complete the task at the correct time, the time interval is increased; if they are unable to complete the task without cueing, the time interval is decreased. In addition to varying the length of the time delay, the following variables can be manipulated to make PROMPT easier or more difficult: (a) difficulty of the prospective task (e.g., simple motor task vs. complex multimodality task), (b) presence or absence of a distracter during the time delay (e.g., sitting with no distraction vs. completing another task during the delay), and (c) presence or absence of prompts (e.g., allow the use of a watch alarm vs. independent recall of when to complete the task). Only one variable at a time should be manipulated so that the effects of that variable on the patient's performance can be examined.

Data from a limited number of studies conducted by the authors of PROMPT and their colleagues (Raskin & Buckheit, as cited in D. Raskin & Sohlberg, 2009; S. Raskin & Sohlberg, 1996; Sohlberg et al., 1992) indicated that patients with prospective memory problems subsequent to TBI or stroke improve on trained tasks and may, at least in some cases, display improved recall and completion of untrained real-world tasks, such as completing routine chores at home. Further research is necessary, however, given the weak design of the existing studies (e.g., lack of control groups, inclusion of subjective measures or measures with poor test–retest reliability) (Fish, Wilson, & Manly, 2010). Furthermore, Shum, Fleming, Gill, Gullo, and Strong (2011) recently reported that strategy training had more positive effects on the prospective memory deficits of participants with TBI than a training protocol similar to that described by Raskin and Sohlberg (2009).

Spaced Retrieval

Spaced retrieval is a memory treatment closely related to PROMPT. This technique, like PROMPT, involves patients practicing to recall information or to use a strategy over progressively longer time intervals (Hopper, Drefs, Bayles, Tomoeda, & Dinu, 2010; Mahendra et al., 2011; Piras et al., 2011). Unlike PROMPT, however, in spaced retrieval, cues are provided to the patient (see Table 10-3). For instance, during a session, the patient is asked to recall a piece of information, such as the clinician's name, after a set amount of time (e.g., 30 seconds). If the patient recalls accurately, the time interval is doubled (e.g., 60 seconds); if the patient errs, the clinician provides the correct answer, asks the patient to repeat it, and then reduces the time interval (e.g., 15 seconds). The period during the time delay may remain free from distraction or be filled with related or unrelated activities (e.g., games, conversation). If the patient makes a lot of errors, time intervals may be increased more gradually (vs. doubling the time interval), as ideally the patient should be error-free during training sessions (further information about errorless learning is provided later in this chapter). Spaced retrieval is proposed to facilitate learning and recall by exploiting automatic, implicit memory functions; that is, through this technique's shaping procedures, patients can acquire and subsequently recall trained material or tasks with little effort and, in some cases, little awareness. No generalization to untrained material or tasks is expected.

Numerous studies have found that spaced retrieval is an effective means by which to teach recall of a variety of new or previously known materials (e.g., caregivers' names, the patient's room number and location, stories, songs, recent events) and activities (e.g., compensatory swallowing techniques, use of external memory aids, email, use of a digital camera, paying of bills, taking of medications) to patients with various degrees of memory impairment related to TBI, infection, stroke, or dementia (Bourgeois & Melton, 2004; Haslam, Hodder, & Yates, 2011; Hopper et al., 2010; Mahendra & Arkin, 2003; Mahendra et al., 2011; Malone, Skrajner, Camp, Neundorfer, & Gorzelle, 2007; J. Small, 2012; Turkstra & Bourgeois, 2005). Notably, even patients with progressive forms of dementia, including those with more advanced cognitive deterioration, are able to maintain their recall of trained materials or tasks for extended periods (e.g., several months) following treatment termination. Furthermore, research indicates that paid and unpaid caregivers can easily be trained to implement spaced retrieval to help address memory and behavioral issues encountered in the patients' daily environment (Arkin, 1991; Hunter, Ward, & Camp, 2012; McKitrick & Camp, 1993). The technique may even be used over the phone (Melton & Bourgeois, 2005; Turkstra & Bourgeois, 2005). However, Piras and colleagues (2011) noted in their evidence-based review of the spaced retrieval empirical literature that few studies have examined long-term maintenance of spaced retrieval effects and that there has been limited investigation of functional outcomes (e.g., improved independence in daily activities). Therefore, further evaluation of this instructional technique is warranted.

TABLE 10-3
Steps for Administering Spaced Retrieval Treatment

STEP	EXAMPLE
1. Inform patient that treatment will focus on practicing to remember information/activity. Provide the to-be-remembered information or demonstrate the to-be-remembered activity.	"We're going to work on helping you to remember your room number. Your room number is 183. What is your room number? Good, you remembered it."
2. Pause and take a brief break, and then ask the patient to recall the information/activity.	After five seconds, "Let's try that again. What is your room number?"
3. If the patient correctly recalls the information/activity, move to Step 4. If the patient is unable to recall the information/activity correctly, provide the correct response and have the patient repeat the correct response. Then repeat Step 2. If after three tries the patient cannot complete Step 2 accurately, stop the spaced retrieval session and try at a later date.	
4. Increase the time interval, and fill the pause time with conversation that is or is not related to the therapy activity.	During the 10-second break, say, "That's right. Now we're going to practice remembering your room number several more times so that it will be easy for you to remember where you live in this building. Let's try it again. What is your room number?"
5. If the patient correctly recalls the information/activity, move to Step 6. If the patient is unable to recall the information/activity correctly, provide the correct response and have the patient repeat the correct response. Then return to Step 2.	
6. Increase the time interval again, and fill the pause time with conversation that is or is not related to the therapy activity.	During the 20-second break, say, "You are doing an excellent job of remembering your room number. You are getting it correct and you are remembering it for a longer time. The goal of this practice is to help you remember information for longer and longer periods of time so that, hopefully, you will always remember it. To make sure you remember your room number, we're going to keep on practicing for a while longer today. So, can you tell me what your room number is?"
7. If the patient correctly recalls the information/activity, move to Step 8. If the patient is unable to recall the information/activity correctly, provide the correct response and have the patient repeat the correct response. Then return to the last time interval at which the patient successfully recalled the information/activity.	
8. Continue to ask the patient to recall the information/activity after increasingly longer breaks.	

Chaining Techniques

Like spaced retrieval, several additional memory treatment approaches exploit implicit or procedural memory skills to facilitate learning and recall of new or previously known information and skills. That is, in many neurogenic patient populations (e.g., TBI, certain dementing illnesses such as Alzheimer's disease), implicit or procedural memory appears relatively intact compared to other declarative memory functions and explicit or effortful learning and recall mechanisms (e.g., use of volitional rehearsal, chunking, or other encoding strategies) (Azouvi et al., 2009; Mateer, Kerns, & Eso, 1999). Accordingly, Glisky and colleagues (Glisky, 1992; Glisky & Schacter, 1989; Glisky et al., 1989) developed a "**vanishing cues**" training approach, sometimes referred to as "**backward chaining**," in which patients, particularly during initial sessions, are provided with a level of cueing that will ensure that they recall accurately. As patients progress, the extent of cueing is gradually faded until they can recall the information or task without any cueing.

Glisky (Glisky, 1992; Glisky & Schacter, 1989) and other researchers (Bilda, 2011; Clare, Wilson, Carter, Hodges, & Adams, 2001; J. Dunn & Clare, 2007; Evans et al., 2000; Pitel et al., 2006) have shown that this technique is effective in teaching vocabulary (including people's names), conversational scripts, and a variety of skills, such as the use of a word-processing program or a handheld computer, to patients with memory disorders related to TBI or other acquired neurological disorders, including Alzheimer's disease, encephalitis, stroke, and Korsakoff's disease. Although vanishing cues has proven successful with some patients, even those who are unable to recall participating in therapy, clinicians must keep in mind that learning achieved via this method is typically slow and task or material specific (i.e., gains do not transfer to untrained stimuli or contexts). Research also suggests that the vanishing cues method may not be as effective as other instructional techniques for memory training (Clare et al., 2001; Kessels & de Haan, 2003; Piras et al., 2011). In particular, errorless learning (see next subsection of this chapter) has been found superior to vanishing cues in patients with either static or progressive memory disorders, although thus far, more investigators have utilized the former instructional technique.

Another form of the **chaining technique**, forward chaining, is typically used to train recall of procedures, but can be used for recall of information as well (J. Dunn & Clare, 2007). In forward chaining, the clinician does a detailed analysis of the target procedure to identify all of the steps involved in that procedure. Then, in terms of training, the clinician teaches the patient how to perform the first step in the procedure. Once the patient can perform that first step independently, the second step is introduced, and the patient then practices completing the first two steps. The process is repeated until the patient is completing all steps in the procedure independently. For example, if the target procedure is brewing coffee, the identified steps might be the following:

Step 1: Empty any coffee that might be left over in the coffee pot.
Step 2: Put water in the coffeemaker.
Step 3. Put a filter in the basket.
Step 4. Put coffee in the filter.
Step 5. Turn on the coffeemaker.

The forward chaining procedure would therefore begin by teaching the patient to check the coffee pot for leftover coffee; once that step has been achieved with no guidance from the clinician, the next step—putting water in the coffeemaker—is trained in concert with the first step. Training continues in this manner of adding together these discrete steps. Whereas forward chaining is most frequently used for teaching procedures such as instrumental activities of daily living, it could be used for learning verbal information. For example, it might prove beneficial in helping a patient with aphasia recall a script being trained via conversational coaching (see Chapter 9). In this case, the first step to be trained would be the first piece of information to be shared as part of the conversation script.

Errorless Learning

Another approach based on implicit learning mechanisms is "errorless learning." Advocates of this approach propose that patients who must depend on implicit learning will have difficulty dealing with error responses because if they make a lot of errors, incorrect as well as correct responses will be automatically reinforced over time (Ehlardt et al., 2008; Middleton & Schwartz, 2012; Piras et al., 2011; B. Wilson & Evans, 1996). Therefore, if patients are prevented from making errors during the initial stages of learning, they should acquire the new information or skill more quickly. Accordingly, as the name implies, in **errorless learning,** patients are not allowed to make errors. For example, if they have been asked to recall the name of a person, they will be instructed to give that name only if they are absolutely positive they are correct (i.e., guessing is discouraged). If they are not completely confident in their answer, they are given a letter cue, and again asked to respond only if they are positive they are correct. Cues are provided until patients are certain they can answer accurately (somewhat similar to the previously described backward chaining method). As therapy progresses, patients should require fewer cues and eventually no cues before they can confidently recall the correct information or carry out the action correctly. Note that this contrasts with more traditional training protocols in which patients are allowed to guess and make errors. This traditional approach is sometimes referred to as **effortful learning or errorful learning** because to progress, patients need to remember which was the correct versus incorrect response and thus actively search for a response.

Studies involving patients with TBI, stroke, brain tumor, mild cognitive impairment, and various types of dementia (e.g., semantic dementia, vascular dementia, Alzheimer's disease) indicate that errorless learning is an effective means by which to train learning and recall of specific vocabulary (e.g., names of people or objects), social communication behaviors (e.g., appropriate greetings), information (e.g., a route), or skills (e.g., compensatory strategy use, daily hygiene behaviors) (Cohen et al., 2010; Cotelli et al., 2012; Dechamps et al., 2011; J. Dunn & Clare, 2007; Haslam, Gilroy, Black, & Beesley, 2006; Jokel & Anderson, 2012; Jokel, Rochon, & Anderson, 2010; Lloyd et al., 2009; Mount et al., 2007; Raymer et al., 2012). Whether errorless is superior to effortful learning as a memory training procedure, however, has yet to be resolved (for reviews, see Middleton & Schwartz, 2012; Sohlberg & Turkstra, 2011). Some findings indicate that only when training recall of certain types of information is errorless learning more effectual than errorful learning. For example, Evans et al. (2000) compared the effects of errorless and errorful learning approaches on the memory abilities of patients with neurogenic disorders and found that errorless learning was more effective for teaching face–name associations, but in more functional tasks such as programming a Palm Pilot, errorful learning appeared more useful. Kalla, Downes, and van den Broek (2001) also found a slight advantage for errorless over errorful learning in training face–name associations to memory-impaired patients. In contrast, several other research groups have reported either better outcomes following errorful versus errorless learning or no differential effect, even when training face–name associations (J. Dunn & Clare, 2007; Fillingham, Sage, & Lambon Ralph, 2006; Mount et al., 2007). Variability across individual patients has also been documented with only some patients appearing to learn better via errorless versus errorful learning (Gonzalez Rothi et al., 2009; Haslam et al., 2006; Lloyd et al., 2009). Because errorless learning investigations have varied in terms of the severity and etiology of memory impairment among study participants, the types and complexity of information and tasks trained, the intensity of training provided, and the duration of follow-up, further research is needed to delineate specific errorless learning treatment procedures for specific patient populations.

The above review of memory training approaches indicates that clinicians should expect primarily domain-specific treatment effects (i.e., minimal generalization to untrained stimuli or tasks) unless strategy training is included in the treatment protocol (Cicerone et al., 2011; Ehlardt et al., 2008; Piras et al., 2011). Even in patients with severe or progressive memory deficits, however, maintained recall of trained information or procedures can be achieved with protocols such as spaced retrieval and vanishing cues, which capitalize on implicit memory functioning, There also remains a need to conduct memory training research with stroke populations, as most of the above protocols were developed for TBI and dementia (das Nair & Lincoln, 2008). Additionally, although these various approaches to treating memory were described separately, this does not mean that they cannot be combined in daily clinical practice. On the contrary, findings from several studies support integrating procedures (Clare et al., 2001; Fraas, 2006; Mahendra & Arkin, 2003; C. Wilson & Manly, 2003). For example, Hunkin, Squires, Aldrich, and Parkin (1998) demonstrated that combining aspects of spaced retrieval, errorless learning, and vanishing cues treatments resulted in the successful acquisition of a set of computer skills in their patient with severe memory impairment. Likewise, the memory treatment protocol devised by Thickpenny-Davis and Barker-Collo (2007) involved strategy training, errorless learning, and external devices (i.e., diaries), all provided in a group format.

Finally, it should be noted that in addition to the memory treatments reviewed above, training the use of external supports (e.g., memory books, paging systems, planners, etc.) has proven effective for addressing memory impairments (particularly prospective memory problems) associated with neurogenic language and cognitive disorders (Cicerone et al., 2011; LoPresti, Simpson, Kirsch, Schreckenghost, & Hayashi, 2008; Piras et al., 2011; Radford et al., 2012; S. Raskin & Sohlberg, 2009). These approaches, however, are described elsewhere because they focus on either teaching the use of external aids (see Chapter 12) or addressing executive function deficits such as poor deficit awareness or impaired self-monitoring, which can compromise memory functioning (see the following section of this chapter).

Executive Function Treatments

Over the past decade, there has been a dramatic increase in research aimed at developing treatments for executive function deficits, no doubt a reflection of the ominous consequences such deficits can have on patients' ability to function independently (Poulin, Korner-Bitensky, Dawson, & Bherer, 2012). Effective executive function treatments are also needed, given that progress in other cognitive and linguistic domains will depend on recovery of executive abilities such as error monitoring (e.g., to determine if the correct word was retrieved and produced), inhibition (e.g., to avoid perseveration), and problem solving (e.g., to determine when a compensatory strategy will need to be utilized). The following section of this chapter describes two general approaches for addressing executive function impairments. First, we briefly review a number of environmental adaptations that can be introduced to help support patients' executive functioning (see also Chapter 12). Second, we describe in greater detail treatment techniques that have been developed for specific executive function abilities (e.g., awareness, problem solving).

Environmental Adaptation Approaches

Clinicians may opt to introduce environmental modifications when patients' cognitive impairments are so broad and severe that direct remediation approaches are unlikely to be successful, or when patients are in the earliest stages of recovery, such as the posttraumatic amnesia or confusion phase of TBI, when direct remediation is often inappropriate. Additionally, environmental adaptations can be used effectively to supplement direct remediation approaches.

One frequent environmental modification is to reduce task demands (Mateer, 1999; L. Murray, 2012c; Sohlberg & Turkstra, 2011). For example, to reduce the executive demands of therapy tasks or daily activities, clinicians might (a) simplify tasks by breaking them down into a series of steps, (b) give patients longer to complete tasks, (c) remove or minimize stimuli that elicit inappropriate behavior (e.g., avoid conversational topics that elicit disinhibited arguing and aggressive outbursts), (d) provide breaks to minimize frustration and fatigue, or (e) reduce or eliminate environmental distractions such as noise or visual clutter.

Another approach is to provide external support via cueing or prompting. For example, many patients demonstrate adequate knowledge of what steps or skills are needed to complete complex executive tasks but fail to apply this knowledge online.

When provided cues in the form of verbal reminders, alarm or paging systems, messages on cell phones, or even nonspecific, periodic tones, however, improvements in a variety of executive behaviors, including initiation, planning, and goal management, have been observed in a variety of neurogenic patient populations (Fish et al., 2009; Manly et al., 2004; Martin-Saez, Deakins, Winson, Watson, & Wilson, 2011; Metzler-Baddeley & Jones, 2010; Sohlberg, Sprunk, & Metzelaar, 1988). Further research is needed to evaluate if these types of external modifications can provide long-term support and to determine how environmental modifications might best be combined with direct, behavioral interventions such as those described below.

Treatments for Specific Executive Functions

In addition to or instead of altering the patients' environment, a number of treatments have been developed to address specific executive function impairments by teaching strategies or practicing tasks designed to restore underlying executive abilities. For the most part, these treatment protocols are in the preliminary stages of development, given that further research is still needed to document the reliability of treatment effects, to determine generalization and maintenance of treatment effects, and to delineate which patients are most likely to benefit from the treatment, as with few exceptions, studies have included predominantly participants with TBI (Cicerone et al., 2011; Poulin et al., 2012; Zoccolotti et al., 2011).

Awareness Training

Awareness training targets not only patients' understanding of their current strengths and weaknesses, but also their ability to monitor their performance online. If patients are unaware of certain linguistic or cognitive impairments, awareness training should be the first treatment priority, even before those linguistic or cognitive impairments are treated. Obviously, patients with poor deficit awareness will neither understand nor see the need for treatment, and consequently, even if they can be convinced to attend treatment sessions, they will certainly not be motivated to benefit from treatment. Unfortunately, although researchers and clinicians agree on the importance of addressing awareness deficits, few awareness treatments have been submitted to well-controlled empirical investigation (J. Schmidt et al., 2012). Therefore, without exception, the following approaches require further study to validate treatment effects and to delineate which techniques might produce the most significant and enduring improvements in awareness.

One approach to addressing poor deficit awareness is to educate patients about the nature and implications of their linguistic and/or cognitive impairments. One or more of the following treatment tasks might be used (Kortte & Hillis, 2011; Lundqvist, Linnros, Orlenius, & Samuelsson, 2010; Ownsworth, Turpin, Andrew, & Fleming, 2008; J. Schmidt et al., 2012; Ylvisaker, Szekeres, & Feeney, 1998): (a) Provide in spoken, written, or videotape form a description of their neurological disorder and resulting cognitive and/or linguistic symptoms (e.g., brochures, medical records) (for an example study utilizing this approach, see C. Roberts, Rafal, & Coetzer, 2006), being sure to accommodate for the patients' deficits (e.g., use simple and short sentences for patients with comprehension deficits); (b) have patients educate or describe to others (e.g., family, co-workers, health-care workers, other patients) their neurological disorders and cognitive and/or linguistic symptoms through activities such as giving a presentation, writing a narrative or educational brochure, peer teaching, or creating a self-advocacy videotape (see Table 10-4); (c) compare patients' ratings of their current abilities to those of their family, friends, and/or health-care team to identify and discuss areas of agreement and discrepancy; (d) have patients view, judge, describe, and discuss videotaped, written, or audiotaped samples of other patients who display similar cognitive and/or linguistic symptom profiles; and (e) utilize a game format such as the Road to Awareness board game of Chittum, Johnson, Chittum, Guercio, and McMorrow (1996) to have patients ask and answer questions about their neurological disorder and resulting symptoms.

Another option is to engage patients in activities that help them experience alterations in their abilities and behaviors that have occurred since the onset of their neurological disorder (Cicerone & Giacino, 1992; Kortte & Hillis, 2011; Schlund, 1999; Schmidt et al., 2012). For example, patients might be required to complete tasks that are likely to elicit negative and positive behaviors, but, prior to completing the tasks, also asked to predict their performance. Relatedly, patients might be asked to rate, tally, or track their performance while completing activities. Following task completion, patients compare their predictions or ratings with their actual performance to identify and discuss discrepancies and agreements. Another possible activity is role-playing, in which patients act out one or more of the following: (a) negative symptoms, (b) strategies to avoid or compensate for negative symptoms, or (c) consequences of negative symptoms (e.g., the social reaction of peers when inappropriate language is used).

When completing these and other educational tasks, clinicians must be cognizant to avoid excessive confrontation that might cause a defensive reaction or loss of self-worth in the patient. This can be avoided, at least in part, not only by assuring that awareness training activities focus on increasing awareness of deficits, but also by increasing awareness and appreciation of patients' areas of strength; for instance, clinicians should assure that in addition to being able to identify their errors, patients can accurately judge when they have correctly completed a task. It also is important to note that this educational approach is unlikely to be successful with patients who have profound global unawareness and severe concomitant cognitive deficits (Sohlberg & Mateer, 2001). In these cases, treatment efforts will be more productive if aimed at caregiver education and training (see Chapter 12).

Once patients have a better sense of the presence and nature of their deficits, treatment can focus on addressing difficulties with self-monitoring and, relatedly, strategy decision making (e.g., knowing when and how to implement trained linguistic or cognitive strategies). Generally, treatment involves teaching patients the following: (a) to review functional tasks prior to completing them so that, given their impairments, they can make a prediction regarding task difficulty and thus, their expected performance;

TABLE 10-4
Goals and Procedures for Making Transitional or Self-Advocacy Videotapes
(Adapted from Ylvisaker et al., 1998)

GOALS/PROCEDURES	STEPS
Goals	1. Enhance patients' self-esteem and sense of control. 2. Increase patients' awareness of their cognitive and/or linguistic strengths and weaknesses. 3. Encourage patients' active involvement in their rehabilitation program. 4. Educate family and caregivers about patients' cognitive and/or linguistic strengths and weaknesses. 5. Encourage interdisciplinary collaboration.

Procedures	1. Decide what content the videotape should contain. Regardless of which of the following content areas are included, clinicians must ensure that strengths as well as weaknesses are emphasized.
	  a. Motoric strengths, weaknesses, and rehabilitation issues (e.g., necessary prostheses, types and frequency of cues needed)
	  b. Cognitive strengths, weaknesses, and rehabilitation issues (e.g., types of compensatory behavioral strategies being used, types of external devices being used, helpful environmental modifications, types and frequency of cues needed)
	  c. Linguistic strengths, weaknesses, and rehabilitation issues (e.g., types of behavioral compensatory strategies being used, types of external devices being used, helpful environmental modifications, types and frequency of cues needed)
	  d. Other strengths, weaknesses, and rehabilitation issues (e.g., behavioral problems and modification procedures, emotional well-being, social issues)
	2. Determine how the content will be communicated or demonstrated on the videotape. Possible options include segments with:
	  a. Role-playing of strengths, weaknesses, and/or rehabilitation strategies or procedures
	  b. Samples of actual treatment sessions to demonstrate strengths, weaknesses, and/or rehabilitation strategies or procedures, or to document improvements over time
	  c. Samples of the patient in natural contexts to demonstrate strengths, weaknesses, and/or rehabilitation strategies or procedures, or to document improvements over time
	  d. Patient and clinician conversing about the patient's strengths, weaknesses, and/or rehabilitation strategies or procedures
	  e. Creating a written script or story that the patient will read to describe his or her strengths, weaknesses, and/or rehabilitation strategies or procedures
	  f. Family, caregivers, and/or other health-care team members giving their accounts of the patient's strengths, weaknesses, and/or rehabilitation strategies or procedures
	3. Decide who will do the videotaping and editing.
	4. Ensure that appropriate videotaping release forms have been signed.

(b) based on that review, to make decisions regarding which strategies if any are most appropriate; (c) to apply the strategies; and (d) to monitor the outcome of their strategy use. Throughout each of these steps, the clinician should provide immediate and respectful feedback regarding the patient's performance. Examples of specific procedures that have been used include the following (Golisz, 1998; Ownsworth, Fleming, Desbois, Strong, & Kuipers, 2006; Ownsworth et al., 2008; Schmidt et al., 2012):

- Requiring patients to predict their performance prior to completing treatment tasks (which may include an identification of factors that may or may not make the task difficult), and comparing this prediction to their actual performance
- Requiring patients to estimate or rate how well they did following completion of treatment tasks, particularly after a delay versus immediately after task completion, and comparing this estimation to their actual performance
- Encouraging patients to use verbal mediation or self-questions prior to or while completing treatment tasks (e.g., Will I need to take notes during this listening task to help my understanding? Did I check that the oven was turned off?)
- Using video- or audiotape feedback following completion of treatment tasks so that patients can make off-line judgments about task difficulty, their strategy use, and their task performance
- Identifying situations or materials for which trained strategies or behaviors will and will not be appropriate

These types of activities, particularly when used in combination with the previously described educational and experiential methods and within a group therapy context, have been found to help improve patients' understanding of and/or use of strategies for their motor, memory, attention, communication, and/or executive functioning abilities (Fasotti et al., 2000; Fotopoulou, Rudd, Holmes, & Kopelman, 2009; Lundqvist et al., 2010; Ownsworth et al., 2006, 2008; Schlund, 1999; Toglia, Johnston, Goverover, & Dain, 2010). Most previous research, however, has been conducted with patients whose cognitive problems are a product of TBI, and maintenance of effects has been infrequently examined (Zoccolotti et al., 2011). Consequently, further study is needed to determine the following: (a) how other patient populations respond to these treatment activities, (b) whether these activities are similarly effective for addressing impaired monitoring and application of strategies for the range of linguistic deficits possible in neurogenic language and cognitive disorders, and (c) whether awareness gains are stable over time. Additionally, clinicians must keep in mind that patients often have reduced awareness of a number of symptoms (see Chapter 2 for a description of anosognosia) and that awareness training may produce task- or symptom-specific effects; that is, patients may show improved awareness of the target symptom or improved self-monitoring during trained activities, but fail to generalize these improvements to other symptoms or during other activities (Ownsworth et al., 2006). Accordingly, the above procedures may need to be repeated when patients need to improve their awareness of a number of cognitive-linguistic problems.

Treatment of Perseveration

Although perseveration commonly accompanies a variety of neurogenic language and cognitive disorders, few formal treatments have been developed to ameliorate the linguistic and cognitive problems that may result from this executive function deficit. An exception is *Treatment for Aphasic Perseveration* (TAP; Helm-Estabrooks, Emery, & Albert, 1987; Helm-Estabrooks & Albert, 2004). As the name indicates, TAP aims to reduce verbal perseveration in patients with aphasia so as to increase their spoken lexical-retrieval accuracy and fluency. The first step to TAP is to determine if it is appropriate for a given patient by calculating that patient's perseveration severity rating. This rating is computed by having the patient complete the Confrontation Naming subtest of the *Boston Diagnostic Aphasia Examination* (BDAE), and then analyzing the percentage of items on which the patient perseverated: Patients who perseverate on 20% or more of the items are considered appropriate TAP candidates. Next, a stimulus hierarchy is developed so that easier semantic categories and stimuli are presented at the beginning of each therapy session, and more difficult ones are presented later. Categories and items are generated directly from the BDEA Confrontation Naming subtest. For example, if during testing the patient showed the least perseveration and best accuracy while naming body parts, body parts are targeted first within a TAP session; if most perseveration and least accurate naming occurred while the patient was naming letters, letter naming would not be trained until later in the TAP program.

The final steps of TAP involve carrying out the actual therapy sessions. First, patients are educated about perseveration and why TAP is being administered. Next, sessions focus on training confrontation naming by stimulating spoken lexical–semantic retrieval via semantic, phonological, orthographic, or other cues (for cue options, see Table 9-5), by increasing the patient's awareness of their perseveration, and by teaching strategies to minimize perseverations. That is, if the patient cannot name an item, up to three cues are provided to facilitate retrieval of the spoken label. If the patient perseverates while attempting to name the item, the clinician points out the perseverative response to the patient (e.g., writes the perseveration on a piece of paper and then rips up the paper and leaves the pieces as a reminder in case the patient makes the same perseverative error again), and then slows the stimulus presentation rate or provides an overt break before presenting the next stimulus (e.g., introduce that a new item is being given, have the patient complete a distracter task between items). Additionally, patients are taught to try to avoid perseveration by waiting before answering or, when they feel like they might perseverate, by not responding and instead asking for help.

Currently, only one empirical investigation of TAP has been completed (Helm-Estabrooks et al., 1987). In this study, the effects of TAP were compared to those of other traditional language treatments (e.g., auditory comprehension or stimulation therapy, Voluntary Control of Involuntary Utterances [VCIU]) in three patients with varying aphasia types. Whereas all patients showed greater decreases in perseveration following TAP versus the alternative treatment, generalization to untrained tasks, stimuli, or language modalities was not explored, leaving the need for additional examination of this treatment approach.

The only other option described in the research literature to address perseveration is to introduce stimulus or environmental manipulations that will decrease the likelihood of perseveration, keeping in mind that not all patients will necessarily respond to these manipulations (Corbett, Jefferies, & Lambon Ralph, 2008; Frankel & Penn, 2007; Gotts, Incisa della Rocchetta, & Cipolotti, 2002; Moses, Nickels, & Sheard, 2004). The types of variables that may be manipulated to help decrease perseverative responses include:

- Stimulus presentation rate, with a longer inter-stimulus interval less likely to evoke perseveration
- Word or target frequency, with high-frequency targets less likely to evoke perseveration
- Semantic relatedness among stimuli, with unrelated stimuli less likely to evoke perseveration
- Repetition of stimuli, with stimuli that are repeated throughout a task more likely to evoke perseveration
- Extrinsic cues such as phonemic, whole word, or sentence completion cues, with the provision of a cue less likely to evoke perseveration
- Interactional/conversational style of the communication partner (e.g., ignoring perseverations and then reorienting to the appropriate conversational topic is less likely to evoke further perseveration)

It should be noted that these potentially influential variables have been identified via experimental tasks. Therefore, research is needed to determine how to incorporate the manipulation of these variables into a treatment protocol and to identify which patients are responsive to these types of stimulus and task manipulations.

Treatment of Disinhibition

Difficulty inhibiting impulsive or inappropriate behavior can have calamitous consequences on social functioning and completion of daily activities. Only a limited number of treatment approaches, however, have been described to address this type of executive dysfunction (Cattelani, Zettin, & Zoccolotti, 2010). Instead, in the treatment literature, disinhibition is often targeted in comprehensive behavioral management programs designed to minimize a number of problematic behavioral symptoms (e.g., aggression, irritability); for comprehensive reviews of behavioral interventions, see Cattelani and colleagues (2010) or Ylvisaker and colleagues (2007).

With respect to treatments specific to disinhibition, Blake and colleagues (as cited by Mateer, 1999) developed a protocol to treat their patient's impaired inhibition of interruptive behavior. In this treatment, the patient was first taught those individuals with whom he was allowed to interact and those he was not. To aid his discrimination of appropriate and inappropriate conversational partners, staff members he was allowed to approach wore large green squares and those he was not to approach wore large red squares. Appropriate discrimination (i.e., approaching only staff with green squares) was rewarded with extended conversation, whereas inappropriate discrimination (i.e., approaching staff with red squares) was addressed by ignoring the patient. As the patient's inappropriate interruptive behavior began to decrease, the saliency of the external cues was reduced by shrinking the size of the staff's badges. Eventually, staff reported minimal disruption by this patient while on the rehabilitation unit, even when the visual cues had been completely faded.

Alderman and colleagues (Alderman, 1996; Alderman, Fry, & Youngson, 1995) have similarly shown that other behavioral modification approaches, in particular response cost programs, may be effective in increasing inhibitory control. In response cost paradigms, patients are given a set number of tokens, which after a certain period of time can be exchanged for a reward. Each time they display a targeted negative behavior, however, one or more of their tokens are taken away, and they are reminded why they are losing the tokens; consequently, having fewer tokens results in a smaller number or variety of rewards when tokens are eventually exchanged. Alderman et al. (1995) found that this behavioral approach was effective in reducing improper verbalizations in a patient with brain damage related to encephalitis. Whereas the patient displayed improved inhibitory control in a variety of contexts on her rehabilitation unit following the response cost treatment, generalization to settings outside of her rehabilitation environment did not occur. Accordingly, primarily context-specific training effects should be expected with this type of behavioral technique.

Treatment of Goal Setting, Planning, and Problem-Solving Impairments

Disorganized behavior is a frequent executive function deficit subsequent to TBI and other forms of brain damage, particularly those that compromise neural circuits involving the frontal lobe (Alvarez & Emory, 2006; Stuss, 2011). This disorganization has been linked to problems implementing and maintaining goal-directed behavior and is known to negatively affect occupational outcomes. Accordingly, treatment protocols have been developed to teach systematic goal setting, and, relatedly, planning and problem solving, to patients with executive problems, primarily subsequent to TBI.

One approach involves teaching task-specific routines (Martelli, 1999; Sohlberg & Mateer, 2001). That is, complex daily behaviors such as maintaining personal hygiene, getting to work, shopping, household cleaning, and operating household appliances or electronic equipment, which patients are unable to complete independently, are taught via the following therapy procedures: (a) The behavior or routine is analyzed and divided into a series of simple steps; (b) a checklist is developed and reviewed with patients so they can see what steps need to be completed, in what order the steps should be completed, and how to record what steps have been completed; (c) extensive practice is provided to help automate checklist use and completion of the complex behavior or routine; and (d) even after the target behavior appears habitual, periodic "retraining" sessions may be necessary, particularly if there are alterations in patients' daily environments or schedules. In selecting which behavior or behaviors to target, clinicians should consider the functional impact of training the patient's independent completion of the routine; which behavior caregivers recommend training; and, perhaps most importantly, which behavior the patient recommends training (to maximize his or her motivation during the exhaustive training sessions that are often needed to habituate the behavior) (Ylvisaker et al., 1998). Additionally, because generalization is not expected with this type of treatment, training should be conducted in the same context in which the routine will take place (Sohlberg & Mateer, 2001). Despite limited generalization, this approach to remediating executive problems is recommended for patients with severe memory and/or awareness deficits, or who do not benefit from other self-instructional techniques such as those described next.

Other treatment approaches are similar to teaching task-specific routines in that they focus on breaking down complex behaviors into sequences of simpler steps. They differ, however, in that they also train patients to adopt one or several strategies that may help them complete a variety of complex behaviors (Kennedy et al., 2008). For example, Robertson (1996) developed the five-stage **Goal Management Training (GMT)** program depicted in Figure 10-1. Initial sessions teach patients about each stage by describing what the stage is, giving examples of what happens when there is a breakdown at that stage, and demonstrating appropriate completion of the stage using examples from everyday tasks. In the original program, patients then practiced applying these steps while completing a series of paper-and-pencil versions of everyday, complex tasks (e.g., proofreading, how to deal with a power outage). In more recent modifications of GMT or programs similar to it (e.g., Goal-Plan-Do-Review strategy training; Dawson et al., 2009), practice has also been provided in virtual environments (e.g., Rand, Weiss, & Katz, 2009) as well as via interactive computer software (e.g., Man, Soong, Tam, & Hui-Chan, 2006). Final sessions of the program involve using the steps, with a visual reminder or flowchart of the steps if necessary, to complete real-life activities (e.g., setting up an answering machine) in typical, daily environments. Across training sessions, cues from the clinician regarding implementing the GMT steps should be faded while the complexity of the target tasks or problems should be increased.

Levine et al. (2000) found that even following a single hour of GMT, a group of patients with TBI completed a set of everyday tasks significantly more accurately and more slowly, indicating more attention to task completion. These researchers also provided a more comprehensive GMT program to a post-encephalitic patient to address her difficulties with daily meal preparation. Following five GMT sessions, which included specific instructions and a checklist regarding how to apply GMT steps to meal preparation, the patient achieved and maintained improved performance of everyday paper-and-pencil tasks, and reductions in problem behaviors that impeded her ability to complete meal preparation. She also reported fewer difficulties with meal preparation following treatment, as quantified by her entries into the self-report diary she was required to keep during the study. Several other researchers have reported positive outcomes when GMT or treatments similar to GMT were utilized to address problems in completing other real-world activities (e.g., math assignments, use of memory diary, shopping, manuscript editing, social-behavioral scenarios) in both individual therapy settings (Dawson et al., 2009; Man et al., 2006; Metzler-Baddeley & Jones, 2010; Ownsworth & McFarland, 1999; Rand et al., 2009; von Cramon & Mattes-von Cramon, 1992) and group therapy settings (Hickey & Saunders, 2010; Langenbahn et al., 2008;

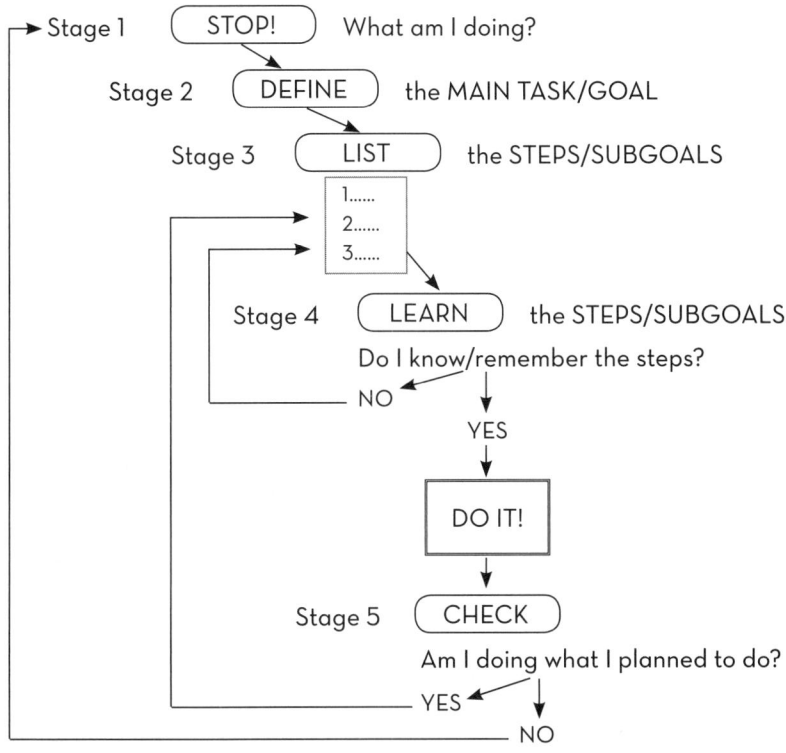

Figure 10-1. The five stages of Robertson's (1996) Goal Management Training. *Note.* From "Rehabilitation of Executive Functioning: An Experimental-Clinical Validation of Goal Management Training," by B. Levine, I. Robertson, L. Clare, G. Carter, J. Hong, B. Wilson, J. Duncan, and D. Stuss, 2000, *Journal of the International Neuropsychological Society, 6*(3) p. 300. Copyright 2000 by the International Neuropsychological Society. Reprinted with permission of Cambridge University Press.

Rath, Simon, Langenbahn, Sherr, & Diller, 2003) with a variety of patient populations (e.g., stroke, TBI, tumor, infection).

A few approaches that incorporate strategy training have been developed to address planning difficulties. One approach focuses on **verbal mediation** training, in which patients are taught to talk themselves through the planning and execution of tasks (Cicerone & Giacino, 1992; Cicerone & Wood, 1987). As training progresses, patients move from talking out loud to covert verbalization of the steps. Preliminary findings indicate that verbal mediation training can lead to decreases in task-related and perseverative errors, as well as decreases in off-task behaviors. The second approach involves teaching patients to self-cue their recall of past planning experiences when undertaking a new planning experience (Hewitt, Evans, & Dritschel, 2006). In the study describing this self-cue approach, two groups of TBI patients were first asked to describe how they would plan eight common, unstructured activities. Next, one group received 30 minutes of training that involved learning about and practicing the self-cue strategy while the other group had the half-hour off. Subsequent to the training session, both groups were asked to describe again a plan for those same eight activities: Only the treatment group demonstrated improvements in that their post-training plans were more effective and included a larger number of relevant steps. These initial, promising results for these planning treatment approaches deserve follow-up to examine the reliability of the findings and to examine their maintenance and generalization potential.

Finally, given that positive outcomes have been reported with each of the executive function treatment approaches reviewed, recently developed protocols now include aspects of several of these approaches. For example, in the multifaceted treatment program of Spikman, Boelen, Lamberts, Brouwer, and Fasotti (2009), a number of executive functions were targeted via (a) awareness training that included psycho-education, as well as prediction and self-monitoring protocols; (b) goal-setting and planning-strategy training that was similar in content and format to GMT (described above); and (c) practice of goal-setting and planning strategies in daily settings and activities with the addition of external devices (e.g., diaries, alarms) if needed. Compared to a control group who only received practice with a cognitive software program, the treated patients demonstrated greater gains on executive function tests, as well as on measures of activity and participation (e.g., increases in amount and quality of social interactions and leisure activities).

General Cognitive Stimulation Approaches

Although treatments for each cognitive domain have been described separately thus far in this chapter, it is important to keep in mind that most patients with neurogenic language and cognitive disorders have difficulties with a variety of linguistic and nonlinguistic cognitive functions. Therefore, it is quite common to utilize multicomponent treatment protocols that target in concert a number of cognitive abilities. In fact, there is a rather large literature documenting the effects of general cognitive stimulation programs, during which patients practice an array of tasks designed to address multiple cognitive-linguistic functions (e.g., short-term recall of visual and verbal information, sustained and selective attention, verbal and visual reasoning or problem solving, processing speed, visuoperception) (Ciancarelli, Cofini, & Carolei, 2010; Cotelli et al., 2012; Herrera, Chambon, Michel, Paban, & Alescio-Lautier, 2012; L. Murray, 2012c; Viola et al., 2011; Zientz, Rackley, Bond-Chapman, Hopper, & Mahendra, 2007). Such programs have been provided in a variety of contexts (e.g., individual and/or group sessions; in the clinic under the direction of a clinician and/or at home under the direction of a caregiver trained by a clinician to administer the program), and are now considered the treatment of choice for the individuals in the early stage of dementia (National Institute for Health and Clinical Excellence, 2006).

Following completion of these programs, which are frequently computerized, improvements on trained tasks, as well as tests similar to the trained tasks, have been documented and appear well maintained in both healthy and patient populations (e.g., TBI, dementia, mild cognitive impairment, stroke, schizophrenia). Similar to stimulation programs for more specific cognitive functions, the functional consequences of these programs have not yet been adequately documented, often because functional outcome measures have not been included in the empirical investigations. It should be noted that when functional gains (e.g., increases in daily living activities, decreased caregiver burden) or transfer to untrained tasks that are dissimilar to training activities have been reported (e.g., Herrera et al., 2012; Viola et al., 2011), the treatment protocols have typically extended beyond stimulation tasks and included other intervention approaches (e.g., strategy training, alternative approaches such as exercise or relaxation therapy [see Chapter 12], patient and caregiver education; for an example, see below).

Activities Included in the Multicomponent Intervention Program Developed by Viola et al. (2011) for Individuals with Alzheimer's Disease and Their Caregivers:

Cognitive Stimulation Procedures

- Paper-and-pencil tasks
- Computerized games
- Board games
- Strategy training

Art Therapy

Occupational Therapy

- Practice completing basic and instrumental activities of daily living
- Strategy training for completing basic and instrumental activities of daily living
- Environmental/household adaptations

Physical Therapy

- Balance and fall-prevention exercises

Exercise Therapy

- Strength training
- Group walking and stretching sessions

Speech-Language Therapy

- Communication strategy training

Caregiver Training

- Education regarding strategies and environmental adaptations
- Education regarding Alzheimer's disease symptoms and progression
- Counseling

Use of Commercially Available Workbooks and Computer Software for Treating Cognitive Disorders

Similar to the workbook and computer software materials for targeting language abilities reviewed in Chapter 9, there is an ever-increasing corpus of such materials available for cognitive disorders (see Table 10-5). Like with language materials, cognitive workbooks and software programs vary from those designed to address a variety of cognitive disorders (e.g., *Results for Adults: Cognition*; M. Baker & Johnson, 2010) to those suitable for working on a limited number of problems (e.g., *Left Visual Inattention Workbook*; Knauss, 1998). Whereas many contain contrived activities (e.g., canceling out filled-in circles to target visual scanning), others include more functional exercises (e.g., time management scenarios to target planning and problem solving). With respect to software programs, clinicians might also consider some of the products that are currently available for current gaming platforms and systems. Many of these games require players to exploit a number of cognitive abilities (e.g., remembering which route was a dead end vs. led to a new level of a game; visually scanning the entire screen for a target) and, thus, may be more fun and motivating for patients.

The same set of advantages (e.g., encourage at-home practice) and disadvantages (e.g., suspect validity) associated with workbook or computerized activities discussed with respect to language materials in Chapter 9 applies to these cognitive materials. Although there is some empirical support for the use of computerized activities when targeting attention (S. H. Chen, Thomas, Glueckauf, & Bracy, 1997; Niemann, Ruff, & Baser, 1990; Webster et al., 2001) and memory (S. H. Chen et al., 1997; Niemann et al., 1990), further research is needed to specify which patients are most likely to respond positively to workbook or software activities, and to determine whether practice of these activities produces enduring gains or generalizes to completion of everyday interactions and activities. Use of workbooks or computer programs without the input of a clinician is *not* recommended (Cornis-Pop et al., 2012).

Cognitive Training for Everyone!

Traditionally, cognitive training software programs were developed solely for clinical populations by educational or rehabilitation publishing companies. In the past few years, however, there has been a surge in marketing such software to the general population as a means to improve "brains—and lives" (Lumos Labs, 2013). Given that these products have the same strengths and limitations as software programs described in this chapter and in Chapter 9, interested consumers might be advised to do their own cost-benefit analysis before purchasing a program or a subscription to a program.

TABLE 10-5
Examples of Workbooks and Software Programs for Treating Cognitive

MATERIAL	PRIMARY TARGET AREA(S)	AUTHOR(S)
Workbooks		
Attention Workbook Volume 1	Attention	Evanofski (1997)
Brainwave-Revised	Various cognitive skills	Malia, Bewick, Raymond, & Bennet (2002)
Cognition: Functional Rehabilitation Activity Manual	Various cognitive skills	Messenger & Ziarnek (2004)
Critical Thinking for Activities of Daily Living and Communication	Pragmatics and executive functioning	Daly & Fouche (1999)
Left Visual Inattention Workbook	Visual neglect	Knauss (1998)
Results for Adults: Cognition	Various cognitive skills	M. Baker & Johnson (2010)
The Source for Executive Function Disorders	Various cognitive skills	Keeley (2003)
Workbook of Activities for Language and Cognition 3: Everyday Problem Solving	Problem solving	Bowers, Huisingh, Johnson, LoGiudice, & Orman (2003)
Software		
Captain's Log	Various cognitive skills	BrainTrain (2002-2010)
Generations Trivia: Interactive Game Shows for Recall and Deductive Reasoning	Memory and reasoning	Linguisystems (2009)
Luminosity	Various cognitive skills	Lumos Labs (2010)
Moriarty Mystery Dinner	Reasoning and problem solving	Bungalow Software (2005)
Parrot Software	Various cognitive and linguistic skills for English and Spanish speakers	Parrot Software (various publication dates)
PSSCogRehab	Various cognitive skills	Psychological Software Service (2012)

Cognitive Approaches to Treating Linguistic Disorders

Researchers have begun to explore whether directly treating cognition or utilizing cognitive instructional techniques such as errorless learning will positively affect the linguistic abilities of patients with neurogenic language and cognitive disorders. In terms of direct cognitive treatments, the effects of attention, memory, and executive function interventions have been examined in a growing, albeit still somewhat limited, number of studies. The theoretical impetus for this line of research relates to models that acknowledge the close relationship between linguistic and extra-linguistic cognitive abilities and that assert that deficits in these extra-linguistic functions may produce or exacerbate linguistic impairments (Alexander, 2006; R. Martin & Allen, 2008; L. Murray & Kean, 2004; see also Chapters 1 and 2).

Addressing Language via Direct Cognitive Treatments

Several investigators have provided attention training to patients with neurogenic language and cognitive disorders to determine whether such training reduces language symptoms (Coelho, 2005; Evans et al., 2009; L. Murray et al., 2006; Sinotte & Coelho, 2007; Wilson & Robertson, 1992). Whereas in most studies, language improvements were observed subsequent to attention intervention (e.g., Coelho, 2005), L. Murray and colleagues (2006) observed negligible improvements in the auditory comprehension abilities of their patient with aphasia after the patient was provided *Attention Process Training–II*. Given variation in the training protocols, participant characteristics, and language profiles, resolution of discrepant findings awaits further research.

The effects of short-term and working memory treatments on neurogenic language disorders have also been explored (for a review see L. Murray, 2012a). Francis et al. (2003) and Koenig-Bruhin and Studer-Eichenberger (2007) used sentence repetition tasks to target short-term memory or the buffer component of working memory (see Chapter 1) in patients with aphasia. Both sets of researchers reported improvements in their study participant following treatment: The participant in the former study demonstrated gains in auditory comprehension, and the participant in the latter study achieved spoken language improvements. Similarly, Kalinyak-Fliszar, Kohen, and Martin (2011) and Salis (2012) reported positive cognitive-linguistic outcomes in their aphasic patients who completed a word and nonword repetition protocol or listening span training (i.e., deciding if two lists of words were the same or different), respectively. Other researchers have used training protocols designed to target the buffer as well as the executive components of working memory (Mayer & Murray, 2002; Vallat et al., 2005). For instance, the participant in the study by Vallat and colleagues practiced tasks such as the following: (a) naming a word that had been spelled orally but with a missing letter; (b) naming a word that had been presented in the form of spoken scrambled syllables; and (c) given a list of spoken words, coming up with the word that could be spelled from the first letter of each word in that list (e.g., for the list "bird," "under," and "grin," naming the word "bug"). The positive language outcomes reported following these treatments that focused on strengthening maintenance and manipulation aspects of working memory are encouraging, and hopefully spur future memory training research.

Although there has been nominal examination of whether direct training of executive functions might by itself reduce linguistic symptoms in patients with neurogenic disorders, some investigators have included executive function tasks (e.g., problem-solving and categorizing tasks) in their general cognitive training protocols (Kohnert,

2004; Mahendra & Arkin, 2003; Ramsberger, 2005). Although in all of these investigations concomitant improvements in cognitive task performances and language abilities were reported, none had strong study designs, and, again, executive function tasks were provided in concert with other cognitive tasks (i.e., it cannot be determined whether training all or just select cognitive domains evoked language changes).

Addressing Language via Cognitive Instructional Approaches

Researchers also have investigated adapting cognitive instructional approaches to train linguistic skills directly. For instance, Abel, Schultz, Radermacher, Willmes, and Huber (2003) reported that both a vanishing cues and a traditional cueing hierarchy approach were effective in improving confrontation naming in a group of patients with aphasia. Although none of their patients appeared to profit from just the vanishing cues approach, and several only improved with the traditional approach, these researchers noted that their alternating treatment design might have interfered with implicit learning, upon which the vanishing cues approach is based. More recently, Bilda (2011) described a computerized conversational-script treatment, which incorporated aspects of vanishing cues into the protocol. For example, in the initial training step, participants watched and listened to videotaped conversations that included pictures of target words and concepts. In later training steps, the pictures of target words and concepts were not shown, and some of the conversational dialogue was missing; in these steps, participants were required to fill in the missing dialogue.

Fillingham, Sage, and Lambon Ralph (2005, 2006) found similar rates of naming improvement when errorless versus errorful learning were used as part of anomia treatment. These researchers noted that although their patients with aphasia preferred the errorless learning approach, those with more intact memory and attention skills responded best to the errorful approach. Variable response to errorful versus errorless learning among patients with aphasia has also been reported by Wierenga and colleagues (2006) when these instructional techniques were used during mapping therapy, a syntax treatment described in Chapter 9.

Spaced retrieval has been implemented during anomia treatment (Fridriksson, Holland, Beeson, & Morrow, 2005; Morrow & Fridriksson, 2006): Faster acquisition and better maintenance of word retrieval improvements were observed when spaced retrieval was used to train target words compared to a more traditional cueing hierarchy. Fridriksson and colleagues also found that both fixed and random inter-stimulus interval schedules resulted in similar improvement patterns. In contrast, spaced retrieval did not have any advantage over simple repetition when used in concert with a word retrieval treatment for semantic dementia (Bier et al., 2009).

Addressing Language via a Cognitive Stimulation Strategy

Another cognitive approach is similar to a strategy used to alleviate neglect, that is, limb activation. Crosson and colleagues (Crosson, 2008; Crosson et al., 2007; Richards,

Singletary, Gonzalez Rothi, Koehler, & Crosson, 2002) required patients with nonfluent aphasia to perform either complex left limb movements designed to encourage activation of right hemisphere areas dedicated to response initiation or intention, or a head and gaze turn toward their left side that was designed to promote more general attention mechanisms within the right hemisphere during traditional phonological naming treatment. They found that both the limb and head movements produced positive outcomes, with a trend toward better improvement with the intention treatment (i.e., left limb activation). Further research is necessary to determine whether improvements associated with the intention or attention treatment should be attributed to the additional limb or head movement, respectively, or simply to phonological stimulation, given that a direct comparison of intention/attention treatment outcomes to traditional naming treatment outcomes has not yet been completed.

The above cognitive approaches to treating linguistic impairments appear to hold promise. Recommendations regarding which direct or indirect cognitive treatment protocols are most effective, which patients (e.g., acute vs. chronic, TBI vs. stroke) are most likely to benefit from cognitive treatment, or which linguistic symptoms (e.g., lexical–semantic retrieval vs. syntactic processing) are most amenable to a cognitive approach cannot be forwarded until the completion of further empirical investigation.

Generalization and Transfer of Learning

The same factors that have been found to enhance maintenance and generalization of linguistic treatment effects (see Chapter 9) have also proven influential for cognitive treatments (Ehlardt et al., 2008; Golisz, 1998; Piras et al., 2011; Sohlberg & Turkstra, 2011; Wressle et al., 2002). Clinicians are again reminded that they cannot just hope that patients will transfer use of trained behaviors and strategies to contexts outside of the therapy room. Rather, from the initial treatment session, clinicians must consider manipulating the following factors when devising therapy procedures and materials.

Variation is a key characteristic of cognitive treatments with outcomes that endure and generalize. Whenever possible, variation should pervade all aspects of the treatment, including, but not limited to, stimuli (e.g., objects vs. pictures), stimulus and response modality (e.g., spoken vs. written), therapy context (e.g., individual vs. small group), physical environment (e.g., at-home practice in kitchen vs. living room, inside vs. outdoors), and therapist (e.g., familiar vs. unfamiliar). Clinicians must also consider the *ecological validity* of treatment targets, regardless of whether they are more information-based or activity-/procedure-based. Functional and personally relevant treatment targets will have both motivational and emotional meaning for patients (as well as caregivers) and, consequently, result in better recall of the targets, as well as better therapy compliance. Finally, comprehensive reviews of the cognitive treatment literature indicate that *extensive and intensive practice* (i.e., greater than two training sessions per week) will foster both maintenance and generalization of treatment effects (e.g., Ehlardt et al., 2008; Piras et al., 2011).

Summary

Clinicians have many options when designing treatment programs to address the cognitive limitations of their patients with neurogenic language and cognitive disorders. As mentioned throughout this chapter, however, several areas pertaining to cognitive intervention for neurogenic patient populations are in need of further research. First, the vast majority of these treatments have been developed for the TBI patient population, with far less inclusion of individuals with aphasia, RHD, or progressive disorders (with the exception of Alzheimer's disease) in empirical evaluations of cognitive interventions. Second, guidance for clinicians working with acute or subacute patient populations is lacking, as most cognitive treatment research has involved patients who are beyond one year postonset of brain damage. Third, for some cognitive deficits (e.g., perseveration), only a limited number of treatment protocols have been developed. Fourth, and similar to the linguistic treatment literature reviewed in Chapter 9, further documentation of the maintenance and generalization of cognitive treatment effects is needed; in particular, future studies must include outcome measures that will allow documenting the effects of these treatments on performance of daily activities and participation in typical environments. Lastly, although there is growing support for the benefit of combining treatment approaches (e.g., retraining plus strategy training plus external support), research to quantify and qualify the benefits (both behavioral and economic) of these cognitive treatments used in concert with pharmacotherapy versus by themselves (see Chapter 11) is needed.

Discussion Questions

1. Describe the strengths and weaknesses of structured retraining programs (e.g., Attention Process Training) for attention and memory impairments.
2. Identify one neglect treatment approach that would and one neglect treatment that would not be expected to produce meaningful generalization of treatment effects to untrained tasks or contexts.
3. Identify a memory training approach that would be appropriate for a patient with mild to moderate Alzheimer's disease. Outline the specific treatment steps that would be used to facilitate this patient's recall of information pertaining to his upcoming vacation to Europe.
4. Develop a treatment activity that would be appropriate for addressing a patient's poor awareness of her auditory comprehension deficits.
5. Design two treatment programs for addressing the planning deficits of a patient who suffered a traumatic brain injury but is hoping to return to his job as a restaurant manager. The activities and procedures for one treatment should be developed so that only task-specific effects would be expected, whereas the activities and procedures for the other treatment should be developed so that generalization of treatment effects to untrained stimuli and contexts would be possible.

Remediation of Body Structure and Function: Pharmacotherapy Approaches

chapter 11

Learning Objectives

After reading this chapter, you should be able to:

- Identify pharmacotherapies that may be used to address linguistic disorders in patients with neurogenic language or cognitive disorders
- Identify pharmacotherapies that may be used to address cognitive disorders in patients with neurogenic language or cognitive disorders
- Discuss future research needs pertaining to pharmacotherapy for patients with neurogenic language or cognitive disorders

Key Terms

- acetylcholine
- agonists
- amphetamines
- antagonists
- bromocriptine
- catecholamine system
- cholinergic system
- donepezil
- dopamine
- memantine
- methylphenidate
- neurotransmitters
- norepinephrine/noradrenalin
- pharmacotherapy
- selective serotonin reuptake inhibitors

Introduction

In contrast to the behavioral treatments reviewed in Chapters 9 and 10, which require practice of target linguistic or cognitive behaviors or strategies, **pharmacotherapy**, or drug treatment, aims to replace or augment behavioral practice with medications. Pharmacotherapy focuses on direct remediation of physiological deficits (i.e., the International Classification of Functioning, Disability, and Health [ICF; WHO, 2001] level of body structure), which in turn should result in the resolution of problematic linguistic and/or cognitive behaviors at the ICF level of body function. Over the past few decades, extensive research funds have been spent on developing and evaluating medications that will prevent or remediate a variety of diseases and medical conditions known to cause neurogenic language and cognitive disorders. Although researchers have most frequently examined the effects of these medications on the memory and attention abilities of patients with neurogenic language and cognitive disorders related to Alzheimer's disease or traumatic brain injury, there is increasing interest in exploring drugs that will alleviate the linguistic and cognitive problems of other patient populations.

Whereas it is clearly beyond the purview of speech-language pathologists to prescribe medications (see Chapter 4 for a description of the various health-care team members), they are responsible for identifying positive as well as negative changes in the linguistic and cognitive abilities of their patients who take these medications. That is, clinicians' observations are essential to helping health-care teams monitor the effects of medications in terms of changes in target behaviors or the onset of negative side effects and, relatedly, whether patients should continue with a given medication or whether a new medication or dosage level is needed. Accordingly, knowing what behavioral outcomes have been associated with specific medications will help clinicians direct their observational focus when providing services to patients receiving pharmacotherapy; this knowledge also will empower clinicians to make suggestions to the medical team regarding the prescription of certain medications as possible treatment options.

The purpose of this chapter is to review the variety of medications that have been effective at, or show promise for, remediating linguistic and cognitive impairments in neurogenic patient populations. Before describing these drug treatments, however, it is important to have some basic understanding of how medications affect brain functioning. Therefore, this chapter begins with a brief discussion of neurotransmitters and their role in pharmacotherapy.

The Basics of Pharmocotherapy: Neurotransmitters

Both static (e.g., stroke, traumatic brain injury, hypoxic-ischemic brain injury) and progressive forms (e.g., tumors, Parkinson's disease, Alzheimer's disease) of brain damage result in injury not only to brain tissue, but also to the **neurotransmitter** systems that underlie communication among neurons (Arciniegas, 2011; Berthier, Pulvermuller, Davila, Casares, & Gutierrez, 2011; J. Young, 2011). More specifically, neurotransmitters are chemicals that facilitate message transmission among neurons. For example, in some cases, neurotransmitters may be excitatory and increase the activity of neurons; in other cases, neurotransmitters are inhibitory and decrease neuronal activity. Following the onset of brain damage or disease, the availability of certain neurotransmitters (see Figure 11-1), the sensitivity of neurons to certain neurotransmitters, or both may be compromised. Impairment of two neurotransmitter systems, the **catecholamine** and **cholinergic systems**, have been posited to underlie many of the linguistic and cognitive symptoms associated with neurogenic language disorders. Consequently, the goal of most drug treatments for neurogenic language or cognitive disorders is to restore these disrupted neurotransmitter systems, which in turn should enhance functioning of the neural circuits, which support language and other cognitive abilities. Thus, pharmacotherapy should facilitate linguistic and cognitive recovery in the case of static brain injury, or slow linguistic and cognitive deterioration in the case of progressive brain disorders.

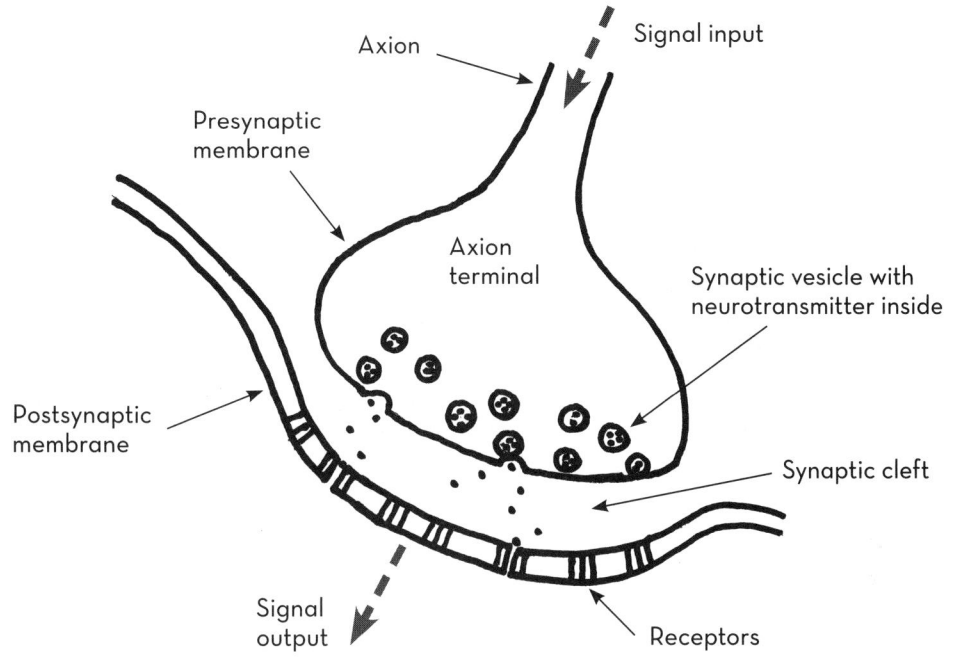

Figure 11-1. A simplified illustration of a synapse in which neurons use neurotransmitters to communicate with each other.

Medications can affect neurotransmitter systems in two basic ways: They may facilitate the effects of one or more neurotransmitters, or they may inhibit the effects of one or more neurotransmitters. Drugs designed to increase the amount or efficiency of neurotransmitters are referred to as **agonists**; for example, a drug that increases levels of dopamine, a neurotransmitter essential to a variety of cognitive functions, would be called a dopamine agonist. In contrast, drugs that reduce the amount or efficiency of neurotransmitters are called **antagonists**. Therefore, dopamine antagonists decrease levels of dopamine or interfere with the ability of neurons to utilize dopamine. Information about specific agonists and antagonists used to manage neurogenic language and cognitive disorders is provided in the following sections of this chapter.

Finding the "Language Neurotransmitter": A Possible or Impossible Challenge?

Without question, neuroscientists have determined that the neural areas that support linguistic and cognitive functioning utilize a certain set of neurotransmitters, including dopamine, acetylcholine, and noradrenalin. Have they, however, yet found that specific neurotransmitters uniquely support specific linguistic or cognitive functions? The answer is that currently there are no known exclusive relationships between a neurotransmitter and circumscribed linguistic or cognitive abilities. That is, as of yet, there is no "language neurotransmitter." Instead, the neurotransmitters that have been identified to underlie linguistic and cognitive functioning are known to sustain not only a variety of linguistic and cognitive abilities, but also a number of additional skills. For example, dopamine has been associated with verbal fluency, emotional functioning, and motor performance, as well as several cognitive functions, including attention and working memory. Likewise, other neurotransmitters such as noradrenalin and serotonin have also been associated with at least some of these linguistic, emotional, cognitive, and motor abilities. Therefore, when a patient is given a drug designed to increase levels of a certain neurotransmitter in the hopes that it will help resolve certain linguistic or cognitive symptoms, it is important to realize that other neurotransmitter levels may still need to be adjusted to resolve those symptoms and that other abilities may inadvertently be altered.

Pharmacological Treatment of Linguistic Impairments

To date, pharmacotherapy for linguistic impairments has focused primarily on remediating aphasic symptoms with drugs that increase activity within the catecholamine or cholinergic systems. These drugs also have been prescribed to patients with other neurogenic disorders, including those with traumatic brain injury (TBI), right hemisphere brain damage (RHD), or dementia. Research and clinical focus with these patient populations, however, has been primarily confined to these drugs' effects on cognitive, emotional, or behavioral outcomes rather than linguistic deficits (see the "Pharmacological Treatment of Cognitive Impairments" section of this chapter). Furthermore, when language skills have been evaluated in TBI, RHD, and dementia pharmacotherapy research, outcome measures have examined a restricted range of linguistic abilities (e.g., confrontation naming, verbal fluency). Consequently, our review in this section will concentrate on drug treatments that may facilitate linguistic recovery in patients with aphasia.

Enhancing the Catecholamine System

The catecholamine system includes two neurotransmitters, **dopamine** and **norepinephrine** (which also is sometimes referred to as **noradrenalin**). Both of these neurotransmitters have been linked to a number of cognitive and linguistic functions (Arciniegas, 2011; Berthier, 2005; Berthier et al., 2011; J. Young, 2011). Accordingly, researchers have explored whether dopamine and noradrenergic agonists positively affect language recovery in patients with aphasia when administered alone or in concert with behavioral treatments (see Table 11-1).

TABLE 11-1

Drugs Used to Treat Linguistic and Cognitive Deficits in Adults With Neurogenic Language or Cognitive Disorders

DRUG GROUP	GENERIC (AND COMMERCIAL) DRUG NAMES	PHYSIOLOGICAL MECHANISM	POSITIVE BEHAVIORAL EFFECTS	TARGET NEUROGENIC DISORDER
Stimulants	Amphetamines (Dexedrin)	Dopamine agonist Noradrenergic agonist	↑ memory, language, attention; ↓ apathy, disinhibition	Aphasia, traumatic brain injury, stroke, frontotemporal dementia
	Methylphenidate (Ritalin)	Dopamine agonist Noradrenergic agonist	↑ attention, language, initiation, memory, nonverbal fluency; ↓ apathy, neglect, depression, perseveration	Aphasia, traumatic brain injury, right hemisphere stroke, vascular dementia, Alzheimer's disease
	Amantadine (Symmetrel)	Dopamine agonist Noradrenergic agonist Cholinergic antagonist	↑ attention, learning, alertness, information-processing speed, executive functions; ↓ fatigue, agitation, perseveration	Aphasia, traumatic brain injury, multiple sclerosis, Alzheimer's disease, Parkinson's disease
	Bromocriptine (Parlodel)	Dopamine agonist	↑ memory, motivation, executive functions, verbal fluency, reading; ↓ apathy, neglect	Nonfluent aphasia (particularly transcortical motor aphasia), traumatic brain injury, right hemisphere stroke
	Selegiline (Eldepryl)	Dopamine agonist	↑ memory, attention, learning, ADL; ↓ depression, apathy, behavioral symptoms	Traumatic brain injury, Alzheimer's disease, frontotemporal dementia, Human immunodeficiency virus (HIV)-associated dementia
	Carbidopa-Levodopa (Sinemet); levodopa	Dopamine agonist	↑ attention, arousal, verbal fluency, repetition; ↓ neglect	Traumatic brain injury, aphasia, right hemisphere stroke
	Bifemelane hydrocholoride	Dopamine agonist Cholinergic agonist	↑ auditory comprehension, naming, repetition, memory, reading, writing	Aphasia, multi-infarct vascular dementia
	Tacrine (Cognex)	Cholinergic agonist	↑ memory, naming, general cognitive abilities	Alzheimer's disease, traumatic brain injury, Parkinson's disease
	Donepezil (Aricept)	Cholinergic agonist	↑ memory, ADL, attention, auditory comprehension, verbal fluency; ↓ general cognitive decline, apathy, visual hallucinations	Alzheimer's disease, multi-infarct vascular dementia, frontotemporal dementia, right hemisphere stroke, multiple sclerosis, traumatic brain injury, aphasia, Parkinson's disease, dementia with Lewy bodies

(continues)

TABLE 11-1 (continued)

DRUG GROUP	GENERIC (AND COMMERCIAL) DRUG NAMES	PHYSIOLOGICAL MECHANISM	POSITIVE BEHAVIORAL EFFECTS	TARGET NEUROGENIC DISORDER
Stimulants (continued)	Rivastigmine (Exelon)	Cholinergic agonist	↑ memory, ADL, attention, general cognitive abilities; ↓ apathy	Alzheimer's disease, vascular dementia, Parkinson's disease, Huntington's disease, frontotemporal dementia, dementia with Lewy bodies
	Galantamine (Reminyl)	Cholinergic agonist	↑ memory, ADL, naming, auditory comprehension, verbal fluency; ↓ behavioral symptoms	Alzheimer's disease, vascular dementia, aphasia, Parkinson's disease, primary progressive aphasia
	Physostigmine	Cholinergic agonist	↑ naming, attention, memory	Alzheimer's disease, aphasia, traumatic brain injury
	Memantine (Namenda)	Glutamate receptor Antagonist	↑ language, behavior, general cognitive abilities	Aphasia, primary progressive aphasia, Alzheimer's disease, vascular dementia, frontotemporal dementia, Parkinson's disease, dementia with Lewy bodies
	Modafinil (Provigil)	Possible dopamine, noreadrenergic, serotonin and/or glutamateine agonist	↓ fatigue; ↑ attention	Multiple sclerosis, stroke, Alzheimer's disease, Parkinson's disease, traumatic brain injury
SSRIs (selective serotonin reuptake inhibitors)	Fluvoxamine	Serotonin agonist	↑ naming, memory; ↓ depression, perseveration, behavioral symptoms	Fluent aphasia, traumatic brain injury, frontotemporal dementia
	Sertraline (Zoloft)	Serotonin agonist	↑ memory, attention; ↓ depression, perseveration, disinhibition, aggressiveness	aphasia, traumatic brain injury, frontotemporal dementia
Neuroleptics/antipsychotics	Haloperidol (Haldol)	Dopamine antagonist	↓ irritability, agitation, hyperactivity, hostility; ↑ social interaction, alertness	Dementia, traumatic brain injury
Nootropics	Piracetam	Cholinergic agonist Glutamate agonist cerebral metabolism	↑ language, memory, attention; ↓ general cognitive decline	Aphasia, stroke, Alzheimer's disease, traumatic brain injury
	Nimodipine	Calcium antagonist	↑ learning, memory	Subcortical vascular dementia, traumatic brain injury, HIV-associated dementia

Note. ADL = activities of daily living.

The effects of **bromocriptine**, a dopamine agonist, on the language abilities of patients with aphasia have been examined in a number of studies. A predominance of dopamine projections have been identified in the frontal cortex and left hemisphere; thus it has been proposed that certain language functions, such as language initiation and verbal fluency, which are dependent on functioning of left frontal regions, may be supported by this neurotransmitter (Gold, VanDam, & Silliman, 2000; Tanaka & Bachman, 2007). Whereas some investigations have obtained null or mixed findings (Ashtary, Janghorbani, Chitsaz, Reisi, & Bahrami, 2006; Ozeren, Sarica, Mavi, & Demirkiran, 1995; Reed, Johnson, Thompson, Weintraub, & Mesulam, 2004), others have reported positive outcomes in terms of improved verbal fluency, word retrieval, or both (Albert, Bachman, Morgan, & Helm-Estabrooks, 1988; Berthier, 2005; Bragoni et al., 2000; Gold et al., 2000; Raymer, 2003; Raymer, Bandy, & Adair, 2001). Unfortunately, many of these studies had methodological weaknesses, including inadequate control of placebo or practice effects (e.g., Albert, Bachman, et al., 1988) and the lack of a drug withdrawal phase (e.g., Gupta & Mlcoch, 1992). Furthermore, the vast majority of studies utilizing bromocriptine have only involved patients with nonfluent aphasia profiles, and thus the effects of this drug on fluent aphasia profiles have not yet been sufficiently examined. There have also been inconsistencies across the studies in terms of doses (e.g., varying from a low of 10 mg daily to as high as 60 mg daily) and time post-onset (e.g., acute vs. chronic aphasia recovery phase). Finally, with the exception of Bragoni et al.'s work (2000), bromocriptine in the above-cited studies was prescribed in the absence of behavioral aphasia treatment.

Accordingly, whether more substantial and enduring improvements can be obtained when dopaminergic agonists and behavioral treatment are provided in concert has been the focus of more recent drug trials. For example, Seniow, Litwin, Litwin, Lesniak, and Członkowska (2009) utilized a randomized double-blind, placebo-controlled study design to examine the effects of providing a single dose of levodopa prior to every session of language therapy. Their aphasic participants, particularly those with frontal lesions, demonstrated greater improvements in their verbal fluency and repetition abilities with levodopa versus the placebo. However, Leemann, Laganaro, Chetelat-Mabillard, and Schnider (2011) did not find significant differences in the amount of improvement achieved when levadopa versus placebo were combined with aphasia therapy. Again, procedural differences between the studies (e.g., Seniow et al. [2009] included only participants with chronic stroke-induced aphasia vs. Leeman et al. [2011], who included participants in the subacute phase of recovery from a variety of etiologies, including stroke and TBI) confound interpreting the inconsistent outcomes reported thus far for levodopa.

Amphetamines also mediate the catecholamine system, particularly noradrenergic functioning, and have been administered to patients with various types and severities of aphasia. Both negative (F. L. Darley, Keith, & Sasanuma, 1977) and positive (McNeil, Small, Masterson, & Fossett, 1995; Walker-Batson, Curtis, Wolf, & Porch, 1996; Walker-Batson et al., 1992, 2001; Whiting, Chenery, Chalk, & Copland, 2008) outcomes have been reported. As with the bromocriptine findings, significant improvements were noted only in studies in which amphetamines were used to complement behavioral aphasia treatments (e.g., McNeil et al., 1995; Walker-Batson et al., 2001; Whiting et al., 2008). Similar to findings reported for motor recovery in stroke patients when amphetamines are combined with physical therapy (Harbeck-Seu et al., 2011; Lokk, Salman Roghani, & Delbari, 2011), amphetamines appear to be most effective when provided during acute stages of aphasia recovery (e.g., McNeil et al., 1995; Walker-Batson et al., 2001).

Collectively, aphasia studies examining the effects of dopaminergic and noradrenergic agonists indicate these drugs must be paired with language treatment to have a significant effect (e.g., Barrett & Eslinger, 2007; Seniow et al., 2009; Whiting et al., 2008). Further research is required to explore the long-term effects of combining these drugs and behavioral treatment, and to determine optimal dosage and patient selection criteria (e.g., age, concomitant symptoms, aphasia characteristics, time postonset).

Enhancing the Cholinergic System

The cholinergic system relies upon **acetylcholine**, a neurotransmitter that has been linked to several linguistic and cognitive functions (e.g., naming, attention, learning and memory) and, when deficient, to certain neurogenic disorders (e.g., Alzheimer's disease) (Berthier et al., 2011; Hughes, Jacobs, & Heilman, 2000; Tanaka & Bachman, 2007). Likewise, in healthy individuals, greater cholinergic activity has been observed in the left versus right temporal lobe, and acetylcholine has been posited to enhance signal-to-noise ratios within cortical regions. Accordingly, researchers have speculated that providing cholinergic agonists should facilitate language abilities such as naming or word-finding skills.

As predicted, improvements in general as well as specific language abilities—in particular, naming, auditory comprehension, and repetition—have been reported when cholinergic agents such as galantamine, physostigmine, bifemelane hydrochloride, or piracetam have been administered to patients with dementia (Farlow et al., 1992) or acute or chronic aphasia (De Deyn, De Reuck, Orgogozo, Vlietinck, & Deberdt, 1997; Hughes et al., 2000; D. Jacobs et al., 1994; Kabasawa et al., 1994; Pashek & Bachman, 2003), including primary progressive aphasia (Kertesz et al., 2008) (see Table 11-1). For example, in a few randomized double-blind, placebo-controlled investigations, patients with aphasia who received piracetam plus traditional language treatment displayed significantly greater improvements in their overall aphasia severity, compared with patients who received a placebo plus traditional language treatment (Enderby, Broeckx, Hospers, Schildermans, & Deberdt, 1994; Huber, Willmes, Poeck, Van Vleymen, & Deberdt, 1997; Kessler, Thiel, Karbe, & Heiss, 2000). More specifically, the piracetam group achieved higher gains in their naming, writing, auditory comprehension, repetition, and phonological, semantic, and syntactic aspects of their spontaneous verbal output than the placebo group did. Less positive long-term outcomes for piracetam, however, have more recently been reported. Güngör, Terzi, and Onar (2011) found that across several language measures, only auditory comprehension scores showed greater improvement in their piracetam versus placebo groups following six months of treatment (with both groups also receiving traditional language therapy). The participants in this study, however, had larger lesions and more severe levels of aphasia than those in early studies (e.g., Enderby et al., 1994) had.

Donepezil is another cholinergic agonist that has been the focus of several recent aphasia studies (Berthier, Hinojosa, Martín, & Fernandez, 2003; Berthier et al., 2006; Y. Chen, Li, Wang, Xu, & Shi, 2010; Pashek & Bachman, 2003). Positive outcomes have been identified among patients in both the acute (e.g., Y. Chen et al., 2010) and chronic (e.g., Berthier et al., 2006) phases of aphasia recovery. Although the types and amounts of language and communication gains have varied across these aphasia studies, improvements in naming and repetition have been consistently reported.

In summary, further exploration of cholinergic agonists is needed as many of the above cited studies had weak designs. That is, many studies failed to control for a number of confounds, including spontaneous recovery, placebo, experimenter bias, and practice effects; neglected to indicate whether or not the cholinergic agonist was provided by itself or in concert with behavioral language treatment; or both (e.g., Berthier et al., 2003; Y. Chen et al., 2010; Pashek & Bachman, 2003; Tanaka, Miyazaki, & Albert, 1997).

Summary of Pharmacotherapy for Linguistic Impairments

The study of pharmacotherapy for linguistic impairments is still in the initial stages of development. Not only have a limited number of investigations been completed, but those that have been completed often have produced disparate findings. These conflicting data can be attributed, at least in part, to one or more of the following methodology differences across the studies: (a) varying patient selection criteria, such as whether patients who had or did not have concomitant emotional disorders were included or whether patients were in the acute or chronic stage of aphasia recovery; (b) use of different study designs, such as a blind design (i.e., test examiners did not know which patients were receiving the drug treatment) versus an open-label design (i.e., test examiners are aware of which patients were receiving the drug treatment); (c) inclusion of different outcome measures, such as using different aphasia tests or including versus excluding patient or caregiver feedback; and (d) amount and type of language treatment provided, such as when language treatment was used in concert with pharmacotherapy, and minimal details regarding that language treatment were provided (e.g., Güngör et al., 2011; Seniow et al., 2009).

Although definitive conclusions regarding the efficacy of pharmacotherapy for linguistic impairments cannot yet be made, findings from the existing literature do suggest that drug treatments will not replace more traditional, linguistic treatments, but rather serve to enhance the extent of recovery achieved with these behavioral treatments. Numerous avenues of research remain to be explored, including determining (a) optimal dosages to maximize positive effects and minimize negative side effects, (b) whether drugs directly affect language abilities or affect them indirectly via their influence on other cognitive functions (e.g., attention, working memory) or emotional status (e.g., depression, anxiety), (c) whether the linguistic impairments of patients with neurogenic language disorders other than aphasia (e.g., RHD, TBI) respond to pharmacotherapy, (d) if certain types and/or severities of linguistic deficits or particular sites and/or sizes of brain lesions are more or less ameliorable to pharmacotherapy (e.g., morphosyntactic and pragmatic measures have been infrequently included when examining drug effects), (e) long-term stability effects of drug treatments on linguistic abilities or response to behavioral language treatments once the drug has been discontinued, and (f) the effects of combination drug therapies (e.g., dopaminergic + cholinergic agonist drug treatment; cholinergic agonist + glutamate receptor antagonist drug treatment).

Pharmacological Treatment of Cognitive Impairments

There has been a recent surge of research exploring whether certain drugs may help ameliorate the cognitive deficits associated with a variety of acquired neurogenic disorders. As with pharmacotherapy for linguistic deficits, drug treatments for cognitive impairments have been designed primarily to manipulate catecholamine and/or cholinergic neurotransmitter systems because of their documented involvement in a number of cognitive functions and their vulnerability in many neurological disorders (Berthier, 2005; Harbeck-Seu et al., 2011; J. Young, 2011).

Enhancing the Catecholamine System

A number of dopaminergic and noradrenergic agonists have been used to treat a spectrum of cognitive problems associated with TBI; progressive neurological disorders such as Alzheimer's and Parkinson's diseases; and, to a lesser extent, stroke (see Table 11-1). For example, **methylphenidate**, more commonly known as Ritalin, has been the focus of numerous investigations with a variety of neurogenic patient populations. In patients with stroke, methylphenidate has been found useful in treating left neglect, depression, and apathy (Hurford, Stringer, & Jann, 1998; Watanabe et al., 1995; J. Young, 2011), but ineffective for treating memory problems (Tiberti, Sabe, Jason, Leiguarda, & Starkstein, 1998). Whereas some studies report that this drug positively affects aspects of attention, memory, and executive functioning in patients with TBI (Chew & Zafonte, 2009; Frankel & Penn, 2007; J. Young, 2011), others observed minimal effects, particularly when patients with TBI were in the more chronic stages of recovery (Speech, Rao, Osmon, & Sperry, 1993; S. E. Williams et al., 1998). These mixed findings have led researchers to conclude that in TBI, methylphenidate may be most effective in assisting acute recovery of cognitive abilities or may be ineffective as a long-term medication (Kajs-Wyllie, 2002; J. Young, 2011). Further studies are needed to examine methylphenidate's long-term efficacy, and thus specify at what point or dosage this drug may no longer augment cognitive recovery subsequent to TBI.

Another dopaminergic agonist—amantadine—also has been shown to assist in the acute and chronic cognitive recovery of patients with TBI, including those in a vegetative or minimally conscious state (Chew & Zafonte, 2009; Sawyer, Mauro, & Ohlinger, 2008; Wu & Garmel, 2005; J. Young, 2011). For example, Wu and Garmel (2005) presented a case report of a woman who was unresponsive for three days following a motor vehicle accident. Following six doses of amantadine, improvements were noted in terms of spontaneous eye opening and her response to a variety of external stimuli (e.g., pain, her name); a week following her TBI, she was completing activities of daily living with minimal assistance. Amantadine also has been found to enhance general cognitive functioning in patients with Alzheimer's disease, even those in the end stages of the disease (Erkulwater & Pillai, 1989), and patients recovering from stroke or infection (Patrick, Buck, Conaway, & Blackman, 2003; J. Young, 2011). In contrast, amantadine effects scant change in the cognitive impairments associated with Huntington's disease (Krishnamoorthy & Craufurd, 2011).

Collectively, initial findings suggest that dopamine agonists may be particularly useful in enhancing cognitive functions in acute or severely impaired neurogenic patient populations. Further empirical investigation is necessary, however, as much of this research has been limited to studies with weak designs (e.g., Wu & Garmel, 2005) or has produced disparate findings (Portugal, Marinho, & Laks, 2011; Sawyer et al., 2008).

The Roles of Speech-Language Pathologists in Pharmacotherapy

At the beginning of this chapter, we mentioned two important ways that speech-language pathologists can contribute to the process of pharmacotherapy. First, if they keep abreast of pharmacotherapy research, they may make suggestions to the medical team about drugs that may prove to positively affect the linguistic and/or cognitive symptoms of their patients. Second, they can provide important observational data pertaining to the effects of prescribed medications on the linguistic and cognitive abilities of their patients. Another possible contribution can be providing behavioral treatments (see Chapters 9-10) or training compensatory strategies (see Chapter 12) that will help ensure that patients take their medications on a regular basis in order to optimize pharmacotherapy effects. For example, the clinician might add the times at which a patient with TBI is to take his medication to that patient's memory book. Treatment might then focus on several of the following: (a) making sure the patient knew where he could find this medication information within his memory book, (b) training the patient to consult this section of his memory book on a regular basis, (c) training caregivers to cue the patient to consult this section of his memory book on a regular basis, and (d) monitoring how frequently the patient independently or with cueing took his medication at the right time.

Enhancing the Cholinergic System

Substantial research indicates that cholinergic agonists such as rivastigmine, donepezil, galantamine, and piracetam can enhance recovery or delay progression of cognitive and behavioral symptoms in a variety of patient populations with static or progressive neurogenic disorders, respectively (Atri, 2011; Chang et al., 2011; Levine & Langa, 2011; Portugal et al., 2011; D. Wilkinson et al., 2010; Winnicka, Tomasiak, & Bielawska, 2005) (see Table 11-1). Because of its longer-acting properties and lower risk of negative side effects compared with other cholinergic agents such as tacrine and rivastigmine, **donepezil** has become one of the most frequently prescribed cognitive enhancing medications (Howland, 2011; Rhodes-Kropf et al., 2011; D. Wilkinson et al., 2010). For instance, in patients in the acute or chronic stages of TBI recovery, gains in attention, short- and long-term verbal memory, visuoperception, alertness, social interaction, and activities of daily living have been reported following administration of donepezil (Chew & Zafonte, 2009; S. Griffin, van Reekum, & Masanic, 2003; Larner, 2010). In one of the few studies exploring pharmacotherapy for RHD, Chang and colleagues (2011) reported improvements in general cognitive status (that were maintained at a follow-up assessment one-month post-treatment) among their patients taking donepezil in concert with their behavioral rehabilitation therapies. Likewise, patients ranging from the early to late stages of dementing diseases such as Alzheimer's disease, vascular dementia, frontotemporal dementia, Parkinson's disease, and dementia with Lewy bodies have been found to display significant improvements in their general cognitive abilities, slowing or stabilizing in their rates of cognitive and functional decline, or both when taking donepezil, compared with those receiving placebo treatment (Atri, 2011; Howland, 2011; Levine & Langa, 2011; Portugal et al., 2011; Rhodes-Kropf et al., 2011; D. Wilkinson et al., 2010), often these positive outcomes are sustained for several years with continuous donepezil use (Atri, 2011; D. Wilkinson et al., 2010). Unfortunately, neither cognitive nor motor impairments in Huntington's disease or progressive supranuclear palsy respond to donepezil (Krishnamoorthy & Craufurd, 2011; Larner, 2010). Likewise, galantamine failed to improve behavioral, language, or functional impairments in patients with the behavioral variant of frontotemporal dementia (Kertesz et al., 2008).

Although further investigation of the long-term effects of cholinergic agonists is needed, the positive findings reported to date are particularly encouraging given the strong research designs of many previous studies. Additionally, whereas the improvements identified in dementia studies frequently prove statistically significant, the clinical significance of these improvements has been questioned, particularly given the costs of cholinergic agonists (Levine & Langa, 2011; Rhodes-Kropf et al., 2011).

Summary of Pharmacotherapy for Cognitive Impairments

As concluded in our review of pharmacological treatments for linguistic impairments, further investigation of the efficacy of pharmacotherapy for cognitive impairments is warranted to rectify the methodological weaknesses of some previous studies (e.g., reliance on subjective vs. objective measures, failure to control for placebo or practice effects, failure to specify the amount and type of behavioral treatment provided in concert with the pharmacotherapy), as well as to explore issues that have yet to be addressed. For example, nominal research has compared the effects of drug treatment alone to a combined drug and behavioral treatment approach. An exception is a study by Chapman, Weiner, Rackley, Hynan, and Zientz (2004). These investigators found slower rates of decline in emotional well-being, discourse production and comprehension, and completion of daily activities in patients with Alzheimer's disease who received donepezil *and* cognitive-linguistic treatment, compared with those who received only the drug treatment. Given these encouraging, albeit preliminary, results and the positive outcomes associated with integrating drug and behavioral therapies to treat language impairments (e.g., Seniow et al., 2009), it is predicted that the combined treatment approach holds promise as an effective approach to managing cognitive problems associated with a spectrum neurogenic disorders.

Other research avenues to pursue in the area of pharmacotherapy for cognitive impairments include examining the effects of combination drug treatments, such as prescribing cholinergic agonists in concert with SSRIs. Future studies should also include outcome measures that evaluate a broader range of cognitive abilities, in particular executive functions, and ensure that more patients with aphasia, RHD, and dementing diseases other than Alzheimer's disease are represented in the subject samples. Finally, there remains a need to determine which patient characteristics (e.g., age, dementia type and severity, concomitant symptoms) can help health-care teams predict which patients will most likely benefit from pharmacotherapy for cognitive impairments.

DANGER! Some Communication- and Cognition-Unfriendly Drugs

There are some drugs prescribed for medical and psychiatric conditions that have been shown to have negative consequences on communication and cognitive abilities (de Boissezon et al., 2007). For example, some cancer drugs have been reported to induce dysarthria and aphasia. Likewise, psychiatric drugs such as certain antipsychotic (e.g., haloperidol) and antidepressant (e.g., tricyclics) medications may compromise language as well as cognitive abilities (Atri, 2011; Vigen et al., 2011).

Other Pharmacological Approaches

As shown in Table 11-1, a number of drugs with effects other than or in addition to modulating the catecholamine or cholinergic systems have been found to ameliorate the linguistic, cognitive, or emotional-behavioral problems that frequently coexist with neurogenic language and cognitive disorders. For example, neuroleptic or antipsychotic medications, which affect brain functioning by reducing activity within dopaminergic systems (i.e., dopaminergic antagonists), have been successfully used to reduce negative behaviors such as agitation and aggressiveness and to enhance alertness and responsiveness to rehabilitation in patients with dementia or TBI (Atri, 2011; Chew & Zafonte, 2009; Rhodes-Kropf et al., 2011).

With respect to aphasia, **memantine** (a glutamate receptor antagonist that may enhance the activity of neural circuits; Berthier et al., 2011) has been shown to enhance language and communication outcomes when combined with intensive language therapy (Berthier et al., 2009); trends toward decreasing the rate of language and cognitive decline in primary progressive aphasia have also been reported (Boxer et al., 2009; N. Johnson et al., 2010). Positive cognitive and functional (e.g., completion of activities of daily living) outcomes have also been documented when memantine has been prescribed to individuals with vascular dementia (A. Lee, 2011; Levine & Langa, 2011). This drug is also FDA-approved as a treatment for moderate to severe Alzheimer's disease (Atri, 2011; Howland, 2011; Rhodes-Kropf et al., 2011).

Researchers also have begun to explore the effects of **selective serotonin reuptake inhibitors (SSRIs)**—such as sertraline and fluvoxamine—on a variety of linguistic and cognitive disorders associated with acquired brain damage or disease (Chew & Zafonte, 2009; Portugal et al., 2011; Stone et al., 2011; Tanaka & Bachman, 2007). Rationales for prescribing SSRIs include the following: (a) serotonin levels are reduced in certain neurological disorders; (b) the serotonergic system affects functioning of neural areas crucial to a number of cognitive functions, including attention or arousal (i.e., reticular formation) and memory (i.e., hippocampus); and (c) SSRIs are commonly used to treat depression, which is a frequent concomitant symptom in neurogenic language or cognitive disorders. Some initial SSRI studies have produced positive findings, including reduced perseveration and improved naming in aphasia (Tanaka et al., 2004; Tanaka & Bachman, 2007), improved attention and memory in TBI (Chew & Zafonte, 2009; Meythaler, Depalma, Devivo, Guin-Renfroe, & Novack, 2001), decreased disinhibition in frontotemporal dementia (Portugal et al., 2011; Swartz, Miller, Darby, & Schuman, 1997), and decreased cognitive decline in Alzheimer's disease and vascular dementia (Levine & Langa, 2011; Stone et al., 2011). Another benefit of SSRIs is that they produce minimal negative side effects (Meythaler et al., 2001).

Lastly, modafinil (a drug initially used to treat narcolepsy) is now being investigated regarding its potential to reduce fatigue, sleepiness, and depression and, consequently, to enhance attention and other cognitive abilities in a spectrum of neurological disorders. Some initial positive findings have been reported for patents with stroke, TBI, or Alzheimer's or Parkinson's diseases (Chew & Zafonte, 2009; Cochran, 2001; Kajs-Wyllie, 2002; J. Young, 2011).

Summary

A relatively new approach to resolving the linguistic and cognitive impairments associated with neurogenic disorders involves prescribing medications. These medications are designed to remediate the alterations in neurotransmitter systems that occur subsequent to the onset of brain damage or disease. The majority of drugs that have been investigated to date affect the catecholamine or cholinergic neurotransmitter systems because these systems have been shown to have important ties to a number of linguistic and cognitive functions. Indeed, a growing research base indicates that pharmacotherapies that target these neurotransmitter systems can produce positive changes in the linguistic and/or cognitive functioning of patients with static brain damage (e.g., stroke, TBI) or progressive brain damage (e.g., Alzheimer's disease). Importantly, however, the most consistently positive findings have been reported when the drugs are used to supplement behavioral treatments. It is anticipated that adults with neurogenic language or cognitive disorders will benefit greatly from future research designed to identify additional pharmacotherapy and behavioral treatment combinations, to specify which patients are most likely to respond positively to these treatment regimens, or both.

Discussion Questions

1. Select one of the cholinergic agonists mentioned in this chapter and identify the following:
   (a) Linguistic and/or cognitive abilities that may be affected by taking this medication
   (b) Side effects associated with taking this medication
   (c) Patient populations for whom this medication may be effective
   (d) Patient populations for whom this medication would likely be ineffective
2. In light of the International Classification of Functioning, Disability, and Health, why would you expect to have better language and cognitive outcomes when medications are used in concert with other, non-pharmacologic treatments, rather than when used by themselves?
3. Based on the research needs identified in this chapter, develop a study that would allow examining the effects of a stimulant drug plus behavioral treatment on:
   (a) Discourse production symptoms associated with right hemisphere brain damage
   (b) Episodic memory problems associated with Alzheimer's disease
   (c) Word retrieval deficits associated with aphasia
   What variables influence your selection of outcome measures and the type and amount of drug and behavioral treatment?

Remediation of Activity and Participation: Approaches for Linguistic and Cognitive Disorders

chapter 12

Learning Objectives

After reading this chapter, you should be able to:

- Compare and contrast body structure and function versus activity/participation remediation strategies
- Identify a variety of compensatory strategies that may enhance the communication or cognitive functioning of patients with neurogenic language or cognitive disorders
- Describe treatment approaches that target the use of multiple modalities to enhance communication effectiveness
- List augmentative communication options for individuals with linguistic and cognitive impairments
- List external devices that may be used to help patients compensate for their linguistic and/or cognitive impairments
- Describe training procedures for fostering patients' effective use of compensatory strategies or external devices
- Discuss the benefits of group treatment and identify characteristics of effective group intervention strategies
- Identify a variety of strategies for modifying the environment to enhance communication effectiveness and cognitive functioning
- Describe how training caregivers and volunteers may facilitate the life participation of patients with neurogenic language or cognitive disorders
- Discuss the issues surrounding the chronicity of neurogenic language and cognitive disorders, including the role of speech-language pathologists in providing counseling and education and identifying other community resources available to assist patients and their caregivers in participating fully in desired activities and social roles
- Describe alternative treatment approaches that have been used to alleviate the effects of neurogenic language and/or cognitive disorders

Key Terms

- acupuncture
- augmentative or alternative communication (AAC)
- authentic context
- biofeedback
- compensatory strategies
- complementary and alternative medicine
- guided imagery
- interaction
- multimodal communication
- progressive muscle relaxation
- relaxation therapy
- sensory stimulation
- text-to-speech capability
- transaction
- transcutaneous electrical nerve stimulation

Introduction

With respect to the International Classification of Functioning, Disability, and Health (ICF) model (WHO, 2001), the body structure and function level treatment strategies discussed in Chapters 9, 10, and 11 will often result in observable changes in communicative and cognitive activities and life participation (e.g., Best, Greenwood, Grassly, & Hickin, 2008). As the underlying impairments contributing to neurogenic language and cognitive disorders are remediated, it is anticipated that patients will be more effective communicators in daily situations and will resume participation in many previously enjoyed personal, social, and professional activities, which is the ultimate goal of treatment. In addition to these body structure and function level strategies, however, clinicians also may select treatments that directly target communicative and cognitive effectiveness, participation, or both. Activity and participation level treatments may help facilitate carryover of improved linguistic and cognitive capabilities to functional communicative and cognitive effectiveness functioning (and thus be used in concert with procedures described in Chapters 9–11), may serve to "fill the gap" when underlying cognitive and/or linguistic functions are not completely restored, and can be implemented from the outset of treatment. Because these treatment activities tend to involve daily, functional communicative and cognitive behaviors, patients with neurogenic language or cognitive disorders and their caregivers may find them more intrinsically reinforcing and thus help them stay motivated to participate actively in treatment (Manochiopinig, Reed, Sheard, & Choo, 1997). Finally, because activity and participation level treatments are not necessarily specific to underlying impairments, many of the strategies are appropriate for individuals affected by aphasia, dementia, or cognitive-communicative disorders related to traumatic brain injury or right hemisphere brain damage.

Activity-Focused Treatments

The first section of this chapter reviews a number of strategies for targeting the ICF level of activity. Most of these strategies emphasize modifying the patients' communicative or cognitive behaviors, whereas others aim to enhance their communicative and cognitive effectiveness by modifying their environment, training their communication partners and caregivers, or both.

Compensatory Strategies

Instruction in the use of **compensatory strategies** is a common component of intervention for many neurogenic language and cognitive disorders. Compensatory strategies allow patients to communicate or to complete daily activities more effectively in spite of the presence of significant linguistic and/or cognitive impairments. In general, patients compensate by exploiting intact linguistic and cognitive skills to circumvent the limitations imposed by underlying impairments. Some strategies rely primarily on the patient utilizing readily available communication modalities (e.g., drawing, gesturing) or more deliberate cognitive functioning (see included DVD: Patient 6c, 6d), whereas other strategies incorporate external devices that serve to cue or replace verbal output, or to support problematic cognitive functions.

Multimodal Communication Approaches

Although a hallmark of aphasia is language impairment evident across communication modalities (i.e., speaking, listening, reading, writing, and gesturing), many patients experiencing neurogenic language or cognitive disorders will demonstrate areas of relative strength in one or more communication modalities. **Multimodal communication** approaches help patients exploit the stronger modalities to compensate for weaker ones.

Drawing. The use of drawing to compensate for linguistic impairment has intuitive appeal, as visuospatial skills often remain relatively intact following damage to the language-dominant hemisphere and most patients retain at least a basic ability to draw and interpret drawings (e.g., Sacchett & Black, 2011). Anyone who has played the popular games Pictionary or DrawSomething, however, knows that communicating complex ideas graphically can be very difficult. Nonetheless, clinicians can help patients with neurogenic language or cognitive disorders develop drawing as an effective mode of communication (see included DVD: Patients 3b, 6d).

An obvious factor influencing the potential effectiveness of drawing as a communication modality is drawing ability, which may be compromised by motor impairments affecting limb movements (e.g., hemiparesis, limb apraxia; see Chapter 5 for a description of confounding motor symptoms). Moreover, many patients with aphasia will be forced to use their non-dominant hand for drawing, which may have a significant impact on drawing speed, coordination, and legibility. Visual problems such as those reviewed in Chapters 2 and 5 also may impede drawing legibility. Accordingly, clinicians must carefully assess the patient's drawing ability (see Chapters 5 and 6) with consideration of motoric and visuospatial limitations.

If drawing appears to have communicative potential, clinicians may consider "Back to the Drawing Board" (Morgan & Helm-Estabrooks, 1987) or its more recent revision, "Communicative Drawing Program" (CDP; Helm-Estabrooks & Albert, 2004), as treatment approaches to develop basic drawing skills for communicative purposes. CDP involves ten sequential steps, beginning with activities targeting foundational conceptual skills and progressing to drawing complete scenes. The authors recommended that patients master each step (i.e., 100% accuracy) before proceeding to the next step in the program.

- **Step #1: Semantic-Conceptual Knowledge**—Given a selection of ten pictured items, the individual must identify which five items belong together (share relevant semantic features). Although the clinician selects the pictures based on common superordinate categories, this information is not made available to the individual.

- **Step #2: Knowledge of Object Color Properties**—The individual must select appropriate colored markers for nine line drawings of objects generally associated with specific colors (e.g., flag, witch's hat). They then color in the line drawing with the selected marker.
- **Step #3: Outlining Pictures of Objects With Distinct Shape Properties**—The individual uses a pen to outline (draw around the outside lines of) line-drawn pictures (e.g., church, apple).
- **Step #4: Copying Geometric Shapes**—The individual copies geometric shapes from line drawings, with instruction to match the target with respect to size, shape, and three-dimensional properties.
- **Step #5: Completing Drawings With Missing Features**—The individual identifies missing features from line drawings and then completes the drawings with his or her own pen.
- **Step #6: Drawing Characteristic Shapes from Memory**—The individual is asked to study pictures of common objects (e.g., hammer) and then to draw the item from memory once the picture has been removed from view.
- **Step #7: Drawing Objects From Stored Representations**—The individual draws items that are presented verbally or by printed word, but without a picture or drawing.
- **Step #8: Drawing Objects Within Categories**—The individual is presented with a verbal stimulus that is an exemplar (e.g., tulip) of a superordinate category (e.g., flower). The individual is then instructed to draw another exemplar of that category.
- **Step #9: Generative Drawing of Animals and Modes of Transportation**—The individual draws as many exemplars as possible from these two superordinate categories.
- **Step #10: Drawing Cartooned Scenes**—The individual is asked to study paneled cartoons and then draw the scene from memory. This step begins with single-paneled cartoons and progresses to multiple-paneled cartoons.

Once basic drawing ability has been established, patients must develop strategies for effectively using drawing as a communication modality; that is, they must be able to transfer basic drawing skills to daily communicative interactions. Clinicians may be pleasantly surprised to learn that the strategies used in Pictionary apply very well to graphic communication. Although a specific time limit is not generally imposed in typical communication interactions, communication is enhanced when message exchange occurs at a reasonable pace. Accordingly, because drawing usually requires more time than is typically needed to speak a message, patients must learn to convey their drawn messages as efficiently as possible. Figure 12-1 provides examples of inefficient and efficient drawings. Several strategies for improving efficiency of graphic communication are listed below:

- Avoid producing one drawing for each word in a sentence. Use one or two drawings of the most relevant concepts to capture the gist of the message.

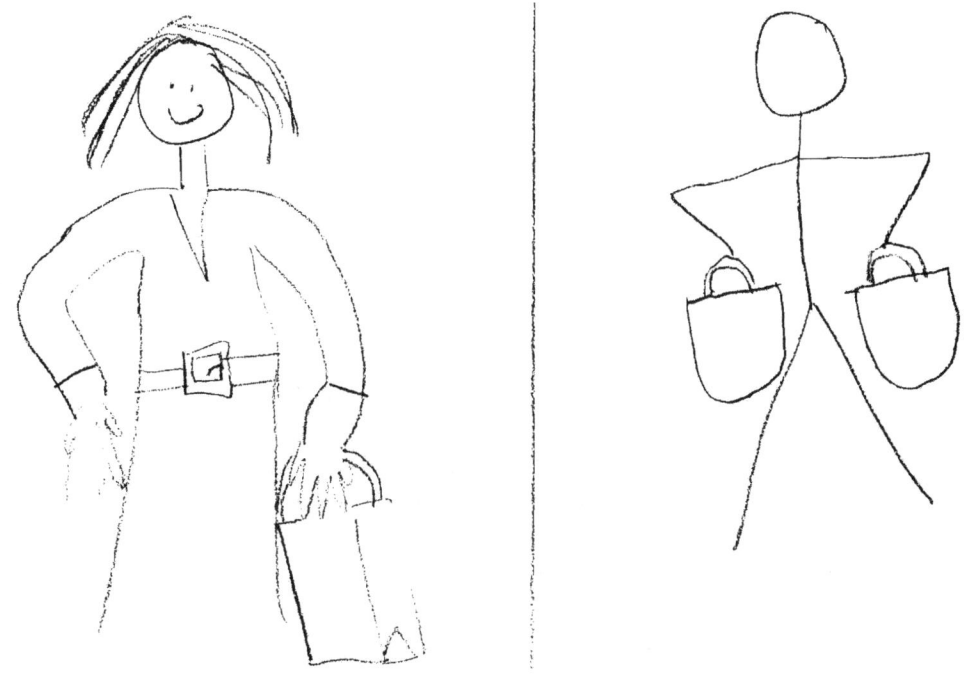

Figure 12-1. Examples of inefficient (left) and efficient (right) drawings.

- Use arrows and other icons to convey relationships among pictures.
- Avoid unnecessary detail and discontinue detailing a picture once it has been appropriately identified by the communication partner.
- Point to previous drawings rather than redrawing pictures if a concept is repeated in subsequent messages.
- Use color only if meaning is unclear without it.

As with most communication modes, graphic communication will be enhanced if the drawer is sensitive to the receiver's comprehension and can employ repair strategies. These strategies may include adding detail to help receivers differentiate similar concepts (e.g., house vs. school vs. store), or drawing additional pictures if receivers overlook or need elaboration of a key concept (e.g., adding a car between pictures if the intent is to communicate a mode of transportation). Likewise, Lyon and Helm-Estabrooks (1987) recommended training communication partners to utilize certain spoken and graphic prompts that serve to elicit these types of drawing strategies and thus enhance successful communicative interactions. Also, clinicians should keep in mind that just as drawing can aid patients' message production, it can also aid their message comprehension (Brennan, Worrall, & McKenna, 2005), and thus caregivers in addition to patients might be trained to use drawing in the same ways described for patients.

Importantly, several case and small-group studies support the use of drawing programs with patients who have severe spoken and written language production deficits (Beeson & Ramage, 2000; Sacchett, Byng, Marshall, & Pound, 1999), including those with concomitant hemiparesis (e.g., Rao, 1995) or progressive disorders (e.g., L. Murray, 1998). Moreover, drawing has the potential to facilitate verbal expression (Farias, Davis, & Harrington, 2006), further enhancing communicative success. Additional investigations with stronger research designs are needed not only to replicate and validate previous findings, but also to specify further which patients are most likely to benefit from drawing therapy and which treatment procedures result in the greatest generalization of trained drawing skills to daily communicative interactions. Whether computerized tablet devices, which allow users to draw, hold any advantage over paper-and-pencil methods should also be examined.

Gesturing. Unlike drawing, gesturing is a communication mode that is used regularly by many speakers for such purposes as clarifying meaning, adding emphasis, or even replacing speech (e.g., waving hello, pointing in response to "where" questions) (Rose, 2006). Moreover, many gestures are universally recognized by communicators of a given language or dialect (e.g., the "OK" gesture, wiping the hand across the forehead to express relief). Because patients likely used gestures to enhance communication prior to the onset of their neurogenic language or cognitive disorder, they often are willing to expand their use of gestures to further enhance communicative effectiveness (see included DVD: Patients 3b, 6a, 6d, 8g, 8h, 9b). As with drawing and writing, however, it is important to keep in mind that many patients will be attempting to use this communication mode in the presence of motor deficits affecting one or both limbs.

Although many conventional gestures exist to communicate a great variety of meanings, most patients with neurogenic language or cognitive disorders will need to develop a more elaborate gesture system to communicate the complex messages characteristic of adult life. Several gestural codes have been suggested as potentially effective communication modes for patients with neurogenic language or cognitive disorders, in particular those with severe aphasia. Although highly developed sign systems are used by deaf cultures, these systems have several disadvantages for patients with aphasia. First, many sign languages, including American Sign Language (ASL), are unique languages with word forms and syntax dissimilar from English or other spoken languages. Accordingly, it is unreasonable to expect that patients with an impaired language system will learn an entirely new language such as this, even if individual signs might be successfully acquired (S. Anderson et al., 1992; Sardina, 2010). Signed Exact English (SEE) partially addresses this problem by using ASL signs with standard English syntax. Both ASL and SEE utilize bimanual signs, however, which can be difficult for patients with hemiplegia or hemiparesis to produce. Moreover, the communicative effectiveness of ASL or SEE will be limited by the number of potential communication partners familiar with the language.

A potentially better choice, therefore, is Amer-Ind, a gestural code based on American Indian hand talk (Skelly, 1979). This system can be used with one hand and utilizes gestures that are relatively transparent (i.e., understandable to individuals unfamiliar with the code) (Campbell & Jackson, 1995; Daniloff et al., 1986). Because of these features, Amer-Ind has been more widely recommended than any other gestural system for patients with aphasia, and indeed some research supports this endorsement. For instance, several studies have reported that patients with moderate, severe, and even progressive forms of aphasia have been able to acquire, use, and, in some cases, even sequence three or more Amer-Ind signs to improve their communication success (Dowden, Marshall, & Tompkins, 1981; Heilman, Rothi, Campanella, & Wolfson, 1979; S. L. Schneider, Thompson, & Luring, 1996).

For some patients with profound deficits of language, other aspects of cognition, or both, even relatively simple gestural systems such as Amer-Ind may be inappropriate (Coelho & Duffy, 1987). These patients may instead benefit from instruction in using **pantomime**, a form of gestural communication that involves a series of relatively transparent movements that are associated with a given activity or situation. For example, to pantomime pouring a glass of milk, an individual might pretend to hold a glass in one hand while holding the other hand in an open posture and tipping that hand toward the hand "holding the glass."

The use of pantomime can be considered augmentative (see section below) as a means of supplementing speech or such gestures can be used a means of cueing spoken word retrieval (J. Marshall et al., 2012, Raymer et al., 2006; Rose & Douglas, 2002, 2006). The findings of controlled treatment studies have been mixed, with some patients demonstrating improved spoken word retrieval after pantomime-focused treatment and others improving only in their ability to use pantomime to augment speech.

One approach to training pantomime use as a communication modality is Visual Action Therapy (VAT; Helm-Estabrooks, Fitzpatrick, & Barresi, 1982; Helm-Estabrooks & Albert, 2004; Ramsberger & Helm-Estabrooks, 1989). The steps in VAT are designed to help patients first comprehend how pantomimed movements represent ideas or concepts, and then to learn to produce a set of pantomimes. The program begins with training pantomimes that involve proximal gestures (i.e., those using gross limb movements, such as waving a flag), then progresses to pantomimes that involve distal gestures (e.g., dialing a telephone), and finally progresses to pantomimes that involve oral gestures (e.g., sipping from a straw). When all three phases are mastered, Helm-Estabrooks and colleagues have recommended expanding the gesture repertoire by incorporating Amer-Ind signs. Below are the steps of the Visual Action Therapy Program (Helm-Estabrooks & Albert, 2004; Helm-Estabrooks et al., 1982):

- **Step #1: Matching Pictures and Objects**—This step is further broken down into smaller steps of placing objects on pictures, placing pictures on objects, pointing to objects when presented with the picture, and pointing to pictures when presented with the object.
- **Step #2: Object Use Training**—The individual must demonstrate the ability to use each object appropriately.
- **Step #3: Action Picture Demonstration**—The clinician selects an object and then provides the individual with an action picture incorporating that object. Then the clinician manipulates the object in the manner that is depicted on an action picture.

- **Step #4: Following Action Picture Commands**—The individual must select the appropriate object from a group of objects and manipulate it in the manner that is depicted on an action picture.
- **Step #5: Pantomimed Gesture Demonstration**—The clinician identifies an object and then models the pantomime of the gesture associated with that object.
- **Step #6: Pantomimed Gesture Recognition**—The individual must identify from a selection the object that corresponds to a pantomime produced by the clinician.
- **Step #7: Pantomimed Gesture Production**—The individual produces the appropriate pantomime when provided with the corresponding object.
- **Step #8: Representation of Hidden Objects Demonstration**—The clinician models pantomimes associated with objects that are known to the individual but out of immediate view.
- **Step #9: Production of Gestures for Hidden Objects**—The individual produces a pantomime to request an object that is known to both participants but out of immediate view.

The training protocol described by Raymer and colleagues (2006) does not emphasize the physical characteristics of the pantomime (i.e., proximal vs. distal), but instead progresses through a cueing hierarchy, similar to cueing strategies described in Chapter 9. Both approaches to training are progressive, starting with less sophisticated cues and/or responses and moving toward more sophisticated responses. Initial evidence suggests that gestural training programs may be beneficial (e.g., Daumuller & Goldenberg, 2010); additional research is needed to determine how to best promote generalization to untrained communication contexts.

Augmentative Communication

Although both graphic and gestural communication are typically "augmentative" to spoken communication, the term **augmentative or alternative communication (AAC)** is generally used to denote a communication system whereby the speaker points to or otherwise selects written words or pictured symbols to communicate meaning. AAC can facilitate communication in a number of ways. Most obviously, AAC provides a modality of expression when speech or verbal expression is limited (see included DVD: Patient 6c, 6d). Expression may be enhanced for both "online" and "offline" purposes (van de Sandt-Koenderman, 2004). Online responses are those that are composed during the actual communicative exchange. In contrast, "offline" refers to when patients with neurogenic language or cognitive disorders use these devices to prepare for future communication encounters (e.g., a repairperson coming to fix a home appliance, a telephone call to make an appointment, a parent–teacher conference) by preselecting and/or preprogramming messages. Beyond expression, however, AAC strategies can also facilitate comprehension. For instance, communication partners might augment their speech by pointing to pictures on a patient's augmentative system to emphasize key points of their message.

AAC systems range from the very simple (e.g., a single sheet of paper with the words "yes" and "no" in large print) to the very complex (e.g., computer-synthesized voice activated by eye-blink switches). The applications of AAC are much broader than neurogenic language and cognitive disorders; thus, a thorough discussion of the principles guiding the development of AAC systems is beyond the scope of this text. Instead, readers are referred to Beukelman and Mirenda (2013) for an in-depth review of AAC and its broad applications and to Koul (2011) for discussion of AAC specifically for adults with aphasia. In this chapter, we will explore some of the issues that should be considered when developing AAC systems for patients with neurogenic language and cognitive disorders and review briefly the growing literature supporting AAC in this context.

The nature of neurogenic disorders dictates that AAC systems selected for these patients should not rely heavily on linguistic processing (Lasker, 2008). For example, whereas some patients demonstrate adequate reading skills to use print (at least at the letter or word level), others may benefit from graphic symbols or photographs. Multimodal systems, such as Visual Scene Displays (VSD; Beukelman, Dietz, Hux, McKelvey, & Weissling, 2007), involve a combination of highly contextual images and text. Such interfaces reduce cognitive demands and provide a rich context that facilitates message exchange (McKelvey, Hux, Dietz, & Beukelman, 2010).

The *Multimodal Communication Screening Task for Persons With Aphasia* (MCST-A; K. Garrett & Lasker, 2005b) can be used to help identify the types of items that will be most useful, the cues that best facilitate responses, and the complexity of communicative tasks that benefit from multimodal and/or augmentative communication strategies (Lasker & Garrett, 2006). The MCST-A is composed of eight tasks that require the patient to select symbols in response to a communicative prompt provided by the examiner. The sections are as follows: (a) symbol messages to request basic needs or respond to biographical information questions; (b) combining two to three symbols; (c) categorizing; (d) using environmentally stored phrases in a specific context; (e) story telling using a descriptive scene sequence; (f) story retelling (from a model) using a descriptive scene sequence; (g) telling about locations from a map; and (h) spelling (first letter, partial word, or complete word). For each item, the examiner notes the types of cues necessary for accurate responses, such as repetition or directing the patient's attention. A summary sheet allows the examiner to compile a profile of the patient's performance, thus informing AAC planning and training. The MCST-A website (http://aac.unl.edu/screen/screen.html) further includes tools for screening visuoperception and attention (see below and Chapter 5), identifying communication needs, and characterizing the skills of conversation partners.

As noted above, clinicians also must be sensitive to the presence of deficits of visuoperception, attention, or both that will influence the size and/or placement of items (Purdy & Dietz, 2010). For instance, if a patient with aphasia has concomitant right neglect, items may need to be placed in a vertical rather than horizontal array so that the patient is able to view readily all item choices. Similarly, motor deficits such as hemiplegia or limb apraxia may limit access options, in that patients may need to access the system with their non-dominant or a weak hand. Memory and executive function abilities also must be considered, particularly in terms of the amount and organization of information to be contained within the system, and in terms of the complexity of the operational skills that will be necessary for independent system use. For example, a patient with severe cognitive and motor speech deficits related to traumatic brain injury (TBI) may be able to select items on a high-tech, dynamic screen device when provided with clinician prompting, but without guidance be unable to find these same items because of memory limitations. Finally, clinicians should be diligent in selecting age- and culturally appropriate symbols and/or photographs and should consult with patients and their caregivers regarding which words and phrases should be included within the AAC system.

A growing body of literature describes different ways individuals with aphasia and other neurogenic disorders may benefit from AAC (e.g., Hough & Johnson, 2009). Some of the earliest studies examined the use of dedicated AAC devices or specialized software programs for desktop or laptop computers. These studies demonstrated that patients with moderate to severe forms of nonfluent aphasia improved their lexical-retrieval and syntax formulation abilities via the Computer-Assisted Visual Communication system (C-VIC; Shelton, Weinrich, McCall, & Cox, 1996), Lingraphica (Aftonomos et al., 1999), or C-Speak Aphasia (Nicholas & Elliott, 1999; Nicholas, Sinotte, & Helm-Estabrooks, 2011). A more recently developed program, SentenceShaper (Linebarger & Schwartz, 2005), also has demonstrated benefit for communicative informativeness (M. Bartlett, Fink, Schwartz, & Linebarger, 2007; Fink, Bartlett, Lowery, Linebarger, & Schwartz, 2008; True, Bartlett, Fink, Linebarger, & Schwartz, 2010).

In recent years, portable and handheld devices have become more powerful, more affordable, and available to the general public through familiar retailers. Technologies such as the iPad, Kindle Fire, and smartphones are commonly used by people of all ages and are thus a minimally obtrusive technology that can be exploited for communication purposes. Importantly, a number of AAC applications are available for handheld devices that may facilitate communicative function for individuals with neurogenic language and cognitive disorders.

Some of the applications that facilitate communication are marketed broadly as productivity tools. Such applications tend to be relatively inexpensive and typically require minimal training to use. For example, **text-to-speech capability** allows individuals who can use the written modality to have spoken output. Word prediction further facilitates text to speech, as the user does not need to spell words in their entirety or with complete accuracy (Dietz et al., 2011; for an example of how word prediction software can be incorporated into an aphasia treatment, see L. Murray & Karcher, 2000). Text-messaging (texting), which does not necessarily involve speech generation, also allows users to take advantage of word prediction, making another commonly used communication modality accessible to individuals with verbal expression limitations. Applications for speech to text are also widely available to assist those with writing deficits (e.g., acquired dysgraphia).

A number of handheld applications were designed specifically with the needs of individuals with aphasia in mind. One of the first systems developed for handheld devices is the Personal Communication Assistant for Dysphasic People (PCAD; van de Sandt-Koenderman, 2004). This system included modules such as (a) hierarchically represented vocabulary; (b) digitized or synthesized speech output; (c) options allowing the patient to draw or type information into the device; and (d) phonemic cueing, in which the initial sound of a word or phrase is generated by the device. Early studies indicated that patients with aphasia could learn to operate the device and a majority of patients employed the device in daily communicative settings and activities. Successful use of PCAD was reported up to two years post-treatment. The PCAD underwent refinement and is now marketed as TouchSpeak (van de Sandt-Koenderman, Wiegers, & Hardy, 2005). Individuals with aphasia who use the TouchSpeak device reportedly do so most often in trained situations but may also incorporate the device into everyday situations (van de Sandt-Koenderman, Wiegers, Wielart, Duivenvoorden, & Ribbers, 2007).

The Lingraphica system, which began as a computer-mediated program, has also incorporated handheld applications. SmallTalk is an application that can be used as an independent system or be synchronized to the computer-based AllTalk system. Both the computer and handheld systems offer options for text- and icon-based touch screens, but only the AllTalk can be personalized. Research examining outcomes associated with these systems is limited, although a preliminary study reported by the developer suggested that individuals with Broca's or global aphasia benefitted from the Lingraphica system (Steele, 2006).

A large number of handheld applications have been developed in recent years, with more becoming available almost daily. These applications vary greatly in cost from free or nearly so to well over $100. The nature and availability of these tools changes so rapidly that a detailed review of them in a textbook is not feasible. Instead, a non-exhaustive list of handheld applications that may facilitate communication follows:

> First Ten Visual Schedule (goodkarmaapplications.com)
> Lingraphica SmallTalk (aphasia.com)
> MyVoice (myvoiceaac.com)
> Pictello (assistiveware.com)
> Predictable (tboxapps.com)
> Proloquo2go (assistiveware.com)
> SceneSpeak (goodkarmaapplications.com)
> SimplifiedTouch (simplifiedtouch.com)
> SpeakinMotion (speakinmotion.com)
> TalkTablet (gusinc.com)

At the time of this writing, the most extensive range of applications is for iPad/iPhone products, but it is anticipated that applications for other platforms will become available as the market demands. Research is needed to identify the features of applications that are most beneficial for individuals with specific linguistic and cognitive impairments, the most effective methods for training individuals to use the applications, and the outcomes associated with use of these technologies. Although we have incorporated the discussion of AAC into the discussion of activity and participation treatments, use of these systems may effect changes at other levels of the ICF as well (van de Sandt-Koenderman, 2011). Likewise, many of these applications are similar in nature, and thus similar in strengths and weaknesses, to the workbooks and computer software training programs described in Chapters 9 and 10; accordingly, clinicians should have input before patients and their caregivers purchase any of these applications.

Individualized AAC systems may play an important role in maximizing communication effectiveness for patients with neurogenic language and cognitive disorders. Additionally, many patients may benefit from impromptu augmentative communication systems. For example, patients with limited verbal expression may point to items on a menu to facilitate ordering in a restaurant. Store catalogs and newspaper inserts may be used to develop shopping lists and/or request assistance from store clerks. Importantly, all patients with aphasia, even those with mild linguistic deficits, should carry a small card listing important personal information and providing a brief description of aphasia so that if they find themselves in an emergency, this card can be used to augment their spoken output, which will no doubt be affected negatively by the stress of the situation (Wallace & Bradshaw, 2011). Conveniently, these types of cards can be obtained for free from the National Aphasia Association (www.aphasia.org). Creative clinicians will be on the alert for other readily available and low-cost products and materials that can augment the communication abilities of the adult with a neurogenic language or cognitive disorder.

Additional Issues

Whereas drawing, gesturing, or using AAC may serve as the principal communication mode for some patients with neurogenic language disorders, even patients whose primary output modality is speech may effectively exploit these other modalities. In fact, there is evidence that pairing another modality with speech may actually enhance verbal output (e.g., Faria et al., 2006; Hanlon, Brown, & Gerstman, 1990; Lyon & Helm-Estabrooks, 1987). Nonetheless, clinicians should be sensitive to the fact that some patients, their caregivers, or both may be reluctant to adopt multimodality and/or AAC strategies. Some may perceive drawing or gesturing to be juvenile or judge their own drawing ability to be inadequate. Others may be embarrassed by their need for gesturing or pointing to pictures to assist their comprehension or expression abilities, whereas others may perceive that accepting use of AAC is the same as accepting that the patient will never talk (Beukelman & Mirenda, 2013; Weissling & Prentice, 2010). In these situations, clinicians must help patients and caregivers appreciate that the benefits of enhanced communication usually outweigh the potential disadvantages. Allowing multiple opportunities for patients to explore various forms of multimodal communication strategies may give patients a greater sense of control of their communication options, which may ultimately lead to better outcomes (Pattee, Von Berg, & Ghezzi, 2006).

A valuable feature of multimodality approaches is that they can be introduced at nearly any point in recovery. Many patients may benefit from using gestures or AAC very early post onset, when deficits tend to be most severe. Acceptance of multiple modalities at this stage may be enhanced because patients and their family members may perceive the alternate modality as a temporary strategy that will be discontinued when patients regain their ability to understand and/or use verbal communication. During the chronic stage of the neurogenic language disorder is another time when patients may be more willing to explore alternative modes of communication. Patients and caregivers who have lived with a neurogenic language or cognitive disorder for a more extensive time period are more likely to have a realistic understanding of the nature of language and cognitive impairments and the impact of these impairments on daily communication. They also may be more cognizant of the chronicity of the disorder, often having undergone many hours of rehabilitation yet still experiencing communication difficulties. Additionally, patients and caregivers living with chronic neurogenic language or cognitive disorders may have discovered for themselves the benefits of multimodal communication but are in need of instruction in effective use of these strategies. Finally, the use of multimodal strategies in the context of progressive disorders should not be overlooked (see included DVD: Patient 6c, 6d), with empirical support for their use with several neurogenic patient populations (Fried-Oken, 2008; L. Murray, 1998; Pattee, Von Berg, & Ghezzi, 2006).

Funding Treatment After the Acute Phase of Recovery

It was once commonly believed that little could be done to help individuals with residual impairments months to years after onset of a neurogenic language or cognitive disorder. Thus, third-party payers such as Medicare and private insurance traditionally have been unwilling to fund speech-language therapy once a condition is considered chronic (i.e., three to six months postonset). If necessary, clinicians may advocate for the individual's right to appropriate services, regardless of time postonset, keeping in mind that the vast majority of studies documenting the efficacy of neurogenic language and cognitive treatments have involved patients with chronic disorders (i.e., greater than six months postonset). If third-party funding cannot be secured, some individuals with neurogenic language or cognitive disorders may choose to fund their own services, particularly if they perceive that treatment will significantly impact their functional communication and participation in desired activities.

Cognitive Strategies

A number of strategies are available that can be taught to patients with neurogenic language and cognitive disorders to augment direct retraining of their cognitive abilities or to help them compensate for cognitive impairments that do not appear amenable to direct retraining. At least some of these strategies are similar to those already described with respect to communication. For instance, utilizing multimodality communication can benefit patients with deficits of attention, memory, or executive functioning (e.g., organization deficits). As an example, these patients might be taught to take notes during daily activities (e.g., telephone conversations, business meetings) as a strategy to help them attend throughout the activity, recall information being conveyed during the activity, or outline or organize information pertaining to the activity.

Other cognitive strategies differ from communication strategies in that they involve teaching patients to utilize their linguistic skills to guide or support their compromised cognitive abilities. In particular, verbal mediation has proven to be an effective strategy to help patients compensate for a number of cognitive impairments, including attention, memory, and executive function deficits (Cicerone & Giacino, 1992; Spikman et al., 2009). For example, Ylvisaker and Feeney (1998) described a case study of a patient with TBI who was taught to utilize successfully the self-cue of "Gotta check it out, man" (p. 18). This patient used this verbal cue to assist himself in making plans and decisions throughout his daily schedule and social interactions, which in turn helped him to reduce confusion and his inappropriate responses to that confusion (i.e., verbal aggression and social withdrawal). He was taught to use the self-cue by having those with whom he interacted remind him to "check it out" before he completed a task or gave a response, or alternately after he completed a task or response, ask him whether or not he had "checked it out" with his caregivers or certain peers. The patient also was provided with the opportunity to review periodically videotaped samples of himself completing everyday tasks and in social interactions to determine if he was appropriately utilizing this verbal mediation strategy.

Cognitive strategies also are available for particular cognitive deficits (Ptak et al., 2010; Sohlberg & Mateer, 2001; Sohlberg & Turkstra, 2011; Tompkins, 1995). For memory problems, there are several internal or covert strategies, such as mental rehearsal, covert self-instruction, imagery, and elaboration (see Chapter 10 for a discussion of these strategies); more overt memory strategies train patients to ask for information to be repeated or restated, or to repeat aloud information several times as part of the rehearsal process (note that these strategies would also benefit patients with auditory comprehension problems). Patients with fatigue or sustained attention problems might benefit from pacing strategies. These include learning to take rest breaks on a regular basis throughout the day at predetermined time intervals (e.g., every 20 minutes) or after completing a certain amount or set number of activities (e.g., after writing one paragraph, after completing morning hygiene activities). Another form of pacing involves teaching patients to identify what times of the day are most or least productive for them, and then to adjust their daily schedules accordingly. For instance, a patient with TBI returning to a university might use the strategy of scheduling classes in the morning and study sessions in the late afternoon because he is most fatigued and easily distracted in the early afternoon after lunch and in the evening. Finally, a few strategies for addressing neglect include teaching patients the following: (a) to sit with their trunks turned to their neglected side, (b) to select and place anchors on their neglected side prior to completing a task, and (c) to use their neglected hand to complete tasks when possible.

Clinicians should keep in mind that extensive practice is necessary to help patients automate strategy use. Therefore, strategy training should begin as early as possible, even while patients are receiving direct and intensive cognitive retraining. That is, it might be tempting to incorporate strategy training only after patients have plateaued in treatment activities designed to stimulate or re-establish cognitive functioning. It is more useful, however, to consider strategy training a complement to these types of treatment activities, as strategies offer patients a means by which to compensate for cognitive deficits that are still being directly retrained.

External Devices

Numerous external devices are available to help patients compensate for their linguistic and/or cognitive impairments (see Table 12-1). As with AAC, external aids can vary from simple, low-technology sticky notes to sophisticated, high-technology handheld devices (Ptak et al., 2010; Sohlberg, 2011). They also can vary in that some devices are helpful in a variety of settings (e.g., computerized personal planner), whereas others provide assistance while completing only certain tasks (e.g., key finder). Given the number of device options available, selection of which aids are most appropriate for a given patient should be based on factors such as the following:

- The patient's linguistic abilities (e.g., if a patient is unable to read, devices such as written to-do lists would be inappropriate)
- The patient's cognitive abilities (e.g., if a patient has severely impaired learning abilities, devices that require multiple steps to use may be inappropriate)
- The patient's motor abilities (e.g., if a patient has impaired fine motor skills, a device such as a smartphone that requires precise, complex manual manipulations would be inappropriate)
- The patient's sensory and perceptual skills (e.g., a patient with a concomitant hearing loss may have difficulty using devices that provide only auditory cues or feedback)
- Cost, particularly if the patient must pay for the device(s) out-of-pocket
- Strategies or devices that the patient used premorbidly, and thus may already be familiar with and already own
- The patient's preference, as when the patient likes the device, he or she will be more motivated to use the device
- Caregivers' preference, as when they like the device, they will be more likely to encourage the patient to use it, and thus help with generalization and maintenance of device use
- The patient's daily needs (e.g., one external memory device may be suitable for use in the patient's home, but another external memory device is needed when the patient is driving)
- Availability of support (e.g., family member, co-worker) if the patient is unable to independently program the device or trouble-shoot if the device is not working properly

Additionally, it is particularly important for clinicians to determine whether patients present with anosognosia, or impaired awareness of their deficits. External devices are

TABLE 12-1
Examples of External Devices

DEVICE	POTENTIAL USES
Calendar/appointment book	• Record important dates and appointments to aid memory, organization, and planning • Orient to day, week, month, and year
To-do list	• Record daily or weekly chores or schedule to aid memory, organization, and planning • Rank items in chronological order or in order of importance • Place in each room of the house to aid recall of daily activities to be completed in that room (e.g., brush teeth, wash face, shave, etc., on list placed on bathroom mirror)
Photograph album (hard copy and/or electronic version)	• Include labeled pictures and labels of important people and events to aid memory and language abilities, such as word finding or story telling
Memory or communication book/wallet/box	• Include labeled pictures, short poems, small items, maps, books/wallets/boxes, etc., to aid memory, attention, word finding, and conversational skills
Electronic speller	• Aids in correcting plausible spelling errors
"Windowed" cover sheet	• Covers all other words or lines of text on a page to reduce visual distractions and thus aid reading
Daily/weekly pillbox	• Aids in recall for taking medications
Digital camera/smartphone	• Take pictures of people, events, objects, etc., to aid recall of or communication about daily activities
Visual cues	
Labels/flags	• Place on appliances to aid recall of turning appliance on/off • Place on cupboards/drawers/closets to aid recall of what is in them or to aid word retrieval
Instructions	• Place list of simple instructions (laminated will last longer) on appliances or other electronic devices (e.g., DVD player) used on a regular basis to aid recall of how to use device or problem-solving if device is not working
Alarms (kitchen timers, alarm clocks, alarm watches, electronic/computerized planners, smartphones)	• Set alarms to remind about when tasks should be initiated and/or completed to aid memory, initiation, and planning
Ear plugs/headset	• Aid in reducing auditory distractions and thus facilitate attention
Electronic and computerized planner/smartphone	• Program important dates and appointments to aid memory, initiation, organization, and planning • Program names, contact information, birthdates, and other important information pertaining to family, friends, business associates, etc., to aid memory and word finding
Pagers/cell and smartphones	• Aid in recall, initiation, and completion of daily activities

typically inappropriate for patients with poor deficit awareness, as such individuals will not recognize the need for the device and consequently will lack the motivation to use the device (Ownsworth & McFarland, 1999; Ptak et al., 2010; Svoboda & Richards, 2009).

Not only are there many devices from which to choose, there also are several options in terms of how these devices can be used, and thus, how patients can be trained. For example, the goal of training may be that (a) patients will be responsible for using the device independently, (b) caregivers will assist patients with device use, or (c) caregivers will be responsible for implementing device use. Some patients with severe memory and/or executive function impairments are often unable to use external devices independently because they forget to use the device, lose the device, or cannot problem-solve to determine under what circumstances they will need to use the device (Ptak et al., 2010). Consequently, for these patients, training will focus on teaching the caregivers when and how to use the device to facilitate the patients' cognitive and/or linguistic abilities. Generally, training the use of an external device will involve treatment sessions focused on teaching patients and/or caregivers how to use the device (e.g., steps necessary to program and consequently access information in a pocket-sized computerized planner) and when (e.g., in what physical and social settings will device use be necessary and appropriate), as well as sessions focused on practice with the device in a variety of situations so as to foster independent and maintained device use outside of the therapy room (Sohlberg, 2011). For more specific descriptions of training procedures, see DePompei et al. (2008), Sohlberg and Turkstra (2011), and Svoboda and Richards (2009) (see included DVD: Patient 2b, 2c, 6c).

External devices are commonly used in clinical practice, and a growing research literature supports their use to help patients compensate for impaired linguistic and/or cognitive abilities (DePompei et al., 2008; LoPresti et al., 2008; Ptak et al., 2010; Shum, et al., 2011; Svoboda & Richards, 2009; Svoboda, Richards, Polsinelli, & Guger, 2010). One device that has been the focus of several investigations is the Neuropage system (Evans, Emslie, & Wilson, 1998; Fish et al., 2009; Martin-Saez et al., 2011; T. Teasdale et al., 2009; B. Wilson, Emslie, Quirk, & Evans, 2001; B. Wilson, Evans, Emslie, & Malinek, 1997). Neuropage (available as PageMinder in North America) consists of both computer and paging devices. Reminders of a given patient's needs are entered into the computer and uploaded to the paging company at appropriate times to send those reminders to the patient's pager. The pager is equipped with an auditory or vibratory alarm to notify patients that they need to look to see what reminder has been sent; more recently, Neuropage has been adapted so that patients may opt to have reminders sent to their cell phone versus a pager. Several studies have shown that patients of varying age, etiology (i.e., TBI, stroke, progressive neurological disease), and degree of cognitive impairment may benefit from this or similar paging systems. Importantly, these benefits have included greater levels of independence while completing daily activities such as using public transportation, taking medications, and carrying out self-care and hygiene activities. Furthermore, some patients have been able to maintain their improvements even when they are no longer using the pager or receiving the reminders.

This device has not proven helpful, however, for patients with poor insight who did not understand why they needed the device and thus were reluctant to utilize the system. Similar benefits also have been reported when patients with severe memory disorders were trained to use a Sony IC Recorder (ICD-50), a small, portable electronic device that can present approximately 300 spoken messages at preprogrammed times on a daily or weekly basis (Yasuda et al., 2002). Because the ICD-50 provides spoken cues, it is appropriate for patients who have reading or visual impairments that can interfere with their ability to read pager messages. The text-messaging feature of standard cell phones can be exploited in a similar fashion as described for Neuropage (e.g., Culley & Evans, 2010). Many smartphones have text-to-speech functions that can provide spoken reminders for patients with reading or visual impairments. Indeed, the technologies available to support these types of alerts change rapidly, but the principles guiding their use should generalize across devices.

Another device that has been used frequently in both clinical and research settings is a memory or communication book, which also can be provided in alternate forms such as a memory or communication wallet or box (Bourgeois, 2007; Ptak et al., 2010). A typical memory or communication book will contain sentence and picture stimuli that represent events, people, pets, hobbies, and places that are important to the patient (see included DVD: Patient 8l). Other pages to incorporate into the book include a calendar (e.g., weekly, monthly), map (e.g., city, state, and/or country; [see included DVD: Patient 6c]), and blank pages on which patients and/or caregivers can record daily activities (see Figure 12-2). When these books are being used primarily to assist communication abilities, pages that list the alphabet and numbers also are often appropriate. All stimuli are placed into a three-ring binder with page protectors and tabs to divide the book into information categories (e.g., family, hobbies, "my past").

Steps to creating a memory book include first interviewing patients and caregivers (i.e., family as well as other health-care providers, such as therapists, nursing assistants, etc.) to determine what information should be included and how best to organize that information. Next, to make the actual book, the clinician must consider that patient's motoric, sensory, cognitive, and linguistic abilities to determine the size of the book (e.g., a small, wallet-sized book may be more appropriate for a patient who is mobile and does not want to carry around a large, cumbersome binder), the size of the pictures and written stimuli (e.g., for patients with visual impairments, large font, enlarged pictures, and/or line drawings are most appropriate), the complexity of written stimuli (e.g., for patients with aphasia and/or dementia, single words or short phrases with simple grammar are often most appropriate), and the amount of information to be included (e.g., patients with memory and/or attention impairments may be unable to learn what information is in their book and where that information is located within their book if the book contains too much information or too many information categories or pages).

The next step is to train patients and/or caregivers how and when to use the book. First, patients and caregivers should be oriented to what information has been included and where that information is located within the book. Second, patients and caregivers should be shown how to utilize the information. For example, patients with aphasia

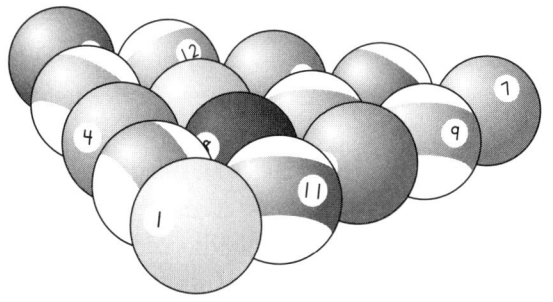

I was a competitive billiards player. I won the regional championship in 1978.

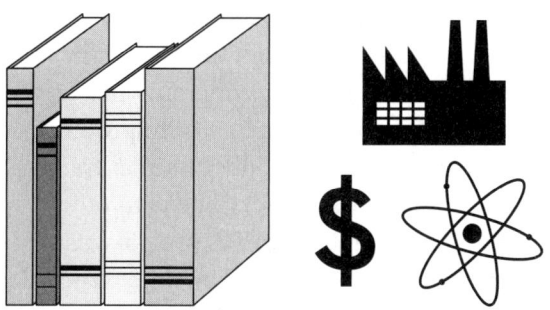

I like to read biographies of important figures in industry, banking, and science.

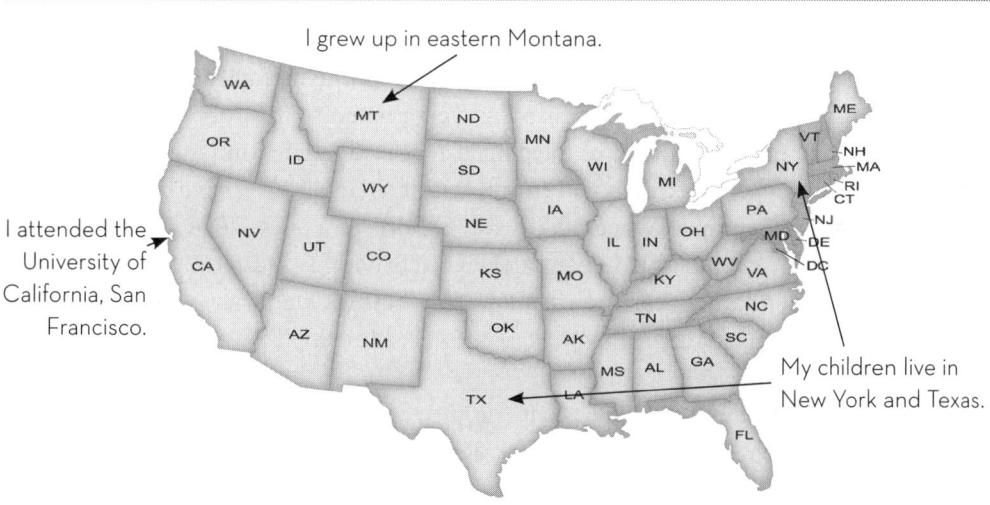

Figure 12-2. Sample Memory Book pages.

should be shown how the book can help them with their word-retrieval difficulties. Similarly, patients with TBI, right hemisphere brain damage (RHD), or mild dementia should be shown how to use the book to compensate for their short- and long-term memory problems. For patients with severe linguistic and/or cognitive deficits, training will focus more on the caregivers so that they can learn how to use the book to facilitate conversations with the patients (e.g., avoid quizzing and grilling about information in the book). When the goal of training is to facilitate the patient's independent use of the memory or communication book, clinicians must assure that sufficient practice sessions are provided, and must additionally incorporate a variety of activities and communication partners into these practice sessions so as to encourage device use in a variety of settings (see included DVD: Patient 8l).

Bourgeois and colleagues (Bourgeois, 1992; Bourgeois, Dijkstra, Burgio, & Allen-Burge, 2001; Bougeois et al., 2003; Hoerster, Hickey, & Bourgeois, 2001) as well as other researchers (Andrews-Salvia, Roy, & Cameron, 2003; Mahendra, Scullion, Hamerschlag, 2011; Schmitter-Edgecombe et al., 2008) have conducted a series of studies supporting the use of memory books, wallets, and boxes with patients who have varying types and severities of dementia. Positive outcomes include increases in the frequency and quality of dementia patients' daily social interactions, improvements in the informativeness of patients' verbal output, and decreases in patients' depression symptoms and repetitive behaviors (e.g., perseverative questions or comments). Importantly, improvements have been observed even when caregivers were provided with only minimal training. Other researchers have evaluated the effects of providing memory books to other patient populations, such as those with memory problems related to TBI or stroke (Campbell, Wilson, McCann, Kernahan, & Rogers, 2007; McKerracher, Powell, & Oyebode, 2005; Ownsworth & McFarland, 1999; Squires, Hunkin, & Parkin, 1996). The results of these studies indicate that when these patients were provided with adequate training and support regarding device use, gains in their daily communication, memory, attention, and executive function abilities (e.g., organization, deficit awareness), as well as their emotional well-being (e.g., decreased distress related to memory problems), were achieved. Similar positive outcomes have been reported when computerized memory "books," such as pocket-sized personal computers or smartphones, have been used with patients with TBI (Gentry, Wallace, Kvarfordt, & Bodisch Lynch, 2008; Svoboda et al., 2010; P. Wright et al., 2001) or dementia (DeLeo, Brivio, & Sautter, 2011; Meiland et al., 2012), and when larger tabletop displays (e.g., TalkingMats) have been used with patients with dementia (Murphy, Gray, & Cox, 2007; Murphy, Tester, Hubbard, Downs, & MacDonald, 2005).

In summary, research indicates that the provision of external devices represents an effective approach for compensating for acquired linguistic and/or cognitive deficits. Further research remains necessary, however, to help determine (a) which devices might be most appropriate for which patients or symptoms, (b) long-term effects of device use (e.g., can improvements be maintained following withdrawal of the device or withdrawal of training with the device?), and (c) which methods (e.g., errorful vs. errorless learning; see Chapter 10) are most efficient for training device use.

Practicing Compensatory Strategies

Once effective compensatory strategies are identified, clinicians should structure treatment to allow patients with neurogenic language or cognitive disorders to practice using their strategies during interactions and activities that mimic typical daily situations. Such practice provides patients with an opportunity to explore which strategies are best applied under which circumstances, as well as to develop confidence and, hopefully, automaticity in using the strategies for functional communication and daily activities.

Strategy and External Device Training. Carryover and maintenance of strategy or external device use to untrained contexts is unlikely if clinicians do not properly teach patients how to use the strategy or device. Research indicates that successful strategy and external device use is most likely when training stresses the following (Mateer, 2009; O'Connell, Mateer, & Kerns, 2003; Singer & Bashir, 1999; Sohlberg et al., 2007; Svoboda et al., 2010): (a) developing the patient's motivation to use the strategy or device and, relatedly, caregivers' motivation or approval of the strategy so that they will encourage the patient's strategy use in settings outside of the therapy room; (b) ensuring that the patient knows how and when to use the strategy or device; and (c) providing intensive and extensive practice (e.g., as long as two years has been recommended in some cases). Clinicians should keep in mind that the following procedures should also be adhered to when training caregivers on the use of strategies (see Conversation Partner section of this chapter).

A few procedures can be implemented to ensure adequate motivation to use the strategy or device (DePompei et al., 2008; Sohlberg & Turkstra, 2011; Tompkins, 1995). First, patients and caregivers should be allowed to participate in selecting possible strategies and devices. To help them make their choice, patients might try using a number of strategies, and then the patient, caregiver, and clinician can discuss which one or ones they felt were most helpful. Alternately, the clinician, patient, and caregiver might interview other patients already using a strategy or device regarding their perceptions of strategy or device benefits. Second, there should be some discussion about how prevalent strategy and device use is, even among people who do not have neurogenic language or cognitive disorders. Such a discussion may help allay fears of social stigma or concern that strategy or device use is a sign of weakness or giving up on communicative or cognitive recovery.

The next treatment step involves teaching patients how to execute the strategy or use the external device (see included DVD: Patient 2b, 2c). This can be achieved through activities such as clinician- or peer-modeling, extensive hands-on patient practice to help automate strategy or device use, and review of video- or audiotaped samples of the patient's performance when using (as well as not using) the strategy or device, to further the patient's understanding of the benefits of the strategy or device (O'Connell et al., 2003; Sohlberg & Turkstra, 2011; Tompkins, 1995). Clinicians should keep in mind that because use of many strategies and devices involves several abilities or steps, a task analysis may be necessary to determine how to break down strategy or device use into smaller and distinct task components (Sohlberg & Turkstra, 2011; Svoboda et al., 2010). Treatment then proceeds by training the first subcomponents and adding subsequent steps when the patient has mastered the initial steps. For example, the initial steps for training use of an electronic planner might include establishing where the planner will be kept (e.g., shirt pocket, purse, pants pocket), learning how to turn the device on and off, and finding the calendar display on the device. Later training steps might include programming in upcoming events and setting the alarm so that the patient can receive an auditory reminder about these events.

To ensure transfer and maintenance of strategy or device use, training should include having the patient identify situations or activities in which the strategy or device would and would not be appropriate (Sohlberg & Turkstra, 2011; Tompkins, 1995); this will help foster the patient's ability to predict what task or situations will necessitate strategy or external device use. Additionally, involving caregivers (e.g., family, peers, other medical team members) in treatment sessions will provide patients with practice in variable contexts, and encourage caregivers' understanding and reinforcement of the patients' strategy or device use.

For patients with severe cognitive deficits, device or strategy use might be trained using the errorless learning (see included DVD: Patient 2b, 2c), spaced retrieval, or vanishing cues techniques described in Chapter 10 (e.g., Svoboda et al., 2010). Because skills acquired via these training procedures are not typically expected to generalize (i.e., they result in primarily task-specific learning), this approach is most appropriate when patients will need the strategy or device for only a small set of activities or contexts (e.g., uses a watch alarm as a reminder for taking medication only). With severely impaired patients, it also is often necessary to make caregivers responsible for prompting patients to use their strategy or device, as these patients often lack the executive skills (e.g., self-monitoring, problem-solving, initiation) essential to independent strategy or device implementation.

Promoting Aphasics' Communicative Effectiveness. *Promoting Aphasics' Communicative Effectiveness* (PACE; G. Davis & Wilcox, 1985; G. Davis, 2005) is a clinical protocol that provides practice for communication strategies. The goal of PACE is to structure treatment so that the communication interactions share characteristics with customary daily communication (see included DVD: Patient 6d). For example, the classic PACE activity involves using cards with information printed on one side placed face down on the table. The content of the cards is unknown to *both* the clinician and the patient. The clinician and the patient take turns selecting a card and attempting to communicate the content of the card to the other person. Similar PACE activities can be incorporated into a variety of similar task scenarios (e.g., role playing, barrier tasks), as well.

Four principles of PACE are applied during treatment interactions. The first principle is equal participation: Taking turns as sender and receiver of messages is thought to be similar to the turn taking typical in conversational interactions. Another benefit of equal participation is that the "power" of the communicative interaction is shared more evenly between the participants (i.e., clinician and patient) than is characteristic of most therapy interactions.

The second principle is that there is an exchange of new information between the participants. In many typical therapy activities, clinicians already know the information patients are trying to convey and thus are in a position to evaluate the "correctness" of patients' communication attempts. Further, when one communication partner (usually the clinician) can predict what the other is trying to convey, the validity of the communication interaction is diminished. By practicing barrier activities (see Chapter 9) and using picture cards or other stimuli that are unknown to the clinician, the patient, or both, the information being communicated will be new or, at least, indefinite to both participants. Structuring the activity so that clinicians are truly unaware of card content can be a challenge for clinicians, as typically they have to supply the stimuli. Nonetheless, if the selection of cards is large enough and well shuffled, there is less risk that clinicians will be able to guess what is being communicated based on familiarity with the stimuli. Alternately, clinicians might elicit the assistance of caregivers in providing stimuli (e.g., family photographs) so that they are truly naïve about at least some of the treatment stimuli.

The third, and arguably most important, principle of PACE interactions is that both clinicians and patients are free to use any mode available to communicate the message. Clinicians do not direct patients to use a particular mode, even if one or two specific modes (e.g., drawing and gesturing) were previously practiced during therapy drills and determined effective. Instead, clinicians may model the use of potentially effective modes when it is their turn to send a message. This principle highlights the emphasis on effective communication, rather than skill in using a specific communicative strategy.

The final principle of PACE is that "feedback" occurs naturally as listeners indicate their understanding of the message. This feature of PACE activities is significantly different from most impairment-level treatments, during which clinicians typically provide feedback regarding specific aspects of the patients' responses (e.g., linguistic accuracy, promptness), provide cues for more "accurate" responses, or both. Once again, because in PACE, clinicians are not in the authoritative role of determining the quality of patients' communicative attempts, the power in treatment interactions is more balanced.

Although PACE activities are not perfect simulations of natural conversation, they do provide an opportunity for patients with neurogenic language or cognitive disorders to apply compensatory strategies in a more natural communicative interaction. Such exchanges afford practice of both comprehension and expression strategies (Kurland et al., 2010; Marini, Caltagirone, Pasqualetti, & Carlomango, 2007). These activities also provide an opportunity for patients to explore metacommunicative and pragmatic aspects of interactions, such as recognizing communication breakdowns and using repair strategies (Davis, 2005, 2007). The principles of PACE may be incorporated into most therapeutic interactions to facilitate generalization of compensatory strategies and external devices into functional daily communication.

The effectiveness of PACE or of treatment protocols that incorporate PACE principles has been evaluated in several aphasia treatment studies (e.g., Kempler & Goral, 2011; Li, Kitselman, Dusatko, & Spinelli, 1988; Maher et al., 2006; L. Murray, 1998). The results of these investigations consistently indicate that this treatment approach positively affects the communicative abilities of patients with aphasia, particularly in terms of their communicative flexibility (i.e., they use a greater variety of communication modalities) and success (i.e., regardless of whether linguistic accuracy improved, communication partners were able to understand and respond to more of the patients' communication attempts). Although this approach clearly has clinical applications for other neurogenic language disorders (e.g., pragmatic difficulties of patients with TBI or RHD), treatment research involving patient populations other than those with aphasia has yet to be conducted.

Group Treatment

There is little question that patients with neurogenic language or cognitive disorders benefit from one-on-one interactions with a speech-language pathologist. Individual treatment sessions provide an opportunity for clinicians and patients to focus on specific communicative or cognitive skills in a relatively risk-free context. Group treatment, however, offers several advantages that are not easily achieved by individual treatment (Downs & Bowers, 2008; Elman, 2007). For example, given increasing demands on health-care funding (see Chapter 13) and clinicians' time, group treatment represents a cost-effective therapy approach. Group treatment provides an opportunity for patients to communicate with and receive feedback from non-professionals in a supportive atmosphere. Not only is the clinician available for support, but so are the other group members who are experiencing similar communicative and/or cognitive challenges. Patients participating in group treatment also have the opportunity to observe their peers' use of compensatory strategies and general progress over time, which may provide an avenue for insightful assessment of their own communicative or cognitive strategies and recovery, respectively. A growing body of evidence supports the use of group treatment for a variety of patient populations, reporting (in addition to improvements in cognitive or communicative functioning) benefits such as increased socialization, decreased depression, and improved life satisfaction (Cicerone, Mott, Azulay, & Friel, 2004; M. Davis, Guyker, & Persky, 2012; Goff, Hinckley, & Wingo, 2011; Huckans et al., 2010; E. Kim et al., 2006; Lin, Dai, & Huang, 2003; Rath et al., 2003; A. Ross, Winslow, & Marchant, 2006; Simmons-Mackie & Elman, 2011; Vickers, 2010). Accordingly, clinicians will want to be familiar with some of the unique aspects of this intervention approach.

Selecting Group Members

Several factors have been suggested as entry criteria for group membership (R. Marshall, 2007). Some groups might be organized according to severity of linguistic or cognitive impairment or personality (Bernstein-Ellis & Elman, 2007) or stage of recovery (Gillis, 2007). Groups organized in this way may be particularly useful if the clinician intends to use group treatment to address specific communicative or cognitive strategies. Because group treatment relies heavily on conversation among participants, designing groups with related interests also may facilitate quality interactions. Because it may be difficult to determine the interests of patients before the groups are formed, a simple way to address this issue is to group members by age, as contemporaries often share similar historical knowledge as well as current life issues (e.g., raising a family, job concerns, retirement). Of course, practical concerns such as availability of transportation, jobs, and family responsibilities may also serve to establish group membership. It is recommended that groups be limited to 5 to 10 members, as larger groups may not allow ample opportunity for every member to participate (Bernstein-Ellis & Elman, 2007).

Group Process

A strength of group treatment is that it can easily be adapted to meet the needs of almost any group of patients with neurogenic language or cognitive disorders. For example, group sessions may be scheduled daily, weekly, or at longer intervals and may vary in duration (e.g., 60 vs. 90 minutes), depending primarily on the treatment setting and each individual participant's goals. Similarly, the group process or function will arise from the group's goals. For instance, groups to address specific communicative or cognitive strategies will likely include more structure and more direct clinician support. Such group sessions may include activities similar to what have been described for individual treatment sessions, with the modification that all group members may serve as the "speakers" and the "listeners" during the activities. Other groups focusing on realistic practice and generalization of communicative or cognitive strategies may be conversation-oriented or incorporate completion of real-world activities (e.g., a group outing to a concert, mock job interviews); given the nature of the activities in these groups, the clinician's role may differ significantly from what is typical of individual treatment sessions (Ewing, 2007).

Bernstein-Ellis and Elman (2007) described group treatment strategies that may address group goals. Because group members may come to rely on the clinician to direct group interactions, it may be helpful to devise strategies that allow group members to assume leadership roles. For example, group members might take turns serving as facilitator for a given conversation or activity. Alternatively, members might take turns within a single conversation or activity, prompting participation from other members at the end of their conversation or activity turn. As the group process becomes more established, group members themselves can be responsible for monitoring participation by all members and planning group activities. For example, group members might facilitate communication in much the same way that the clinician may have during the initial stages of treatment, by encouraging multimodality communication, reminding members about trained strategies (e.g., word-retrieval or memory techniques), and perhaps even cueing other group members to facilitate communication or activity completion. Group members may also provide feedback to participants who tend to dominate the conversation or activity or who are unsupportive of the group goals.

If the group chooses to explore activities other than conversation, a variety of other activities are easily incorporated into a group treatment setting (Bourgeois & Hickey, 2009; A. Holland & Beeson, 1999; Lin et al., 2003). For example, traditional PACE activities such as those described previously in this chapter can be implemented in a small group. Clinicians may find it useful to have a variety of PACE materials available so that the activities can be carried out in pairs or in larger groups. Because group treatment sessions provide a safe environment in which to practice communicative and cognitive strategies, clinicians may wish to incorporate role-plays and scenarios to simulate real-life situations. For patients practicing communicative strategies, group members may find it helpful to develop scripts for specific communication situations (e.g., refusing phone solicitation) and then practice those scripts in role-plays (akin to the conversational script training described in Chapter 9). Script development may also be useful for group members practicing executive function strategies, such as those to facilitate problem solving, planning, or organization. Group participants should be encouraged to identify relevant role-plays, scenarios, or other stimuli, and to give feedback to group members as they apply communicative and cognitive strategies during these activities.

Some real-life activities can be incorporated into group sessions without the need for simulation. For instance, card and board games are a common recreational activity for which patients with neurogenic language or cognitive disorders may wish to develop or maintain communicative and cognitive strategies. It is recommended that games requiring the exchange of ideas or information (e.g., bridge, Pictionary, charades) be selected over those that are inherently less communicative (e.g., rummy, Yahtzee, dominoes, Old Maid) when group treatment goals are more focused on communication (Holland & Beeson, 1999). Alternately, if the goal of the group activity is to allow practice of cognitive strategies such as use of memory or problem-solving techniques, these other games may still be appropriate (K. Johnson & Bourgeois, 1998). Reminiscence activities also are popular in both cognitive and communicative therapy groups (M. Davis et al., 2012; Kim et al., 2006). These activities usually involve reviewing materials such as old photographs, songs, newspapers, or magazines to encourage group participants to share their memories of typically distant past experiences.

Does Group Treatment Pay?

One of the potential advantages of group treatment is reduced cost. That is, the cost of one hour of the therapist's time could theoretically be shared by all members of the group. Imagine the SLP charges $110 per hour for individual therapy and $25 per hour for group therapy. If the group has at least five individuals, the therapist will earn no less for the group session than for an individual session, yet each of the group participants will pay less than 25% of what they would pay for an individual session. But what if one or more of the patients receiving group treatment have Medicare as their funding source (see Chapter 13)? Medicare's reimbursement rate for group speech-language treatment is roughly 30% of the reimbursement for individual treatment (ASHA, 2012a). Therefore, the SLP will almost "break even" as long as the group has at least three participants. Medicare and other insurance companies may set specific limits on how many individuals can be billed for the same group treatment session. Medicare, for example, specifies that group treatment can include up to four patients. In essence, the reimbursement rate in combination with any "maximums" set by the insurance company will determine whether group treatment "pays" from the perspective of the SLP. For patients, the value of group treatment will almost certainly be determined by whether it helps them meet their goals.

Considerations for Specific Patient Groups

A key feature of activity- and participation-level treatments is that their application is not dependent on specific underlying impairments. However, treatment groups made up of patients experiencing particular impairments may have unique goals or group processes, even if the activities addressing the goals are quite similar across treatment groups.

Aphasia Groups. Although patients with cognitive-communicative disorders due to dementia and TBI may experience auditory comprehension difficulties, such deficits are likely more common and pronounced in patients with aphasia. Thus, the group process in aphasia groups may emphasize strategies and activities addressing comprehension, as well as appropriate group interaction (Kearns & Elman, 2008). In particular, patients in aphasia groups can be encouraged to develop independence in monitoring their own comprehension and initiating clarification strategies (e.g., requesting repetitions, asking communication partners to write down or draw what was being said). Language expression difficulties common to patients with aphasia are easily targeted during the general group treatment activities described in the previous sections of this chapter. Although not typically the primary focus of group treatment, there is evidence that even impairment-focused treatments such as semantic feature analysis can be successfully implemented in a group treatment format (Falconer & Antonucci, 2012).

RHD and TBI Groups. Group treatment for patients with RHD and TBI often incorporates goals addressing the unique cognitive or communicative impairments (e.g., disorientation, inattention, pragmatic disruptions) or needs of these patients (e.g., because patients with TBI are often younger than other neurogenic patient populations, they often have more needs related to vocational or educational issues). However, the group activities addressing these issues often may be the same as those incorporated into aphasia groups. The difference will be primarily with respect to which compensatory strategies each patient will need to use to participate effectively in the group interaction or activity.

Many patients with RHD and TBI will benefit from group treatment addressing orientation and attention, particularly during the early stages of recovery (Cherney & Halper, 2007; Corrigan, Arnett, Houck, & Jackson, 1985; Gillis, 2007). These "reality orientation" groups can involve activities such as making crafts for an upcoming holiday, singing songs that pertain to the time of year, and reviewing orientation facts such as the day's date and the group's location. Daily reality orientation groups are particularly appropriate for residential care centers, as orientation to time, place, and person will be common to all patients. Sharing of personal biographical information and discussion of current news events can also be incorporated into orientation groups. These group sessions are typically shorter and more frequent than groups designed for other purposes, but still provide an opportunity for patients to practice orientation strategies such as attending to environmental cues (e.g., checking outside to identify visual cues regarding time of day or season), or using external devices (e.g., checking the date on one's watch).

Group treatment also is an appropriate venue for practicing compensatory strategies addressing higher level cognitive skills, such as memory, time management, organization, goal setting, and problem solving (Bertisch, Rath, Langenbahn, Sherr, & Diller, 2011; Hickey & Saunders, 2010; R. Marshall, 2007; Niemeier, Kreutzer, & Taylor, 2005). The types of activities discussed previously (e.g., conversation, role-playing, PACE-like interactions, reminiscence) provide a context for targeting a variety of cognitive abilities, including recalling and sequencing of information, inhibition, problem solving, planning, initiation, awareness of deficits, and self-monitoring. Because pragmatic skills are often impaired in patients with RHD or TBI, group treatment for these patients (as reviewed in Chapter 9) may have a greater emphasis on appropriate interaction in a variety of contexts (e.g., giving impromptu speeches, debating, role-playing service encounters), as opposed to effective transaction, which may more often be of concern for aphasia groups (Appleton et al., 2011; Braden et al., 2010; Gillis, 2007).

Dementia Groups. Although group treatment for patients with dementia poses unique challenges, those with milder deficits may benefit from the opportunity to practice compensatory strategies in a group treatment setting; accordingly, for these dementia patients, group treatment goals and activities may be similar to those described previously for aphasic, RHD, and TBI patient populations (Bourgeois & Hickey, 2009; Johnson & Bourgeois, 1998; Lin et al., 2003). For example, Santo Pietro and Boczko (1998) have developed and successfully implemented a Breakfast Club treatment protocol in which a group of patients living in an extended care facility come together to prepare, serve, eat, and then clean up breakfast under the supervision of a clinician; during these breakfast-related activities, patients are encouraged through multi-modality cues to use their cognitive and communicative strategies.

For patients with more severe dementia, group treatment may provide a context for clinician-facilitated group interaction with less emphasis on patients' ability to use compensatory strategies (Bourgeois & Hickey, 2009). L. Clark and Witte (1995) suggested several strategies for enhancing the effectiveness of group treatment in advanced dementia. First, perhaps more so than is necessary for other treatment groups, topics of discussion should be concrete, related to common life experiences, or both. The clinician may frequently be required to redirect the conversation to maintain topical cohesion, and to restate, rephrase, and/or simplify expressed concepts in terms of vocabulary and syntactic complexity to ensure comprehension by all group members. Stimulation techniques and scaffolding strategies (see Chapter 9) may also be incorporated to facilitate richer contributions from the group members. Reality orientation activities, similar to those described for RHD and TBI groups, are another common component of group treatment for patients in middle to later stages of dementia (Akanuma et al., 2011; Hickey & Bourgeois, 2003; Knapp et al., 2006).

Assessing Group Outcomes

As suggested above, although group treatment can be structured to address underlying linguistic and cognitive impairments contributing to neurogenic language and cognitive disorders, more often group treatment focuses on activity-level function. Thus, clinicians may find it useful to incorporate measures of functional communication, as well as participation and quality of life, such as those described in Chapter 8, when evaluating the effectiveness of group treatment (K. Garrett, 1999; Togher, 2012; Vickers, 2004). The feedback provided by group members and their communication partners throughout the group treatment process, although not formal measures of outcome, also may help clinicians identify the most useful aspects of group treatment (Togher, 2012).

Reimbursement for Group Treatment

Most common third-party payment sources, including Medicare, Medicaid, and private insurers, usually cover group treatment services for patients with neurogenic language or cognitive disorders (C. Busch, 1999), provided the groups involve four or fewer patients (ASHA, 2012b). As is true for reimbursement of any speech-language service, the clinician must clearly demonstrate to the payer that the service was necessary, was provided in a manner consistent with established practice patterns, and resulted in desired outcomes (see Chapter 13). The group treatment that is provided should be clearly related to the patient's treatment plan. In some cases, clinicians may need to provide a thorough rationale to third-party payers regarding how the group treatment addresses the functional goals of the treatment plan, as well as provide evidence that such treatment has been shown to be beneficial for other patients with similar communicative or cognitive impairments.

When group treatment is a part of service addressing the long-term impacts of neurogenic language or cognitive disorders (e.g., Life Participation Approach to Aphasia—see below), third-party payment may be harder to secure. In such cases, patients may choose to fund their group treatment personally (i.e., private-pay). Because group treatment costs are shared by all group members, the cost to individual participants is typically lower than the cost of individual treatment, making private-pay affordable to many individuals. Clinicians should be careful to ensure patients that although the lower fee makes group treatment a better value, it in no way means that group treatment is less valuable than individual treatment.

Modifying the Environment

It is likely that most speech-language pathologists focus the greater part of their treatment efforts on remediating underlying linguistic and cognitive impairments and training individuals with neurogenic language or cognitive disorders to use compensatory strategies. However, as the ICF emphasizes, the degree to which patients are able to participate in desired activities depends also on contextual factors, some of which are external to patients. Thus, clinicians may effect positive changes in communicative and cognitive success and in overall participation and quality of life by addressing these external, environmental factors.

Training Communication Partners

As human communicators, we are all aware that effective communication depends on both the senders and receivers of messages. This applies to neurologically intact communicators as well as patients experiencing neurogenic language and cognitive disorders. Communication partners unfamiliar with neurogenic language and cognitive disorders may be reluctant to interact with patients experiencing these communication and/or cognitive difficulties, in many cases, due to the assumption that these patients lack the ability to communicate, lack intellectual competence, or both (Holland & Fridriksson, 2001; Laroi, 2003; Parr, 2007). For elderly patients, communication interactions may be further limited in terms of quantity or quality by partners with misconceptions or a lack of awareness of age-related changes in communication and cognition (L. Armstrong & McKechnie, 2003; K. N. Williams, Herman, Gajewski, & Wilson, 2009). Additionally, given the increasing frequency with which volunteers are incorporated into treatment programs for patients with neurogenic language and cognitive disorders (Hickey, Bourgeois, & Olswang, 2004; McVicker, Parr, Pound, & Duchan, 2009; Meinzer, Streiftau, et al., 2007; Rayner & Marshall, 2003), many potential communication partners are being identified who are enthusiastic about interacting with patients but are uncertain how to ensure that these interactions are positive. Even partners who understand the nature of neurogenic language and cognitive disorders or age-related communication-cognition changes may still lack skill in facilitating communication in the presence of significant language deficits (Brereton, Carroll, & Barston, 2007; Rayner & Marshall, 2003; K. N. Williams et al., 2009; Zientz et al., 2007). However, just as both participants in a typical conversation must take responsibility for effective communication, communication partners of patients with neurogenic language and cognitive disorders can develop skill in "maintaining the integrity of the conversational process" (Kagan, Black, Duchan, Simmons-Mackie, & Square, 2001, p. 625).

One approach to training communication partners involves identifying communicative behaviors that disrupt communication and then working to eliminate those behaviors (L. Murray, 1998; Orange & Colton-Hudson, 1998; Simmons-Mackie, Raymer, Armstrong, Holland, & Cherney, 2010; R. Wilkinson et al., 1998; Zientz, Rackley, Bond-Chapman, Hopper, & Mahendra, 2007). This method has the greatest potential for success when the clinician is familiar with the partners' communication patterns during interactions outside of the clinical setting so that the most disruptive behaviors can be targeted. Unfortunately, many clinicians do not have an opportunity to assess naturally occurring interactions. An alternative approach, providing structured training in the behaviors that support successful interactions, may ultimately have the same effects as the first approach, as there is evidence that "poor" speaking partners fail to demonstrate the facilitative communicative behaviors exhibited by "good" speaking partners (Simmons-Mackie & Kagan, 1999). Moreover, positive communication skill training has the advantage that trained partners will develop skills that will enable them to interact effectively in different settings, as well as with other individuals experiencing neurogenic language disorders (Hickey et al., 2004; Kagan et al., 2001; McVicker et al., 2009; Rayner & Marshall, 2003; Togher, McDonald, Tate, Power, & Rietdijk, 2009).

In studies of conversations between patients with neurogenic language and cognitive disorders and volunteers or health-care workers, several communicative behaviors have been identified as facilitating effective communication (E. Armstrong et al., 2011; Simmons-Mackie & Kagan, 1999; Sundin, Jansson, & Norberg, 2000) (see Table 12-2). For example, conversation can be enhanced when the communication partner acknowledges the communication attempts of the patient with a neurogenic language or cognitive disorder. This acknowledgment may be verbal (e.g., "I see") or nonverbal (e.g., nodding the head) and indicates to the patient that the partner is actively engaged in the interaction. Positive communicators also provide sufficient time for patients to process conversation, as well as formulate and produce their contributions to the conversation; if patients feel rushed, they are likely to feel stressed, which in turn can negatively affect their communication abilities, lead to decreased conversational participation, or both. A third facilitating behavior that serves a similar acknowledgment function is "congruent overlap." When the partner's response is simultaneous with and reinforces what the patient is expressing, it communicates a sense of unity between the conversation participants. The use of disjunct markers, or cues that what is about to be communicated is incongruent with the previous exchange, also appears to facilitate communication. These markers serve as a polite and respectful means of disagreeing with or modifying a previous contribution made by the other conversation participant. For example, in the following exchange, the marker "Well . . ." signals to the patient that the communication partner is declining the request for her to stay for dinner.

> PATIENT: "Gonna stay . . . dinner stay."
> PARTNER: "Well, I am having dinner at my sister's tonight."

Effective communication partners also demonstrate accommodation to nonstandard communication modalities (Hickey et al., 2004; Simmons-Mackie & Kagan, 1999; Sundin et al., 2000). Previous sections of this chapter explored the potential benefits of multimodality communication for patients with neurogenic language or cognitive disorders, but clearly these strategies can be effective only to the extent they are accepted by conversation partners. Simmons-Mackie and Kagan (1999) described a communication partner who demonstrated understanding of the patient's gestures, but still requested that the patient try to say the appropriate words. The authors pointed out that the partner was not trying to be unkind, but apparently perceived talking to be the only acceptable communication modality. With appropriate training, partners can facilitate the effectiveness of multimodal communication, perhaps as did another partner described

TABLE 12-2
Examples of Strategies for Facilitating Communication With Patients With Neurogenic Language or Cognitive Disorders (Beukelman & Mirenda, 2013; Simmons-Mackie & Kagan, 1999)

DESCRIPTION OF STRATEGY	EXAMPLE
Introduce/confirm the topic: When communication partners are aware of the topic, it is easier to predict what is being communicated.	"Are we talking about your visit to Atlanta?"
Be aware of turn-taking signals: Patients with nonfluent aphasia may be slow to initiate speech and may have difficulty getting a turn in conversation. Patients with fluent aphasia and "press of speech" may continue speaking long after they have expressed their "main point."	Indications a turn is desired: • Prolonged eye contact • Leaning forward or other anticipatory posture • Deep inhalation Requesting a turn: • Holding up a hand • Saying, "Excuse me."

Provide sufficient time for the patient to formulate a response. Attend to and acknowledge communication attempts: Give the speaker your attention and acknowledge communication attempts. Attend to and acknowledge all communication modes and cues.	• Nodding
	• Saying, "I see."
	• Asking, "Is that so?"
	• Possible communication modes and cues:
	  ~ Verbal
	  ~ Intonation
	  ~ Gesture
	  ~ Context

Manage communication breakdown: Signal the individual as soon as you fail to understand, then identify specifically what you misunderstood, and utilize previously agreed-upon clarification strategies based on those practiced during treatment (the patient should be aware of and be comfortable with identified strategies—finishing the sentence, guessing, providing additional time).	Signal misunderstanding: • Lifting a finger • Raising eyebrows or using other facial expression to signal confusion Identify misunderstanding: • Saying, "I didn't catch who you are talking about." • Asking, "This happened when?" • Asking, "Do you want this one or that one?"
Incorporate face-saving strategies: Minimize the interactional cost of the communication breakdown by reinforcing the competence of the patient and your relationship with him or her.	• Saying, "Whew! We really worked at that one, didn't we?" • Saying, "I see where you're going with this." • Saying, "I'm glad we figured that out."

in this study, who not only accepted alternate communication modalities but also adopted some of the alternative communicative behaviors in his own contributions to the conversation.

The final characteristic of good conversation partners described by Simmons-Mackie and Kagan (1999) is the use of "face-saving" repair strategies. These authors reported that whereas nearly all the conversation partners in their study asked clarification questions, some did so in such a way as to acknowledge the competence of the patient with the neurogenic language or cognitive disorder. For example, one partner closed a long repair sequence by acknowledging the information that was successfully communicated. In contrast, another partner repeatedly asked the same clarification question even after a feasible response had been provided by the patient. The authors pointed out that this second behavior can be interpreted as a lack of confidence in the patient's response, and thus communicates a lack of appreciation for the patient's inherent competence.

> ### The Importance of Supporting Written as Well as Spoken Communication
>
> Considering the ever-increasing number of people who regularly utilize social media venues such as Facebook and Twitter, clinicians must not overlook the importance of training strategies that can facilitate patients' ability to both understand and send written messages. Improving access to written communication within these social media contexts is clearly consistent with the other treatment approaches reviewed in this chapter designed to effect positive change in activities and participation. Consequently, it is important to point out that many of the strategies reviewed in this chapter, which focus on spoken communication, may also be used when training communication partners to "converse" via writing with neurogenic patients (e.g., using familiar vocabulary, paraphrasing repetition of important information). For a review of a number of techniques to support patients' reading and writing (e.g., pairing email text with contextual pictures, ensuring access to word prediction software), see Dietz and colleagues (2011).

The intervention program "Supported Conversation for Adults With Aphasia" (SCA; Kagan et al., 2001) evolved out of research into the behaviors of effective conversation partners. The philosophy of SCA is that effective conversation partners both acknowledge and reveal the competence of patients with neurogenic language or cognitive disorders through appropriate communicative behaviors. Behaviors that acknowledge competence include using "natural adult talk" with tone and style appropriate for the context, and demonstrating sensitivity to the conversation partner. Sensitivity may be demonstrated by acknowledging attempts to communicate, providing encouragement, listening respectfully, avoiding rushing the patient, and bearing an appropriate amount of the communicative burden so that the patient feels neither overburdened nor patronized. SCA trains conversation partners to reveal competence in three main ways: (a) ensure that the patient understands what is being communicated, (b) ensure that the patient has a means of responding, and (c) verify that the message received was that intended by the patient. Each of these goals can be accomplished using verbal strategies (e.g., redundancy, providing fixed choice options), nonverbal approaches (e.g., using and receiving multimodal messages; providing tangible or graphic conversational aids such as maps, newspaper headlines or articles, calendars), or both. In each case, SCA encourages conversation partners to be responsive to communicative cues provided by the patient (e.g., facial expressions, inconsistent responses).

The developers of SCA have created online training modules that include examples of positive and negative communicative behaviors (http://www.aphasia.ca/cop/). Training in SCA is appropriate for family members, health-care providers, and community members. Importantly, Kagan et al. (2001) found that when volunteers were provided with SCA training, the communication skills of both the trained volunteers and the patients with neurogenic language or cognitive disorders improved, as evidenced by more effective interactional (i.e., interpersonal) and transactional (i.e., informational) exchanges. Similar programs developed by Hickey et al. (2004), Rayner and Marshall (2003), and McVicker et al. (2009) also have been found to produce positive changes in not only the volunteers' communication style but also the patients' participation levels and accuracy during conversations. A recent systematic review (Simmons-Mackie et al., 2010) concluded that communication partner training is effective in improving measures of communicative activities and participation of the trained partner and probably has similar effects for individuals with chronic aphasia when they converse with trained partners. The review further concluded that the evidence regarding the benefits of conversation partner training for patients with acute aphasia is insufficient. Additional research is also needed to explore outcomes for language impairment, psychosocial adjustment, and quality of life. Moreover, there is evidence that the use of positive communicative behaviors by trained volunteers declines over time (Rayner & Marshall, 2003), suggesting that maintenance training may be necessary.

Communication partners of patients with cognitive-communicative disorders due to RHD, TBI, or dementia may benefit from instruction in different, or at least additional, strategies for facilitating effective communication than those described above for aphasia, as the communication breakdowns of these patients may involve other aspects of language (e.g., pragmatics, suprasegmental phonology), stem from different underlying impairments (e.g., attention or memory deficits, impaired emotion perception), or both and can lead to problematic behavior (Gitlin, Winter, Dennis, Hodgson, & Hauck, 2010; Tompkins, 2008, 2012). For example, a variety of verbal and nonverbal communication strategies have been recommended to encourage and facilitate the activity and social participation of patients with TBI or dementia (Appleton et al., 2011; Orange & Colton-Hudson, 1998; J. Small & Perry, 2005; Togher et al., 2009; R. Wilson, Rochon, Mihailidis, & Leonard, 2012; Zientz et al., 2007). In addition to the communication strategies consistent with SCA, caregivers of patients with dementia should be trained to use consistent words or phrases to communicate recurrent concepts (e.g., mealtimes, leaving the home). Further, the caregivers' nonverbal communication (i.e., facial expression, intonation, gestures, and other body language) should be both calming and congruent so that all cues are communicating the same meaning, adding to communication redundancy. Additional strategies for which there is empirical support, at least for the dementia population, include avoiding analogies and other figurative or complex language structures (see included DVD: Patient 8l), providing explicit conversational topic introductions and indications of when topic changes are occurring (e.g., "Let's talk about planning dinner . . . okay, now let's switch and talk about the phone bill"), asking questions or giving directions one at a time, eliminating distractions, providing paraphrased (vs. verbatim) repetitions, asking closed- rather than open-ended questions, and encouraging patients to circumlocute when they are experiencing word-finding difficulties (Kemper & Harden, 1999; Orange & Colton-Hudson, 1998; J. Small & Gutman, 2002; J. Small & Perry, 2005; Wilson et al., 2012). Although it has often been recommended that caregivers speak slowly to enhance the comprehension of patients with dementia, research indicates that this strategy is ineffective (Wilson et al., 2012), and in fact viewed as patronizing by patients with dementia (Kemper & Harden, 1999). Accordingly, this strategy should not be recommended, and clinicians should observe patient–caregiver interactions to determine if this is a negative caregiver communication behavior that needs to be addressed. Importantly, there is some evidence indicating that providing dementia caregivers with information pertaining to communication symptoms and strategies may also improve quality of life in the dementia patient (Zientz et al., 2007).

Communication partners of patients with RHD or TBI may benefit from strategies addressing the communicative behaviors common in these conditions. For both RHD and TBI, pragmatic deficits commonly contribute to communication breakdown. Because disruptive pragmatic behaviors such as interrupting or inappropriate proxemics (e.g., standing too close to communication partners) may be interpreted as rudeness (as opposed to a reflection of a disability), instructing communication partners about the nature of the pragmatic deficits accompanying RHD and TBI may foster greater understanding and, thus, patience with the communication behaviors of these patients (Laroi, 2003; Togher et al., 2009). Instruction in specific strategies for facilitating communication in the presence of pragmatic or other cognitive-communicative deficits specific to these patient populations may also be provided. Table 12-3 lists several disruptive cognitive-communicative impairments and the partner responses that may improve communication effectiveness.

Additionally, communication partners should be made aware of cognitive deficits such as visuoperceptual, attention, and memory impairments that may disrupt communicative interactions with these patients. Again, disruptive behaviors related to these cognitive impairments can be misinterpreted by family members and caregivers (Laroi, 2003). For instance, families might assume that patients' failure to complete daily chores represents resistance to authority when it is actually a product of memory difficulties. Likewise, decreased arousal and initiation may be inappropriately attributed to depression, laziness, or poor motivation. Accordingly, education about these symptoms can foster families' and caregivers' patience and acceptance of patients, which in turn will lead to increased socialization with the patients, participation in patients' treatment programs, or both. Information about specific strategies also may be provided. For example, partners may be instructed on where best to stand or present visual information to ensure perceptual awareness when interacting with patients with neglect.

TABLE 12-3
Example Communication Strategies Addressing Specific Cognitive-Communicative Deficits

COGNITIVE-COMMUNICATIVE DEFICIT	STRATEGY FOR COMMUNICATION PARTNER
Failure to maintain appropriate eye contact	Model appropriate contact, positioning yourself in the patient's line of sight.
Lack of conversation initiation	Introduce a broad topic, or offer choices of topic.
Inappropriate social greetings	Model appropriate greetings.
Interrupting or impaired turn taking	Use a nonverbal signal (e.g., raising a finger or hand) to indicate your turn is not over and that the patient should wait until you have completed your turn. A similar signal may be used to indicate a turn has been inappropriately long.
Inappropriate proxemics	Reposition yourself to a more comfortable proximity, and if necessary explain why you have moved.
Failure to monitor listener responses	Use a verbal or nonverbal signal to convey a lack of understanding or a need to respond. Minimize environmental distractions.
Poor topic maintenance or perseveration	Redirect the conversation to the appropriate topic. This can be done with disjunctive markers such as "What I was saying a minute ago...?" or "I think we reached closure on that issue. What did you think of...?"
Inappropriate topic initiation	Redirect the conversation to an appropriate topic. Disjunctive markers such as "I'd rather talk about that later" or "We probably shouldn't talk about that now" may be used.
Difficulty interpreting prosodic cues (e.g., emphatic stress, emotional intonation)	Match your linguistic content and prosody to provide redundant cues regarding the meaning of your verbal output. Ask the patient to summarize his or her interpretation of what's been said to ensure appropriate understanding.
Difficulty interpreting figurative and indirect language	Avoid using figurative and indirect linguistic devices, or, if these devices are used, provide redundant cues and ask the patient to summarize his or her interpretation of what's been said to ensure appropriate understanding.
Difficulty with prosody production	Encourage the patient to select words that will cue you regarding what parts of the message are most important or that will explicitly tell you his or her feelings.

Maintaining eye contact, periodically saying the patient's name or touching his or her arm, and reducing or eliminating environmental distractions (visual, auditory, or both) may help maintain or redirect attention. Finally, providing periodic summaries of what has been discussed may compensate for short-term memory deficits. Whenever possible and appropriate, communication partners also may wish to provide reminders or cues to patients to use their own compensatory strategies for addressing these impairments.

Before leaving the discussion of training communication partners, it may be helpful to consider techniques clinicians may employ when instructing communication partners. Bayles and Kaszniak (1987) suggested the following steps: First, provide oral and written descriptions of the strategy, followed by demonstration with the patient. Multimedia strategies can be incorporated into this step as well (Irvine, Ary, & Bourgeois, 2003). The communication partner should practice the strategy with the clinician and, when skilled in using the strategy, practice with the patient (Zientz et al., 2007). Bayles and Kaszniak (1987) further recommended that practice interactions be videotaped so that the communication partner can review and evaluate the effectiveness of the interaction. Additionally, group treatment sessions provide an opportunity for communication partners to practice communication enhancement strategies in a more natural communication setting (Clark & Witte, 1995; K. Garrett, Staltari, & Moir, 2007). Practice of these skills in group treatment also serves to emphasize the interactional nature of communication and to extend the responsibility for effective communication to all communication partners. Sorin-Peters (2004) additionally advocated that when training communication partners, clinicians apply adult learning principles such as considering the partners' individual learning styles (e.g., do they learn better by doing or by observing?), encouraging partners to evaluate their own progress, and collaborating with partners to establish target communicative behaviors. Finally, clinicians should not overlook the wisdom that may be provided by patients and their families regarding the most valuable aspects of the conversation training process (Togher, 2012). The insights provided by the "consumers" of such training are invaluable in refining the services we provide.

Medical professionals are another category of conversation partners who may benefit from training in facilitating communication (Burns, Baylor, Morris, McNalley, & Yorkston, 2012; Welsh & Zhabo, 2011; K. N. Williams et al., 2009; Zientz et al., 2007). Because it is unlikely that health-care workers would be able to attend individual or group therapy sessions on a regular basis, workshops may be a more appropriate means by which to educate these possible communication partners about effective cognitive and communicative strategies to enhance their interactions with patients with neurogenic language or cognitive disorders. The content of these workshops may include description and examples (e.g., videotape samples) of the types of cognitive and communicative impairments that their patients may display, as well as review of the types of strategies covered in the preceding paragraphs of this chapter. Inclusion of a practical skills training component within these workshops (e.g., role-playing and/or disability simulation exercises) and the provision of handouts or booklets that can be referred to after the workshop also are effective means by which to train these types of caregivers. Fortunately, there are a few commercially available workshop programs that provide guidelines for which content and activities to include (e.g., Jordan, Bell, Bryan, Maxim, & Axelrod, 2000; Ripich, 1996). Several studies have confirmed that providing these types of workshops can produce significant increases in health-care workers' knowledge of neurogenic language or cognitive disorders, use of positive communication strategies, and empathetic awareness of the effects of neurogenic language or cognitive disorders on the lives of patients and their loved ones (Maxim, Bryan, Axelrod, Jordan, & Bell, 2001; Pentland, Hutton, MacMillan, & Mayer, 2003; Rayner & Marshall, 2003; Shaw & May, 2001; K. Williams, Kemper, & Hummert, 2005; Zientz et al., 2007).

Modifying the Physical Environment

With the advent of the Americans With Disabilities Act (1990) and other manifestations of the disability movement, our society has a broadened awareness of how modifying the physical environment can greatly improve accessibility of products, services, and activities for individuals with physical disabilities. Curb cutouts, buildings equipped with ramps and automatic doors, Braille markings on elevator doors, auditory signals at crosswalks, closed captioning, and TTD phone lines are commonplace and expected. Unfortunately, society remains less sensitive to how the physical environment may influence the ability of individuals with more invisible disabilities, such as neurogenic language and cognitive disorders, to participate in desired life activities (Bourgeois & Hickey, 2009; Howe, Worrall, & Hickson, 2008; Pryor, 2004).

Accordingly, an important component of speech-language intervention is teaching patients and their caregivers how to alter their physical environment to maximize patients' cognitive and communicative abilities. An initial step is for the clinician to assess the physical environment to determine if modifications are necessary and, if so, which modifications will facilitate effective communication and efficient completion of daily activities. This evaluation is a part of the assessment of activity and participation (see Chapter 8) and includes considering the arrangement of the home, work, or classroom setting, mobility options, and sensoriperceptual factors such as lighting and noise levels (Gitlin, Liebman, & Winter, 2003; Lubinski, 2001; Pryor, 2004).

Probably the most obvious environmental characteristic influencing communicative effectiveness and cognitive functioning is the acoustic environment. Patients with neurogenic language and cognitive disorders often experience auditory comprehension deficits that are exacerbated by hearing loss related to age, noise exposure, or trauma (e.g., blast injury). Patients with compromised attention abilities also will be easily distracted, and thus have problems with communication and other activities in the presence of noise. Furthermore, potential communication partners also may demonstrate hearing difficulties. Accordingly, the clinician can help patients, their family members, or health-care-facility workers arrange the physical environment to facilitate clear transmission of auditory signals. An obvious strategy for enhancing the acoustic environment is reducing background noise (e.g., television and stereo sounds) that may compete with spoken auditory signals or cause distraction while patients are completing daily activities (Bourgeois & Hickey, 2009; Calkins, 2009; Gitlin et al., 2003; Sohlberg, 2002). Other, less apparent sources of noise include appliances, clocks, and traffic and other sounds that may be coming from outside of the home or work setting. It is not always necessary or even desirable to eliminate these noise sources, because they can be stimulating and provide a source of conversation (Lubinski, 1991). However, the clinician can help patients and their family members identify areas in the environment where the noise level is low or controllable. The placement of sound-absorbing materials (e.g., curtains, carpet, ceiling tiles) may further reduce noise levels (Bourgeois & Hickey, 2009; Calkins, 2009; Calkins & Brush, 2003). If patients or their communication partners demonstrate hearing loss, the clinician should collaborate with an audiologist to ensure that suitable amplification devices are available and used appropriately.

Another aspect of the environment that influences communicative effectiveness and daily activity performance is lighting, along with other aspects of the visual environment. Consideration of lighting is particularly important given that many patients with neurogenic language and cognitive disorders have impairments (e.g., vision field cut, visuospatial neglect, glare sensitivity, decreased light accommodation, visuoperceptual limitations) that limit their visual access (Barton, 2011; Gitlin et al., 2003; Rowe et al., 2011; see also Chapter 5 for a description of these visual problems). Adequate lighting facilitates conversation by allowing the communication partners to observe facial expressions and other nonverbal cues and to attend to contextual cues. Other, less obvious characteristics of the visual environment may also influence the communication interactions of and daily activity completion by patients with neurogenic language and cognitive disorders. For example, visual stimuli serve as a primary source of conversation topics and as an initiative to complete many daily activities. If patients do not have the same visual access to these stimuli as other individuals in the environment, they will be less able to participate in interactions or activities. The clinician can assist families and health-care providers by identifying key features of the visual environment that serve as meaningful stimuli (e.g., weather, television news, photos, magazines, etc.). Visual access to these stimuli may then be enhanced by thoughtful arrangement of the communication environment. Potential environmental modifications that may facilitate visual access to promote effective communication and successful activity participation include the following:

- Use visual contrasts (e.g., dark against light colors).
- Reduce glare by covering shiny surfaces, using indirect lighting, and/or adding window shades.
- Position important visual information at eye level, with consideration for the patient's most typical position (e.g., wheelchair vs. standing). Visual information includes clocks, calendars, photographs, sculptures, magazines, room numbers, and other items in the environment that contribute to orientation or communication.
- Provide even and adequate but not excessive lighting, allowing the patient control of lighting intensity whenever possible.
- If appropriate, position the patient so he or she has visual access to the most common sources of communication topics and activities (e.g., television, window, kitchen or other common center of activity).

A number of additional environmental modifications may enhance orientation to person, place, and time (Bourgeois & Hickey, 2009; Brush, Sanford, Fleder, Bruce, & Calkins, 2011; Calkins, 2009; Gitlin et al., 2003; Lubinski, 2001). Enhancing personal orientation may be most important for patients with severe dementia and primarily involves personalizing the environment. Placement of personal items (e.g., photographs) is a common way of facilitating orientation and can be extended to include personal furniture, clothing, bedding, and small appliances. Allowing the patient to participate in selecting room colors or arranging items in the room can also serve to personalize the environment. Orientation to time can be heightened via natural environmental cues, such as those provided by windows (e.g., day vs. night, seasonal cues such as leaves on or off the trees), or visual access to normal daily activities (e.g., meals, regularly scheduled television programs). Clocks and calendars as well as other seasonal props (e.g., seasonal floral arrangements, holiday decorations) may also enhance temporal orientation. Finally, maintaining a consistent routine may facilitate orientation, as the patient associates specific activities (e.g., bathing, shopping) with a certain caregiver, time of day, or day of the week.

Spatial orientation is most easily enhanced by maintaining a consistent physical environment. Placing additional cues in the environment, such as personal items or graphic signs, may also facilitate orientation. For patients with severe deficits, color-coded pathways may facilitate independence in moving from one location to another (e.g., bedroom to dining room) within a given area. These will be particularly helpful in environments where traditional spatial cues are lacking (e.g., most homes have only one hallway that leads to bedrooms and bathrooms, whereas assisted care facilities often have many hallways that may lead nearly anywhere).

Environmental modifications also may be useful in reducing the frequency and severity of certain behavioral disturbances (Bourgeois & Hickey, 2009; Calkins, 2009; Chavin, 2002; Gitlin et al., 2003; E. Kong, Evans, & Guevara, 2009). For example, patients who are easily agitated may respond positively to calming background music or simulated-presence audiotapes (e.g., audiotape of a loved one talking to the patient) or videotapes (e.g., videotape of the patient's family completing daily activities). Wandering and exiting problems may be minimized by covering doorknobs with cloth, storing keys to doors and vehicles in out-of-sight locations, installing a home alarm system, placing motion detector lights near exits, creating an area or clear pathway where patients may wander or pace safely (e.g., establishing a walking route in an assisted-care facility, rearranging furniture to provide a clear path), and disguising exit doors with curtains, posters, or murals.

Patients with higher level cognitive deficits may also benefit from environmental modifications. Parenté's and Herrmann's (2010) five basic principles for organizing the environment to compensate for memory and other cognitive deficits are as follows:

- Consistency
- Accessibility
- Grouping
- Proximity
- Separation

The first principle is consistency, which refers not only to the arrangement of the environment but also to how various items in the environment are used. For example, these authors recommended that a receptacle inside the main entrance to the house be used for keys. Likewise, a specific area could be identified where any items to be taken to work or school (e.g., lunch bag, tote, etc.) will be placed, and another area could be designated for dirty laundry. The intent of this principle is to allow habits to compensate for disruptions in memory or attention that impede a patient's ability to navigate an inconsistent environment.

The second principle is accessibility. Parenté and Herrmann (2010) recommended that the environment be organized so that items used frequently are located in the most physically accessible areas and less frequently used items are placed in less accessible areas. This principle is one most individuals adopt to some extent, but may need to be carefully and systematically applied in the environments of patients with visuoperceptual, attentional, memory, and/or planning or problem-solving deficits. This principle is closely related to two other principles, those of grouping and proximity. By arranging the environment so that related items are located together (i.e., grouping), with the most commonly used items most accessible within the grouping (i.e., accessibility) and maintained near the area in which they are used (i.e., proximity), patients may rely less on their own organization skills to identify needed items, or on their own visuoperceptual, attention, and memory skills to locate those items. For example, the area most accessible to the bathroom sink might include items such as soap, towels, comb, and toothbrush. Other bathroom items used less frequently and thus placed in less accessible areas might include tweezers or a hair dryer.

Separation, the final principle of organization, refers to arranging the environment so that conceptually separate items are placed in discrete locations (Parenté & Herrmann, 2010). Examples include arranging clothes according to purpose (e.g., work vs. leisure clothing) or by season, or arranging the pantry so that breakfast items are on one shelf, lunch and dinner items on another shelf, and baking items on still another shelf. Parenté and Herrmann pointed out that each patient may benefit from different organization strategies, and that careful observation over time may be the best method for identifying the most effective environmental organization.

Participation-Focused Treatments and Community Resources

The last decade has seen a growing awareness of the life changes that often accompany chronic neurogenic language and cognitive disorders. Because communication is so endemic to human interactions, the impact of these disorders extends beyond the ability to exchange information (Hilari, Needle, & Harrison, 2012; Lyon, 1998). Patients coping with neurogenic language and cognitive disorders may find themselves "disconnected" from their social networks, or even from their spouse or close family members. The psychosocial impacts of neurogenic language and cognitive disorders are not limited to the patients experiencing the disorder, but extend to those around them as well

(Alzheimer's Association, 2012; Bakas et al., 2006b; Neugroschl & Wang, 2011; Vangel et al., 2011). As communication and other health and social service professionals have become more aware of the chronicity of neurogenic language and cognitive disorders (Lyon, 1998; E. Miller et al., 2010), systematic attempts to alleviate the life disruption of these disorders have emerged. This section will review treatments that focus primarily on improving the patients' participation in life activities, irrespective of their communicative effectiveness or the integrity of their cognitive abilities.

Life Participation Approach to Aphasia

A relatively recent movement in the delivery of services to patients with neurogenic language or cognitive disorders is the Life Participation Approach to Aphasia (LPAA; Chapey et al., 2008). Although this approach was originally conceived as a service delivery model for patients with aphasia, the philosophy driving the LPAA is applicable to the management of all neurogenic language and cognitive disorders, and several existing treatment approaches for TBI and dementia contain elements consistent with LPAA tenets (e.g., Mahendra & Arkin, 2004; Ylvisaker, Szerkeres, & Feeney, 2008). The LPAA does not prescribe specific clinical methods, but rather encompasses a set of values that guide the management of neurogenic language or cognitive disorders.

One core value of the LPAA is that the primary goal is the enhancement of life participation by patients experiencing neurogenic language or cognitive disorders. This includes appropriate assessment of life participation and the impact of a neurogenic language or cognitive disorder on participation, as well as the identification of strategies for improving life participation. Inherent to this tenet is the importance of outcome measures that address participation and quality of life (see Chapter 8). Further, the LPAA acknowledges that the effects of neurogenic language or cognitive disorders are broader than those experienced by the individual with the condition, and, thus, a third core value is to provide support for family and other individuals who interact with the patients. Relatedly, the LPAA recognizes that improving life participation for patients may include targeting personal and environmental factors, as well as the underlying functional impairments contributing to participation limitations. Finally, the LPAA emphasizes providing service at all stages of recovery or disease progression. Patients with neurogenic language or cognitive disorders experience life changes common to many individuals, changes such as moving to a new home, changes in marital status, gaining family members through birth and marriage, employment changes (e.g., retirement), financial changes, and health changes. Such changes may alter the degree to which a neurogenic language or cognitive disorder is impacting the patient's life participation, and thus may warrant intervention. The LPAA embraces the notion that the primary criteria for treatment eligibility be need and potential benefit rather than time post onset.

Because the LPAA reflects a philosophical perspective rather than specific treatment procedures, conventional efficacy data for this approach are not readily available.

Instead, empirical support for this approach is provided by studies examining the benefits of treatments consistent with LPAA values, many of which are reviewed in the following sections.

Participation Treatments Expand the Role of the Speech-Language Pathologist

In Chapter 8, we introduced Ray, who sought assistance with regaining his driver's license. Ray had received impairment-level treatment in the days and weeks following his stroke, but these services had been discontinued when he was discharged from the rehabilitation center. The severe aphasia Ray continued to experience a year after his stroke minimally impacted his participation in independent living and social interactions, but his lack of a driver's license was a significant impediment.

The focus of Ray's treatment was preparation for the written examination that was required to regain his driver's license. Intervention activities included reviewing the DMV driving handbook, developing strategies for comprehending the questions and response choices, and identifying reliable response modes for expressing choices of the correct response. Ray participated in 16 treatment sessions before attempting the written test. The test center offered several accommodations during the written test, including reading the questions aloud and yes/no responses to each of the choices. Additionally, a speech-language pathologist assisted in administering the test to help facilitate Ray's comprehension and expression.

Consistent with the LPAA, Ray received services during a period of time post onset when intervention has traditionally not been offered. Additionally, treatment focused on compensatory techniques and environmental modifications expressly for the purpose of improving a specific aspect of life participation, with little concern for improving underlying language ability.

To complete the story, Ray passed the written test and went on to pass the driving portion of the test as well. He was issued a restricted driver's license that allowed him to drive on non-interstate highways within 50 miles of his home. The restriction was imposed because of Ray's inability to read printed road signs. However, this restriction did not pose a significant barrier to Ray's participation in desired activities, so his goals for treatment were met.

Social Model

Social models (Byng & Duchan, 2005) embrace a philosophy closely related to the LPAA. Specifically, social models emphasize how the presence of a neurogenic language or cognitive disorder affects patients' communication in social contexts, as well as how social contexts facilitate or inhibit patients' participation. Simmons-Mackie (2008) identified several principles embraced by social models. First, social models recognize that communication serves purposes beyond the exchange of information, or **transaction**. Although transaction is an important function of communication, another equally important function is reciprocal activity to establish and maintain relationships, or **interaction**. Social models recognize the importance of adequate communication for accomplishing social goals and emphasize the need to address this aspect of communication during intervention.

Second, similar to the LPAA, social models emphasize the need to address communication and cognition in relevant contexts. Traditional impairment-level treatments, including many of those reviewed in Chapters 9 and 10, often involve highly structured communicative or cognitive tasks targeting specific linguistic or cognitive processes, disconnecting the processing from its typically occurring or **authentic context**. For example, a common communicative context is conversation; thus, treatment within a social model emphasizes practicing communication strategies in the context of conversation. To ensure that the context is realistic, clinicians can involve patients and caregivers in generating conversational topics or target activities of daily living (see included DVD: Patient 6b), and should encourage practice in settings outside of the therapy room (Sorin-Peters, 2004). Relatedly, social models acknowledge that communication in authentic contexts is rarely "perfect," but rather is characterized by disfluencies, interruptions, and corrections (Simmons-Mackie, 2008). Because these imperfections are accepted as normal aspects of daily communication, patients with neurogenic language or cognitive disorders and their caregivers are encouraged to focus less on perfect word choices or grammar and more on successful transactions and interactions.

Social models also are consistent with the LPAA in acknowledging that neurogenic language and cognitive disorders affect individuals in addition to the patients who are experiencing the disorders, and that the effects extend beyond the immediate home environment to the larger social context. Thus, intervention within social models may include training communication partners and modifying the environment, as discussed earlier in this chapter. The emphasis within the framework of social models is on enabling patients with neurogenic language and cognitive disorders, as well as other individuals affected by these disorders, to participate fully in the communicating society.

Intervention programs designed within a social model will incorporate a common set of goals: enhanced communication, increased participation, development of support systems, increased confidence and positive identity, and improved advocacy (Simmons-Mackie, 2008). Thus, the conversation-based treatments, including conversational coaching or conversational script training (e.g., Bilda, 2011; Cherney & Halper, 2008), discussed in Chapter 9, are among the interventions consistent with social models. Supported Conversation for Adults With Aphasia (Kagan et al., 2001) and conversation partner training, described earlier in this chapter, are also consistent with both LPAA and social models. The final areas of intervention embraced by social models are the development of support systems and improved advocacy.

Support Groups, Community Resources, and Advocacy

The treatment approaches discussed in Chapters 9 and 10, as well as in this chapter, highlight the important role speech-language pathologists and other professionals play in the management of neurogenic language and cognitive disorders. Nonetheless, it would be both immodest and naïve for professionals to underestimate the contribution of non-professional support systems to participation and well-being. When neurogenic language and cognitive disorders (or their causes) are well known (e.g., Alzheimer's disease), patients and family members are likely to either be aware of community resources or at least presume such resources exist and can be sought out. Other neurogenic language and cognitive disorders (e.g., aphasia and RHD), though not uncommon, are not well known; many people experiencing or affected by these impairments know very little about the nature and impact of these conditions until they themselves are experiencing them. Thus, a sense of being the only one coping with these conditions may be more common than it is for individuals with more well-known and visible disabilities (Rosenthal, 2004). Support groups consisting of patients affected by neurogenic language and cognitive disorders can be very helpful in assisting patients in adjusting to and coping with the presence of a communicative or cognitive disability. Similarly, support groups for caregivers of those with neurogenic language and cognitive disorders can play an important role in helping caregivers adjust to and accept the many changes that accompany the onset of a neurogenic language or cognitive disorder.

Several types of support groups exist for patients with neurogenic language and cognitive disorders and their caregivers. These groups typically function to provide information about the neurogenic language and cognitive disorder or disease, discuss coping and management strategies, and help patients and caregivers identify other appropriate community resources (e.g., respite care programs, home health-care services, legal consultants). For example, many communities have established stroke support groups that serve patients experiencing a variety of the impairments common in stroke. Although not every member of the group is affected by neurogenic language and cognitive disorders, group members may share experiences related to changes in health status, employment, navigation of health-care systems, and securing of funding for rehabilitation costs. Groups established for specific neurogenic language or cognitive disorders—such as aphasia, progressive aphasia, RHD, dementia (in particular, Alzheimer's disease), and TBI—and for caregivers of patients with these disorders also are available in many communities.

In addition to local support groups, many national associations serve patients affected by neurogenic language and cognitive disorders. Most of these associations have as their primary mission the direct support of patients affected by neurogenic language and cognitive disorders by providing easily understood information about the condition and contact information for local support groups and association representatives. Often the organizations maintain websites that include discussion forums and other avenues for connecting with other patients or caregivers affected by the condition (see Table 12-4). These organizations also often seek to educate the public and health-care

TABLE 12-4
List of Example Internet Resources

Sites for Individuals Affected by Stroke	
National Stroke Association	www.stroke.org
American Stroke Association (a division of the American Heart Association)	www.strokeassociation.org
	www.heart.org
American Stroke Foundation	www.americanstroke.org
Washington University Internet Stroke Center	www.strokecenter.org

Sites for Individuals Affected by Aphasia	
National Aphasia Association	www.aphasia.org
Aphasia Hope Foundation	www.aphasiahope.org

Sites for Individuals Affected by RHD	
ASHA Public Information about RHD	www.asha.org/public/speech/disorders/RightBrainDamage.htm

Sites for Individuals Affected by TBI	
Brain Injury Association of America	www.biausa.org
North American Brain Injury Society	www.nabis.org

Sites for Individuals Affected by Dementing Diseases	
Alzheimer's Association	www.alz.org
Alzheimer's Disease International	www.alz.co.uk
Alzheimer's Disease Education & Referral Center	www.alzheimers.org
Dementia Advocacy and Support Network	www.dasninternational.org
Dementia Information from the Neurology Channel	www.healthcommunities.com/dementia/dementia-overview-types.shtml
National Parkinson Foundation	www.parkinson.org
The Michael J. Fox Foundation for Parkinson's Research	www.michaeljfox.org
Huntington's Disease Society of American	www.hdsa.org
National Multiple Sclerosis Society	www.nationalmssociety.org

Note. RHD = right hemisphere brain damage; TBI = traumatic brain injury.

providers about the condition, as well as to fund research related to the condition. Clinicians may wish to refer to the American Speech-Language-Hearing Association website, which includes a comprehensive and up-to-date list of these organizations.

In addition to specific groups and organizations serving to support patients and caregivers affected by neurogenic language and cognitive disorders, many other community resources may be useful as patients resume their participation in usual activities. Each state operates a department of vocational rehabilitation that assists patients with disabilities as they re-enter the workforce. Services provided by vocational rehabilitation centers include identifying and facilitating the implementation of appropriate accommodations (including financial support for augmentative communication or external cognitive devices) so that patients can return to their previous occupations. If necessary, patients also can receive education and/or training in a new field.

Older patients with neurogenic language and cognitive disorders may benefit from attending a senior center or related program that provides social programs for elderly individuals. Not only are these centers generally supportive of patients with disabilities, but many older adults without disabilities attend activities at the center, providing a rich social context for patients with neurogenic language and cognitive disorders. These centers may be particularly useful in helping patients identify hobbies and other recreational activities that are compatible with their current physical, cognitive, and communicative abilities. Larger communities may have similar centers for young adults and professional-aged individuals.

Complementary and Alternative Treatments

Complementary and alternative medicine (CAM) represents one of the most rapidly growing approaches to preventing and treating a spectrum of medical and psychological problems, including neurogenic language and cognitive disorders, with approximately 38% of the U.S. adult population utilizing CAM (P. Barnes, Bloom, & Nahin, 2008). The National Center for Complementary and Alternative Medicine (NCCAM; 2013) describes CAM as a diverse collection of health-care systems (e.g., traditional Chinese medicine, folk healing), therapies (e.g., hypnosis, natural environment therapy, massage), and products (e.g., herbal medications, homeopathic preparations) for maximizing, restoring, or maintaining physical and mental well-being that have been developed and primarily utilized outside of conventional medical institutions. Despite the heterogeneity of these approaches, all focus on providing individualized treatment of patients and on emphasizing "holistic" treatment in terms of not only remediating medical or physical ailments but also fostering mental and spiritual well-being (P. Barnes, Powell-Griner, McFann, & Nahin, 2004). Accordingly, many of these treatments aim to go beyond effecting change at only the ICF level of body structure and function, and strive to enhance patients' recovery at ICF activity and participation levels as well. Because of increased consumer interest in CAM techniques, and because of growing empirical support for the use of at least some of these techniques, a brief description of a few CAM approaches that have been used with neurogenic patient populations is provided below.

Relaxation Therapy

Relaxation therapy, which includes meditation, progressive muscle relaxation, and biofeedback, is one of the most commonly practiced forms of CAM (P. Barnes et al.,

2004; NCCAM, 2013) and has become more widely used in recent years (P. Barnes et al., 2008). Very generally, these therapies involve sustaining attention to a verbal (e.g., word, phrase, prayer) or nonverbal (e.g., tone, mental image) stimulus or muscle activity while concurrently inhibiting thoughts or sensory input that may interfere with the attentional focus on the target stimulus or activity (L. Murray & Kim, 2004). Practice of these relaxation techniques can produce physiological changes (e.g., reduced heart and breathing rates) to counter stress, and has been found to address a variety of conditions (e.g., chronic pain, anxiety, depression, cardiovascular disease) that commonly coexist with neurogenic language or cognitive disorders (V. Busch et al., 2012; Jorm, Christensen, Griffiths, & Rodgers, 2002; Tekur, Nagarathna, Chametcha, Hankey, & Nagendra, 2012; Wetherell, 1998). Moreover, evidence suggests that relaxation therapy can have positive effects on non-cognitive/communicative symptoms of neurologic disease (Sutherland, Andersen, & Morris, 2005; van Kessel et al., 2008; for a review of additional relaxation research involving neurogenic populations, see Murray, 2008a).

Initial research indicates that relaxation therapy might help ameliorate the linguistic and cognitive symptoms associated with a number of neurological disorders. For example, meditation has been used in combination with other CAM or conventional (e.g., memory strategy education) procedures to enhance the cerebral blood flow, word retrieval, memory, and attention abilities of patients with aphasia (Ince, 1968; Orenstein & Shisler, 2009), mild cognitive impairment (Belleville et al., 2006; Newberg, Wintering, Khalsa, Roggenkamp, & Waldman, 2010; S. Rapp, Brenes, & Marsh, 2002), multiple sclerosis (Tesar, Bandion, & Baumhackl, 2005), or TBI (C. Wilson & Robertson, 1992). **Guided imagery (GI)** also has been used with neurogenic patient populations. This relaxation technique requires patients to select a pleasant and calm location or event, and then imagine being at that location or event (P. Barnes et al., 2004). When combined with other CAM or conventional treatments, GI has been found to improve social interaction (Welden & Yesavage, 1982), quality of life (Bédard et al., 2002), and the informativeness of verbal output (Murray & Ray, 2001) in patients with dementia, TBI, or aphasia. More substantial positive effects have been associated with **progressive muscle relaxation (PMR)**, which involves successively contracting and relaxing certain muscle groups (P. Barnes et al., 2004). For example, both R. Marshall and Watts (1976) and Suhr, Anderson, and Tranel (1999) found that PMR by itself facilitated the linguistic (i.e., naming, verbal fluency, and other spoken language abilities) and cognitive (i.e., memory) abilities of patients with aphasia or Alzheimer's disease, respectively. Another relaxation therapy that has proven effective with neurogenic patient populations is **biofeedback**. This technique involves teaching patients conscious self-regulation of physiological functions (e.g., brain wave activity, skin temperature) that are related to stress levels by connecting patients to simple electronic devices that monitor the target physiological functions (P. Barnes et al., 2004). Whereas most biofeedback research has focused on motoric changes in patients with neurogenic disorders (e.g., Yoo, Park, & Chung, 2001), a study by D. Holland, Witty, Lawler, and Lanzisera (1999) indicated that two TBI patients with severe cognitive-communicative disorders not only learned how to utilize biofeedback, but also consequently exhibited decreased anxiety and increased therapy compliance and achieved faster therapy progress while using this CAM technique.

It is also noteworthy that relaxation therapy has been successfully used to alleviate stress and other negative symptoms in caregivers of patients with neurogenic language and cognitive disorders. For example, Mizuno, Hosaka, Ogihara, Higano, and Mano (1999) enrolled one group of caregivers of dementia patients in a five-week intervention program consisting of education (e.g., information about dementia, associations between stress and disease), group discussions on caregiving problems, and relaxation therapy, while another group of caregivers on their waiting list served as controls. Caregivers who completed the intervention program displayed significantly improved emotional and immune functioning compared to the control group. Additionally, caregivers who continued to use relaxation techniques at home were able to maintain or make additional improvements at two months post-treatment. Similar findings have been reported by other researchers (Khan & Curtice, 2011; Lavretsky et al., 2012) and for caregivers from a variety of cultures (Y. Lee, Sung, & Kim, 2012; Llanque & Enriquez, 2012), suggesting that relaxation techniques may be a valuable component of caregiver training programs.

Sensory Stimulation

Of the various CAM approaches tried with neurogenic patient populations, **sensory stimulation** techniques have been utilized most frequently both clinically and in the research literature. As shown in Table 12-5, there are a variety of sensory stimulation treatments, all of which are based on exposing patients to, and allowing them to interact with, often in a non-directive manner, stimuli that will excite one or more senses. The rationale for sensory stimulation is that patients with neurogenic disorders often not only present with disease- and/or age-related declines in their sensory and perceptual abilities but also may live in sensory-deprived environments, particularly those who reside in long-term-care facilities (Bourgeois & Hickey, 2009; Chung & Lai, 2009; Kovach, 2000). These biologically and environmentally related sensory deficiencies can lead to a state of sensory deprivation, which in turn has been found to evoke or aggravate behavioral, social, cognitive, and psychiatric problems. Accordingly, preventing or ameliorating sensory deprivation should have beneficial effects on patients' physical and mental well-being.

Indeed, several sensory stimulation treatments, including light (e.g., McCurry et al., 2011; Yamadera et al., 2000), toy (e.g., L. Murray, Dickerson, Lichtenberger, & Cox, 2003), music (e.g., Guétin et al., 2009; Raglio et al., 2008; Vink, Bruinsma, & Scholten, 2011), robotic pet (e.g., Libin & Cohen-Mansfield, 2004), and pet (e.g., Chitic, Rusu, & Szamoskozi, 2012; Richeson, 2003) therapies have been successfully utilized with neurogenic patients. Most research, however, has focused on the provision of multisensory stimulation, which is also referred to as Snoezelen (Chung & Lai, 2009; Lancioni, Cuvo, & O'Reilly, 2002). In this treatment approach, patients are exposed to an environment or collection of stimuli designed to stimulate all sensory channels. For example, a long-term-care facility may have a Snoezelen room that contains spot lights, mirror balls, and/or optic fiber sprays to stimulate vision, music equipment to stimulate audition, essential oil samples to stimulate smell, vibrating chairs and/or fabric samples to

TABLE 12-5
Sensory Stimulation Treatments

TYPE OF THERAPY	BRIEF DESCRIPTION AND EFFECTS
Multisensory stimulation or Snoezelen	Structured or unstructured exposure to visual (e.g., colored lights), auditory (e.g., music), tactile (e.g., fabric samples with different textures), olfactory (e.g., scented oils), proprioceptive (e.g., a swinging chair), and/or gustatory (e.g., different flavored candies) stimuli to decrease disruptive behaviors and to increase communicative output, cognitive functioning, socialization, and emotional well-being
Toy stimulation	Provision of toys, in particular plush animal toys or baby dolls, which patients care for and interact with to decrease disruptive behaviors and to increase communicative output and emotional well-being
Pet or animal-assisted therapy	Inclusion of trained pets (e.g., dog, cat) in traditional behavioral treatment to enhance linguistic and/or cognitive abilities, to improve emotional functioning, and to decrease disruptive behaviors
Music therapy	Patients produce or listen to music to facilitate their linguistic and/or cognitive abilities, to decrease disruptive behaviors, and to improve emotional functioning
Light therapy or phototherapy	Structured exposure to bright light emitted from light boxes, light rooms, or light visors to improve sleep/wake cycle regularity and consequently improve general cognitive, behavioral, and emotional functioning
Robotherapy	Provision of robotic pets that patients care for and interact with to decrease disruptive behaviors and to increase communicative output and emotional well-being
Natural environment therapy	Exposure to objects, colors, sounds, and so forth that are indigenous to patients' daily environments prior to being admitted to an acute or chronic care facility

stimulate touch, and food samples to stimulate taste. A key component to this approach, particularly when it is provided to patients with dementia, is that patients are given the choice to interact with whatever stimuli appeal to them. Positive outcomes reported in studies involving patients with varying forms of moderate to severe dementia (e.g., Alzheimer's disease, Huntington's disease, multi-infarct dementia) include decreases in disruptive behaviors, apathy, negative emotions (e.g., anxiety), and perseveration, and increases in socialization, memory, attention, communicative output and fluency, mobility, activities of daily living, quality of life, and caregiver morale when even brief periods of multisensory stimulation were provided (Chung & Lai, 2009; Cornell, 2004; Leng et al., 2003; Milev et al., 2008). These improvements are typically temporary, but even transient positive changes have clinical significance for those caring for these patients.

Multisensory stimulation also has been provided to patients who have suffered a severe stroke or TBI in an attempt to increase the rate and extent of recovery from coma and persistent vegetative state (Meyer et al., 2010). Treatment procedures for this patient population differ from those described above for patients with dementia in that the sensory stimuli are selected and applied by the clinician or caregiver on typically a more intensive schedule (e.g., one- to two-hour sessions per day) and in a more structured manner. Positive outcomes such as increased levels of cognitive functioning and decreased coma lengths and severity have been frequently reported (e.g., Noda, Maeda, & Yoshino, 2004; Oh & Seo, 2003; Urbenjaphol, Jitpanya, & Khaoropthum, 2009; S. L. Wilson, Powell, Elliot, & Thwaites, 1993). However, despite the predominance of encouraging findings for patients with dementia, severe TBI, or stroke, most previous studies had weak research designs (e.g., use of unstandardized measures, biased observers, failure to include a control group, small or imprecisely described subject samples). Therefore, more methodologically rigorous investigations must be completed before definitive conclusions regarding the effectiveness of multisensory stimulation can be made (Chung & Lai, 2009; Lombardi, Taricco, De Tanti, Telaro, & Liberati, 2002; Meyer et al., 2010).

Acupuncture

Acupuncture involves stimulating the skin, and consequently the nerves, at designated anatomic locations or acupoints in order to reestablish blocked or intermittent flow of body energy, referred to as "chi" or "qi" (Barnes et al., 2004; L. Murray & Kim, 2004). There are numerous forms of acupuncture that vary in terms of stimulation method (e.g., needling/manual or electric needle insertion, finger pressure/acupressure, heat application/moxibustion) and location and number of acupoints. Empirical studies have verified that stimulation of these peripheral acupoints does indeed activate higher levels of the nervous system (e.g., spinal cord, midbrain, cortical regions), as well as cause the release of neurotransmitters and neurohormones (e.g., enkephalines, serotonin) (Lo & Cui, 2003).

Whereas the use of acupuncture to treat certain medical conditions (e.g., chronic pain, nausea) has a long history of empirical support (Fouladbakhsh, 2012; Rabinstein & Shulman, 2003), application of this CAM technique to remediate neurogenic language and cognitive disorders has been studied with greater interest only in recent years. Early studies produced mixed findings (L. Murray & Kim, 2004). For instance, in several studies conducted by Chinese researchers to evaluate the effects of acupuncture on aphasia, it is not clear whether the positive changes reported reflected improved motor speech versus improved motor speech and spoken language, or whether the positive changes were maintained over time (Zhang, 1989; Zhang & Zhao, 1990). A more recent systematic review conducted by Chinese researchers (Y. Pang, Wu, & Liu, 2010) considered findings from 11 randomized controlled trials. The reviewers concluded that although acupuncture in isolation may be beneficial, acupuncture combined with language therapy resulted in the best outcomes with respect to "cure rate," language function score, and oral expression. Of interest, recent studies have attempted to explain the benefit of acupuncture. Chau, Fai Cheung, Jiang, Au-Yeung, and Li (2010) examined the effects of eight weeks of acupuncture on individuals with chronic aphasia who were receiving no other rehabilitation. They reported improved language performance, as well as increased metabolism in Wernicke's area, and the increase in metabolism correlated with the increase in language performance. Additional research is needed to determine the mechanisms by which acupuncture affects language performance and the nature of behavioral treatments that are most effectively paired with acupuncture.

Research with TBI or Parkinson's disease patients has primarily evaluated changes in motor symptoms and has failed to include linguistic or cognitive outcome measures (L. Murray & Kim, 2004). Moreover, a recent systematic review of the literature examining the role of acupuncture in the rehabilitation of TBI concluded that insufficient evidence is currently available to support this approach (Wong, Cheuk, Lee, & Chu, 2011).

More encouraging findings, however, have been reported when **transcutaneous electrical nerve stimulation (TENS)** has been used with neurogenic patient populations. TENS is similar to electro-acupuncture, as it involves stimulating the skin at certain frequencies and skin sites (which tend to overlap with acupoints). TENS has been shown to reduce left neglect in patients with RHD (Beschin, Cocchini, Allen, & Dela Sala, 2012; Polanowska et al., 2009; Vallar, Rusconi, & Bernardini, 1996). Early studies also demonstrated improvements in memory, verbal fluency, and emotional-behavioral symptoms in patients with Alzheimer's disease following TENS (Scherder, Bouma, & Steen, 1992, 1995). More recent investigations, however, have reported less impressive effects (Scherder, Vuijk, Swaab, & van Someren, 2007; Van Dijk et al., 2006). Further research is thus needed to clarify the benefits of TENS and to determine optimal stimulation schedules, to examine how long these positive changes are maintained, and to explore, as has been done with acupuncture, whether pairing TENS with behavioral interventions might result in more positive and enduring outcomes.

Exercise

Augmenting conventional behavioral linguistic or cognitive treatments with physical exercise has been found to benefit patients representing a range of static and progressive neurological disorders (Hammer & Chida, 2009; Lorenzen & Murray, 2008a), as well as their caregivers (Thom & Clare, 2011). Various forms of exercise have been incorporated into treatment, including yoga, tai chi, dancing, walking, biking, and strength/weight training. The addition of exercise to linguistic and cognitive rehabilitation programs is supported by several lines of research, including the following: (a) the prevalence of suboptimal levels of physical activity among the elderly, particularly those with neurological disorders (e.g., Roger et al., 2011); (b) the fact that in animal and some human studies, exercise has been found to enhance cerebral blood flow (Ding, Vaynman, Souda, Whitelegge, & Gomez-Pinilla, 2006), increase brain volume (Colcombe et al., 2006), promote immune system functioning, and evoke structural and neurochemical changes in brain regions that are known to support linguistic and cognitive functioning, including the hippocampus and prefrontal cortex (e.g., Rogers, Schroeder, Secher, & Mitchell, 1990; Vaynman, Ying, & Gomez-Pinilla, 2003); and (c) that exercise has been found to help healthy adults, as well as those with a variety of medical conditions (e.g., depression, anxiety, diabetes mellitus, osteoarthritis, incontinence), improve or maintain their physical, cognitive, and emotional status (e.g., Brazzelli, Saunders, Greig, & Mead, 2011; Keogh & MacLeod, 2012).

A body of literature has developed examining the benefits of exercise for individuals with neurogenic language and cognitive disorders (e.g., McDonnell, Smith, & McIntosh, 2011). Early studies documented the benefits of exercise on the physical well-being of individuals with TBI, particularly in terms of reductions in fatigue (A. Moran, 1976; Wolman, Cornall, Flucher, & Greenwood, 1994), which in turn may positively affect cognitive and linguistic functioning (Merritta, Cherian, Macaden, & John, 2010). For example, Grealy, Johnson, and Rushton (1999) directly examined the effects of exercise on the cognitive abilities of patients in the acute or chronic stages of recovery from TBI. Two groups of patients with TBI were involved in this study: one group that only received traditional rehabilitation procedures and one that received both traditional rehabilitation procedures as well as a virtual reality exercise program. The four-week exercise program consisted of riding a virtual reality exercise bicycle at least three times per week for up to 25 minutes per session. The virtual reality component consisted of a color monitor that displayed graphics pertaining to a bicycle ride on an island, in a town and countryside, or on a snowy mountain; patients were also provided kinesthetic stimulation (e.g., bike seat would tilt when they did a turn), tactile stimulation (e.g., a fan would blow on them to simulate air flow), and auditory stimulation (e.g., they heard sounds relating to the pictured scenes). A comparison of the treatment and control group's pre- and post-treatment test performances indicated that the treatment group displayed superior improvements on tests of verbal and visual learning that were attributed to improved working memory abilities, as well as significantly faster reaction times. The effect of exercise on cognitive function in TBI continues to be of great interest to rehabilitation researchers. Systematic reviews (e.g., Devine & Zafonte, 2009) can assist clinicians in determining the best candidates for exercise programs and the types of cognitive behaviors that are best facilitated by exercise.

The results of several investigations have established that exercise can enhance cognitive functioning in patients with mild to severe forms of dementia (Ahlskog, Geda, Graff-Radford, & Petersen, 2011; Bonner & Cousins, 1996; Thom & Clare, 2011). For example, Arkin (2003; Arkin & Mahendra, 2001; Mahendra & Arkin, 2004) has published a series of studies on the positive effects of the Elder Rehab program on the linguistic, cognitive, physical, and emotional functioning of community-dwelling patients in the early to middle stages of Alzheimer's disease. Arkin's treatment program includes the following: (a) two to three weekly exercise sessions consisting of aerobic exercise (i.e., walking, stationary biking), strength training, and flexibility and balance exercises; (b) one weekly volunteer work session at which patients help out at community agencies; (c) one weekly recreational activity such as going to a museum or concert; and (d) language exercises (e.g., providing opinions and advice concerning controversial topics, generating the pros and cons of situations and issues, object description tasks) and memory exercises (i.e., listening to tape-recorded narratives about their life and family and answering questions pertaining to these tapes) completed either during or prior to exercise sessions. For all components of the program, either student volunteers or caregivers accompany the patients. Comparisons of pre- and post-intervention assessment results have indicated that patients with dementia show significant improvements in their physical fitness and depression levels, and they have higher or maintained general cognitive abilities, as well as improved or maintained spoken language production (e.g., informativeness levels) and comprehension (i.e., proverb interpretation) skills. Similar findings have been reported in other studies examining cycling exercise (Anderson-Hanley et al., 2012), as well as yoga (Fan & Chen, 2011) and tai chi (Lam et al., 2011). Unfortunately, most research has involved only patients with Alzheimer's disease; thus, how patients with other dementing illnesses (e.g., frontotemporal dementia) respond to exercise needs to be examined.

Although it seems likely that positive outcomes with physical exercise could also be achieved in patients with aphasia or cognitive-communicative disorders related to RHD, research to support this contention is only beginning to emerge. Lorenzen and Murray (2011) have presented some initial positive findings: Their patients with anomic or Broca's aphasia demonstrated greater improvements in aphasia severity, processing speed, and executive functioning following six weeks of recombinant bike exercise (one session/week) versus six weeks of a control treatment (simply conversing with an undergraduate student). Such data are encouraging and highlight the need for additional research with aphasic as well as RHD patients.

In summary, despite growing empirical support for using CAM to supplement more traditional behavioral linguistic or cognitive treatments for neurogenic language and cognitive disorders, further research is required to resolve a number of issues. First, it is not yet known whether certain CAM approaches might prove more suitable for certain neurogenic patient populations or certain linguistic or cognitive symptoms. Second, investigation of the long-term effects of CAM is needed (e.g., Are positive effects maintained following termination of the CAM technique? How much CAM intervention is needed to foster maintenance of positive treatment effects?). Third, many previous studies had weak designs (e.g., failed to control for placebo or practice effects, relied on subjective measures), and thus investigations with strong, controlled designs are still needed. Finally, future research should focus on extending our understanding of the effects of CAM to a broader range of neurogenic disorders and linguistic and cognitive abilities. Almost certainly, CAM approaches will be most effective when paired with body structure and function- and/or activity/participation-focused treatments targeting specific communicative and/or cognitive behaviors.

Counseling and Education

It is somewhat misleading to introduce the topic of counseling and education in Chapter 12, as this aspect of service to patients and caregivers affected by neurogenic language and cognitive disorders is crucial from the moment speech-language pathologists meet patients and their families (McFarlane, 2012). Although neurogenic language or cognitive disorders are relatively common, many individuals know very little about these conditions and may experience considerable anxiety related to the "unknown." Moreover, physicians and other members of the care team may be more concerned or familiar with immediate physical health concerns, and thus fail to address issues related to communication and cognition. Therefore, it is important that clinicians be prepared to provide information, along with other components of counseling (e.g., allowing patients and caregivers an opportunity to state concerns or vent frustrations related to the neurogenic disorder or treatment program), to patients and their caregivers or families immediately upon meeting them, as well as throughout the recovery process, or, in the case of progressive disorders (e.g., Alzheimer's disease, Huntington's disease), throughout disease evolution.

The amount and type of information individuals need vary according to a variety of factors, so clinicians will need to be sensitive to relevant cues (e.g., signs of confusion, fatigue, and/or impatience) when providing information (A. Holland, 2007; Paul & Sanders, 2010). During the days early postonset or immediately following diagnosis with a progressive disease, most families will benefit from basic information about the neurogenic language or cognitive disorder, explanation of professional jargon, and description and demonstration of simple strategies for facilitating communicative interactions with their loved ones. It is likely that this information will need to be provided more than once, as the stress associated with medical crisis affects individuals' ability to understand and retain the vast amount of information that will be presented to them by a variety of different medical professionals (Hinckley, 2000). Providing written material in addition to verbal explanations is highly recommended, as it may help individuals comprehend the information being presented and will allow them to reread and refer back to the information as often as they need (E. Miller et al., 2010; Sorin-Peters, 2004; Togher, 2012); additionally, they will be able to share this written material with family members and significant others who are unable to speak directly with the health-care team. In addition to considering the modality of information presentation, clinicians should attend to how they format other counseling techniques (e.g., types of questions and affirmations used by the clinician). Interested readers can consult counseling articles (e.g., McFarlane, 2012) and books (e.g., A. Holland, 2007) for descriptions and applications of key counseling skills not covered in this or other chapters of our book.

When the immediate health crisis has passed, family members will likely request information about when communication or cognition will return to normal (A. Holland, 2007; A. Holland & Fridriksson, 2001). In the case of progressive disorders, patients and families will want to know how quickly abilities will deteriorate. Often clinicians will be unable to provide a prognosis so early in recovery or the disease process, but it may be possible to discuss the factors that influence the rate and degree of recovery or disease progression (see Chapters 6 and 7 for a description of linguistic and cognitive prognostic indicators, respectively) and begin to explore treatment options with patients and their families. Because status changes are common in the early days of recovery from static disorders (e.g., stroke, TBI), clinicians also should be prepared to explain variability so that patients, their caregivers, or both do not become discouraged or overly optimistic when communication or cognitive abilities change temporarily.

As patients continue through the recovery process, they may benefit from more detailed information about treatment options (see included DVD: Patient 2b). Similarly, family members may request information about the treatments their loved ones are receiving. In particular, the purpose of many treatment activities or compensatory strategies may not be obvious to non–speech-language pathologists. For patients experiencing degenerative conditions, counseling and education should include information to help the patient and family members prepare for the inevitable decline in cognitive and communicative abilities and, accordingly, for continual changes in therapy goals (which, it should be emphasized, focus on maintaining rather than necessarily improving current functioning) and procedures. When discussing treatment procedures and progress, clinicians should always ensure that they not only identify linguistic and cognitive areas in need of remediation, but also emphasize areas of strength (see included DVD: Patient 8l) by describing how patients' abilities have progressed or been maintained over the course of treatment (A. Holland, 2007; A. Holland & Fridriksson, 2001; McFarlane, 2012; E. Miller et al., 2010).

At every stage in the clinical process, the clinician should provide referrals to appropriate resources, including support groups, which were discussed in greater detail in an earlier section of this chapter. Clinicians also may wish to provide a printed list of key internet resources, with the understanding that additional resources may be identified through an internet search. Table 12-4 includes a sample list of sites clinicians might include. Given the relative speed with which internet resources appear and disappear, it is recommended that these lists be updated at least annually. A variety of print resources also are available. For example, a very useful resource developed specifically for patients affected by neurogenic language disorders is *Coping With Aphasia* (Lyon, 1998). In language appropriate for non-communication professionals, this book addresses a plethora of concerns experienced throughout the various stages of recovery. Although this book focuses on aphasia, much of the information is applicable to any condition of sudden onset. Also available are a number of personal accounts written by individuals affected by neurogenic language and cognitive disorders (see Table 12-6).

Finally, clinicians should be cautioned that because the speech-language pathologist may be the health-care professional with whom individuals have the greatest contact, patients and their families may request information and/or counseling outside the scope of practice of the speech-language pathologist. It is not uncommon to receive questions related to insurance, medication, other symptoms (e.g., sexual dysfunction, psychiatric disorders, family adjustment issues), other therapies, or even laboratory test results. In these cases, the clinician should be prepared to refer patients and their families to the appropriate professional. More specifically, clinicians should develop a list of health-care professionals who are experienced not only in their own area (e.g., family therapy, counseling, social work, psychiatry) but also in issues specific to neurogenic language and cognitive disorders (e.g., how aphasia may affect a marriage, how TBI

TABLE 12-6
Examples of Published Personal Accounts of Individuals With Neurogenic Language and Cognitive Disorders

TITLE	AUTHOR	PUBLISHER
Stroke, Aphasia		
A Mind of My Own: Memoir of Recovery From Aphasia	Mills (2004)	Authorhouse
Crossing the Void: My Aphasic Journey	Schultz (2010)	CreateSpace
My Stroke of Insight: A Brain Scientist's Personal Journey	J. Taylor (2008)	Viking
Pathways: Moving Beyond Stroke and Aphasia	Ewing & Pfalzgraf (1991)	Wayne State University Press
The Invaluable Guide to Life After Stroke: An Owner's Manual	Josephs (1992)	Amadeus Press
Return to Ithaca	Newborn (1997)	Element
Stroke: From Crisis to Victory	Lavin (1985)	Scholastic Library
My Stroke of Luck	K. Douglas (2003)	HarperCollins
RHD		
Right Hemisphere Stroke: A Victim Reflects on Rehabilitative Medicine	F. Johnson (1990)	Wayne State University Press
TBI		
Gabby: A Story of Courage and Hope	Giffords & Kelly (2011)	Scribner
Brain Storm: A Journey of Faith Through Brain Injury	Allen & Allen (2012)	Vintage
Where Is the Mango Princess? A Journey Back From Brain Injury	Crimmins (2001)	WestBowPress
Over My Head	Osborn (2000)	Andrews McMeel
In an Instant: A Family's Journey of Love and Healing	Woodruff & Woodruff (2007)	Random House
I'll Carry the Fork! Recovering a Life After Brain Injury	Swanson (1999)	Rising Star
Surviving Black Ice: A Survivor's Insight to Life After Head Injury	Fierce (2002)	Writer's Block Press
Dementia		
Alzheimer Diary: A Wife's Journal	Montgomery (2010)	CreateSpace
Alzheimer's From the Inside Out	R. Taylor (2006)	Health Professions Press
My Journey in Alzheimer's Disease	R. Davis (1994)	Tyndale House
Living in the Labyrinth: A Personal Journey Through the Maze of Alzheimer's	McGowin (1994)	Dell
Living With Alzheimer's: Ruth's Story	Danforth (1986)	Prestige Press

can impact a patient's ability to fulfill her parental role, how to assess depression in the presence of severe language impairment), including previous familiarity with adapting their services to meet patients' communicative and cognitive strengths and weaknesses (e.g., the professional is experienced in using multimodality communication strategies; for patients with memory problems, the professional provides information in a written format to serve as a reminder of what transpired during the session).

Summary

In this chapter, a number of strategies for assisting patients with neurogenic language and cognitive disorders in communicating effectively and participating fully in desired activities, even in the presence of significant impairments, have been reviewed. It should be clear to the reader that managing neurogenic language and cognitive disorders extends not only beyond remediation of the impairments in body function and structure exhibited by the patient, but also beyond even the patient: Clinicians may effect significant changes in a patient's activity and participation by directing efforts toward the communication and cognitive context, including communication partners and the larger social and even physical environment. A beginning literature supports the benefits of activity and participation level treatments, and as the ICF framework becomes more widely applied in American health care, it is likely that reimbursement for these treatments will be more commonplace. In the meantime, clinicians must continue to advocate on a case-by-case basis for the most appropriate intervention plans.

Discussion Questions

1. How will you determine which compensatory strategies will be most effective for any given patient?
2. How does the use of AAC by individuals with neurogenic language and cognitive disorders differ from that of other populations (e.g., children with cerebral palsy, adults with dysarthria)?
3. Explain how communicative strategies are similar to and different from cognitive strategies. Could any one patient use both communicative and cognitive strategies?
4. How will you likely collaborate with other professionals to help patients and their families implement environmental modifications?
5. How would your professional approach to training conversation partners differ from that of intervening directly with patients? Consider your communication style, methods of assessment, and training strategies.
6. How will you respond to patient, family, or other professional inquiries regarding the potential benefit of complementary and alternative approaches for improving communication or cognition?

The Context of Care: Legislative and Economic Influences

chapter 13

Learning Objectives

After reading this chapter, you should be able to:

- Identify key legislation affecting services to individuals with neurogenic language and cognitive disorders
- List funding models for services provided to individuals with neurogenic language and cognitive disorders
- Discuss influences of health-care economics on provision of services to individuals with neurogenic language and cognitive disorders
- Describe how speech-language pathology (SLP) services vary across the continuum of care

Key Terms

- acute care
- adaptive
- caps or limits
- capitation systems
- case-mix adjustment
- case rate
- continuum of care
- diagnosis-related group (DRG)
- fee-for-service
- health-care reform
- home health
- home health resource group (HHRG)
- intensive care unit (ICU)
- long-term care
- managed care
- Minimum Data Set (MDS)
- outpatient
- per diem
- preferred providers
- primary care
- prospective payment
- quality assurance
- rehabilitation
- resource utilization group (RUG)
- restorative
- secondary care
- skilled nursing facility
- tertiary care
- third-party payers

Introduction

In the preceding chapters, we have used the constructs of the International Classification of Functioning, Disability, and Health (ICF; WHO, 2001) to characterize the complexity of neurogenic cognitive and language disorders. Of note, we have considered the importance of contextual factors that influence the impact of neurogenic disorders on the individual and his or her family. In this chapter, we consider additional contextual factors informing the management of neurogenic language and cognitive disorders. The factors discussed in previous chapters were those that often require assessment to determine their presence and influence (e.g., availability of communication partners). The factors reviewed in this chapter tend to vary across health-care systems or broad population groups rather than across individuals. It is typically not necessary, therefore, to assess these factors for individual patients. Instead, the issues discussed in this chapter are those that clinicians must understand to provide the most appropriate care and to conduct a successful clinical practice. By necessity, this discussion will emphasize the legislative and economic influences on health care in the United States. We readily acknowledge that the information we include may not be applicable to all readers' practices, but we hope that our review may alert non-U.S. readers to the types of contextual factors with which they should become familiar.

Continuum of Care: Health-Care Delivery

Health-care delivery models vary widely internationally. The focus of this chapter will be care in the United States, while acknowledging that even within the United States, practices may vary considerably (e.g., at the state level). The phrase "**continuum of care**" refers to matching an individual's changing needs with the appropriate level and type of care. The continuum of care is employed judiciously in two main contexts: The first relates to how individuals access various levels of medical expertise, whereas the second refers to the levels of care individuals receive during and following hospitalization. These contexts will be discussed in turn, but keep in mind that the care for most individuals takes places across these contexts (Figure 13-1).

The continuum of care can be considered with respect to points of access to general and special services. **Primary care** (WHO, 1978) is typically the first and most frequent point of contact individuals have with the health-care system. In the United States, adult primary care is delivered in the community by general practitioners, internists, gerontologists, and nurse practitioners. Preventative care and care for common illnesses and injuries are typically managed through primary care. Individuals who experience gradual onset of language or cognitive symptoms will likely first seek evaluation through their primary care provider. Referral to SLP and related disciplines (e.g., neuropsychology, occupational therapy) from primary care providers is not uncommon, particularly if a medical diagnosis has been established.

> ### The Role of Speech-Language Pathologists (SLPs) in Prevention
>
> The importance of SLP services for individuals experiencing neurogenic cognitive or language disorders is emphasized throughout this text. But what role can SLPs play in the prevention of these difficulties? In a position statement issued 25 years ago, ASHA (1988) characterized a number of primary prevention activities within the scope of practice for SLP. These activities include raising awareness about neurogenic cognitive and language disorders and the conditions with which they are associated. "May Is Better Speech and Hearing Month," "Brain Awareness Week," and "Aphasia Awareness Month" are annual events that pro-

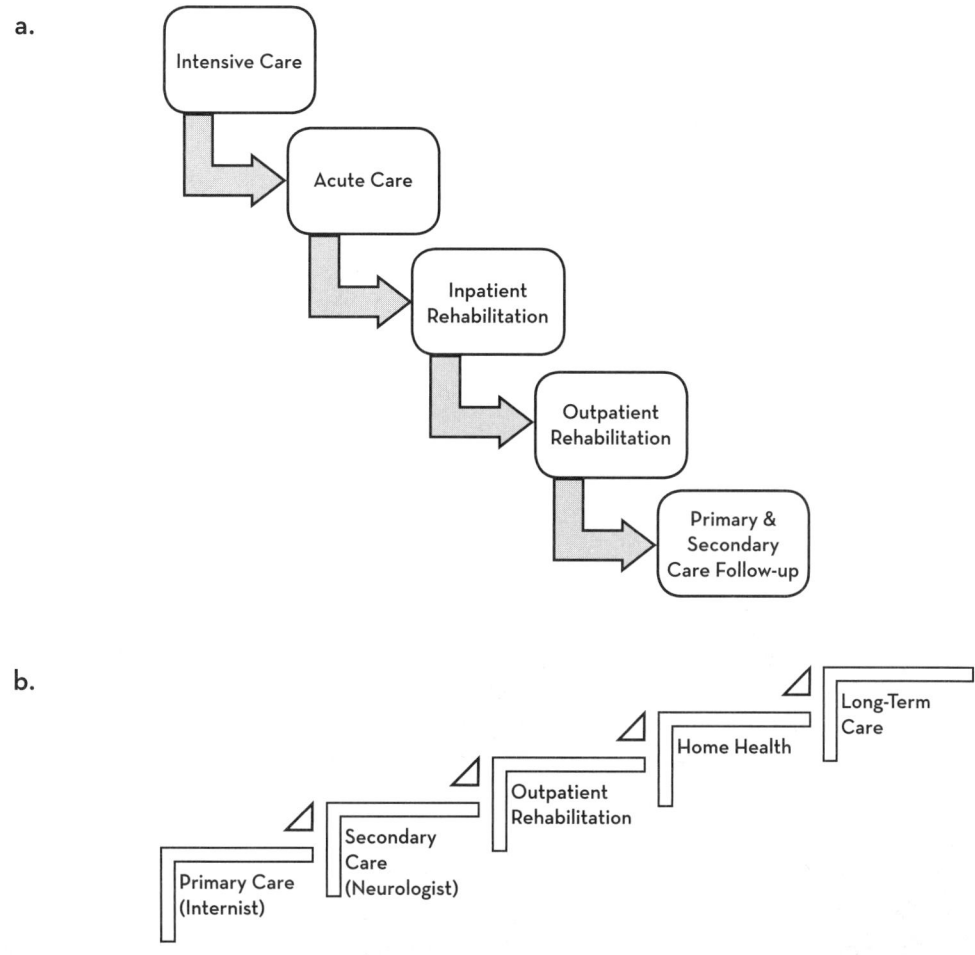

Figure 13-1. Examples of how the continuum of care may be employed by an individual with (a) an acute event (e.g., stroke, TBI) or (b) a progressive condition (e.g., Parkinson disease). Keep in mind that it is possible to skip a level of care or to return to a previous level of care in the context of changing function.

vide ready avenues for primary prevention activities. Flyers, brochures, banners, and public service announcements reminding the public about the importance of helmets and seat belts, risk factors for stroke, descriptions of aphasia and communication strategies, and warning signs of head injury or cognitive decline not only provide important prevention information but also raise awareness of communication and cognitive difficulties as well as the services SLPs can provide to individuals with these difficulties and to their families and communities.

Prevention and wellness activities should target individuals across the lifespan (H. Clark, 1999), in recognition that it is not just adults who experience acquired neurogenic language and cognitive problems. Clinicians also may promote wellness through educational programs designed to teach individuals how to cope with existing cognitive and/or communicative impairments. These programs might target individuals with the impairments, their families, friends, co-workers, and employers (see Chapter 12). These programs may have as great an impact on patients' participation as any direct treatment provided.

Many individuals with neurogenic language and cognitive disorders will be referred by their primary care provider for additional assessment by a **secondary care** professional or specialist. Neurologists are, not surprisingly, the most likely specialist to be consulted to address such difficulties. In the case of dementing diseases, psychiatry is a common secondary care profession. If not already completed, a referral to SLP services often occurs at this point in the continuum of care, perhaps even as the medical evaluation process is ongoing. Some neurologists consult SLPs to assist in establishing a differential diagnosis. More common, however, are SLP referrals for behavioral rehabilitation of cognitive and linguistic impairments.

Beyond secondary care is **tertiary care**, which is delivered through hospitals and specialty centers employing subspecialists with expertise in very particular disorder areas. Subspecialties typically involved in the assessment and management of neurogenic language and cognitive disorders include physiatry, behavioral neurology, cerebrovascular neurology, and neurosurgery, among others. Tertiary care is most often employed when a medical diagnosis is not easily established, in the context of complicating comorbidities, and when a condition does not respond as expected to standard treatment. SLPs may be consulted in the context of tertiary care to provide input informing differential diagnosis and to provide management strategies.

The continuum of care can also refer to the intensity and type of care provided in the event of an acute illness or injury. SLP services may be delivered across the continuum of care, from the intensive care unit to the home health setting, and even palliative care (E. Miller et al., 2010). The medical status of the patient, the length of treatment, and the availability of support (health-care providers and family) and funding all impact how services are delivered across the continuum of care. The care settings described in this section are those included in traditional U.S. health-care models, but readers are reminded that services also may be provided in nontraditional settings (e.g., life participation approaches; see Chapter 12).

Intensive Care

The **intensive care unit (ICU)**, also called the "critical care unit," is often the setting of care for the most critically ill or injured patients. Larger medical centers may employ separate intensive care units for different medical problems (e.g., cardiac intensive care, neonatal intensive care). Patients with traumatic brain injury, severe infections (e.g., meningitis), or hemorrhagic stroke, or who are undergoing neurosurgery, may be admitted to the neurosurgical or neurologic intensive care unit. Patients who receive rtPA (recombinant tissue plasminigen activator) intervention for ischemia (see Chapter 3) typically are also admitted to the intensive care unit for 24 hours because of the risk of secondary hemorrhage (H. Adams et al., 2007). Both general and specialized units hold life preservation as the primary health-care goal. Depending on the nature of a patient's medical conditions, he or she may undergo a variety of diagnostic tests or receive a multitude of treatments (Silbergleit & Basha, 2007). For example, a stroke patient will likely undergo several imaging studies during the first few hours to days following admission to determine the nature and extent of the stroke. A patient with head trauma may require orthopedic or neurosurgery and may have additional complications, such as the presence of a tracheostomy and mechanical ventilation. Length of stay in the ICU depends on the nature and severity of the illness or trauma, but a stay of one to two days would not be uncommon following an ischemic stroke, and head trauma or hemorrhagic stroke may warrant ICU stays of five to seven days or longer.

Referrals to SLP for patients in the ICU are not uncommon, and the clinician's role in this setting is rather unique. Perhaps in this setting more than any other, communication with the referring physician is critical, so that the SLP clearly understands what is being requested. Some physicians will request that clinicians address swallowing function in the ICU but defer communication services until the patient is transferred to the medical floor, whereas other physicians will request communication assessment immediately. Frequently, physicians are seeking additional information that will help inform differential diagnosis, and other times the request is to begin rehabilitation.

If the request is to provide information to assist in differential diagnosis, then careful assessment of all modalities at the impairment level is warranted. Keep in mind that the clinician, as the communication expert, may have the best understanding of the potential relationships between observed behaviors and neurogenic pathology. Although it is inappropriate to make a medical diagnosis, it is quite appropriate to suggest possible pathologies, such as "The patient exhibits anosognosia concurrent with a gross left neglect. She demonstrates a flat affect and responds inappropriately to indirect requests. . . . These characteristics are consistent with damage to the nondominant hemisphere."

An important aspect of care during this critical time is ongoing assessment. When a patient's medical status is poor and rapidly changing, the most telling signs of improvement or decline may be changes in communication, swallowing, or cognitive function. The astute clinician will continually assess the patient for evolution of symptoms that might indicate a change in medical status, the need for additional medical intervention, or both. The clinician should feel comfortable alerting the physician or the attending nurse to changes in status, and must be able to describe specifically the nature of these changes and the cause for concern or, hopefully, optimism. It has been our experience that as other health-care providers see the relevance of the observations SLPs make, a greater respect for our services develops.

For some patients, it will be appropriate to begin rehabilitation in the ICU, especially if the patient appears aware of his or her surroundings but is unable to communicate. In this case, establishing a communication system as soon as possible will have an immeasurable impact on the patient's well-being, the family's anxiety, and even the care the patient receives, as the physicians and other care providers have a means of communicating with the patient (G. Bartlett, Blais, Tamblyn, Clermont, & MacGibbon, 2008; Downey & Hurtig, 2006; Joint Commission, 2010). In some cases, the first communication system developed will be nonverbal, perhaps using eye-gaze or pointing. Equally important is educating family and health-care providers on the reliability of patients' yes/no responses and comprehension accuracy, as well as appropriate communication (e.g., for a patient with auditory comprehension problems, keeping their sentences short with simple syntax and pairing their speech with gesture or writing) and cognitive strategies (e.g., for a patient with neglect, presenting information on the non-neglected side). The reader is encouraged to review Chapter 12 and explore additional sources on augmentative and alternative communication systems in health-care settings (e.g., Hurtig & Downey, 2009) for more information on this aspect of care.

The Risks of Miscommunication

Patients with aphasia are often excellent at hiding or minimizing the severity of their communication impairments. Consequently, families as well as health-care professionals who are naïve about aphasic symptoms may easily misperceive the extent of patients' communication difficulties. For example, a spouse of one of the patients in our aphasia support group recently related an incident that occurred while her husband was in the hospital immediately following his stroke. One day she entered his hospital room while a nurse was collecting medical information from her husband. The nurse appeared to know that he had aphasia, as she was relying on primarily yes/no questions to complete his case history (i.e., avoiding the need for him to provide extensive verbal responses); however, the nurse was not aware that he had an unreliable yes/no response and significant auditory comprehension problems that compromised his understanding even at the single-word level. If his wife had not entered his hospital room when she did, this patient could have received inappropriate medical treatment, as the nurse was asking about whether or not he had any allergies—he responded no, when indeed he did have allergies, including some with respect to certain medications. Accordingly, educating all potential communication partners about patients' cognitive and communicative strengths and weaknesses is an essential component of treatment for any neurogenic language disorder.

Acute Care

"**Acute care**" generally refers to the services provided on a typical hospital ward. Most patients in acute care are no longer considered to be in a life-threatening condition, although they may still be quite ill or injured. A typical stay in acute care following stroke is three to seven days (DeFrances, Lucas, Buie, & Golosinskiy, 2008) and up to nine days or longer when SLP services are indicated (ASHA, 2008). The medical goals at this time are differential diagnosis and stabilization of the patient's medical status so that he or she can be discharged.

SLP referrals during this stage are typically for differential diagnosis of the cognitive and/or communicative impairments and to provide recommendation for discharge plans (J. Duffy et al., 2011). It is not likely that the patient will remain in acute care long enough for the development and/or execution of a formal treatment plan; thus, the role of SLPs in this setting can be considered "consultative" (J. Duffy et al., 2011; A. Johnson et al., 2006). Likewise, in the case of patients with TBI who might still be demonstrating post-traumatic amnesia (see Chapter 2), formal assessment is inappropriate at this stage of recovery because of patients' significant confusion, low frustration tolerance, and significant day-to-day if not moment-to-moment variability. Relatedly, during this time, even though patients may be medically stable or, in the case of TBI, out of the post-traumatic amnesia phase, patients with neurogenic language or cognitive disorders may have decreased alertness and reduced stamina; thus, sessions with patients are often only 10 to 20 minutes in length. This is not an extensive period of time in which to conduct a comprehensive assessment, so clinicians must learn to be creative in their assessment strategies. One way to work effectively within these time restrictions is to schedule short but frequent visits throughout the day. This has an advantage of increasing contact time and also allows the clinician to observe variations in performance related to time of day, fatigue, medication schedule, the presence of family members, and other factors.

Another way to maximize time with acute-care patients is to modify assessment tools to meet the time restrictions inherent to this setting. Recall from Chapters 4, 6, and 7 that most assessment batteries and tests for assessing more specific aspects of communication and cognition may take up to 60 minutes to administer to patients who can maintain alertness and attentional focus. Therefore, in the acute-care setting, it is usually better to select screening measures or informal instruments such as those described in Chapters 4 through 7 that, although less time-consuming, may provide the information needed in this assessment context (J. Duffy et al., 2011).

Clinical Dilemmas: Balancing "Real-World" Constraints With Established Clinical Principles

In Chapters 4 through 8 of this text, we have emphasized the importance of selecting clinical assessment procedures based on the best available evidence, including considering psychometric properties (e.g., validity and reliability) of standardized tools. Yet some clinical contexts pose constraints that preclude the use of tools with established evidentiary support. For example, consider a patient who is intubated and able to respond only by nonverbal means, or a patient who maintains alertness for 10 minutes or less. Is it acceptable, under these circumstances, to use assessment procedures that have not been standardized or to modify the administration of standardized tools?

Although this issue may be somewhat debatable, it is a simple statement of fact that validated, standardized, clinical procedures are not available for every conceivable variation of clinical practice. Instead, sound clinical decision making must be employed to determine which behaviors must be sampled to answer the primary clinical questions, as well as the procedures and materials that are most likely to elicit the behaviors of interest. The following cases will serve as an illustration.

I was asked to evaluate a patient who had undergone left hemispherectomy for treatment of intractable (unresponsive to medication) seizures. Two days post-surgery, she remained nonverbal and followed commands only sporadically, according to reports by the neurosurgeon and the nursing staff. Contrast this patient with a gentleman who experienced sudden onset of right-sided weakness and difficulty speaking. Imaging revealed blockage of the M1 segment of the left middle cerebral artery. He underwent thrombectomy and his symptoms quickly improved. The neurology staff could detect no difficulty with comprehension, repetition, or expression. The patient, however, insisted his expression was sluggish.

These patients arguably reflect the extremes of the aphasia severity continuum. In the first case, standardized assessment would likely have been unfruitful given the patient's overall lack of responsiveness. Instead, I utilized tasks and materials with the goal of identifying any conditions under which the patient could produce intentional nonverbal or verbal communication. This ultimately involved utilizing familiar items from her immediate surrounding and providing repeated, elaborated cues. In the second case, standardized aphasia assessment likely would have revealed "normal" performance. Instead, I had the patient complete tasks typical of his workday, including checking his email and role-playing providing instructions to his assistant. In addition to my own observations, I asked the patient to identify when he felt that his performance was inaccurate or inefficient.

Utilizing non-standardized procedures introduces potential confounds to the assessment process, making it all the more critical for the clinician to document the nature of the assessment tasks utilized and the behaviors observed. However, depending on the purposes of assessment and the interpretations to be made, non-standardized observations may be not only necessary but preferred.

In addition to differential diagnosis, another important goal of assessment in acute care is to develop discharge recommendations. Health-care economics dictate that services be provided with the goal of restoring the greatest amount of function for the least cost, or in the least expensive setting along the continuum of care. The SLP assessment should lead to recommendations regarding the need for cognitive and/or communication treatment, the environment in which the treatment would be best provided, and the prognosis for functional improvement. The prognostic factors discussed in Chapters 6 and 7 should be among those considered by the clinician when making discharge recommendations.

As was discussed for the ICU, rehabilitation in acute care should begin as soon as it is appropriate, especially if the patient requires an augmentative communication system. Clinicians should further provide family members and care staff with instruction in the use of any developed systems, including modifications they might need to adopt when communicating with patients or assisting them with daily activities. The importance of patient and family education at this point cannot be understated (J. Duffy et al., 2011; A. Holland & Fridriksson, 2001). In the immediate aftermath of a neurologic event requiring emergency or intensive care, family members may be so concerned about whether the patient will survive that the impact of any cognitive or communicative impairments is not considered. Thus, it is often in the acute care period when the patient and family begin to realize that communication or cognition has not returned to normal and may not do so for some time, if ever. The clinician should provide as much information as possible about the nature of the patient's impairments—highlighting strengths and needs—and provide a reasonable prognosis, if possible, based on the information available. It is often hard to make a confident prognosis in acute care, especially if the patient is very early postonset, and occasionally the clinician will have to say, "It's too early to tell." At such times, clinicians can share with families the factors that will impact the prognosis, and provide information about the services that will be provided during the patient's stay.

Finally, the importance of ongoing assessment during the acute-care phase is similar to that discussed for ICU. Patients with neurogenic disorders may alternate between the ICU and the acute medical floor as their conditions destabilize, and it is the SLP's responsibility to continue to assess communication and certain cognitive abilities and to provide recommendations as indicated throughout this process.

Inpatient Rehabilitation

Many patients who experience neurologic insult will benefit from intensive **rehabilitation** services, typically provided in an inpatient rehabilitation unit. Patients are transferred to a rehabilitation or "rehab" unit when they are considered medically stable and can participate in two to four hours of treatment per day. Patients may also enter rehabilitation from other settings (e.g., home, long-term care). Inpatient rehabilitation stays for patients with acute neurologic disease are often 10 to 28 days in length (E. Miller et al., 2010; Rinere O'Brien, 2010; Roth & Lovell, 2003), during which the goal is to regain function.

It is not unusual for patients with neurologic diagnoses to receive their first SLP services in the inpatient rehabilitation setting (ASHA, 2011a). However, even when the patient has been evaluated in another setting, SLP services in rehab typically begin with assessment. Unlike the acute phase, when assessment is often necessarily abbreviated, assessment procedures in the rehabilitation phase are typically more comprehensive to best direct treatment efforts. SLP treatment in rehab settings is intense, with most patients receiving therapy five or more times per week, with sessions lasting up to 30 minutes or more (ASHA, 2011a). Most patients will be receiving therapies in addition to SLP (e.g., occupational therapy [OT] plus physical therapy [PT] plus SLP); thus, the total number of hours of therapy per day for a patient in rehab is usually quite high.

Rehabilitation for individuals with neurologic insult is a team effort. Treatment goals are often jointly developed and progress toward these goals is discussed regularly during multidisciplinary rounds. In some cases, it may be advantageous to implement joint treatment sessions with other disciplines, for example when goals are vocationally focused (e.g., "The patient will use his augmentative communication device to access the computer network at his place of employment").

Treatment in rehab settings is often both **restorative** (i.e., targeting the impairment) and **adaptive** (i.e., targeting activity and participation), although the goal in both cases is to improve overall function. Treatment may be individual, group, or both. Patients will typically make large gains while in rehab, as the benefits of spontaneous recovery and intensive treatment are exploited.

Patients are discharged from the rehabilitation unit when it is judged that their rehabilitation needs have been met or when additional treatments can be provided more efficiently in a less expensive setting. As was true in acute care, the SLP will provide input regarding the most appropriate disposition from rehab, including recommendations for additional treatment.

Skilled Nursing Facilities

Patients who are medically stable enough to be discharged from acute care but who cannot tolerate the intensive treatment regimen characteristic of inpatient rehabilitation units may be admitted to a **skilled nursing facility** (**SNF**). Patients in an SNF require skilled nursing care and may receive rehabilitation services, although typically not as intensely as what is provided in rehab. Stays in SNFs average 30 days but tend to be more extended for individuals with dementia (E. Miller et al., 2010; Sabbagh et al., 2003). The goal of care in SNFs is to continue to improve the patient's medical status and functional abilities.

For patients who are recovering from acute neurological illness, communication and cognitive services in SNFs are very similar to those provided in rehab units, although perhaps with different intensity (ASHA, 2011c). Some patients are admitted to SNFs because of a decline in function due to degenerative disease (e.g., Alzheimer's disease or Parkinson's disease). For these patients, the focus of services may be maintenance rather than improvement of function. When this is the case, the clinician will need to not only address current function, but also plan for future declines in function. For patients with degenerative disease, treatment in SNFs is nearly always adaptive rather than restorative. As was true with acute care and rehab, it will be necessary for clinicians in SNF settings to participate in discharge planning and to provide education to the family and paid caregivers in how to best facilitate communication and completion of daily activities with the patient.

Long-Term-Care Facilities

When individuals can no longer live independently or be cared for in the home, they may be admitted to a facility for **long-term care** (**LTC**). Unlike SNFs, where patients receive skilled nursing care, LTC facilities typically provide limited nursing and rehabilitation services. The goal in LTC is to maintain medical stability and facilitate quality of life (E. Miller et al., 2010). Many patients admitted to LTC facilities will remain there until death, which can be months or even years after admission. Most patients in LTC are not expected to make substantial gains in function, so SLP services typically focus on maintaining functional cognitive and communicative abilities. Treatments are almost always adaptive in nature.

Because many patients in LTC often suffer from degenerative disease, it will be necessary for the SLP to provide ongoing assessment of communication, swallowing, and cognition in order to recommend changes in care as needed. Often ongoing assessment in this setting takes the form of systematic screening of all residents, with special consideration given to those with relevant admitting diagnoses. Periodically, patients in LTC facilities will experience an acute neurologic insult, such as a stroke or TBI. In that event, the SLP will be responsible for assessing and treating the patient, always keeping in mind baseline function when developing a prognosis and treatment plan.

Treatment in LTC facilities often involves environmental manipulation and staff education rather than, or in addition to, direct intervention with individual patients. Many patients in LTC cannot benefit from direct intervention, even adaptive strategies, because of severe cognitive deficits. In such cases, the clinician may still impact the patient's functional abilities by targeting contextual factors: modifying surroundings and instructing families and caregivers in how to best facilitate communication and cognitive functioning. Group treatment is another possible treatment option, at least for some patients, particularly given the social and emotional benefits associated with group participation (see Chapter 12).

Home Health

Some patients will benefit from nursing and rehabilitation services provided in the home (i.e., **home health** services). Typically, home health rehabilitation services are offered to individuals who have been discharged from acute care, rehab, or skilled nursing. Patients who might benefit from additional treatment but who are unable to leave their homes to receive the services may be eligible for home health care. Additionally, individuals with degenerative disease who continue to live at home may also benefit from home health services. The goal of home health care is to maintain or improve medical status while maintaining or improving functional abilities. For most individuals, home health rehabilitation services may last 14 to 30 days, although some people retain skilled home nursing care for longer durations (E. Miller et al., 2010).

Services in home health settings range from daily intensive restorative treatment (e.g., for individuals recovering from acute illness) to weekly or monthly adaptive treatment focusing on environmental modification and caregiver training (e.g., for individuals at the end stages of degenerative disease). Home health services offer the advantage of being provided in the environment that is typically most conducive to the patient's function and will often involve the caregiver more directly than is generally possible in other settings. However, these same factors can be disadvantages if the home environment and/or the caregiver do not facilitate communication or cognitive functioning. In such cases, the clinician would likely target these contextual factors, as well as those directed at modifying the patient's cognitive or communicative behaviors.

Intentional coordination of services with other disciplines is particularly important in the home health setting. Because many different therapists and caregivers may be going in and out of the home at different times throughout the week, it is often difficult for the patient or the family to keep track of goals, treatment schedules, or both. Treatment in home health will be most successful if the various care providers are aware of all the services the patient is receiving (e.g., to avoid duplicating or omitting assessment and/or treatment of certain symptoms) and if all of these services are coordinated and targeted toward common functional goals.

Outpatient Services

The final setting to be discussed in this chapter is the **outpatient** setting. Patients who live at home and have transportation to a treatment facility may receive outpatient services. Most patients receiving outpatient services are medically stable but exhibit functional deficits. Outpatient rehabilitation services typically last 4 to 12 weeks (E. Miller et al., 2010), or potentially longer if the patient continues to show functional gains and has the financial resources to pay for continued services. Most patients receive two therapy sessions per week for up to an hour each session (ASHA, 2011b).

Outpatient services may be recommended for individuals discharged from other facilities following acute episodes or for individuals in the early stages of degenerative disease. In both cases, it is likely that a thorough evaluation of communication and cognitive function is warranted before the initiation of treatment. In the first case, information will be gained regarding current status and amount of recovery experienced since the onset of the condition. In the second case, a baseline will be established from which it will be possible to compare future rate and amount of decline in function.

Treatment of cognitive and communicative problems in outpatient settings is usually both restorative and adaptive in nature. Outpatient services can be very beneficial because at this point in their recovery, most patients and caregivers are in a position to incorporate strategies introduced into their home or work settings, taking advantage of the opportunity to discuss the successes or failures during subsequent sessions. Outpatient treatment sessions may involve family members and can specifically target educational or vocational goals. Outpatient services also have the advantage of being the least expensive of all care settings (particularly when services are provided at a university clinic), so many patients can often afford more treatment than could be obtained in other settings.

Legislation

Health-care reform may seem a very contemporary concept, but in fact it has been the subject of debate in the United States since the early 1900s. In this section, we will review key federal legislation influencing the current status of health-care practices in the United States. Readers are cautioned, however, that legislation impacting health care is enacted almost continually and that any textbook is likely to contain outdated information. The ASHA website (http://www.asha.org/advocacy) is a good resource for up-to-date information on health-care legislation impacting SLP services.

Medicare, the federally funded health insurance for older Americans, was originally enacted in 1965. Since its inception, Medicare legislation has undergone numerous policy changes with respect to the types of goods and services provided, the processes for authorizing services and receiving reimbursement, and the models used for determining the amount of reimbursement. Although such legislation technically applies only to Medicare services to older Americans, changing policies often have more widespread impact because other funding systems (e.g., private insurance) typically model their own policies after Medicare.

Currently, the insurance provided by Medicare is categorized into several "parts" that cover costs associated with different health-care services. Medicare Part A is hospital insurance that covers a portion of the cost of inpatient care in hospitals, skilled nursing facilities, hospice, and home health care. Part A is free to Americans over age 65 (and disabled individuals under age 65) who paid Medicare taxes while they were working. Part B Medicare is insurance that covers outpatient care, medical equipment, and preventative services. Unlike Part A, Part B involves a monthly premium that is paid by subscribers. Medicare Part C, also known as Medicare Advantage, is an alternative to Plans A and B. With Part C, hospital and medical insurance is administered by Medicare-approved private insurance companies. Part C plans may also cover services beyond those of Parts A and B, such as vision and dental services. Subscribers pay premiums to the private insurer, who receives supplemental funding from the federal government. Finally, Medicare Part D provides prescription drug coverage. Similar to Part C, this coverage is typically administered through a private insurance company; many subscribers use the same company for both Parts C and D. Readers are referred to www.Medicare.gov for updated, patient-friendly information on Medicare insurance plans.

Medicaid, created by the same federal legislation that enacted Medicare, is jointly funded by state and federal governments. Although generally considered to be an insurance program for individuals with low income, "not all of the poor are eligible, not all those covered are poor" (Herz et al., 2005, p. 2). It is beyond the scope of this chapter to explain the intricacies of Medicaid eligibility, particularly since each state sets unique criteria. In general, however, individuals qualifying for Medicaid are those who are eligible for other financial assistance programs (e.g., welfare, food stamps, disability). Most states provide inpatient hospital care, outpatient medical services, nursing facilities, therapies, and medical devices through Medicaid funding. Providers of Medicare and Medicaid services must be approved by the Centers for Medicare and Medicaid Services. A more detailed discussion of how providers receive payment through these funding sources is included in a later section on health-care economics.

In 2010, the Patient Protection and Affordable Care Act was passed by Congress and signed into law. Subsequent review by the Supreme Court in 2012 upheld the legislation. The primary features of the Affordable Care Act are provisions for rights and protections of health-care consumers, insurance choices and managing insurance costs, expanded services to Medicare enrollees, quality-of-care monitoring for facilities receiving Medicare payments, and tax credits for small employers (U.S. Department of Health and Human Services, 2012). At the time of writing of this textbook, many of the Affordable Care Act provisions had only recently taken effect; the impact of the Act is not fully understood. The section below discussing the impact of legislation and health-care financing on SLP services will address the ways the Affordable Care Act is predicted to most directly impact the services provided to individuals with neurogenic disorders of language and cognition by SLPs.

Although the federal legislation pertaining to Medicare and Medicaid has the greatest and most direct impact on the SLP services provided to most individuals with neurogenic language or cognitive disorders, other legislation is also relevant to this discussion. The Americans With Disabilities Act (ADA; 1990) does not provide funding for medical or rehabilitative services, but does include provisions requiring employers to provide reasonable accommodation for individuals whose language or cognitive disorders impact their ability to perform job duties. The ADA mandates are most commonly applied to accommodate physical disabilities, but may also apply to environmental modifications described in Chapter 12. The Rehabilitation Act (1973) funds Vocational Rehabilitation agencies, which may assist in the coordination of accommodations made to the workplace and/or retraining in new skills if language or cognitive disorders preclude individuals from returning to their previous work.

Finally, the Health Insurance Portability and Accountability Act (HIPAA; 1996) mandates procedures for ensuring patient privacy and maintaining confidentiality of each patient's identifiable health information. HIPAA regulations are intended to primarily impact practice management, but do hold some implications for clinical procedures. Most relevant to the management of neurogenic language and cognitive disorders is the need for the clinician to maintain patient confidentiality within the context of patient assessment and treatment. Information about the patient's communication and/or cognitive status should be shared only with those individuals who have been authorized to receive such information. Held to the letter of this law, family education about specific aspects of the patient's condition likely would be limited to the patient's spouse. In practice, however, it is generally sufficient to consult with the patient or family to clarify what information can be shared with the individuals present, and to proceed accordingly.

Health-Care Economics

The previous sections of this chapter highlight that the continuum of care and legislation are closely tied to costs associated with service provision. A thorough discussion of health-care economics is beyond the scope of this chapter, yet successful practice of SLP requires a basic understanding of economic influences. In this section, we will define key concepts of health-care economics and consider various funding models for speech-pathology services. We will further consider how these models affect service delivery from both clinical (i.e., the types of assessment and treatment services provided) and administrative (i.e., the nature of documentation needed to ensure full payment) perspectives.

Although clinicians ideally make clinical decisions based on the needs of the patient and his or her family, funding models have the potential to influence practice patterns by creating financial incentives for specific practice decisions. To better appreciate these influences, it is first necessary to understand the different funding models and the conditions under which each model is likely to be applied (see Table 13-1 for a listing of acronyms related to health-care funding models).

One model is **fee-for-service**, in which health-care providers are reimbursed retrospectively (i.e., after the fact) for services based on per-visit or per-procedure rates. This is the funding model that applies to many consumer exchanges (e.g., oil changes, haircuts, dry cleaning). In the context of health-care financing, many **third-party payers**

TABLE 13-1
Common Acronyms Associated With Health-Care Financing

ACRONYM	REFERENCE	DEFINITION
DRG	Diagnosis-Related Group	Designates the reimbursement rate for patients receiving Medicare Part A coverage in acute-care settings, based on the diagnosis or diagnoses of individual patients
CMS	Centers for Medicare and Medicaid Services	Agency of the federal government responsible for administering Medicare and Medicaid
HHRG	Home Health Resource Group	Prospective payment system funding home health services
MDS	Minimum Data Set	Assessment and outcome assessment system determining RUG
OASIS	Outcome and Assessment Information Set	Outcome and assessment system determining HHRG
PPS	Prospective Payment System	Providers are paid a predetermined rate based on the patient's diagnosis or rehabilitation needs
RUG	Resource Utilization Group	Designates the reimbursement rate for patients receiving Medicare Part A coverage for acute rehabilitation centers or skilled nursing facilities, based on the skilled nursing and rehabilitation needs of individual patients

(i.e., insurance companies) that reimburse via fee-for-service incorporate **caps or limits** that dictate the maximum reimbursement that will be paid for any procedure or service (e.g., $65 per hour for therapy) or over a specified period of time (e.g., $1,500 per year or $20,000 over a lifetime) or both. A key economic feature of the fee-for-service model is that providers can increase revenue by increasing services (e.g., increasing the frequency or total duration of treatment). In other words, providers have financial incentives to provide higher levels of care. To help prevent the provision of inappropriate services, many third-party payers require pre-authorization of services, as well as ongoing documentation that the patient is benefiting from services. Medicare, Medicaid, and most private insurers utilize fee-for-service funding models in the context of outpatient primary care. The Balanced Budget Act of 1997 enacted a cap of $1,500 for physical therapy and speech therapy provided in outpatient and skilled nursing settings. Due to a number of congressional moratoriums, these caps have not been consistently enforced since they were first implemented. At the time of this writing, the therapy cap for combined physical and speech therapy is $1,880, although review processes are in place to consider exceptions to the caps when continued services are deemed medically necessary (ASHA, 2012a). A common variation of fee-for-service funding is **discounted fee-for-service**. In this funding scheme, providers agree to provide services to specified groups of individuals at reduced reimbursement rates. Typically, discounted fee-for-service arrangements are part of **managed care** systems that designate **preferred providers**. Within this model, financial incentives apply to both patients and providers. For the patient, managed care plans provide higher levels of coverage (i.e., lower out-of-pocket expenses) for care obtained from preferred providers. When a preferred provider contracts with managed care systems to accept discounted fee-for-service rates, it is with the expectation that higher patient volume will make up for any potential reductions in revenue.

An Illustration of Preferred Provider Systems

Sally's insurance company incorporates a preferred provider model of funding. Her insurance company provides a list of health-care providers that are designated "in-network." If she obtains care from in-network providers, her out-of-pocket expenses are limited to nominal co-payments for some services (e.g., office visits are $25) or a percentage of the overall cost for other services (e.g., 20% of the cost of outpatient surgery). However, if Sally obtains care from providers designated as "out-of-network," she is required to pay higher amounts (e.g., office visits are $40, 50% of other services). It is to Sally's financial advantage to utilize the in-network services, but she retains at least some insurance coverage if she chooses out-of-network providers.

John is an SLP who owns a private practice. His customary rates are $250 per hour of evaluation and $120 per hour of therapy. However, the largest employers in his community subscribe to managed care plans incorporating preferred provider funding systems. To join the preferred provider network, John must agree to provide services to subscribers at a reduced rate ($150/hr for evaluation and $75/hr for treatment).

John's dilemma is that if he does not agree to the lower rates and thus does not become an in-network provider, he will risk losing business to SLPs who are preferred providers. Remember, Sally will pay only $25 for each therapy session with an in-network SLP, but $40 for out-of-network. By becoming a preferred provider, John is gambling that he will get more business from network customers, and that the extra business will make up for the reduced rates.

An alternative to fee-for-service funding is **prospective payment**. Under prospective payment systems (PPSs), providers are paid a preset fee that is determined by the diagnosis of the patient, the amount/intensity of specialty services required, the socioeconomic status of the community, and/or whether care is provided in the context of medical training (Centers for Medicare & Medicaid Services, 2012). PPSs differ significantly from fee-for-service in that compensation is *not* based on the actual services provided, thus there is no incentive to provide additional, perhaps unnecessary, services as a means of increasing income.

A PPS takes three primary forms: case rate, per diem, and capitation. In a **case rate** system, providers are compensated according to the patient's diagnosis. **Per diem** funding compensates providers based on the number of days the patient is receiving care. **Capitation systems** compensate providers based on the number of people subscribed to a managed care plan. In all three PPS funding schemes, the financial risk lies primarily with the provider. The following case rate example will serve to illustrate this point.

Imagine two individuals who present to the emergency room with a left hemisphere stroke. Under a PPS, the funding agency will pay the acute care hospital to which they are admitted a set amount (e.g., $10,000) for each patient's care, regardless of the number of services the patient actually utilizes. Thus, if Patient A has a typical hospital course, undergoing the standard diagnostic tests and treatment protocols, she may be discharged after 48 hours and incur $6,800 (for example) of actual costs. For Patient A, the hospital would earn a profit of $3,200, because the cost of caring for her is less than what is paid by the third-party funding agency. Imagine that Patient B, however, had a nonstandard hospital course, perhaps related to a particularly severe or unfortunately located lesion resulting in dense hemiparesis, global aphasia, right neglect, and significant dysphagia. This patient may undergo numerous diagnostic tests, including additional x-rays and a neurosurgical consult. His severe dysphagia may result in aspiration pneumonia and subsequent placement of a feeding tube. Therefore, his stay in acute care may extend to six days or more before being discharged to the skilled nursing facility. For the sake of illustration, assume the total cost for Patient B's care is $23,000. Fortunately for the patient, he is not responsible for paying the $13,000 that the insurance company will not cover. Unfortunately, the hospital would incur a loss of $13,000, as the cost of this patient's care exceeded the prospective payment. Most funding models are more complex than suggested by these examples (e.g., the third-party payer may provide additional funds if additional diagnoses are implicated), but the implication is clear: Providers have incentives to provide *less* rather than *more* care.

Medicare Part A case rate prospective payments are based on **diagnosis-related groups (DRGs),** which are determined by the average resources required to treat patients with a given diagnosis. Similarly, Medicare funds home health services according to **home health resource groups (HHRGs)** and rehabilitation and skilled nursing services according to **resource utilization groups (RUGs)**. HHRGs and RUGs differ slightly from DRGs in that resource groups are determined not only by medical diagnosis but also by rehabilitation and skilled care needs. This funding strategy is known as **case-mix adjustment**. The determination of how the patient's needs dictate the funding rate is made through specialized documentation systems developed by the Centers for Medicare and Medicaid Services (CMS). For example, the **Minimum Data Set** (**MDS**; see Chapter 8) determines the RUG classification determining the per diem rate paid to skilled nursing facilities. A similar system, the Outcome and Assessment Information Set (OASIS) instrument, is used to determine the HHRG classification.

Implications of Health-Care Legislation and Economics

Current health-care legislation and economics have direct and indirect implications for individual clinicians and patients. Many patients seeking SLP services for neurogenic language and cognitive disorders will depend on third-party funding for at least a portion of the cost of care. This may limit their options with respect to who provides their care (e.g., preferred provider contracts), the type of services they can receive (e.g., individual, group, family-based), and the amount of treatment they can receive (e.g., number of visits, total cost of care). Unfortunately, not all patients who are subject to these restrictions are fully aware of the limits of their policies or understand how the limitations can be mitigated. Moreover, some of these policies may be changed by the Patient Protection and Affordable Care Act (2010). Professional medical social workers are uniquely equipped to help patients understand the benefits to which they are entitled through their insurance plans. It is the role of the SLP to help the patient and family understand options for best utilizing available benefits. For example, if a patient with a degenerative condition has an insurance policy with a lifetime cap on benefits, the SLP might recommend that funds be held in reserve to allow for appropriate services as function declines.

Health-care economics also affect SLPs in ways that extend beyond the restrictions imposed on any given patient. Almost without exception, SLPs provide care in settings in which financial incentives are apparent. A common manifestation of these incentives is productivity targets, which are institutionally determined expectations for the proportion of minutes in the workday that will be spent in billable activities (J. E. Brown

& Pietranton, 2007). Clinicians may also have incentives to select specific assessment strategies (e.g., endoscopic swallowing assessments are compensated at a higher rate than clinical exams) and treatment schedules (e.g., patients receiving higher frequency of treatment may qualify for care in a setting with higher prospective rates). Economic influences on clinical care are a reality, yet quality SLP services can be provided to patients with neurogenic language and cognitive impairments within the constraints imposed by funding models. ASHA provides a number of resources related to the economics of SLP practice, including web resources (http://asha.org/practice), continuing education materials (e.g., Health Plan Coding and Claims Guide; McCarty & White, 2012), and special sessions at the Annual ASHA Convention.

Another impact of health-care economics on SLP services is the use of SLP assistants (SLPAs). Although the roles and responsibilities of SLPAs were first described by ASHA in 1996, with the more recent position statement published in 2004, many healthcare providers have not yet incorporated the services of these individuals (ASHA, 2002), possibly due to the ambivalence with which the field of SLP, at least in the United States, has received the concept of SLPAs (ASHA, 2009). Although it is not our intention to advocate one way or another on this issue, it is important to point out that the utilization of SLPAs has the potential to reduce treatment costs. It is clear that a paraprofessional working at a rate of $20 per hour can provide more treatment hours for $100 than can the professional working at a rate of $45 per hour. However, the cost savings is maintained only if quality treatment is administered and the patient demonstrates functional gains as a result. When SLPAs provide treatment, it is the responsibility of the supervising SLP to ensure quality care by carefully assessing the patient, developing an appropriate treatment plan, and providing appropriate supervision to the SLPA (ASHA, 2004b). Ideally, the use of SLPAs will improve the efficiency of services and help maintain the livelihood of the profession in the current health-care environment.

One caution regarding the use of SLPAs in medical settings is noteworthy. ASHA policies, as well as some state legislation, significantly limit the services SLPAs can provide in the area of dysphagia (ASHA, 2000; North Carolina Board of Examiners, 1999). Stated another way, *only* SLPs can provide most dysphagia services, whereas screening and treatment of other disorder areas (including neurogenic language and cognitive disorders) *can* be carried out by SLPAs if under the supervision of a licensed SLP. A likely, although probably unintended, result of this mandate is that the most highly skilled professional services will be provided to individuals with dysphagia, whereas support personnel will carry out services to individuals with other impairments. The efficacy of therapy services provided by SLPAs has not been sufficiently studied, either generally or specifically within the context of neurogenic language and cognitive disorders (although there is some empirical literature pertaining to training volunteers or caregivers to carry out treatments for neurogenic language and cognitive disorders under the supervision of an SLP; e.g., Togher et al., 2009). Nonetheless, recent efforts by ASHA to more fully integrate SLPAs and audiology assistants into the professions may lead to greater awareness of the roles SLPAs may play and thus facilitate a richer research base pertaining to efficacy and efficiency of services provided by assistants.

The policies and procedures governing Medicare have a particularly strong influence on the documentation SLPs must provide regarding the care they provide. It is beyond the scope of this chapter to review in detail clinical documentation policies in the context of third-party payment, but a few key issues will be discussed. More detailed and up-to-date information regarding reimbursement documentation is provided on the ASHA website (http://www.asha.org/practice).

One aspect of clinical documentation relates closely to the ICF framework that has guided the organization of this textbook. Specifically, reports should describe the patient's status at the levels of body structure and function, as well as activity and participation. Disruptions in activity and participation are often referred to as "functional deficits" and are considered an important justification for intervention. Moreover, changes in functional status must be documented to warrant continued intervention. Therefore, instead of writing goals or reporting progress in terms of impairments that make sense only to other clinicians (e.g., "Mr. Smith will produce embedded clauses with third-person reflexive pronouns during idiom descriptions with 95% accuracy"), clinicians should document goals, progress, and outcomes in ways that indicate how patients' activity and participation should change or have changed as a result of intervention (e.g., "Mr. Smith will obtain billing information from three local businesses utilizing the strategies practiced during treatment sessions: scripts, alphabet cueing, and drawing") (see Table 13-2). In essence, clinicians must highlight the effects of services on the patient's daily activities and participation, rather than on underlying impairments. Impairments may improve subsequent to treatment, but clinicians must show that those are not the *only* positive effects of treatment.

An issue closely tied to clinical documentation is outcome assessment for **quality assurance** purposes. Not only is there a focus on functional measures (see Chapter 8), but also there is an incentive to show how SLP services contribute to overall reduced cost of care. For example, a medical center or health-care system studying its own service statistics might observe that patients undergoing rehabilitation for TBI who re-

TABLE 13-2
Clinical Goals Under Managed Care

ACTIVITY/PARTICIPATION-LEVEL (FUNCTIONAL) GOALS/OUTCOMES	IMPAIRMENT-LEVEL GOALS/OUTCOMES
Ms. Jones will independently use target strategies to complete written tasks involving both left and right hemispace.	Ms. Jones will reduce hemispatial neglect.
Mr. Smith will participate in a 10-minute discussion of work-related topics, using target strategies to maintain topics and repair communication breakdowns.	Mr. Smith will improve the length and syntactic complexity of spoken sentences.
Ms. Harris will successfully use a public transportation system to attend a cultural event.	Ms. Harris will improve reasoning skills.

ceived group SLP therapy had average lengths of stay that were shorter than those who did not participate in group therapy. The institution would thus likely be supportive of resources for group treatment, as it reduces the overall cost of care. Similar data analyses are common for determining the factors that contribute to reduced rates of rehospitalization following discharge, decreased errors in medication, and improved customer satisfaction. Although cost effectiveness is not the only consideration in quality assurance, it is highly valued and thus closely scrutinized. The contribution of SLP services to improved patient outcomes and reduced health-care costs will become only more important as provisions of the Patient Protection and Affordable Care Act (2010) take effect.

Related to the issues discussed above is the need for clinicians to market actively the services provided to individuals with communication and/or cognitive difficulties. Clinicians must ensure that physicians, nurses, social workers, other health-care providers (e.g., OTs, neuropsychologists), case managers, and, perhaps most important, patients and their caregivers understand how neurogenic language and cognitive disorders impact activity and participation and how our services positively influence the lives of the patients we serve. Marketing may be particularly important in relation to specific services. For example, as mentioned in other chapters of this book (e.g., Chapter 4), physicians and other health-care providers may be unfamiliar with SLP services to individuals with dementia or other cognitive-communicative disorders, or of the role of SLPs in the management of the progressive disorders. This can be accomplished in a variety of ways. The following suggestions are not meant to be exhaustive, but instead provide a place to start and will perhaps inspire even more creative ideas.

More Than a Swallow-ologist

The need for marketing is illustrated quite clearly by the following two situations. First, early in my clinical career, after I had evaluated the swallowing function of an individual who had experienced a stroke, I spoke to the physician about addressing the patient's communication deficits. The physician asked for more information, and when I explained how the patient was having difficulty understanding and expressing himself and how I could help the patient with these difficulties, the physician replied, "Huh, I didn't know you guys did anything except swallowing."

Later in my career, I was conducting a study comparing the language abilities of patients with Parkinson's disease to those of patients with Huntington's disease. Significant empirical and clinical evidence indicates that these diseases can cause significant motor speech and swallowing problems and dementia; likewise, an emerging empirical literature has documented language problems subsequent to the onset of either disease. However, only 2 out of more than 30 patient participants had received SLP services (both for swallowing vs. cognitive-communicative issues) prior to their participation in the study, even though many demonstrated significant dysarthria and cognitive problems. At a workshop I was giving several years after data collection for this study, patients with Parkinson's disease and their families reported that little had changed, as few were aware of the services SLPs could provide them, had yet to receive an SLP referral despite being in the middle or later stages of the disease, or both.

The first example shows how, because our services in the area of dysphagia are in such high demand, our expertise in the areas of communication and cognition is becoming de-emphasized, and perhaps overlooked completely (for a description of a similar situation in Great Britain, see Code & Petheram, 2011). The second example indicates that we need to not only increase health-care professionals' understanding of the breadth of services provided by SLPs, but also improve the general public's awareness of the field of speech-language pathology so that they can request our services.

Perhaps the most effective way of marketing services is to speak directly to potential referral sources, preferably face to face. When professional colleagues know the SLP and the services he or she provides, simply seeing the clinician in the hallways might spark a referral. Professional relationships will only be strengthened as colleagues become aware of the professional and effective care that SLPs provide, as well as the impact of services for communicative and cognitive disorders on the patient's overall health and wellness.

Patient and professional advocacy is another activity that is becoming increasingly important in the advent of managed care. Advocacy is particularly important with respect to patients with neurogenic language and cognitive disorders, given that these patients are often less able than other patient groups to self-advocate for appropriate services and financial coverage. Many prevention, marketing, and education activities may also serve the purpose of advocacy as referral sources become more aware of the value of SLP services. Clinicians may find it necessary to advocate for specific patient needs (e.g., comprehensive assessment, continued treatment, augmentative communication systems and other assistive devices), which may involve speaking directly with primary care physicians, administrators, and/or third-party payment providers. Useful resources for clinicians practicing patient advocacy can be found on the Advocacy section of the ASHA website (http://www.asha.org/advocacy).

Finally, we cannot leave the topic of health-care legislation and economics without highlighting the role of evidence-based practice (EBP), which was discussed in detail in Chapter 1. Although outcome assessment plays a role in EBP, there is increasing pressure for clinicians to demonstrate *a priori* that an assessment tool or treatment procedure they plan to use has documented efficacy for the types of communicative and/or cognitive problems for which it will be prescribed. The EBP strategies described in Chapter 1 will help clinicians justify the nature, intensity, and duration of assessments and treatments they recommend, thereby reducing the likelihood of reimbursement denials by third-party payers.

Looking Ahead

The goal of this chapter was to provide a picture of the "real-world" clinical environments in which clinicians often provide care to patients with neurogenic language and cognitive disorders. The contextual factors discussed here are often viewed as unfortunate limitations. Indeed, many beginning clinicians express frustration that health-care legislation and economic influences do not allow them to implement clinical practices that they have been taught as being most appropriate. Nonetheless, there are many factors that have positive influences on the context of care to individuals with language and cognitive disorders. As indicated in Chapter 1, the research base documenting the benefits of treatment for neurogenic language and cognitive disorders continues to expand, providing SLPs with the information necessary to appropriately select, implement, and obtain reimbursement for management strategies. As highlighted in this chapter, there also are several approaches that clinicians can adopt to increase public awareness of not only neurogenic language and cognitive disorders, but also the services that our profession can provide to help prevent, assess, and treat those disorders. Better understanding and appreciation of our field should lead to greater demand for SLP services and, consequently, increased pressure on funding agencies to support SLP clinical services as well as research. Additionally, developing technologies, including functional imaging and genetic mapping, continue to enhance our understanding of the nature and causes of neurogenic language and cognitive disorders, as well as the physiologic mechanisms supporting recovery. Finally, as described in Chapters 9 through 12, the variety of management strategies continues to expand. We look forward to a future in which seemingly divergent treatments (e.g., pharmacotherapy, behavioral intervention, life-participation approaches, and alternative medicine) will be integrated to optimize patient outcomes, even for those battling progressive diseases. As the benefits of such integrated management become evident, concurrent reimbursement strategies should follow.

Discussion Questions

1. Compare and contrast the likely continuum of care for an elderly individual who experiences a stroke and a young individual who develops a brain tumor.
2. How does the role of the clinician differ between the ICU and acute care?
3. How does judicious use of the continuum of care reduce health-care costs?
4. Compare and contrast fee-for-service with prospective payment.
5. Discuss how an SLP assistant (SLPA) might participate in the care of individuals residing in a long-term-care facility.

glossary

acetylcholine A neurotransmitter that is found throughout the brain, spinal cord, and autonomic nervous system.

activities and participation International Classification of Functioning, Disability, and Health (ICF) construct that describes an individual's ability to engage in personal, social, vocational, and recreational activities.

acupuncture A technique involving stimulating the skin, and consequently nerves, at designated anatomic locations referred to as acupoints.

acute care Stage in the continuum of care in which most patients' conditions are not currently life-threatening but in need of daily physician and continual nursing care.

adaptive Treatment strategies that compensate for impairments but do not induce permanent improvements in underlying structure or function.

ageism The systematic stereotyping and discrimination of people on the basis of their age.

agnosia Impairment of recognition; can be limited to specific sensory modalities (e.g., auditory agnosia). Recognition deficit is not a product of a sensory deficit (e.g., auditory agnosia is not due to a hearing loss).

agonists Drugs designed to increase the amount or efficiency of neurotransmitters.

agrammatism The production of short utterances that consist primarily of content words (e.g., nouns and verbs), contain relatively few function words (e.g., articles and conjunctions), have either simplified or incomplete grammatical structure, and represent a restricted range of sentence types or forms.

agraphia Impaired written expression. Also called acquired dysgraphia.

alexia Disruption in written language comprehension. Also known as acquired dyslexia.

allesthesia The misattribution of sensory information from one side of the body (i.e., the unattended or neglected side of the body) to stimulation of the other side of the body.

Alzheimer's disease (AD) The most common cause of irreversible dementia and dementia in general. Its etiology remains unknown, although genetic and other physiological causes are still being investigated. Confirmation of an AD diagnosis can only be made upon autopsy.

amphetamine A drug that increases levels of dopamine and norepinephrine within the brain.

aneurysm A weak or thin spot on a blood vessel that causes the vessel to dilate or balloon.

angular gyrus An area of the brain within the parietal lobe that, with the supramarginal gyrus, contributes to written language comprehension and production.

angular gyrus syndrome A collection of symptoms (i.e., disorientation, anomia, and acalculia) caused by multiple lesions to posterior and inferior parietal regions of the left hemisphere.

anomia Difficulty recalling the names of people, objects, locations, concepts, and actions.

anomic aphasia Aphasia characterized by a relatively isolated impairment of naming, with fluent language output and relatively good comprehension of spoken and written language.

anosognosia An impaired awareness or denial of one's own deficits.

antagonists Drugs that reduce the amount or efficiency of neurotransmitters.

anterograde amnesia A memory problem that relates to difficulties storing and retrieving new long-term memories, or more generally new information, subsequent to the onset of brain damage or disease.

anterograde memories Long-term memories that are stored after brain damage has occurred, or after the onset of the neurological disease process.

anticoagulants Medications such as heparin or warfarin that prevent thrombus formation and release of emboli.

antiplatelet medications Drugs such as aspirin or clopidogrel that help reduce the build-up of plaque on existing thrombotic areas.

apathy A lack of feeling or emotion; indifference.

aphasia A disruption in using and understanding language following neurological injury or disease that is not related to general intellectual decline or sensorimotor deficits.

apraxia of speech A difficulty with volitionally positioning muscles, as well as planning and sequencing muscle movements, for the production of phonemes and phoneme sequences.

arcuate fasciculus Association fibrous tract that connects Wernicke's and Broca's areas.

arteriogram The radiological procedure used to visualize the arteries.

arteriovenous malformation (AVM) A congenital defect in the communication links between arteries and veins that results in weakened arterial walls and may lead to hemorrhagic stroke.

association areas Cortical areas surrounding Broca's and Wernicke's areas and involved in language processing and perception.

ataxia Disturbance in movement accuracy, force, and timing due to lesions of the cerebellum.

attention Cognitive function allowing for allocation of processing of resources to stimuli or tasks.

attention switching The process of moving attentional focus from one task, stimulus, or stimulus property to another.

augmentative communication A communication system whereby the speaker points to or otherwise selects written words or pictured symbols to facilitate language expression or comprehension.

augmentative or alternative communication (AAC) A communication system whereby written words or pictured symbols are selected to facilitate language expression or comprehension.

authentic assessment An assessment based on ethnographic and conversational analysis research methods.

authentic context The typically occurring context of linguistic or cognitive processes.

barrier games Activities used for addressing a variety of pragmatic and discourse goals in which a solid barrier is placed between the patient and the clinician to create a communicative need and which, in the absence of nonverbal cues, require utilization of specific and efficient language output.

basal ganglia Subcortical structure with contributions to linguistic and cognitive processing and motor skills. They include structures such as the caudate nucleus, putamen, globus pallidus, subthalamic nucleus, and substantia nigra.

basement or floor effect Test performance profile in which patients predominantly receive scores of 0.

benign Term for tumors that are non-cancerous and do not spread or metastasize to other parts of the body.

biofeedback A relaxation technique used to teach patients conscious self-regulation of physiological functions that are related to stress levels by connecting patients to simple electronic devices that monitor the target physiological functions.

blast injury An injury sustained from direct or indirect exposure to an explosion; the explosion causes barotrauma (i.e., injury due to exposure to extreme pressure changes).

body function A construct of the ICF that describes the functional integrity of tissues and organs.

body structure A construct of the ICF that describes the integrity of tissues and organs.

bradykinesia Slowed movement associated with Huntington's disease, Parkinson's disease, and other neurological diseases.

brain attacks New term for a stroke introduced to encourage patients experiencing symptoms of stroke to get immediate medical help.

Broca's aphasia Aphasia characterized by nonfluent language output and relatively spared language comprehension compared to output fluency difficulties.

Broca's area Area of the brain in the inferior lateral frontal lobe and generally proposed to play a primary role in language expression.

bromocriptine A drug that increases levels of dopamine within the brain.

canonical A sentence using the active voice.

capitated payment Health-care financing system in which providers agree to serve a given population for a preset fee.

caps or limits Designates a maximum amount of third-party funding available for medical or rehabilitative services.

carotid arterial system Arterial system that begins as the left and right common carotid arteries and supplies most of the cerebral hemispheres.

case-mix adjustment Prospective payment system in which providers are compensated according to a patient's diagnosis and in consideration of their rehabilitation needs.

case rate Prospective payment system in which providers are compensated according to the patient's diagnosis.

catastrophic reaction Difficulty maintaining biologic homeostasis and a form of massive denial. Symptoms include sudden and violent switching into a state of intense negativity.

catecholamine system Consists of a certain group of neurotransmitters and the neurons that release those neurotransmitters. These neurotransmitters are related because they are all made from a common chemical pathway. Dopamine, norepinephrine, and epinephrine are the most common catecholamine neurotransmitters.

ceiling Refers to 100% accuracy on test performance.

chemosensory impairment An impaired ability to smell and/or taste.

choline acetyltransferase A chemical responsible for making acetylcholine, an excitatory neurotransmitter known to be important for learning and memory.

cholinergic system Consists of the neurotransmitter acetylcholine and the neurons that release acetycholine.

chorea A motoric disturbance associated with Huntington's disease and other neurological disorders that is characterized by rapid, involuntary, purposeless movements of the extremities, head, neck, or trunk. These movements are irregular and asymmetrical. A symptom of Huntington's disease.

Circle of Willis A ring of arteries located at the base of brain, which connects the carotid and vertebrobasilar artery systems. Provides the brain with collateral circulation that can help compensate for a blockage in one of the major cerebral arteries.

circumlocution The use of descriptions, definitions, or sound effects for target words.

closed head injury A traumatic brain injury in which the skull is not pierced by the external force and thus stays intact.

coarse coding The activation of a wide-ranging network of secondary or peripheral meanings and features.

cognition The process by which sensory information is transformed, condensed, elaborated, stored, retrieved, and exploited, thus allowing understanding and interaction with the environment.

cognitive flexibility A type of executive function that allows for changing or adapting behavior in the event of failure.

cognitive neuropsychological treatments Aphasia treatments in which models of normal and/or disordered language are used to motivate selection of treatment targets and procedures.

cohesion Refers to the linguistic means by which words and sentences are meaningfully linked to each other within a text or spoken discourse sample.

coma A condition characterized by the lack of or minimal organized or purposeful response to external stimuli within one's environment.

communication A fundamental human behavior involving the exchange of ideas.

compensatory strategies Behavioral strategies developed with the goal of lessening the impact of impairment or deficit, without directly addressing the impairment.

complementary and alternative medicine (CAM) A diverse collection of health-care systems, therapies, and products developed outside of conventional medical institutions; used to prevent and treat a spectrum of medical and psychological problems using a holistic approach.

computerized tomography An imaging technique that allows the identification of brain lesions in live patients. Also known as CT scans.

conduction aphasia Aphasia characterized by disproportionately severe deficits during repetition but with relatively good comprehension and fluent spontaneous speech, and mild to moderate naming deficits.

constraint-induced aphasia therapy Approach to aphasia rehabilitation that requires the individual to produce verbal responses to prevent learned nonuse of spoken language functions; is typically provided in an intense treatment format (e.g., several hours per day).

construct validity A psychometric property that indicates how well a test relates to other measures of the same construct.

content validity A psychometric property that indicates how well a test measures all of the behaviors that it purports to measure.

contextual factors Environmental or personal factors that interact with body structure and function to influence activity and participation.

continuum of care A description of the settings available for the provision of medical and rehabilitation services, varying in cost and intensity of care.

contrecoup effect or injury The term used when cerebral contusions occur both at the site of impact (i.e., "coup") and at the opposite side of the brain (i.e., "contre").

contusions Bruises that form around the site of impact of a traumatic brain injury due to laceration of blood vessels.

conversational script training An approach to therapy that involves practicing planned conversational exchanges that comprise common daily interactions

cortical dementia The dementia associated with Alzheimer's disease, Pick's disease, and other neurological disorders that cause brain damage at primarily cortical levels.

cortical stimulation A method of inferring brain function accomplished by applying electrical stimulation to the brain in order to disrupt typical functioning.

criterion-related validity Also called predictive validity, this psychometric property refers to how well a test predicts whether a patient has a deficit.

critical thinking Thoughtful analysis of information, potentially from several sources, for the purpose of forming hypotheses or conclusions.

crossed aphasia A rare aphasia with varied impairments resulting from lesions to the nondominant, and thus typically right, hemisphere.

cueing hierarchy A technique used to stimulate word retrieval skills in which cues that facilitate word retrieval are arranged in a hierarchy according to level of external support they provide.

declarative memory A form of long-term memory that holds information that can be stored and accessed explicitly or consciously.

dementia A chronic, progressive deterioration of memory and at least one other area such as personality, communication ability, or executive control functioning.

depression A mood disorder characterized by feelings of sadness and worthlessness, sleep disturbances, changes in eating habits, and fatigue.

derivational affix A morpheme that, when added to a word, transforms that word into different word forms (e.g., a noun becomes an adjective).

diagnosis related group (DRG) Designates the reimbursement rate for patients receiving Medicare Part A coverage in acute care settings, based on the diagnosis or diagnoses of individual patients.

diffuse axonal shearing or injury Microscopic damage associated with traumatic brain injury that includes the shearing of axons from their myelin sheath or tearing of the axons themselves, and that frequently affects brain tissue at gray–white matter junctions (e.g., inferior frontal lobe, cerebellar peduncles).

diplopia Double vision, typically associated with brainstem damage.

discourse genre Refers to types of discourse such as traditional narrative, procedural, expository, service encounters, expert interviews, and gossiping.

divided attention A complex attentional skill of attending to and completing concurrently more than one task, or simultaneously attending to and processing multiple stimuli.

donepezil A drug that prevents the breakdown of acetylcholine, and thus increases levels of this neurotransmitter.

dopamine A neurotransmitter that is found in particularly high concentrations within frontal regions of the cortex and numerous subcortical areas. It is part of the catecholamine system.

dose The intensity and duration of an intervention.

dysarthria A motor speech disorder caused by impairments of speech musculature tone (i.e., reduced or excessive tone) and/or control (i.e., incoordination, imprecise movements).

dysphagia Swallowing problems found in patients with neurological diseases such as stroke, Huntington's disease, Parkinson's disease, traumatic brain injury (TBI), and amyotrophic lateral sclerosis (ALS). Without treatment, dysphagia may lead to malnutrition, pneumonia, and other medical complications.

ecological validity A psychometric property that refers to how well patients' test performances predict their behavior in daily real-world settings.

edema Swelling that is the product of increased intra- or extracellular fluid in the brain or other bodily tissues.

effectiveness Evidence that an intervention is beneficial when applied under typical clinical conditions.

efficacy Evidence that an intervention is beneficial when applied under ideal conditions.

efficiency Characteristic of an intervention that encompasses the size of benefit as well as the effort expended.

effortful or errorful learning A traditional training approach in which patients are encouraged to generate responses independently, even if they make errors; requires the patient to make an effortful memory search when attempting to generate a response.

electroencephalography (EEG) A method by which gross electrical activity in the brain is measured.

embolus A clot that forms or a piece of fatty plaque that breaks off from elsewhere in the circulatory system and then travels to block off a smaller artery that supplies blood to the brain.

empty speech Fluent speech lacking in information content.

encoding The process of maintaining information in working memory and then transferring that information to long-term memory stores.

endarterectomy A surgical procedure that removes plaque build-up within the carotid artery system.

environmental factors A construct of the ICF that describes contributions such as assistive mobility devices, physical geography, lighting, support systems, attitudes, and policies as they relate to the individual's ability to participate fully in desired activities.

episodic memory A subdivision of declarative memory that contains context-dependent or autobiographical memories.

errorless learning An approach based on implicit learning mechanisms in which patients are prevented from making errors via the use of cues that are gradually withdrawn.

evidence-based practice The systematic review and appraisal of research evidence as a component of clinical decision making.

executive functioning The set of high-level, inter-related cognitive abilities responsible for generating, selecting, planning, and monitoring goal-directed and adaptive responses that in turn sustain completion of independent, purposeful, and/or novel behavior.

fee-for-service A health-care financing strategy in which providers are reimbursed for individual instances of service provision.

fluency Phrase length in the speech production of patients with aphasia, as well as characteristics of melodic line, articulatory agility, speech rate, and grammatical form.

fluent aphasia Aphasia characterized by ease of speech production with melodic line, rhythm, rate, and flow and adequate phrase length.

focused attention The ability to concentrate on and prioritize certain features of the external or internal environment in the presence of competing features or stimuli. Also called selective attention.

frontotemporal lobar degeneration A cause of dementia involving degeneration of the frontal and temporal lobes, with relative sparing of the parietal lobes and in the absence of neuropathological markers of Alzheimer's diseases. Often produces behavioral symptoms such as socially inappropriate behavior and disinhibition.

functional magnetic resonance imaging (fMRI) Provides images of changes in blood oxygenation within the brain, which are used to identify brain areas that are active during specific cognitive and linguistic tasks.

functional measures Measures of performance obtained during activities typical of daily life, including activities related to personal, social, professional, or recreational pursuits.

glioblastomas Malignant (i.e., cancerous) brain tumors that are treated with chemotherapy, radiation, and/or surgery.

global aphasia A type of aphasia marked by significant impairments in all language modalities and functions.

Goal Management Training An approach to remediating executive function deficits, such as planning and problem-solving impairments, that involves making explicit the steps involved in implementing goal-directed behavior.

guided imagery (GI) A relaxation technique requiring patients to select a pleasant and calm location or event, and then imagine being at that location or event.

healthcare reform Legislation designed to influence the access to, quality of, and cost of health care.

hematoma The buildup of blood that escapes from an artery and then surrounds brain tissue.

hemiakinesia Characterized by underuse or in some cases complete lack of use of one side of their body, even in the absence of hemiparesis. Also referred to as hemihypokinesia or motor extinction, impersistence, or neglect.

hemianesthesia Somatosensory problems (e.g., reduced sense of temperature and pain) on only one side of the body.

hemianopia A visual field cut in which the patient cannot see one half (left or right) of the visual field in each eye.

hemiballismus Sudden, centrifugally spreading throwing movements of extremities on one side. It is caused by lesions to the contralateral subthalamic nucleus.

hemi-inattention A common symptom of neglect syndrome that includes problems such as poor response to or report of stimuli presented contralateral to the side of brain damage in the absence of sensory impairments. It results in poor performance of tasks or activities in the contralateral hemispace that cannot be attributed to motor or sensory impairments.

hemiparesis A muscular weakness on one side of the body.

hemiplegia Paralysis of one side of the body.

hemorrhagic stroke A stroke due to a cerebral artery bursting and causing blood to escape and flood surrounding brain tissue.

home health A stage in the continuum of care in which medical and rehabilitative services are provided in the patient's home.

home health resource group (HHRG) Prospective payment Medicare funding system for home health care.

human immunodeficiency virus (HIV) The virus that causes acquired immune deficiency syndrome (AIDS) and that may invade the brain and cause widespread damage (particularly to white matter and subcortical brain structures) and consequently, dementia (sometimes referred to as HIV encephalopathy).

Huntington's disease (HD) A progressive neurological disease that causes gradual deterioration of the caudate nuclei, and eventually cortical cell loss as well. Frequent symptoms include chorea, dysarthria, gait and posture problems, dysphagia, bradykinesia, and social disinhibition.

hypoxic-ischemic brain injury Brain injury resulting from decreased oxygen in brain tissue.

ideational apraxia Difficulty with completing or demonstrating the series of actions needed to complete tasks involving tools (e.g., preparing for and brushing one's teeth).

ideomotor apraxia Difficulty pantomiming or imitating gestures associated with functional movements.

indefinite substitutions The use of nonspecific words or descriptions for target words.

infarct The area of dead brain tissue that results from ischemia or cerebral blood flow disruption.

inflectional affix A morpheme that provides syntactic information (e.g., verb tense) when added to a word.

Informativeness measures Assessment measures used to quantify lexical–semantic content in spoken or written language samples.

inhibition An executive function requiring the ability to regulate and repress automatic, routine, or extraneous processing or behaviors.

intensive care unit (ICU) The specialized center in a hospital where medically unstable patients receive care and whose primary health-care goal is life preservation.

interaction The establishment and maintenance of relationships as a function of communicative exchanges.

internal capsule Subcortical structure consisting of axons from cortical neurons.

International Classification of Disability, Functioning, and Health (ICF) A model created by the World Health Organization (WHO) for describing the impact of disease or injury on the body and its functions, as well as patients' ability to complete tasks or activities relevant to their personal, social, education, and/or vocational pursuits.

intracerebral hemorrhage A hemorrhage in which blood invades tissue within the brain.

irreversible dementia Dementia in which cognitive symptoms are persistent. Most causes of irreversible dementia are progressive neurologic diseases. Sometimes referred to as primary degenerative dementia.

ischemic stroke A stroke caused by a deficiency in blood flow to the brain due to blockage of cerebral artery.

jargon Production of entire sentences in which all content words, and in some cases functor words as well, are replaced with neologisms.

Korsakoff's disease A disease caused by chronic alcohol abuse that results in damage to diencephalic structures (e.g., hypothalamus, mammillary bodies) and widespread cortical atrophy. It is associated with an irreversible and progressive dementia.

lability A difficulty controlling one's emotions that often occurs following brain damage. May result in unprovoked laughing or crying.

lacunar stroke Blockage of small penetrating arteries that supply blood to structures deep within the brain. Associated with lesions that are 2 to 15 mm^2.

language The primary communication tool that utilizes socially shared, rule-based symbols to represent concepts.

language competence Implies possession of underlying language skills, processes, or representations.

language performance The ability to exhibit access to or execution of intact language rules and contents.

lesion method A technique for studying localization of brain function by which changes in behavior following brain injury and/or disease, are noted and the control of those behaviors is deductively attributed to the injured neural area.

limb activation An approach to remediating attention impairments, particularly neglect, that involves moving a limb contralateral to the side of brain damage while completing attention demanding tasks.

limb apraxia A motoric problem characterized by difficulty executing acquired and volitional movements of the fingers, wrists, elbows, and/or shoulders. It is most frequently observed in patients with left hemisphere brain damage.

long-term care A state in the continuum of care in which basic custodial care is provided in a residential setting.

macular degeneration A progressive breakdown or damage to the macular, a portion of the retina. Symptoms include blurring of vision, dim colors, and difficulty reading.

magnetic resonance imaging (MRI) A non-invasive imaging technique that allows scientists to identify brain lesions in live patients.

magnetoencephalography (MEG) The measurement of the magnetic fields generated by electrical activity of the brain.

malignant A term for brain tumors that are cancerous and often recur despite treatment efforts. They may invade other parts of the body or, themselves, be the product of a cancer elsewhere in the body that has infiltrated the brain.

managed care A general term used to describe the current American health-care system; implies external management of health-care practices and financing.

mania A psychiatric disorder characterized by mental and physical hyperactivity, disorganization of behavior, and elevation of mood.

mapping therapy A theoretically motivated approach to treating deficits of grammatical production and/or comprehension in which patients with aphasia are taught to improve their ability to map the relationship between words' thematic roles and their location within a sentence.

measures of participation Tools employed to assess an individual's ability to participate in desired personal, social, recreational, and/or vocational endeavors.

measures of quality of life Tools employed to assess an individual's sense of well-being and satisfaction.

Melodic Intonation Therapy (MIT) Stimulation treatment developed to improve word retrieval and speech prosody of patients with severe nonfluent aphasia.

memantine Medication for Alzheimer's disease that blocks N-methyl-D-aspartate (NMDA)–type glutamate receptors.

memory Cognitive function allowing individuals to store, retain, and subsequently retrieve processed information.

meningioma A brain tumor that arises from the arachnoid tissue that sheaths the brain.

meningitis An infection that causes inflammation of the pia and arachnoid tissues that cover the brain.

metacognitive abilities Cognitive function allowing individuals to think and talk about one's own memory abilities, language abilities, or overall cognitive functioning.

metacognitive training Therapy targeting an individual's ability to think and talk about his or her own cognitive functioning.

methylphenidate A drug (more commonly known as Ritalin) that increases levels of dopamine and norepinephrine within the brain.

micrographia A mechanical disruption of writing that results in extreme reductions in letter size. It is a frequent symptom of Parkinson's disease.

mild cognitive impairment Cognitive decline that is greater than that expected, given an individual's age and level of education.

minimally conscious state A level of consciousness, often subsequent to coma or vegetative state, when there are minimal but distinct intermittent periods of self- and environmental awareness.

Minimum Data Set (MDS) Framework for guiding the assessment process for the purpose of assigning an appropriate resource utilization group.

mnemonic strategies Techniques to enhance memory encoding (or storing) and retrieval skills.

multimodal communication Strategies that can be taught to patients with neurogenic language disorders to augment direct retraining of their spoken language abilities or to help them compensate for attention, memory, or executive functioning impairments.

Multiple Oral Rereading (MOR) Treatment designed to increase use of whole-word reading, which utilizes repeated oral reading of a pre-selected text to increase reading rate.

neglect dysgraphia Writing difficulty related to neglecting the left side of words or the left side of the page.

neglect dyslexia Reading difficulty related to not attending to the left side of words or the left side of the page.

neglect syndrome A set of attention problems associated with predominantly right hemisphere damage (although it can also occur following left hemisphere damage) in which patients are slow or inaccurate at reporting, reacting to, orienting to, or seeking out stimuli that are presented contralateral to the side of their brain damage.

neologisms Substitution of nonwords.

neurofibrillary tangles Unusual triangular and looped fibers in the cytoplasm of neurons that are a pathological marker of Alzheimer's disease.

neurogenic stuttering Disruption in speech fluency, including hesitations, sound and syllable repetitions, and prolongations that arise from neurologic insult.

neuroprotective agents Drugs such as nimodipine (i.e., a calcium blocker) and citicoline (i.e., an acetylcholine precursor) that are designed to protect brain tissue directly adjacent to the infarct (i.e., penumbra) from the fatal chemical changes that occur when its blood flow is reduced.

neuropsychologists Professionals who assess cognitive abilities, including perception, attention, memory, executive functions, and sometimes language.

neurotransmitters Chemical substances that are released by neurons to facilitate message transmission among neurons. They may also facilitate communication between neurons and muscles or neurons and glands.

noncanonical A sentence using the passive voice.

nondeclarative memories A form of long-term memory that can be evoked and, in some cases, stored unconsciously.

nonfluent aphasia Aphasia characterized by speech produced haltingly and with great effort.

norepinephrine/noradrenalin A neurotransmitter that is found throughout the cortex, cerebellum, spinal cord, and autonomic nervous system. It is part of the catecholamine system.

no responses A type of error associated with word-retrieval problems.

nystagmus An involuntary, rapid, and rhythmic movement of the eyeball, which may be horizontal, vertical, rotatory, or mixed.

occupational therapists Professionals who assess fine motor and sensorimotor abilities, skills involved in completing activities of daily living, and sometimes the cognitive abilities of perception, attention, and problem solving.

open head injury A traumatic brain injury in which the skull is fractured or penetrated by an external force and the contents of the skull are exposed.

organization The executive process by which one structures or categorizes incoming information, as well as a response to that information.

orientation A type of cognitive function in which a person demonstrates the ability to orient himself or herself to time, people, and places.

outcome The results of program efforts, specifically, changes in patients' communicative and cognitive functioning.

outcome measurement The process of assessing the result of an intervention.

outcome process measures Procedures that allow individuals or systems to assess whether policies and procedures designed to maximize patient outcomes have been followed.

outpatient A stage in the continuum of care in which patient care is provided at a centralized non-residential setting (e.g., clinic).

pantomime A form of gestural communication that involves a series of relatively transparent movements that are associated with a given activity or situation.

paragrammatism Speech characterized by substitution of inappropriate syntactic elements.

paraneoplastic syndromes Relatively rare disorders that result when one's immune system reacts abnormally to a cancerous tumor, attacking healthy tissue.

paraphasia Error in naming.

Parkinson's disease (PD) A progressive neurological disease associated with deterioration of subcortical structures such as the substantia nigra, and decreased levels of the neurotransmitter dopamine. Common symptoms include dysarthria, bradykinesia, resting tremor, rigidity, gait and posture disturbances, micrographia, and depression.

per diem Funding strategy in which clinicians are compensated on a daily or per-patient basis.

personal factors Aspects of an individual, such as race, age, life experiences, personality and other characteristics, that influence the impact of health conditions.

pharmacotherapy A treatment approach in which medications are used to resolve physiological problems, such as decreased levels of certain chemicals in the brain, that are proposed to underlie behavioral symptoms associated with brain damage or disease.

phonemic paraphasia Sound errors involving substitutions, additions, omissions, and/or rearrangements of target word phonemes. Also known as literal paraphasia.

Pick's disease A relatively rare disease that typically occurs between the ages of 40 and 60 years and affects women more frequently than men. Causes progressive deterioration of primarily frontal regions of the brain and produces an irreversible dementia.

planning A type of executive function that allows for devising the strategies and sequencing the steps of those strategies to achieve intended goals.

positron emission tomography (PET) An invasive imaging technology utilizing injected radioactive isotopes to track blood flow in the brain.

post-traumatic amnesia (PTA) An acute and commonly temporary phase of recovery from traumatic brain injury in which patients who have typically just emerged from coma are extremely confused, distractible, and disoriented. Also referred to as post-traumatic confusion.

practice-based evidence The process of using empirical methods to track clinical progress; provides an additional source of evidence to support future clinical decisions.

preferred provider A care provider who participates in a managed care program, typically providing services at discounted rates.

premorbid abilities Patients' skill levels (e.g., motoric, sensory, cognitive abilities) prior to the onset of brain damage or disease.

presbycusis Progressive deterioration of hearing sensitivity, especially in the high frequencies, due to aging.

presbyopia A deficit of vision due to aging. Specific symptoms include increased sensitivity to glare, and difficulty with accommodation and recession of the near point of vision, so that objects very near the eyes cannot be seen distinctly without the use of convex glasses.

primary care The point in the continuum of care at which individuals typically make first contact with care providers.

primary progressive aphasia (PPA) A degenerative condition generally associated with left hemisphere pathology and characterized by progressive impairment of comprehension, naming, speech fluency, and reading and writing skills, but relative sparing in other areas of cognition.

prism lenses Corrective lenses that were originally designed to improve vision by facilitating the joint focus of both eyes to address double vision; now also used to shift visual focus in patients with visual neglect.

problem solving Executive function processes that include problem identification, as well as generation, selection, and implementation of solutions.

procedural memory A form of nondeclarative, long-term memory that holds memory for motor and cognitive skills that are habitual and that require little effort to recall.

progressive muscle relaxation (PMR) A type of relaxation therapy that involves sustaining attention to the activity of successively contracting and relaxing certain muscle groups while concurrently inhibiting thoughts or sensory input that may interfere with the attentional focus on the target.

prospective memory A memory function that allows recalling and carrying out future intentions.

prospective payment A health-care financing system in which the reimbursement rate is determined according to an estimate of cost of care.

pseudodementia Overt cognitive problems, such as impaired memory and reasoning, which are found in some depressed elderly patients and that may be reversed if patients receive proper and prompt medical treatment for their depression.

pure agraphia Isolated impairments of writing in the absence of any other language impairment.

pure alexia Isolated reading difficulties in the absence of any other language impairment. Also called word blindness.

pure aphasia Isolated impairments of specific language functions.

pure word deafness Profound auditory comprehension deficits without evidence of impairment in other language functions or hearing sensitivity.

qualitative information Information regarding how a patient performs a given task and thus concerns the identification of influential task parameters and patient strategies.

quality assurance Program assessment to optimize clinical processes and outcomes.

random paraphasias Substitutions of words that lack apparent semantic relations to the target words.

reauditorization A treatment technique designed to improve auditory comprehension abilities by having patients first read aloud target items and then repeat aloud these items when provided with a spoken model and a picture stimulus.

rehabilitation A stage in the continuum of care in which patients receive intense rehabilitation services in a residential setting.

relational or closed class words The relatively small set of words, such as prepositions, pronouns, determiners, and conjunctions, that convey primarily morphosyntactic information.

relaxation therapy A form of complementary or alternative medicine that involves sustaining attention to a verbal or nonverbal stimulus or muscle activity while concurrently inhibiting thoughts or sensory input that may interfere with the attentional focus on the target stimulus or activity.

reliability Psychometric property that indicates how similar test results are across repeated administrations of the test under comparable testing conditions.

repetition The ability to repeat words or phrases without processing for meaning.

repetitive transcranial magnetic stimulation A noninvasive method of using electromagnetic induction to cause rapid changes in the depolarization of brain neurons.

resource utilization group (RUG) Designates the reimbursement rate for patients receiving Medicare Part A coverage in acute care settings, based on the rehabilitation/skilled care needs of the patient.

Response Elaboration Training (RET) Program designed to improve utterance length and information content in primarily patients with nonfluent aphasia; it utilizes incidental learning, reinforcement of patient-initiated output, and emphasis on utterance content.

restorative Treatment strategies intended to effect long-lasting improvements in underlying body structure and function.

retrieval The process by which long-term memories are transferred to consciousness.

retrograde amnesia Characterized by continuous or interrupted deficits of long-term memories that were stored prior to the onset of brain injury or disease.

reversible dementia Dementia that can be improved and, in some cases, completely resolved with appropriate medical treatment.

secondary care Care provided by specialists (e.g., neurology), usually initiated by referral from a primary care provider.

segmental phonology Sound elements of words or syllables.

selective or focused attention The ability to concentrate on and prioritize certain features of the external or internal environment in the presence of competing features or stimuli. Also called focused attention.

selective serotonin reuptake inhibitors A class of drugs that prevent the reuptake of serotonin, a neurotransmitter found throughout the brain and spinal cord. By preventing reuptake, these drugs function to increase the level or potency of serotonin. They are commonly used to treat depression and have relatively few side effects.

self-monitoring The executive ability to appraise and adjust one's performance and behavior on the basis of environmental feedback, knowledge of task difficulty, and awareness of one's own strengths and weaknesses.

Semantic Feature Analysis (SFA) Program designed to encourage word generation in patients with aphasia or traumatic brain injury by activating the semantic network (via elicitation of semantic features).

semantic memory A subdivision of declarative memory that holds context-independent, factual memories.

semantic paraphasia Word-choice error that is semantically related to the target word.

senile plaques Aggregations of degenerating neurons and the remains of degenerated nerve fibers that are a pathological marker of Alzheimer's disease.

sensitivity A term applied to the characteristic of an assessment tool or process that relates to its ability to identify individuals with the condition of interest.

sensory stimulation A complementary and alternative medicine approach that exposes patients to and allows them to interact with, often in a non-directive manner, stimuli that will excite one or more senses, such as light or music therapy.

short-term memory The transient store of information for a short time span of a few minutes.

single photon emission computed tomography (SPECT) An invasive imaging technology utilizing injected radioactive isotopes to track blood flow in the brain.

skilled nursing facility A stage in the continuum of care in which continual nursing care is provided in a residential setting.

skull fracture A break or crack in a bone of the skull that can occur following a traumatic brain injury.

social cognition One's knowledge of social rules and conventions, which guides interpretation of others' social actions, as well as generation of our own social actions and responses.

spaced retrieval A memory treatment that involves patients practicing, with the aid of cues, to recall information or to use a strategy over progressively longer time intervals.

specificity A term applied to the characteristic of an assessment tool or process that relates to its ability to identify those individuals who do not have the condition of interest.

speech acts Theoretical units of communication that encompass the various message meanings (intended and actually perceived) by the message-sender and message-receiver and what the rules governing the linguistic utterance are.

standardization Process in which a test is given to a large sample of individuals who represent the cross-section of the population with whom the test will be used in clinical practice.

stimulation treatments Approach to aphasia rehabilitation that emphasizes the role of stimulus factors in a patient's current linguistic abilities. Exposure to stimulus and task hierarchies is the means by which compromised language functions and modalities are rehabilitated.

strategic learning technique A memory strategy that involves identifying relevant and important information and synthesizing that information to determine the overall meaning or gist of the to-be-recalled or -learned information.

stroke Any disruption in blood flow to the brain. Also called a cerebrovascular accident or brain attack.

subarachnoid hemorrhage A hemorrhage in which blood spills into the pia-arachnoid space surrounding the brain.

subcortical aphasia Aphasia resulting from damage to non-cortical sites, such as the thalamus or basal ganglia, and characterized by various language impairments.

subcortical dementia The dementia associated with Parkinson's disease, Huntington's disease, multiple sclerosis, and other diseases that cause brain damage at primarily subcortical levels.

substantive or open class The set of words including verbs, nouns, adjectives, and adverbs that primarily convey lexical–semantic information.

superior longitudinal fasciculus Association fibers that allow intra-hemisphere communication by connecting the frontal cortex with the parietal, temporal, and occipital cortices.

supramarginal gyrus Area of the brain within the parietal lobe that, with the angular gyrus, contributes to written language comprehension.

suprasegmental phonology Intonation, stress, and pauses in speech production.

sustained attention The ability to maintain attention and thus consistent performance over long periods of time.

team approach A treatment approach designed to establish and maintain collaboration among professionals from a variety of health-care disciplines, including speech-language pathology, psychology, audiology, occupational therapy, and physical therapy.

tertiary care A point in the continuum of care during which subspecialty care is provided in a clinical or hospital setting. Tertiary care is typically initiated by referral from secondary care or in the case of acute illness.

text to speech The capability of software interfaces to convert written text to spoken voice.

thalamus Subcortical structure that has been proposed to play a crucial role in a number of cognitive functions, including attention and verbal memory.

theory of mind The ability of an individual to imagine the thoughts and feelings of another.

third-party payers The funding sources (e.g., Medicare, private insurance) that pay for health care provided to individual consumers.

thrombolytic drugs Medicines, such as rtPA (recombinant tissue plasminigen activator), that break up blood clots by speeding up the body's natural clot-dissolving process.

thrombosis An arterial blockage due to a build-up of atherosclerotic or fatty plaque on an artery that provides blood flow to the brain.

tics Involuntary compulsive movements of small-muscle groups of the face.

tinnitus Ringing in the ears.

transaction The communicative exchange of information.

transcortical mixed aphasia Aphasia characterized by severe impairments in comprehension, fluency, and naming, but with repetition ability better than what the other language deficits would suggest. Also known as isolation aphasia.

transcortical motor aphasia Nonfluent aphasia similar to Broca's aphasia and characterized by better verbal output for repeated phrases and sentences than for spontaneous verbal output.

transcortical sensory aphasia Fluent aphasia similar to Wernicke's aphasia and characterized by poor comprehension with better repetition abilities than spontaneous speech abilities.

transcranial direct current stimulation A method of inferring brain function or stimulating neural activity by altering the function of cortical neurons using magnetic fields.

transcutaneous electrical nerve stimulation (TENS) A technique similar to electroacupuncture that involves stimulating the skin at certain frequencies and skin sites to affect brain functioning.

transient ischemic attack (TIA) A small and temporary disruption of blood flow to the brain that does not cause permanent brain damage.

traumatic brain injury (TBI) An insult to the brain produced by external forces that may cause a variety of temporary or permanent physical, cognitive, emotional, and behavioral impairments.

Treatment of Underlying Forms (TUF) A theoretically motivated approach to treating deficits of grammatical production and/or comprehension. Its goal is to remediate patients' ability to process phrase movement by increasing their awareness and understanding of verbs, verb argument structure, and how certain sentence constituents move to form noncanonical sentence types.

tumors or neoplasms Tissue masses that arise from an abnormally fast rate of cell reproduction.

validity The extent to which a measurement tool measures what it purports to measure.

vascular dementia Decline in cognitive function due to diffuse or repeated ischemia in the brain; previously referred to as multi-infarct dementia.

vegetative state A condition when patients appear to waken from coma but demonstrate no willful interaction with their external or internal environments and no communication ability.

verbal mediation A cognitive strategy in which patients are taught to verbalize each step when planning and/or executing tasks.

vertebrobasilar arterial system An arterial system that arises from the left and right subclavian arteries and provides blood supply to the occipital lobes, as well as medial and inferior portions of temporal lobes and subcortical structures such as the thalamus.

visual agnosia A disturbance in recognizing or associating meaning with visual stimuli even though visual sensitivity is adequate to see the stimuli.

Voluntary Control of Involuntary Utterances (VCIU) A treatment program designed to stimulate propositional (i.e., voluntary) verbal output in patients whose current spoken language abilities are restricted to involuntary production of a small set of real words.

watershed areas Lateral areas of the hemispheres that are located where distributions of major cerebral arteries overlap and thus have a back-up blood supply.

Wernicke's aphasia Fluent aphasia characterized by marked comprehension, naming, and repetition impairments.

Wernicke's area The area of the brain located in the posterior aspects of the superior temporal lobe and linked to language comprehension.

working memory The process by which information is temporarily stored while it is concurrently being processed or manipulated.

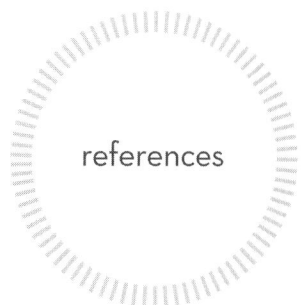

references

Abel, S., Schultz, A., Radermacher, I., Willmes, K., & Huber, W. (2003). Increasing versus vanishing cues in naming therapy. *Brain and Language, 87,* 143–144.

Adair, J., Na, D., Schwartz, R., & Heilman, K. (2003). Caloric stimulation in neglect: Evaluation of response as a function of neglect type. *Journal of the International Neuropsychological Society, 9,* 938–988.

Adamovich, B. B. (1990). *A comparison of FIM evaluations by nurses and speech pathologists.* Paper presented at the Clinical Aphasiology Conference, Santa Fe, NM.

Adamovich, B. B., & Henderson, J. (1992). *Scales of cognitive ability for traumatic brain injury.* Chicago: Riverside.

Adams, H. P., Zoppo, G. del, Alberts, M. J., Bhatt, D. L., Brass, L., Furlan, A., . . . Quality of Care Outcomes in Research Interdisciplinary Working Group. (2007). Guidelines for the early management of adults with ischemic stroke. *Stroke, 38*(5), 1655–1711.

Adams, R., Albers, G., Alberts, M., Benavente, O., Furie, K., Goldstein, L., . . . Schwamm, L. (2008). Update to the AHA/ASA recommendations for the prevention of stroke in patients with stroke and transient ischemic attack. *Stroke, 39,* 1647–1652.

Adams, W., & Sheslow, D. (2003). *Wide range assessment of memory and learning* (2nd ed.). Lutz, FL: Psychological Assessment Resources.

Aftonomos, L. B., Appelbaum, J. S., & Steele, R. D. (1999). Improving outcomes for persons with aphasia in advanced community-based treatment programs. *Stroke, 30,* 1370–1379.

Aftonomos, L. B., Steele, R., Appelbaum, J., & Harris, V. (2001). Relationships between impairment-level assessments and functional-level assessments in aphasia: Findings from LCC treatment programmes. *Aphasiology, 15,* 951–964.

Agranovich, A., Panter, A., Puente, A., & Touradji, P. (2011). The culture of time in neuropsychological assessment: Exploring the effects of culture-specific time attitudes on timed test performance in Russian and American samples. *Journal of the International Neuropsychological Society, 17,* 692–701.

Ahlskog, J. E., Geda, Y. E., Graff-Radford, N. R., & Petersen, R. C. (2011). Physical exercise as a preventive or disease-modifying treatment of dementia and brain aging. *Mayo Clinic Proceedings, 86*(9), 876–884.

Akanuma, K., Meguro, K., Meguro, M., Sasaki, E., Chiba, K., Ishii, H., & Tanaka, N. (2011). Improved social interaction and increased anterior cingulate metabolism after group reminiscence with reality orientation approach for vascular dementia. *Psychiatry Research: Neuroimaging, 192*(3), 183–187.

Al-Aloucy, M., Cotteret, R., Thomas, P., Volteau, M., Benmaou, I., & Della Barb, G. (2011). Unawareness of memory impairment and behavioral abnormalities in patients with Alzheimer's disease: Relation to professional health care burden. *Journal of Nutrition and Health in Aging, 15*(5), 356–360.

Albers, G. W., & Tijssen, J. G. (1999). Antiplatelet therapy: New foundations for optimal treatment decisions. *Neurology, 53,* S25–S31.

Albert, M. L., Bachman, D. L., Morgan, A., & Helm-Estabrooks, N. (1988). Pharmacotherapy for aphasia. *Neurology, 38,* 877–879.

Albert, M. L., Sparks, R., & Helm, N. (1988). Melodic intonation therapy for aphasia. *Archives of Neurology, 29,* 130–131.

Albin, R. L., Young, A. B., & Penney, J. B. (1995). The functional anatomy of disorders of the basal ganglia. *Trends in Neuroscience, 18,* 63–64.

Albright, E., & Purves, B. (2008). Exploring SentenceShaper: Treatment and augmentative possibilities. *Aphasiology, 22*(7–8), 741–752.

Alderman, N. (1996). Central executive deficit and response to operant conditioning methods. *Neuropsychological Rehabilitation, 6*, 161–186.

Alderman, N., Fry, R. K., Youngson, H. A. (1995). Improvement of self-monitoring skills, reduction of behavior disturbance and the dysexecutive syndrome: Comparison of response cost and a new programme of self-monitoring training. *Neuropsychological Rehabilitation, 5*, 193–221.

Alexander, M. P. (2006). Impairments of procedures for implementing complex language are due to disruption of frontal attention processes. *Journal of the International Neuropsychological Society, 12*, 236–247.

Alexander, M. P., & Hillis, A. E. (2008). Aphasia. *Handbook of Clinical Neurology, 88*, 287–309.

Alexander, M. P., Naeser, M. A., & Palumbo, C. L. (1987). Correlations of subcortical CT lesion sites and aphasia profiles. *Brain, 110*, 961–991.

Alexopolous, G. S., Abrams, R. C., Young, R. C., & Shamoian, C. A. (1988). Cornell scale for depression in dementia. *Biological Psychiatry, 23*, 271–284.

Al-Khindi T., Zakzanis, K., & van Gorp, W. (2011). Does antiretroviral therapy improve HIV-associated cognitive impairment? A quantitative review of the literature. *Journal of the International Neuropsychological Society, 17*, 1–14.

Allen, L., & Allen, B. (2012). *Brain storm: A journey of faith through brain injury.* Bloomington, IN: Westbow Press.

Alvarez, J. A., & Emory, E. (2006). Executive function and the frontal lobes: A meta-analytic review. *Neuropsychology Review, 16*(1), 17–42.

Alzheimer's Association. (2012). *2012 Alzheimer's disease facts and figures.* Chicago: Author.

American Brain Tumor Association. (2012). *Facts and statistics, 2012.* Retrieved November 27, 2012, from http://www.abta.org

American Psychiatric Association. (1994). *Diagnostic and statistical manual of mental disorders* (4th ed.). Washington, DC: Author.

American Speech-Language-Hearing Association. (1988). *Prevention of communication disorders* [Position statement]. Available from http://www.asha.org/policy

American Speech-Language-Hearing Association. (2000). *Council on professional standards in speech-language pathology and audiology: Background information and criteria for registration of speech-language pathology assistants.* Rockville, MD: Author.

American Speech-Language-Hearing Association. (2002). *ASHA SLP healthcare survey 2002.* Rockville, MD: Author.

American Speech-Language-Hearing Association. (2003). *National outcomes measurement system (NOMS).* Rockville, MD: Author.

American Speech-Language-Hearing Association. (2004a). *Evidence-based practice in communication disorders: An introduction* [Technical report]. Rockville, MD: Author.

American Speech-Language-Hearing Association. (2004b). *Training, use, and supervision of support personnel in speech-language pathology* [Position statement]. Available from http://www.asha.org/policy

American Speech-Language-Hearing Association. (2005). *Evidence-based practice in communication disorders* [Position statement]. Available from http://www.asha.org/policy

American Speech-Language-Hearing Association. (2007). *Scope of practice in speech-language pathology* [Scope of practice]. Available from http://www.asha.org/policy

American Speech-Language-Hearing Association. (2008). *National Outcomes Measurement System (NOMS): Acute inpatient national data report, 2008.* Rockville, MD: National Center for Evidence-Based Practice in Communication Disorders of ASHA.

American Speech-Language-Hearing Association. (2009). *ASHA SLP healthcare survey 2002.* Rockville, MD: Author.

American Speech-Language-Hearing Association. (2011a). *National Outcomes Measurement System (NOMS): Adults in healthcare—Inpatient rehab national data report 2011.* Rockville, MD: National Center for Evidence-Based Practice in Communication Disorders.

American Speech-Language-Hearing Association. (2011b). *National Outcomes Measurement System (NOMS): Adults in healthcare—Outpatient national data report 2011.* Rockville, MD: National Center for Evidence-Based Practice in Communication Disorders.

American Speech-Language-Hearing Association. (2011c). *National Outcomes Measurement System (NOMS): Adults in healthcare—Skilled nursing facility national data report 2011.* Rockville, MD: National Center for Evidence-Based Practice in Communication Disorders.

American Speech-Language-Hearing Association. (2012a). *2012 Medicare fee schedule for speech-language pathologists.* Rockville, MD: Author.

American Speech-Language-Hearing Association (2012b). *Medicare guidelines for group therapy treatment.* Available from http://www.asha.org/Practice/reimbursement/medicare/grouptreatment/

American Speech-Language-Hearing Association. (2012c). *Overview of documentation for Medicare outpatient therapy services.* Accessed June 17, 2012, from http://www.asha.org/practice/reimbursement/medicare/medicare_documentation/

Americans With Disabilities Act of 1990, 42, U.S.C. § 12101 *et seq.* (1990)

Anderson, C. A., & Arciniegas, D. B. (2010). Cognitive sequelae of hypoxic-ischemic brain injury: A review. *NeuroRehabilitation, 26*(1), 47–63.

Anderson, S. W., Damasio, H., Damasio, A. R., Klima, E., Bellugi, U., & Brandt, J. P. (1992). Acquisition of signs from American sign language in hearing individuals following left hemisphere damage and aphasia. *Neuropsychologia, 30*(4), 329–340.

Anderson-Hanley, C., Arciero, P. J., Brickman, A. M., Nimon, J. P., Okuma, N., Westen, S. C., . . . Zimmerman, E. A. (2012). Exergaming and older adult cognition: A cluster randomized clinical trial. *American Journal of Preventive Medicine, 42*(2), 109–119.

Andersson, S., & Fridlund, B. (2002). The aphasic person's view of the encounter with other people: A grounded theory analysis. *Journal of Psychiatric Mental Health Nursing, 9,* 285–292.

Andrews-Salvia, M., Roy, N., & Cameron, R. (2003). Evaluating the effects of memory books for individuals with severe dementia. *Journal of Medical Speech-Language Pathology, 11,* 51–59.

Angeleri, R., Bosco, F. M., Zettin, M., Sacco, K., Colle, L., & Bara, B. G. (2008). Communicative impairment in traumatic brain injury: A complete pragmatic assessment. *Brain and Language, 107*(3), 229–245.

Anson, K., & Ponsford, J. (2006). Coping and emotional adjustment following traumatic brain injury. *Journal of Head Trauma Rehabilitation, 21,* 248–259.

Antonucci, S. M. (2009). Use of semantic feature analysis in group aphasia treatment. *Aphasiology, 23*(7–8), 854–866.

Aphasia Institute. (2010). *Assessment for living with aphasia.* Toronto, ON: Author.

Appelros, P., Karlsson, G. M., Seiger, A., & Nydevik, I. (2002). Neglect and anosognosia after first-ever stroke: Incidence and relationship to disability. *Journal of Rehabilitation Medicine, 34,* 215–220.

Appleton, S., Browne, A., Ciccone, N., Fong, K., Hankey, G., Lund, M., . . . Yee, Y. (2011). A multidisciplinary social communication and coping skills group intervention for adults with acquired brain injury (ABI): A pilot feasibility study in an inpatient setting. *Brain Impairment, 12*(3), 210–222.

Arciniegas, D. B. (2010). Hypoxic-ischemic brain injury. *International Brain Injury Association Newsletter, 3.* Retrieved from http://www.internationalbrain.org/?q=node/131

Arciniegas, D. B. (2011). Cholinergic dysfunction and cognitive impairment after traumatic brain injury. Part 2: Evidence from basic and clinical investigations. *Journal of Head Trauma Rehabilitation, 26*(4), 319–323.

Ardila, A. (2005). Cultural values underlying psychometric cognitive testing. *Neuropsychology Review, 15*(4), 185–195.

Ardila, A., Rosselli, M., & Strumwasser, S. (1991). Neuropsychological deficits in chronic cocaine abusers. *International Journal of Neuroscience, 57,* 73–79.

Arkin, S. (1991). Memory training in early Alzheimer's disease: An optimistic look at the field. *American Journal of Alzheimer's & Related Disorders Care & Research, 6,* 17–25.

Arkin, S. (1998). Alzheimer memory training: Positive results replicated. *American Journal of Alzheimer's Disease, 13,* 102–104.

Arkin, S. (2003). Student-led exercise sessions yield significant fitness gains for Alzheimer's patients. *American Journal of Alzheimer's Disease and Other Dementias, 18,* 159–170.

Arkin, S., & Mahendra, N. (2001). Discourse analysis of Alzheimer's patients before and after intervention: Methodology and outcomes. *Aphasiology, 15,* 533–569.

Armstrong, E. (Ed.). (2012). Discourse across disorders: Acquired neurogenic conditions. *Seminars in Speech and Language, 33*(1).

Armstrong, E., Ferguson, A., & Simmons-Mackie, N. (2011). Discourse and functional approaches to aphasia. In I. Papathanasiou, P. Coppens, & C. Potagas (Eds.), *Aphasia and related neurogenic communication disorders* (pp. 217–231). Sudbury, MA: Jones & Bartlett.

Armstrong, L., & McKechnie, K. (2003). Intergenerational communication: Fundamental but under-exploited theory for speech and language therapy with older people. *International Journal of Language and Communication Disorders, 38,* 13–29.

Arnold, L. (2003). *Workbook of activities for language and cognition–5: Neuro rehab.* East Moline, IL: Linguisystems.

Asberg, J., & Sandberg, A. (2010). Discourse comprehension intervention for high-functioning students with autism spectrum disorders: Preliminary findings from a school-based study. *Journal of Research in Special Educational Needs, 10*(2), 91–98.

Ashtary, F., Janghorbani, M., Chitsaz, A., Reisi, M., & Bahrami, A. (2006). A randomized, double blind trial of bromocriptine efficacy in nonfluent aphasia after stroke. *Neurology, 66,* 914–916.

Atri, A. (2011). Effective pharmacological management of Alzheimer's disease. *American Journal of Managed Care, 17,* S346–S355.

Auslin, M. S. (2003). *The idioms workbook* (2nd ed.). Austin, TX: PRO-ED.

Azouvi, P., Bartolomeo, P., Beis, J., Perennou, D., Pradat-Diehl, P., & Rousseaux, M. (2006). A battery of tests for the quantitative assessment of unilateral neglect. *Restorative Neurology and Neuroscience, 24,* 273–285.

Azouvi, P., Couillet, J., Leclereq, M., Martin, Y., Asloun, S., & Rousseaux, M. (2004). Divided attention and mental effort after severe traumatic brain injury. *Neuropsychologia, 42,* 1260–1268.

Azouvi, P., Olivier, S., de Montety, G., Samuel, C., Louis-Dreyfus, A., & Tesio, L. (2003). Behavioral assessment of unilateral neglect: Study of the psychometric properties of the Catherine Bergego Scale. *Archives of Physical and Medical Rehabilitation, 84,* 51–57.

Azouvi, P., Samuel, C., Louis-Dreyfus, A., Bernatti, T., Bartolomeo, P., Beis, J., . . . Rousseaux, M. (2002). Sensitivity of clinical and behavioral tests of spatial neglect after right hemisphere stroke. *Journal of Neurology, Neurosurgery, and Psychiatry, 73,* 160–166.

Azouvi, P., Vallat-Azouvi, C., & Belmont, A. (2009). Cognitive deficits after traumatic coma. *Progress in Brain Research, 177,* 89–110.

Babbitt, E. M., & Cherney, L. R. (2010). Communication confidence in persons with aphasia. *Topics in Stroke Rehabilitation, 17*(3), 214–223.

Babikian, T., & Asarnow, R. (2009). Neurocognitive outcomes and recovery after pediatric TBI: Meta-analytic review of the literature. *Neuropsychology, 23,* 283–296.

Babizhayev, M. A., Deyev, A. I., & Yegorov, Y. E. (2011). Olfactory dysfunction and cognitive impairment in age-related neurodegeneration: Prevalence related to patient selection, diagnostic criteria and therapeutic treatment of aged clients receiving clinical neurology and community-based care. *Current Clinics in Pharmacology, 6*(4), 236–259.

Baddeley, A. (2003). Working memory and language: An overview. *Journal of Communication Disorders, 36,* 189–208.

Baddeley, A. (2007). *Working memory, thought, and action.* New York: Oxford University Press.

Baddeley, A., Emslie, H., & Nimmo-Smith, I. (1994). *Doors and people.* Bury St. Edmunds, Suffolk, England: Thames Valley Test Company.

Baines, K. A., Martin, A. W., & Heeringa, H. M. (1999). *Assessment of language-related functional activities.* Austin, TX: PRO-ED.

Bakas, T., Champion, V., Perkins, S. M., Farran, C. J., & Williams, L. S. (2006a). Psychometric testing of the revised 15-item Bakas Caregiving Outcomes Scale. *Nursing Research, 55,* 346–355.

Bakas, T., Kroenke, K., Plue, L. D., Perkins, S. M., & Williams, L. S. (2006b). Outcomes among family caregivers of aphasic versus nonaphasic stroke survivors. *Rehabilitation Nursing, 31*(1), 33–42.

Baker, E. (2012). Optimal intervention intensity. *International Journal of Speech-Language Pathology, 14*(5), 401–409.

Baker, F. A. (2000). Modifying the Melodic Intonation Therapy program for adults with severe non-fluent aphasia. *Music Therapy Perspectives, 18,* 110–114.

Baker, M., & Johnson, C. (2010). *Results for adults: Cognition.* East Moline, IL: Linguisystems.

Bakheit, A., Shaw, S., Carrington, S., & Griffiths, S. (2007). The rate and extent of improvement with therapy from the different types of aphasia in the first year after stroke. *Clinical Rehabilitation, 21,* 941–949.

Balanced Budget Act of 1997. H.R. 2015. 105th Congress (1997). Available at http://www.govtrack.us/congress/bills/105/hr2015

Baldo, J. V., & Dronkers, N. F. (2006). The role of inferior parietal and inferior frontal cortex in working memory. *Neuropsychology, 20*(5), 529–538.

Ball, A. L., Riesthal, M., Breeding, V. E., & Mendozza, D. E. (2011). Modified ACT and CART in severe aphasia. *Aphasiology, 25*(6–7), 836–848.

Ballard, C. G. (2004). Definition and diagnosis of dementia with Lewy bodies. *Dementia and Geriatric Cognitive Disorders, 17,* 15–24.

Ballard, K. J., & Thompson, C. K. (1999). Treatment and generalization of complex sentence production in agrammatism. *Journal of Speech, Language, and Hearing Research, 42,* 690–707.

Banks, S., & Weintraub, S. (2008). Cognitive deficits and reduced insight in primary progressive aphasia. *American Journal of Alzheimer's Disease and Other Dementias, 23*(4), 363–371.

Barca, L., Cappelli, F., Amicuzi, I., Apicella, M., Castelli, E., & Stortini, M. (2009). Modality-specific naming impairment after traumatic brain injury (TBI). *Brain Injury, 23*(11), 920–929.

Bardo, J. V., Delis, D., & Kaplan, E. (2002). *Role of executive functions in language: Evidence from new verbal reasoning test.* Poster presentation at the annual International Neuropsychology Society conference, Toronto, Canada.

Barker, L., Morton, N., Morrison, T., & McGuire, B. (2011). Inter-rater reliability of the Dysexecutive Questionnaire (DEX): Comparative data from non-clinician respondents—All raters are not equal. *Brain Injury, 25*(10), 997–1004.

Barker-Collo, S. L. (2001). The 60-item Boston Naming Test: Cultural bias and possible adaptations for New Zealand. *Aphasiology, 15,* 85–92.

Barker-Collo, S. L. (2007). Boston Naming Test performance of older New Zealand adults. *Aphasiology, 21*(12), 1171–1180.

Barker-Collo, S. L., Feigin, V. L., Lawes, C. M., Parag, V., & Senior, H. (2010). Attention deficits after incident stroke in the acute period: Frequency across types of attention and relationships to patient characteristics and functional outcomes. *Topics in Stroke Rehabilitation, 17*(6), 463–476.

Barker-Collo, S. L., Feigin, V. L., Lawes, C. M., Parag, V., Senior, H., & Rodgers, A. (2009). Reducing attention deficits after stroke using Attention Process Training: A randomized controlled trial. *Stroke, 40,* 3293–3298.

Barkley, R. A. (2011). *Barkley deficits in executive functioning scale (BDEFS for Adults).* New York: Guildford.

Barnes, P. M., Bloom, B., & Nahin, R. (2008). *CDC National Health Statistics Report #12: Complementary and alternative medicine use among adults and children: United States, 2007.* Atlanta, GA: U.S. Department of Health and Human Service.

Barnes, P. M., Powell-Griner, E., McFann, K., & Nahin, R. L. (2004). *Complimentary and alternative medicine use among adults: United States, 2002. Advance data from vital and health statistics, No. 343.* Hyattsville, MD: National Center for Health Statistics.

Barnes, S., & Armstrong, E. (2010). Conversation after right hemisphere brain damage: Motivations for applying conversation analysis. *Clinical Linguistics & Phonetics, 24*(1), 55–69.

Barona, A., Reynolds, C., & Chastain, R. (1984). A demographically based index of premorbid intelligence for the WAIS-R. *Journal of Clinical and Consulting Psychology, 52,* 885–887.

Barrett, A. M., Crucian, G. P., Beversdorf, D. Q., & Heilman, K. M. (2001). Monocular patching may worsen sensory-attentional neglect: A case report. *Archives of Physical Medicine and Rehabilitation, 82,* 516–518.

Barrett, A. M., & Eslinger, P. J. (2007). Amantadine for adynamic speech: Possible benefit for aphasia? *American Journal of Physical Medicine and Rehabilitation, 86,* 605–612.

Barrie, M. A. (2002). Objective screening tools to assess cognitive impairment and depression. *Topics in Geriatric Rehabilitation, 18,* 28–46.

Barthel, G., Meinzer, M., Djundja, D., & Rockstroh, B. (2008). Intensive language therapy in chronic aphasia: Which aspects contribute most? *Aphasiology, 22*(4), 408–421.

Bartlett, G., Blais, R., Tamblyn, R., Clermont, R. J., & MacGibbon, B. (2008). Impact of patient communication problems on the risk of preventable adverse events in acute care settings. *Canadian Medical Association Journal, 178*(2), 1555–1562.

Bartlett, M. R., Fink, R., B, Schwartz, M. F., & Linebarger, M. (2007). Informativeness ratings of messages created on an AAC processing prosthesis. *Aphasiology, 21,* 475–498.

Barton, J. (2011). Disorders of higher visual processing. *Handbook of Clinical Neurology, 102,* 223–261.

Barwood, C., Murdoch, B., Whelan, B., Lloyd, D., Riek, S., O'Sullivan, J., . . . Wong, A. (2011). Improved language performance subsequent to low-frequency rTMS in patients with chronic non-fluent aphasia post-stroke. *European Journal of Neurology, 18,* 935–943.

Bassey, E. J. (2000). The benefits of exercise for the health of older people. Reviews in *Clinical Gerontology, 10,* 17–31.

Basso, A., Cattaneo, S., Girelli, L., Luzzatti, C., Miozzo, A., Modena, L., & Monti, A. (2011). Treatment efficacy of language and calculation disorders and speech apraxia: A review of the literature. *European Journal of Physical Rehabilitation and Medicine, 47,* 101–121.

Bastiaanse, R., & Edwards, S. (2001). Word order and finiteness in Dutch and English Broca's and Wernicke's aphasia. *Brain and Language, 79,* 72–74.

Bastiaanse, R., Edwards, S., & Rispens, J. (2002). *Verb and sentence test.* Bury St. Edmunds, Suffolk, England: Thames Valley Test Company.

Batchelor, S., Thompson, E. O., & Miller, L. A. (2008). Retrograde memory after unilateral stroke. *Cortex, 44*(2), 170–178.

Bate, A. J., Mathias, J. L., & Crawford, J. R. (2001). Performance on the Test of Everyday Attention and standard tests of attention following severe traumatic brain injury. The *Clinical Neuropsychologist, 15,* 405–422.

Bate, S., Kay, J., Code, C., Haslam, C., & Hallowell, B. (2010). Eighteen years on: What next for the PALPA? *International Journal of Speech-Language Pathology, 12*(3), 190–202.

Bates, E. (1976). *Language in context.* New York: Academic Press.

Bayles, K. A. (2003). Effects of working memory deficits on the communicative functioning of Alzheimer's dementia patients. *Journal of Communication Disorders, 36,* 209–219.

Bayles, K., Azuma, T., Cruz, R., Tomoeda, C., Wood, J., & Montgomery, E. (1999). Gender differences in language of Alzheimer's disease patients revisited. *Alzheimer's Disease and Associated Disorders, 13,* 138–146.

Bayles, K. A., & Kaszniak, A. W. (1987). *Communication and cognition in normal aging and dementia.* Boston: College-Hill.

Bayles, K. A., & Kim, E. S. (2003). Improving the functioning of individuals with Alzheimer's disease: Emergence of behavioral interventions. *Journal of Communication Disorders, 36,* 327–343.

Bayles, K., & Tomoeda, C. (1993). *Arizona battery for communication disorders of dementia.* Austin, TX: PRO-ED.

Bayles, K., & Tomoeda, C. (1994). *Functional linguistic communication inventory.* Austin, TX: PRO-ED.

Baylor, C. R. (2003). Structural CT and MRI: The basics. *Special Interest Division 2: Neurophysiology and Neurogenic Speech and Language Disorders Newsletter, 13,* 18–24.

Baylor, C., Burns, M., Eadie, T., Britton, D., & Yorkston, K. (2011). A qualitative study of interference with communicative participation across communication disorders in adults. *American Journal of Speech-Language Pathology, 20*(4), 269–287.

Beats, B. C., Sahakian, B. J., & Levy, R. (1996). Cognitive performance in tests sensitive to frontal lobe dysfunction in the elderly depressed. *Psychological Medicine, 26,* 591–604.

Beaumont, J. G., Marjoribanks, J., Flury, S., & Lintern, T. (1999). A screening test of auditory comprehension for individuals with severe physical disability. *British Journal of Clinical Psychology, 38,* 1–4.

Beaumont, J. G., Marjoribanks, J., Flury, S., & Lintern, T. (2002). *Putney auditory comprehension screening test.* Bury St. Edmunds, Suffolk, England: Thames Valley Test Company.

Beck, A. (1993). *Beck anxiety inventory.* San Antonio, TX: Pearson.

Beck, A. T., Steer, R. A., & Brown, G. K. (1996). *Manual for the Beck Depression Inventory* (2nd ed.). San Antonio, TX: Psychological Corporation.

Bédard, M., Felteau, M., Mazmanian, D., Fedyk, K., Klein, R., Richardson, J., . . . Minthorn-Biggs, M.B. (2003). Pilot evaluation of a mindfulness-based intervention to improve quality of life among individuals who sustained brain injuries. *Disability & Rehabilitation, 25,* 722–731.

Beeke, S., Maxim, J., & Wilkinson, R. (2007). Using conversation analysis to assess and treat people with aphasia. *Seminars in Speech and Language, 28*(2), 136–147.

Beeke, S., Maxim, J., & Wilkinson, R. (2008). Rethinking agrammatism: Factors affecting the form of language elicited via clinical test procedures. *Clinical Linguistics and Phonetics, 22*(4–5), 317–323.

Beeson, P. (1998). Treatment for letter-by-letter reading: A case study. In N. Helm-Estabrooks & A. L. Holland (Eds.), *Clinical decision making in aphasia treatment* (pp. 153–177). San Diego, CA: Singular Press.

Beeson, P. M. (1999). Treating acquired writing impairment: Strengthening graphemic representations. *Aphasiology, 9–11,* 767–786.

Beeson, P. M., & Egnor, H. (2006). Combining treatment for written and spoken naming. *Journal of the International Neuropsychological Society, 12,* 816–827.

Beeson, P. M., & Henry, M. L. (2008). Comprehension and production of written words. In R. Chapey (Ed.), *Language intervention strategies in aphasia and related neurogenic communication disorders* (5th ed., pp. 654–688). New York: Lippincott Williams & Wilkins.

Beeson, P., & Insalaco, D. (1998). Acquired alexia: Lessons from successful treatment. *Journal of the International Neuropsychological Society, 4,* 621–635.

Beeson, P. M., & Ramage, A. E. (2000). Drawing from experience: The development of alternative communication strategies. *Topics in Stroke Rehabilitation, 7*(2), 10–20.

Beeson, P., & Rapcsak, S. Z. (2002). Clinical diagnosis and treatment of spelling disorders. In A. E. Hillis (Ed.), *The handbook of adult language disorders: Integrating cognitive neuropsychology, neurology, and rehabilitation* (pp. 101–120). New York: Psychology Press.

Beeson, P. M., & Rapcsak, S. Z. (2010). Neuropsychological assessment and rehabilitation of writing disorders. In J. Gurd, U. Kischka, & J. Marshall (2010), *Handbook of clinical neuropsychology* (2nd ed., pp. 323–348). New York: Oxford University Press.

Beeson, P. M., Rapcsak, S. Z., Plante, E., Chargualaf, J. Chung, A, Johnson, S. C., & Trouard, T. P. (2003). The neural substrates of writing: A functional magnetic resonance imaging study. *Aphasiology, 17,* 647–665.

Beeson, P. M., Rising, K., Kim, E., & Rapcsak, S. (2010). A treatment sequence for phonological alexia/agraphia. *Journal of Speech, Language, and Hearing Research, 53,* 450–468.

Beeson, P., Rising, K., & Volk, J. (2003). Writing treatment for severe aphasia: Who benefits? *Journal of Speech, Language, and Hearing Research, 46,* 1038–1060.

Behrmann, M., & Lieberthal, T. (1989). Category-specific treatment of a lexical–semantic deficit: A single case study of global aphasia. *British Journal of Disorders of Communication, 24,* 281–299.

Beis, J. M., Andre, J. M., Baumgarten, A., & Challier, B. (1999). Eye patching in unilateral spatial neglect: Efficacy of two methods. *Archives of Physical Medicine and Rehabilitation, 80,* 71–76.

Belanger, H., Scott, S. G., Scholten, J., Curtiss, G., & Vanderploeg, R. D. (2005). Utility of mechanism-of-injury-based assessment and treatment: Blast Injury Program case illustration. *Journal of Rehabilitation Research and Development, 42*(4), 403–412.

Belanger, N., Baum, S., & Titone, D. (2009). Use of prosodic cues in the production of idiomatic and literal sentences by individuals with right- and left-hemisphere damage. *Brain and Language, 110*(1), 38–42.

Belleville, S., Gilbert, B., Fontaine, F., Gagnon, L., Ménard, E., & Gauthier, S. (2006). Improvement of episodic memory in persons with mild cognitive impairment and healthy older adults: Evidence from a cognitive intervention program. *Dementia and Geriatric Cognitive Disorders, 22*(5–6), 486–499.

Bender, H. A., Garcia, A., & Barr, W. (2010). An interdisciplinary approach to neuropsychological test construction: Perspectives from translation studies. *Journal of the International Neuropsychological Society, 16,* 227–232.

Benedict, R. H. B. (1997). *Brief visuospatial memory test–Revised.* Lutz, FL: Psychological Assessment Resources.

Benedict, R., H. B., Motl, R., Foley, F., Kaur, S., Hojnacki, D., & Weinstock-Guttman, B. (2011). Upper and lower extremity motor function and cognitive impairment in multiple sclerosis. *Journal of the International Neuropsychological Society, 17,* 643–653.

Benson, D. F., Cummings, J. L., & Tsai, S. Y. (1982). Angular gyrus syndrome simulating Alzheimer's disease. *Archives of Neurology, 38,* 616–620.

Benton, A. L., Hamsher, K., & Sivan, A. B. (2001). *Multilingual aphasia examination* (3rd ed.). Lutz, FL: Psychological Assessment Resources.

Benton, A. L., Hamsher, K., Varney, N. R., & Spreen, O. (1983). *Contributions to neuropsychological assessment.* New York: Oxford University Press.

Benton, A. L., & Tranel, D. (2000). Historical notes on reorganization of function and neuroplasticity. In H. S. Levin & J. Grafman (Eds.), *Cerebral reorganization of function after brain damage* (pp. 3–23). New York: Oxford University Press.

Benton, E., & Bryan, K. (1996). Right cerebral hemisphere damage: Incidence of language problems. *International Journal of Rehabilitation Research, 19,* 47–54.

Ben-Yishay, Y., & Daniels-Zide, E. (2000). Examined lives: Outcomes after holistic rehabilitation. *Rehabilitation Psychology, 45*, 112–129.

Berg, A., Lonnqvist, J., Palmoaki, H., & Kaste, M. (2009). Assessment of depression after stroke: A comparison of different screening instruments. *Stroke, 40*, 523–529.

Bergh, S., Sebaek, G., & Engedal, K. (2008). Reliability and validity of the Norwegian version of the Severe Impairment Battery (SIB). *International Journal of Geriatric Psychiatry, 23*, 896–902.

Bergner, M., Bobbitt, R. A., Carter, W. B., & Gibson, B. S. (1981). The Sickness Impact Profile: Development and final revision of a health status measure. *Medicare Care, 19*, 787–805.

Bernicot, J., & Dardier, V., (2001). Communication deficits: Assessment of subjects with frontal lobe damage in an interview setting. *International Journal of Language and Communication Disorders, 36*, 245–263.

Bernstein-Ellis, E., & Elman, R. J. (2007). Aphasia group communication treatment: The Aphasia Center of California approach. In R. J. Elman (Ed.), *Group treatment of neurogenic communication disorders: The expert clinician's approach* (2nd ed., pp. 71–94). San Diego, CA: Plural.

Berthier, M. L. (2005). Poststroke aphasia: Epidemiology, pathophysiology and treatment. *Drugs in Aging, 22*, 163–182.

Berthier, M. L., Green, C., Higueras, C., Fernandez, I., Hinojosa, J., & Martín, M. C. (2006). A randomized, placebo-controlled study of donepezil in poststroke aphasia. *Neurology, 67*, 1687–1689.

Berthier, M. L., Green, C., Lara, J. P., Higueras, C., Barbancho, M. A., Dávila, G., & Pulvermüller F. (2009). Memantine and constraint-induced aphasia therapy in chronic poststroke aphasia. *Annals of Neurology, 65*, 577–585.

Berthier, M. L., Hinojosa, J., Martín, M. C., & Fernandez, I. (2003). Open-label study of donepezil in chronic poststroke aphasia. *Neurology, 60*, 1218–1219.

Berthier, M., Pulvermuller, F., Davila, G., Casares, N., & Gutierrez, A. (2011). Drug therapy of post-stroke aphasia: A review of current evidence. *Neuropsychology Review, 21*, 302–317.

Bertisch, H., Rath, J. F., Langenbahn, D. M., Sherr, R. L., & Diller, L. (2011). Group treatment in acquired brain injury rehabilitation. *The Journal for Specialists in Group Work, 36*(4), 264–277.

Beschin, N., Cocchini, G., Allen, R., & Della Sala, S. (2012). Anosognosia and neglect respond differently to the same treatments. *Neuropsychological Rehabilitation*, 1–13. doi: 10.1080/09602011.2012.669353

Best, W., Greenwood, A., Grassly, J., & Hickin, J. (2008). Bridging the gap: Can impairment-based therapy for anomia have an impact at the psycho-social level? *International Journal of Language and Communication Disorders, 43*(4), 390–407.

Beukelman, D., Dietz, A. R., Hux, K., McKelvey, M., & Weissling, K. (2007). Performance of a person with chronic aphasia using personal and contextual pictures in a Visual Scene Display prototype. *Journal of Medical Speech-Language Pathology, 15*(3), 305 - 317.

Beukelman, D., & Mirenda, P. (2013). *Augmentative and alternative communication: Supporting children and adults with complex communication needs*. Baltimore: Brookes.

Beuthien-Baumann, B., Handrick, W., Schmidt, T., Burchert, W., Oehme, L., Kropp, J., ... Franke, W. G. (2003). Persistent vegetative state: Evaluation of brain metabolism and brain perfusion with PET and SPECT. *Nuclear Medicine Communications, 24*, 643–649.

Bhogal, S. K., Teasell, R., & Speechley, M. (2003). Intensity of aphasia therapy, impact on recovery. *Stroke, 34*, 987–993.

Bier, N., Macoir, J., Gagnon, L., Van der Linden, M., Louveaux, S., & Dsrosiers, J. (2009). Known, lost, and recovered: Efficacy of formal semantic therapy and spaced retrieval method in a case of semantic dementia. *Aphasiology, 23*(2), 210–235.

Bilda, K. (2011). Video-based conversational script training for aphasia: A therapy study. *Aphasiology, 25*(2), 191–201.

Binder, J. R., Frost, J. A., Hammeke, T. A., Cox, R. W., Rao, S. M., & Prieto, T. (1997). Human brain language areas identified by functional magnetic resonance imaging. *Journal of Neuroscience, 17*, 353–362.

Binetti, G., Locascio, J., Corkin, S., Vonsattel, J., & Growdon, H. (2000). Differences between Pick disease and Alzheimer disease in clinical appearance and rate of cognitive decline. *Archives of Neurology, 57*, 225–232.

Bird, T., Knopman, D., VanSwieten, J., Rosso, S., Feldman, H., Tanabe, H., ... Hutton, M. (2003). Epidemiology and genetics of frontotemporal dementia/Pick's disease. *Annals of Neurology, 54*, S29–S31.

Bishop, D. (2003). *Test for reception of grammar* (2nd ed.). San Antonio, TX: Pearson.

Bittner, R., & Crowe, S. F. (2006). The relationship between working memory, processing speed and verbal comprehension and FAS performance following traumatic brain injury. *Brain Injury, 20*, 971–980.

Black, S. E., Behrmann, M., Bass, K., & Hacker, P. (1989). Selective writing impairment: Beyond the allographic code. *Aphasiology, 3*, 265–277.

Blomert, L., Kean, M-L., Koster, C., Schokker, J. (1994). Amsterdam-Nijmegen Everyday Language Test: Construction, reliability, and validity. *Aphasiology, 8*, 381–407.

Blomert, L., Koster, C., van Mier, J., & Kean, M-L. (1987). Verbal communication abilities of aphasic speakers: The everyday language test. *Aphasiology, 1*, 463–474.

Blonder, L. X., Bowers, D., & Heilman, K. M. (1991). The role of the right hemisphere in emotional communication. *Brain, 114*, 1115–1127.

Blumstein, S. E. (1998). Phonological aspects of aphasia. In M. T. Sarno (Ed.), *Acquired aphasia* (3rd ed., pp. 157–185). New York: Academic Press.

Blumstein, S. E., Katz, B., Goodglass, H., Shrier, R., & Dworetsky, B. (1985). The effects of slowed speech on auditory comprehension in aphasia. *Brain and Language, 24*, 246–265.

Bogod, N. M., Mateer, C. A., & MacDonald, S. W. S. (2003). Self-awareness after traumatic brain injury: A comparison of measures and their relationship to executive functions. *Journal of the International Neuropsychological Society, 9*, 450–458.

Boland, D., & Stacy, M. (2012). The economic and quality of life burden associated with Parkinson's disease: A focus on symptoms. *American Journal of Managed Care, 18*, S168–S175.

Boman, I., Lindstedt, M., Hemmingsson, H., & Bartfai, A. (2004). Cognitive training in the home environment. *Brain Injury, 18*(10), 985–995.

Bombardier, C. H., & Thurber, C. A. (1998). Blood alcohol level and early cognitive status after traumatic brain injury. *Brain Injury, 12*, 32–48.

Bonakdarpour, B., Eftekharzadeh, A., & Ashayeri, H. (2003). Melodic intonation therapy in Persian aphasia patients. *Aphasiology, 17*, 75–95.

Bonner, A. P., & Cousins, S. O. (1996). Exercise and Alzheimer's disease: Benefits and barriers. *Activities and Adaptation in Aging, 20*, 21–32.

Boo, M., & Rose, M. (2011). The efficacy of repetition, semantic, and gesture treatments for verb retrieval and use in Broca's aphasia. *Aphasiology, 25*, 154–175.

Bourgeois, M. (1992). Evaluating memory wallets in conversations with persons with dementia. *Journal of Speech and Hearing Research, 35*, 1344–1357.

Bourgeois, M. (2007). *Memory books and other graphic cuing systems: Practical communication and memory aids for adults with dementia.* Towson, MD: Health Professions Press.

Bourgeois, M., Camp, C., Rose, M., White, B., Malone, M., Carr, J., & Rovine, M. (2003). A comparison of training strategies to enhance use of external aids by persons with dementia. *Journal of Communication Disorders, 36*, 361–378.

Bourgeois, M., Dijkstra, K., Burgio, L., & Allen-Burge, R. (2001). Memory aids as an augmentative and alternative communication strategy for nursing home residents with dementia. *AAC: Augmentative and Alternative Communication, 17*, 196–210.

Bourgeois, M., & Hickey, E. (2009). *Dementia: From diagnosis to management: A functional approach.* Clifton, NJ: Psychology Press.

Bourgeois, M., & Melton, A. (2004). *Training compensatory memory strategies via the telephone for persons with TBI.* Presentation at the Clinical Aphasiology Conference, Park City, UT.

Bowers, L., Huisingh, R., Johnson, P., LoGiudice, C., & Orman, J. (2003). *Workbook of activities for language and cognition 3: Everyday problem solving.* East Moline, IL: Linguisystems.

Bowers, L., Huisingh, R., & LoGiudice, C. (2007). *Test of problem solving 2: Adolescent.* East Moline, IL: Linguisystems.

Bowers, L., Huisingh, R., & LoGiudice, C. (2009). *Listening comprehension test: Adolescent.* East Moline, IL: Linguisystems.

Bowers, L., Huisingh, R., & LoGiudice, C. (2010). *Social language development test: Adolescent.* East Moline, IL: Linguisystems.

Bowers, L., Huisingh, R., LoGiudice, C., & Orman, J. (2005). *The WORD Test 2: Adolescent.* East Moline, IL: LinguiSystems.

Boxer, A., Lipton, A. M., Womack, K., Merrilees, J., Neuhaus, J., Pavlic, D., . . . Miller, B. L. (2009). An open-label study of Memantine treatment in 3 subtypes of frontotemporal lobar degeneration. *Alzheimer Disease and Associated Disorders, 23*, 211–217.

Boyd, T. M., & Sautter, S. W. (1994). Route-finding: A measure of everyday executive functioning in the head-injured adult. *Applied Cognitive Psychology, 72,* 171–181.

Boyle, M. (2001). Semantic feature analysis: The evidence for treating lexical impairments in aphasia. *Neurophysiology and Neurogenic Speech and Language Disorders, 11,* 23–28.

Boyle, M. (2004). Semantic feature analysis treatment for anomia in two fluent aphasia syndromes. *American Journal of Speech-Language Pathology, 13,* 236–249.

Boyle, M. (2010). Semantic feature analysis treatment for aphasic word retrieval impairments: What's in a name? *Topics in Stroke Rehabilitation, 17*(6), 411–422.

Bracken, B., & Howell, K. (2004). *Clinical assessment of depression.* Odessa, FL: PAR.

Bracy, C. B., & Drummond, S. S. (1993). Word retrieval in fluent and nonfluent dysphasia: Utilization of pictogram. *Journal of Communication Disorders, 26,* 113–128.

Bradburn, N. M. (1969). *The structure of psychological well-being.* Chicago: Aldine.

Braden, C., Hawley, L., Newman, J., Morey, C., Gerber, D., & Harrison-Felix, C. (2010). Social communication skills group treatment: A feasibility study for persons with traumatic brain injury and comorbid conditions. *Brain Injury, 24*(11), 1298–1310.

Brady, M. C., Kelly, H., Godwin, J., & Enderby, P. (2012). Speech and language therapy for aphasia following stroke. *Cochrane Database of Systematic Reviews, Issue 5.* Art. No.: CD000425. doi: 10.1002/14651858.CD000425.pub3

Brady, S., Miserendino, R., & Rao, N. (2004). West Nile virus: A growing challenge for the speech-language pathologist. *ASHA Leader, 9,* 10–13.

Bragoni, M., Altieri, M., DiPiero, V., Padovani, A., Mostardini, C., & Lenzi, G. L. (2000). Bromocriptine and speech therapy in nonfluent chronic aphasia after stroke. *Neurological Sciences, 21,* 19–22.

BrainTrain. *Captain's log* [Computer software]. (2002–2010). Richmond, VA: Author.

Brandt, J., & Benedict, R. H. B. (2001). *Hopkins verbal learning test–Revised.* Lutz, FL: Psychological Assessment Resources.

Brandt, J., & Folstein, M. F. (2003). *Telephone interview for cognitive status: Professional manual.* Odessa, FL: Psychological Assessment Resources.

Braunling-McMorrow, D., Lloyd, K., & Fralish, K. (1986). Teaching social skills to head injured adults. *Journal of Rehabilitation, 52,* 39–44.

Brazzelli, M., Saunders, D. H., Greig, C. A., & Mead, G. E. (2011). Physical fitness training for stroke patients. *Cochrane Database of Systematic Reviews* [Online], (11), CD003316. doi: 10.1002/14651858.CD003316.pub4

Breese, E., & Hillis, A. (2004). Auditory comprehension: Is multiple choice really good enough? *Brain and Language, 89,* 3–8.

Brennan, A., Worrall, L., & McKenna, K. (2005). The relationship between specific features of aphasia-friendly written material and comprehension of written material for people with aphasia: An exploratory study. *Aphasiology, 19*(8), 693–711.

Brereton, L., Carroll, C., & Barnston, S. (2007). Interventions for adult family caregivers of people who have had a stroke: A systematic review. *Clinical Rehabilitation, 21*(10), 867–884.

Brickenkamp, R., & Zillmer, E. (1998). *d2 test of attention.* Lutz, FL: Psychological Assessment Resources.

Brod, M., Stewart, A. L., Sands, L., & Walton, P. (1999). Conceptualization and measurement of quality of life in dementia: The dementia quality of life instrument (DQoL). *Gerontologist, 39*(1), 25–35.

Brooks, J., Fos, L. A., Greve, K. W., & Hammond, J. S. (1999). Assessment of executive function in patients with mild traumatic brain injury. *The Journal of Trauma: Injury, Infection, and Critical Care, 46,* 159–163.

Brookshire, R. H. (1997). *Introduction to neurogenic communication disorders.* New York: Mosby.

Brookshire, R. H. (2007). *Introduction to neurogenic communication disorders* (7th ed.). St. Louis, MO: Mosby.

Brookshire, R. H., & Nicholas, L. E. (1994). Speech sample size and test–retest stability of connected speech measures for adults with aphasia. *Journal of Speech and Hearing Research, 37,* 399–407.

Brookshire, R. H., & Nicholas, L. E. (1995). Performance deviations in the connected speech of adults with no brain damage and adults with aphasia. *American Journal of Speech-Language Pathology, 4,* 118–123.

Brookshire, R. H., & Nicholas, L. E. (1997). *The discourse comprehension test* (Rev. ed.). Minneapolis, MN: BRK Publishers.

Brown, J. E., & Pietranton, A. A. (2007). Current trendings and issues in health care delivery: What speech-language pathologists need to know. In A. F. Johnson & B. H. Jacobson (Eds.), *Medical speech-language pathology: A practitioner's guide* (pp. 213–222). New York: Thieme.

Brown, J. W., Leader, B. J., & Blum, C. S. (1983). Hemiplegic writing in severe aphasia. *Brain and Language, 19*, 204–215.

Brown, K., McGahan, L., Alkhaledi, M., Seah, D., Howe, T., & Worrall, L. (2006). Environmental factors that influence the community participation of adults with aphasia: The perspective of service industry workers. *Aphasiology, 20*(7), 595–615.

Brown, L., Sherbenou, R. J., & Johnsen, S. K. (2010). *Test of nonverbal intelligence* (4th ed.). Austin, TX: PRO-ED.

Brown, V. L., Wiederholt, J. L., & Hammill, D. D. (2009). *Test of reading comprehension* (4th ed.). Austin, TX: PRO-ED.

Brownell, H., Griffin, R., Winner, E., Friedman, O., & Happe, F. (2000). Cerebral lateralization and theory of mind. In S. Baron-Cohen, H. Tager-Flusberg, & D. Cohen (Eds.), *Understanding other minds: Perspectives from developmental cognitive neuroscience* (2nd ed., pp. 306–333). Oxford, UK: Oxford University Press.

Bruck, C., Wildgruber, D., Kreifelts, B., Kruger, R., & Wachter, T. (2011). Effects of subthalamic nucleus stimulation on emotional prosody comprehension in Parkinson's disease. *PLoS One, 6*(4), e19140.

Brumfitt, S., & Sheeran, P. (1999). The development and validation of the Visual Analogue Self-Esteem Scale (VASES). *British Journal of Clinical Psychology, 38*, 387–400.

Bruns, J., & Hauser, A. (2003). The epidemiology of traumatic brain injury: A review. *Epilepsia, 44*(Suppl. 10), 2–10.

Brush, J., Sanford, J., Fleder, H., Bruce, C., & Calkins, M. (2011). Evaluating and modifying the communication environment for people with dementia. *Perspectives on Gerontology, 16*(2), 32–40.

Bryan, K. L. (1995). *The right hemisphere language battery* (2nd ed.). London: Whurr.

Bryant, B. R., Wiederholt, J. L., & Bryant, D. P. (2004). *Gray diagnostic reading tests* (2nd ed.). Austin, TX: PRO-ED.

Buccione, I., Fadda, L., Serra, L., Caltagirone, C., & Carlesimo, G. (2008). Retrograde episodic and semantic memory impairment correlates with side of temporal lobe damage. *Journal of the International Neuropsychological Society, 14*(6), 1083–1094.

Buchman, A. S., Boyle, P. A., Yu, L., Shah, R. C., Wilson, R. S., & Bennett, D. A. (2012). Total daily physical activity and the risk of AD and cognitive decline in older adults. *Neurology, 78*(17), 1323–1329.

Bucks, R. S., Willison, J. R., & Byrne, L. M. T. (2000). *Location learning test*. Bury St. Edmunds, Suffolk, England: Thames Valley Test Company.

Buklina, S. B. (2003). Impairments in premorbid knowledge recall in patients with hemispheric and intraventricular brain damage. *Neuroscience and Behavioral Physiology, 33*, 933–938.

Bungalow Software. *Aphasia tutor* [Computer software]. (2004). Blacksburg, VA: Author.

Burgess, P., Alderman, N., Evans, J., Emslie, H., & Wilson, B. (1998). The ecological validity of tests of executive function. *Journal of the International Neuropsychological Society, 4*, 547–558.

Burgess, P. W., Alderman, N., Forbes, C., Costello, A., Coates, L., Dawson, D. R., . . . Channon S. (2006). The case for the development and use of "ecologically valid" measures of executive function in experimental and clinical neuropsychology. *Journal of International Neuropsychological Society, 12*(2), 194–209.

Burgio, F., & Basso, A. (1997). Memory and aphasia. *Neuropsychologia, 35*(6), 759–766.

Burns, M. I., Baylor, C. R., Morris, M. A., McNalley, T. E., & Yorkston, K. M. (2012). Training healthcare providers in patient–provider communication: What speech-language pathology and medical education can learn from one another. *Aphasiology, 26*(5), 673–688.

Burns, M. S. (1997). *Burns brief inventory of communication and cognition*. San Antonio, TX: Psychological Corporation.

Busch, C. (1999). Group treatment reimbursement issues. In R. J. Elman (Ed.), *Group treatment of neurogenic communication disorders: The expert clinician's approach* (pp. 31–35). Boston: Butterworth-Heinemann.

Busch, C. R., Brookshire, R. H., & Nicholas, L. E. (1988). Referential communication abilities of aphasic speakers. *Journal of Speech and Hearing Disorders, 53*, 475–482.

Busch, V., Magerl, W., Kern, U., Haas, J., Hajak, G., & Eichhammer, P. (2012). The effect of deep and slow breathing on pain perception, autonomic activity, and mood processing—An experimental study. *Pain Medicine, 13*(2), 215–228.

Buschke, H. (1973). Selective reminding for analysis of memory and learning. *Journal of Verbal Learning and Verbal Behavior, 12*, 543–550.

Bush, B. A., Novack, T. A., Malec, J. F., Stringer, A. Y., Millis, S. R., & Madan, A. (2003). Validation of a model for evaluating outcome after traumatic brain injury. *Archives of Physical Medicine and Rehabilitation, 84*, 1803–1807.

Busi, K., & Greer, D. (2010). Hypoxic-ischemic brain injury: Pathophysiology, neuropathology and mechanism. *NeuroRehabilitation, 26*(1), 5–13.

Butcher, J. N., Dahlstrom, W. G., & Graham, J. R. (1989). *Minnesota multiphasic personality inventory–2 (MMPI-2): Manual for administration and scoring.* Minneapolis: University of Minnesota Press.

Butler, J. A. (2002). How comparable are tests of apraxia? *Clinical Rehabilitation, 16*, 389–398.

Butler, O. T., Anderson, L., Furst, C. J., & Namerow, N. S. (1989). Behavioral assessment in neuropsychological rehabilitation: A method for measuring vocational related skills. *Clinical Neuropsychologist, 3*, 235–243.

Butler, R. W., & Copeland, D. R. (2002). Attentional processes and their remediation in children treated for cancer: A literature review and the development of a therapeutic approach. *Journal of the International Neuropsychology Society, 8*, 115–124.

Butt, P. A., & Bucks, R. S. (2004). *Butt non-verbal reasoning test.* Bicester, Oxon, UK: Speechmark.

Butters, N., Delis, D. C., & Lucas, J. A. (1995). Clinical assessment of memory disorders in amnesia and dementia. *Annual Reviews in Psychology, 46*, 493–523.

Butters, N., Lopez, O. L., & Becker, J. T. (1996). Focal temporal lobe dysfunction in probably Alzheimer's disease predicts a slow rate of cognitive decline. *Neurology, 46*, 687–692.

Byatt, N., Rothschild, A. Riskind, P., Ionete, C., & Hunt, A. (2011). Relationships between multiple sclerosis and depression. *Journal of Neuropsychiatry and Clinical Neurosciences, 23*, 198–200.

Byiers, B., Reichle, J., & Symons, F. (2012). Single-subject experimental design for evidence-based practice. *American Journal of Speech-Language Pathology, 21*, 397–414.

Byng, S. (1988). Sentence processing deficits: Theory and therapy. *Cognitive Neuropsychology, 5*, 629–676.

Byng, S., & Duchan, J. F. (2005). Social model philosophies and principles: Their applications to therapies for aphasia. *Aphasiology, 19*(10–11), 906–922.

Cahill, S., Clark, M., O'Connell, H., Lawlor, B., Coen, R., & Walsh, C. (2008). The attitudes and practices of general practitioners regarding dementia diagnosis in Ireland. *International Journal of Geriatric Psychiatry, 23*, 663–669.

Calkins, M. (2009). Evidence-based long-term care design. *NeuroRehabilitation, 25*(3), 145–154.

Calkins, M. P., & Brush, J. A. (2003). Designing for dining. *Alzheimer's Care Quarterly, 4*, 73–76.

Cameron, R., Wambaugh, J., & Mausycki, S. (2010). Individual variability in discourse measures over repeated sampling time in persons with aphasia. *Aphasiology, 24*(6–8), 671–684.

Cameron, R., Wambaugh, J., Wright, S., & Nessler, C. (2006). Effects of a combined semantic/phonologic cueing treatment on word retrieval in discourse. *Aphasiology, 20*(2–4), 269–285.

Campbell, C. R., & Jackson, S. T. (1995). Transparency of one-handed AmerInd hand signals to nonfamiliar viewers. *Journal of Speech and Hearing Research, 38*, 1284–1289.

Campbell, L., Wilson, C., McCann, J., Kernahan, G., & Rogers, R. G. (2007). Single case experimental design study of Carer facilitated Errorless Learning in a patient with severe memory impairment following TBI. *NeurRehabilitation, 22*, 325–333.

Caplan, B. (1987). Assessment of unilateral neglect: A new reading test. *Journal of Clinical and Experimental Neuropsychology, 9*, 359–364.

Caplan, D. (1981). On the cerebral localization of linguistic functions: Logical and empirical issues surrounding deficit analysis and functional localization. *Brain and Language, 14*, 120–137.

Caplan, D. (1993). Toward a psycholinguistic approach to acquired neurogenic language disorders. *American Journal of Speech-Language Pathology, 2*, 59–83.

Caplan, D., & Bub, D. (1990). *Psycholinguistic assessment of aphasia.* Miniseminar presented at the annual convention of the American Speech-Language-Hearing Association, Seattle, WA.

Caplan, D., & Utman, J. A. (1992). Selective acoustic phonetic impairment and lexical access in an aphasic patient. *Journal of the Acoustic Society of America, 95,* 512–517.

Caplan, D., Waters, G. S., & Hildebrandt, N. (1997). Determinants of sentence comprehension in aphasic patients in sentence-picture matching tasks. *Journal of Speech, Language, and Hearing Research, 40,* 542–555.

Caramazza, A., & Berndt, R. S. (1985). A multicomponent deficit view of agrammatic Broca's aphasia. In M. L. Kean (Ed.), *Agrammatism* (pp. 27–63). Orlando, FL: Academic Press.

Caramazza, A., & Miceli, G. (1991). Selective impairment of thematic role assignment in sentence processing. *Brain and Language, 41,* 402–436.

Caramazza, A., Papagno, C., & Ruml, W. (2000). The selective impairment of phonological processing in speech production. *Brain and Language, 75,* 428–450.

Carlomagno, S., Giannotti, S., Vorano, L., & Marini, A. (2011). Discourse information content in nonaphasic adults with brain injury: A pilot study. *Brain Injury, 25*(10), 1010–1018.

Carlomagno, S., Iavarone, A., & Colombo, A. (1994). Cognitive approaches to writing rehabilitation: From single case to group studies. In M. Riddoch & G. W. Humphreys (Eds.), *Cognitive neuropsychology and cognitive rehabilitation* (pp. 485–502). Hillsdale, NJ: Erlbaum.

Carlomagno, S., Pandolfi, M., Martini, A., Di Iasi, G., & Cristilli, C. (2005). Coverbal gestures in Alzheimer's type dementia. *Cortex, 41,* 535–546.

Carmines, E. G., & Zeller, R. A. (1979). *Reliability and validity assessment.* Newbury Park, CA: Sage.

Carrow-Woolfolk, E. (2012). *Oral and written language scales* (2nd ed.). Torrance, CA: Western Psychological Services.

Cary, L. M. (1995). Somatosensory loss after stroke. *Critical Review of Physical and Rehabilitative Medicine, 7,* 51–91.

Cassidy, T. P., Lewis, S., & Gray, C. S. (1998). Recovery from visuospatial neglect in stroke patients. *Journal of Neurology, Neurosurgery, & Psychiatry, 64,* 555–557.

Catroppa, C., & Anderson, V. (2006). Planning, problem-solving and organizational abilities in children following traumatic brain injury: Intervention techniques. *Pediatric Rehabilitation, 9*(2), 89–97.

Cattelani, R., Zettin, M., & Zoccolotti, P. (2010). Rehabilitation treatments for adults with behavioral and psychosocial disorders following acquired brain injury: A systematic review. *Neuropsychological Review, 20,* 52–85.

Centeno, J. (2009). Issues and principles in service delivery to communicatively impaired minority bilingual adults in neurorehabilitation. *Seminars in Speech and Language, 30,* 139–152.

Centers for Disease Control and Prevention. (2012). *Traumatic brain injury.* Accessed November 27, 2012, from: http://www.cdc.gov/TraumaticBrainINjury/index.html

Centers for Medicare & Medicaid Services. (2012). *Prospective payment systems: General information.* Accessed June 17, 2012, from http://www.cms.gov/Medicare/Medicare-Fee-for-Service-Payment/ProspMedicareFeeSvcPmtGen/index.html

Chabok, S. Y., Kapourchali, S. R., Leili, E. K., Saberi, A., & Mohtasham-Amiri, Z. (2012). Effective factors on linguistic disorder during acute phase following traumatic brain injury in adults. *Neuropsychologia, 50*(7), 1444–1450.

Champagne-Lavau, M., & Joanette, Y. (2009). Pragmatics, theory of mind and executive functions after a right-hemisphere lesion: Different patterns of deficits. *Journal of Neurolinguistics, 22,* 413–426.

Chan, A. S., Salmon, D. P., Butters, N., & Johnson, S. A. (1995). Semantic network abnormality predicts rate of cognitive decline in patients with probably Alzheimer's disease. *Journal of the International Neuropsychological Society, 1,* 297–303.

Chan, R., & Manly, T. (2002). The application of "dysexecutive syndrome" measures across cultures: Performance and checklist assessment in neurologically healthy and traumatically brain-injured Hong Kong Chinese volunteers. *Journal of the International Neuropsychological Society, 8,* 771–780.

Chan, R., Shum, D., Toulopoulou, T., & Chen, E. (2008). Assessment of executive functions: Review of instruments and identification of critical issues. *Archives of Clinical Neuropsychology, 23,* 201–216.

Chang, W. H., Park, Y. H., Ohn, S. H., Park, C., Lee, P. K., & Kim, Y. (2011). Neural correlates of donepezil-induced cognitive improvement in patients with right hemisphere stroke: A pilot study. *Neuropsychological Rehabilitation, 21*(4), 502–514.

Chapey, R., Duchan, J., Elman, R., Garcia, L., Kagan, A., Lyan, J., & Simmons-Mackie, N. (2008). Life participation approach to aphasia: A statement of values for the future. In R. Chapey (Ed.), *Language intervention strategies in aphasia and related neurogenic communication disorders* (5th ed., pp. 279–289). Philadelphia: Lippincott, Williams, & Wilkens.

Chapman, S. B., Culhane, K. A., Levin, H. S., Harward, H., Mendelsohn, D., Ewing-Cobbs, L., . . . Bruce, D. (1992). Narrative discourse after closed head injury in children and adolescents. *Brain and Language, 43*, 42–65.

Chapman, S. B., Wanek, A., & Sharpe, S. (1994). *Narrative discourse in pediatric head injury: What a story!* Paper presented at the annual Colorado Speech and Hearing Association convention, Denver, CO.

Chapman, S. B., Weiner, M., Rackley, A., Hynan, L., & Zientz, J. (2004). Effects of cognitive-communication stimulation for Alzheimer's disease patients treated with donepezil. *Journal of Speech, Language, and Hearing Research, 47*, 1149–1163.

Chau, A. C., Fai Cheung, R. T., Jiang, X., Au-Yeung, P. K., & Li, L. S. (2010). An fMRI study showing the effect of acupuncture in chronic stage stroke patients with aphasia. *Journal of Acupuncture Meridian Studies, 3*(1), 53–57.

Chavin, M. (2002). Music as communication. *Alzheimer's Care Quarterly, 3*, 145–156.

Chaytor, N., & Schmitter-Edgecombe, M. (2003). The ecological validity of neuropsychological tests: A review of the literature on everyday cognitive skills. *Neuropsychological Review, 13*, 181–197.

Cheang, H., & Pell, M. (2006). A study of humour and communicative intention following right hemisphere stroke. *Clinical Linguistics and Phonetics, 20*(6), 447–462.

Chen, S. H., Thomas, J. D., Glueckauf, R. L., & Bracy, O. L. (1997). The effectiveness of computer-assisted cognitive rehabilitation for persons with traumatic brain injury. *Brain Injury, 11*, 197–209.

Chen, S. T., Sultzer, D. L., Hinkin, C. H., Mahler, M. E., & Cummings, J. L. (1998). Executive dysfunction in Alzheimer's disease: Association with neuropsychiatric symptoms and functional impairment. *The Journal of Neuropsychiatry and Clinical Neurosciences, 10*, 426–432.

Chen, Y., & Huang, W. (2011). Non-impact, blast-induced mild TBI and PTSD: Concepts and caveats. *Brain Injury, 25*(7–8), 641–650.

Chen, Y., Li, Y. S., Wang, Z. Y., Xu, Q., & Shi, G. W. (2010). The efficacy of donepezil for post-stroke aphasia: A pilot case control study. *Zhonghua Nei Ke Za Zhi, 49*, 115–118.

Chenery, H. J., Copland, D. A., & Murdoch, B. E. (2002). Complex language functions and subcortical mechanisms: Evidence from Huntington's disease and patients with non-thalamic subcortical lesions. *International Journal of Language and Communication Disorders, 37*, 459–474.

Cherney, L. R. (1998). Pragmatics and discourse: An introduction. In L. R. Cherney, B. Shadden, & C. A. Coelho (Eds.), *Analyzing discourse in communicatively impaired adults* (pp. 1–7). Gathersburg, MD: Aspen.

Cherney, L. R. (2002). Unilateral neglect: A disorder of attention. *Seminars in Speech and Language, 23*, 117–128.

Cherney, L. (2004). Aphasia, alexia and oral reading. *Topics in Stroke Rehabilitation, 11*, 22–36.

Cherney, L. (2010a). Oral reading for language in aphasia: Evaluating the efficacy of computer-delivered therapy in chronic nonfluent aphasia. *Topics in Stroke Rehabilitation, 17*(6), 423–431.

Cherney, L. (2010b). Oral reading for language in aphasia: Impact of aphasia severity on cross-modal outcomes in chronic nonfluent aphasia. *Seminars in Speech and Language, 31*, 42–51.

Cherney, L. (2012). Aphasia treatment: Intensity, dose parameters, and script training. *International Journal of Speech-Language Pathology, 14*(5), 424–431.

Cherney, L. R., & Halper, A. S. (2000). Assessment and treatment of functional communication following right hemisphere damage. In L. E. Worrall & C. M. Frattali (Eds.), *Neurogenic communication disorders: A functional approach* (pp. 276–292). New York: Thieme.

Cherney, L. R., & Halper, A. S. (2001). Unilateral visual neglect in right hemisphere stroke: A longitudinal study. *Brain Injury, 15*, 585–592.

Cherney, L., & Halper, A. (2008). Novel technology for treating individuals with aphasia and concomitant cognitive deficits. *Topics in Stroke Rehabilitation, 15*(6), 542–554.

Cherney, L., Halper, A., Holland, A., & Cole, R. (2008). Computerized script training in aphasia: Preliminary results. *American Journal of Speech and Language Pathology, 17*, 19–34.

Cherney, L. R., Patterson, J. P., Raymer, A., Frymark, T., & Schooling, T. (2008). Evidence-based systematic review: Effects of intensity of treatment and constraint-induced language therapy for individuals with stroke-induced aphasia. *Journal of Speech, Language, and Hearing Research, 51*, 1282–1299.

Cherney, L. R., Shadden, B., & Coelho, C. A. (Eds.). (1998). *Analyzing discourse in communicatively impaired adults*. Gathersburg, MD: Aspen.

Cheung, R. W., Cheung, M. C., & Chan, A. S. (2004). Confrontation naming in Chinese patients with left, right or bilateral brain damage. *Journal of the International Neuropsychological Society, 10*, 46–53.

Chevignard, M., Taillefer, C., Picq, C., Poncet, F., Noulhiane, M., & Pradat-Diehl, P. (2008). Ecological assessment of the dysexecutive syndrome using execution of a cooking task. *Neuropsychological Rehabilitation, 18*(4), 461–485.

Chew, E., & Zafonte, R. D. (2009). Pharmacological management of neurobehavioral disorders following traumatic brain injury: A state-of-the-art review. *Journal of Rehabilitation Research and Development, 46*(6), 851–878.

Chiou, K., Carlson, R., Arnett, P., Cosentino, S., & Hillary, F. G. (2011). Metacognitive monitoring in moderate and severe traumatic brain injury. *Journal of the International Neuropsychological Society, 17*, 720–731.

Chitic, V., Rusu, A., & Szamoskozi, S. (2012). The effects of animal assisted therapy on communication and social skills: A meta-analysis. *Transylvanian Journal of Psychology, 13*(1), 1–17.

Chittum, W. R., Johnson, K., Chittum, J. M., Guercio, J. M., & McMorrow, M. J. (1996). Road to awareness: An individualized training package for increasing knowledge and comprehension of personal deficits in persons with acquired brain injury. *Brain Injury, 10*, 763–776.

Chiu, Y. C., Algase, D., Whall, A., Liang, J., Liu, H. C., Lin, K. N., & Wang, P. N. (2004). Getting lost: Directed attention and executive functions in early Alzheimer's disease patients. *Dementia and Geriatric Cognitive Disorders, 17*, 174–180.

Christensen, B. K., Colella, B., Inness, E., Hebert, D., Monette, G., Bayley, M., & Green, R. E. (2008). Recovery of cognitive function after traumatic brain injury: A multilevel modeling analysis of Canadian outcomes. *Archives of Physical Medicine and Rehabilitation, 89*(Suppl. 12), S3–S15.

Christensen, H., Hofer, S. M., MacKinnon, A. J., Korten, A. E., Jorm, A. F., & Henderson, A. S. (2001). Age is no kinder to the better educated: Absence of an association investigated using latent growth techniques in a community sample. *Psychological Medicine, 31*, 15–28.

Christensen, S. C., & Wright, H. H. (2010). Verbal and non-verbal working memory in aphasia: What three n-back tasks reveal. *Aphasiology, 24*(6–8), 752–762.

Christensen, T. A., Lockwood, J. L., Almryde, K. R., & Plante, E. (2011). Neural substrates of attentive listening assessed with a novel auditory Stroop task. *Frontiers in Human Neuroscience, 4*, article 236. doi: 10.3389/fnhum.2010.00236

Christopoulou, C., & Bonvilian, J. (1985). Sign language, pantomime, and gestural processing in aphasic persons: A review. *Journal of Communication Disorders, 18*, 1–20.

Chrysikou, E., & Hamilton, R. (2011). Noninvasive brain stimulation in the treatment of aphasia: Exploring interhemispheric relationships and their implications for neurorehabilitation. *Restorative Neurology and Neuroscience, 29*, 375–394.

Chu, C., & Selwyn, P. (2011). Complications of HIV infection: A systems-based approach. *American Family Physician, 83*(4), 395–406.

Chung, J. C., & Lai, C. K. (2009). Snoezelan for dementia. *The Cochrane Library 2009, 1*, 1–41. doi: 10.1002/14651858.CD003152

Ciancarelli, I., Cofini, V., & Carolei, A. (2010). Evaluation of neuropsychological functions in patients with Friedreich ataxia before and after cognitive therapy. *Functional Neurology, 25*(2), 81–85.

Cicerone, K. D. (2002). Remediation of "working attention" in mild traumatic brain injury. *Brain Injury, 16*, 185–195.

Cicerone, K. D., & Giacino, J. T. (1992). Remediation of executive function deficits after traumatic brain injury. *Neuropsychological Rehabilitation, 2*, 12–22.

Cicerone, K. D., Langenbahn, D. M., Braden, C., Malec, J. F., Kalmar, K., Fraas, M., . . . Ashman, T. (2011). Evidence-based cognitive rehabilitation: Updated review of the literature from 2003 through 2008. *Archives of Physical Medicine and Rehabilitation, 92*, 519–530.

Cicerone, K. D., Mott, T., Azulay, J., & Friel, J. C. (2004). Community integration and satisfaction with functioning after intensive cognitive rehabilitation for traumatic brain injury. *Archives of Physical Medicine and Rehabilitation, 85*(6), 943–950.

Cicerone, K. D., & Wood, J. (1987). Planning disorder after closed head injury: A case study. *Archives of Physical Medicine and Rehabilitation, 68*(2), 111–115.

Cifu, D. X., Kreutzer, J. S., Marwitz, J. H., Rosenthal, M., Englander, J., & High, W. (1996). Functional outcomes of older adults with traumatic brain injury: A prospective, multicenter analysis. *Archives of Physical Medicine & Rehabilitation, 77,* 883–888.

Ciliska, D., Cullum, N., & Marks, S. (2001). Evaluation of systematic reviews of treatment or prevention interventions. *Evidence Based Nursing, 4*(4), 100–104.

Clare, L., Wilson, B., Carter, G., Hodges, F., & Adams, M. (2001). Long-term maintenance of treatment grains following a cognitive rehabilitation intervention in early dementia of Alzheimer type: A single case study. *Neuropsychological Rehabilitation, 11,* 477–494.

Clark, H. M. (1999). *Brain awareness week: Health promotion project for students.* Poster presented at the annual convention of the American Speech-Language-Hearing Association, San Francisco, CA.

Clark, L. W., & Witte, K. (1995). Nature and efficacy of communication management in Alzheimer's disease. In R. Lubinski (Ed.), *Dementia and communication.* San Diego, CA: Singular.

Cleary, S., Donnelly, M., Elgar, S., & Hopper, T. (2003). *Service delivery for Canadians with dementia: A survey of speech-language pathologists.* Poster presented at the Clinical Aphasiology Conference, Orcas Island, WA.

Clifford, D. B. (2000). Human immunodeficiency virus-associated dementia. *Archives of Neurology, 57,* 321–324.

Cobley, C., Thomas, S., Lincoln, N., & Walker, M. (2011). The assessment of low mood in stroke patients with aphasia: Reliability and validity of the 10-item Hospital version of the Stroke Aphasic Depression Questionnaire (SADQH-10). *Clinical Rehabilitation, 26*(4), 372–381.

Cocchini, G., Beschin, N., & Della Sala, S. (2002). Chronic anosognosia: A case report and theoretical account. *Neuropsychologia, 40,* 2030–2038.

Cocchini, G., Gregg, N., Beschin, N., Dean, M., & Della Sala, S. (2010). VATA-L: Visual analogue test assessing anosognosia for language impairment. *The Clinical Neuropsychologist, 24,* 1379–1399.

Cochran, J. W. (2001). Effect of modafinil on fatigue associated with neurological illnesses. *Journal of Chronic Fatigue Syndrome, 8,* 65–70.

Cockerham, G., Goodrich, G., Weichel, E., Orcutt, J., Rizzo, J., Bower, K., & Schuchard, R. (2009). Eye and visual function in traumatic brain injury. *Journal of Rehabilitation Research and Development, 46*(6), 811–818.

Cocks, N., Hird, K., & Kirsner, K. (2007). The relationship between right hemisphere damage and gesture in spontaneous discourse. *Aphasiology, 21*(3–4), 299–319.

Code, C. (2012). Apportioning time for aphasia rehabilitation. *Aphasiology, 26*(5), 729–735.

Code, C., Muller, D. J., & Herrmann, M. (1999). Perceptions of psychosocial adjustment of aphasia: Application of the Code-Muller Protocols. *Seminars in Speech and Language, 20,* 51–63.

Code, C., & Petheram, B. (2011). Delivering for aphasia. *International Journal of Speech-Language Pathology, 13*(1), 3–10.

Coelho, C. A. (1999). Discourse analysis in traumatic brain injury. In S. McDonald, L. Togher, & C. Code (Eds.), *Communication disorders following traumatic brain injury* (pp. 55–79). Hove, UK: Psychology Press.

Coelho, C. (2005). Direct attention training as a treatment for reading impairment in mild aphasia. *Aphasiology, 19,* 275–283.

Coelho, C. (2007). Cognitive-communication deficits following TBI. In N. D. Zasler, D. I. Katz, & R. D. Zafonte (Eds.), *Brain injury medicine: Principles and practice* (pp. 895–910). New York: Demos.

Coelho, C. A., & Duffy, R. J. (1987). The relationship of the acquisition of manual signs to severity of aphasia: A training study. *Brain and Language, 31,* 328–345.

Coelho, C. A., McHugh, R. E., & Boyle, M. (2000). Semantic feature analysis as a treatment for aphasic dysnomia: A replication. *Aphasiology, 14,* 233–242.

Coelho, C. A., Sinotte, M. P., & Duffy, J. R. (2008). Schuell's stimulation approach to rehabilitation. In R. Chapey (Ed.), *Language intervention strategies in aphasia and related neurogenic communication disorders* (5th ed., pp. 403–449). Philadelphia: Lippincott Williams & Wilkins.

Coelho, C. A., Ylvisaker, M., & Turkstra, L. (2005). Nonstandardized assessment approaches for individuals with traumatic brain injuries. *Seminars in Speech and Language, 26*(4), 223–241.

Cohen, M., Ylvisaker, M., Hamilton, J., Kemp, L., & Claiman, B. (2010). Errorless learning of functional life skills in an individual with three aetiologies of severe memory and executive function impairment. *Neuropsychological Rehabilitation, 20*(3), 355–376.

Colcombe, S. J., Erickson, K. I., Scalf, P. E., Kim, J. S., Prakash, R., McAuley, E., . . . Kramer, A. F. (2006). Aerobic exercise training increases brain volume in aging humans. *The Journals of Gerontology. Series A, Biological Sciences and Medical Sciences, 61*(11), 1166–1170.

Cole-Virtue, J., & Nickels, L. (2004). Spoken word to picture matching from PALPA: A critique and some new matched sets. *Aphasiology, 18*, 77–102.

Conklyn, D., Novak, E., Boissy, A., Bethoux, F., & Chemali, K. (2012). The effects of modified Melodic Intonation Therapy on nonfluent aphasia: A pilot study. *Journal of Speech, Language, and Hearing Research, 55*, 1463–1471.

Conley, A., & Coelho, C. A. (2003). Treatment of word retrieval impairment in chronic Broca's aphasia. *Aphasiology, 17*, 203–212.

Conners, C. K. (2013). *Conners' continuous performance test* (3rd ed.). North Tonawanda, NY: MHS.

Constantinidou, F., Werthmeier, J., Tsanadis, J., Evans, C., & Paul, D. (2012). Assessment of executive functioning in brain injury: Collaboration between speech-language pathology and neuropsychology for an integrative neuropsychological perspective. *Brain Injury, 26*(13–14), 1549–1563.

Conway, A. R. A., Cowan, N., Bunting, M. F., Therriault, D. J., & Minkoff, S. R. B. (2002). A latent variable analysis of working memory capacity, short-term memory capacity, processing speed, and general fluid intelligence. *Intelligence, 30*(2), 163–183.

Conway, A. R. A., Kane, M. J., Bunting, M. F., Hambrick, D. Z., Wilhelm, O., & Engle, R. W. (2005). Working memory span tasks: A methodological review and user's guide. *Psychonomic Bulletin & Review, 12*(5), 769–786.

Conway, T. W., Heilman, P., Rothi, L. J. G., Alexander, A. W., Adair, J., Crosson, B. A., & Heilman, K. M. (1998). Treatment of a case of phonological alexia with agraphia using the Auditory Discrimination in Depth Program. *Journal of the International Neuropsychological Society, 4*, 608–620.

Cook, L., DePompei, R., & Chapman, S. (2011). Cognitive communicative challenges in TBI: Assessment and intervention in the long term. *Perspectives on Neurophysiology and Neurogenic Speech and Language Disorders, 21*(1), 33–42.

Coppens, P., Hungerford, S., Yamaguchi, S., & Yamadori, A. (2002). Crossed aphasia: An analysis of the symptoms, their frequency, and a comparison with left-hemisphere aphasia symptomatology. *Brain and Language, 83*, 425–463.

Coppens, P., Parente, M., & Lecours, A. (1998). Aphasia in illiterate individuals. In P. Coppens, Y. Lebrun, & A. Basso (Eds.), *Aphasia in a typical populations* (pp. 175–202). Mahwah, NJ: Erlbaum.

Corbett, F., Jefferies, E., & Lambon Ralph, M. (2008). The use of cueing to alleviate recurrent verbal perseverations: Evidence from transcortical sensory aphasia. *Aphasiology, 22*(4), 363–382.

Cornell, A. (2004). Evaluating the effects of Snoezelen on women who have a dementing illness. *International Journal of Psychiatric Nursing Research, 9*, 1045–1062.

Cornis-Pop, M., Mashima, P., Roth, C., MacLennan, D., Picon, L., Smith Hammond, C., . . . Frank, E. (2012). Cognitive-communication rehabilitation for combat-related mild traumatic brain injury. *Journal of Rehabilitation Research and Development, 49*(7), xi–xxxi.

Corrigan, J. D., Arnett, J. A., Houck, L. J., & Jackson, R. D. (1985). Reality orientation for brain injured patients: Group treatment and monitoring of recovery. *Archives of Physical Medicine and Rehabilitation, 66*(9), 626–630.

Corsten, S., Mende, M., Cholewa, J., & Huber, W. (2007). Treatment of input and output phonology in aphasia: A single case study. *Aphasiology, 21*(6–8), 587–603.

Costa, J., & DeMarco, K. (2011). One center's approach to the assessment and treatment of the pediatric minimally conscious state. *Perspectives on Neurophysiology and Neurogenic Speech and Language Disorders, 21*(1), 6–14.

Cote, H., Payer, M., Giroux, F., & Joanette, Y. (2007). Towards a description of clinical communication impairment profiles following right-hemisphere damage. *Aphasiology, 21*(6–8), 739–749.

Cotelli, M., Manenti, R., Zanetti, O., & Miniussi, C. (2012). Non-pharmacological intervention for memory decline. *Frontiers in Neuroscience, 6*, 46. doi: 10.3389/fnhum.2012.00046

Coull, J. T. (1998). Neural correlates of attention and arousal: Insights from electrophysiology, functional neuroimaging and psychopharmacology. *Progress in Neurobiology, 55,* 343–361.

Cowan, N. (2010). Multiple concurrent thoughts: The meaning and developmental neuropsychology of working memory. *Developmental Neuropsychology, 35*(5), 447–474.

Crary, M. A., Haak, N. J., & Malinsky, A. E. (1989). Preliminary psychometric evaluation of an acute aphasia screening protocol. *Aphasiology, 3,* 611–618.

Crepeau, F., Scherzer, B., Belleville, S., & Desmarais, G. (1997). A qualitative analysis of central executive disorders in a real-life work situation. *Neuropsychological Rehabilitation, 7,* 147–165.

Crerar, M. A., Ellis, A. W., & Dean, E. C. (1996). Remediation of sentence processing deficits in aphasia using a computer-based microworld. *Brain and Language, 52,* 229–275.

Crimmins, C. (2001). *Where is the mango princess? A journey back from brain injury.* New York: Vintage.

Crockford, C., & Lesser, R. P. (1994). Assessing functional communication in aphasia: Clinical utility and time demands of three methods. *European Journal of Disorders of Communication, 29,* 165–182.

Cronbach, L. J. (1990). *Essentials of psychological testing* (4th ed.). New York: Harper and Row.

Crook, T., Ferris, S., McCarthy, M., & Rae, D. (1980). Utility of digit recall tasks for assessing memory in the aged. *Journal of Consulting and Clinical Psychology, 48,* 228–233.

Croot, K. (2002). Diagnosis of AOS: Definition and criteria. *Seminars in Speech and Language, 23,* 267–280.

Crosson, B. (1985). Subcortical functions in language: A working model. *Brain and Language, 25,* 257–292.

Crosson, B. (2000). Systems that support language processes: Verbal working memory. In S. Nadeau, L. Rothi, & B. Crosson (Eds.), *Aphasia and language: Theory to practice* (pp. 399–418). New York: Guilford Press.

Crosson, B. (2008). An intention manipulation to change lateralization of word production in nonfluent aphasia: Current status. *Seminars in Speech and Language, 29*(3), 188–200.

Crosson, B., Fabrizio, K., Singletary, F., Cato, M., Wierenga, C., Parkinson, R., . . . Rothi, L. J. (2007). Treatment of naming in nonfluent aphasia through manipulation of intention and attention: A phase 1 comparison of two novel treatments. *Journal of the International Neuropsychological Society, 13,* 582–594.

Culbertson, W. C., Tanner, D. C., Peck, A. K., & Hopper, A. T. (1998). Orientation testing and responses of brain-injured subjects. *Journal of Medical Speech-Language Pathology, 6,* 93–103.

Culbertson, W. C., & Zillmer, E. A. (2012). *Tower of London DX* (2nd ed.). North Tonawanda, NY: Multi-Health Systems.

Culley, C., & Evans, J. J. (2010). SMS text messaging as a means of increasing recall of therapy goals in brain injury rehabilitation: A single-blind within-subjects trial. *Neuropsychological Rehabilitation, 20*(1), 103–119.

Cummings, J. L. (2000). Cognitive and behavioral heterogeneity in Alzheimer's disease: Seeking the neurobiological basis. *Neurobiology of Aging, 21,* 845–861.

Cummings, J. L., Mega, M., Gray, K., Rosenberg-Thompson, S., Carusi, D. A., & Gornbein, J. (1994). The Neuropsychiatric Inventory: Comprehensive assessment of psychopathology in dementia. *Neurology, 44,* 2308–2314.

Cunningham, R., Farrow, V., Davies, C., & Lincoln, N. (1995). Reliability of the Assessment of Communicative Effectiveness in Severe Aphasia. *European Journal of Disorders of Communication, 30,* 1–16.

Cutica, I., Bucciarelli, M., & Bara, B. (2006). Neuropragmatics: Extralinguistic pragmatic ability better preserved in left-hemisphere-damaged patients than in right-hemisphere-damaged patients. *Brain and Language, 98,* 12–25.

Dabul, B. (2000). *Apraxia battery for adults* (2nd. ed.). Austin, TX: PRO-ED.

Dahlberg, C. A., Cusick, C. P., Hawley, L. A., Newman, J. K., Morey, C. E., Harriszon-Felix, C. L., & Whiteneck, G. G. (2007). Treatment efficacy of social communication skills training after traumatic brain injury: A randomized treatment and deferred treatment controlled trial. *Archives of Physical Medicine and Rehabilitation, 88,* 1561–1573.

Dalemans, R., Wade, D., van den Heuvel, W., & de Witte, L. (2009). Facilitating the participation of people with aphasia in research: A description of strategies. *Clinical Rehabilitation, 23,* 948–959.

Daly, M. P., & Fouche, J. H. (1999). *Critical thinking for activities of daily living and communication.* Austin, TX: PRO-ED.

Damasio, A. R. (1981). The nature of aphasia: Signs and syndromes. In M. T. Sarno (Ed.), *Acquired aphasia* (pp. 51–65). Austin, TX: PRO-ED.

Damasio, A. R. (1995). *Descartes' error: Emotion, reason, and the human brain.* New York: Quill.

Danforth, A. (1986). *Living with Alzheimer's: Ruth's story.* Hampton, VA: Prestige Press.
Daniloff, J. K., Fritelli, G., Buckingham, H. W., Hoffman, P. R., & Daniloff, R. G. (1986). AmerInd versus ASL: Recognition and imitation in aphasic subjects. *Brain and Language, 28,* 95–113.
Dardier, V., Bernicot, J., Delanoe, A., Vanberten, M., Fayada, C., Chevignard, M., . . . Dubois, B. (2011). Severe traumatic brain injury, frontal lesions, and social aspects of language use: A study of French-speaking adults. *Journal of Communication Disorders, 44,* 359–378.
Darley, F. (1982). *Aphasia.* Philadelphia: W. B. Saunders.
Darley, F. A., Aronson, A. E., & Brown, J. R. (1975). *Motor speech disorders.* Philadelphia: Saunders.
Darley, F. L., Keith, R. L., & Sasanuma, S. (1977). The effect of alerting and tranquilizing drugs upon the performance of aphasic patients. *Clinical Aphasiology, 7,* 91–96.
das Nair, R., & Lincoln, N. (2008). Cognitive rehabilitation for memory deficits following stroke. *Cochrane Database of Systematic Reviews, 4.* Art. No.: CD002293. doi: 10.1002/14651858.CD002293.pub2
Dassel, K. B., & Schmitt, F. A. (2008). The impact of caregiver executive skills on reports of patient functioning. *The Gerontological Society of America, 48,* 781–792.
Dau, B., Oda, G., & Holodniy, M. (2009). Infectious complication in OIF/OEF veterans with traumatic brain injury. *Journal of Rehabilitation Research and Development, 46*(6), 673–684.
Daumuller, M., & Goldenberg, G. (2010). Therapy to improve gestural expression in aphasia: A controlled clinical trial. *Clinical Rehabilitation, 24,* 55–65.
Davachi, L., & Dobbins, I. (2008). Declarative memory. *Current Directions in Psychological Science, 17*(2), 112–118.
Davis, C. H., Harrington, G., & Baynes, K. (2006). Intensive semantic intervention in fluent aphasia. *Aphasiology, 20*(1), 59–83.
Davis, G. A. (2005). PACE revisited. *Aphasiology, 19*(1), 21–38.
Davis, G. A. (2007). *Aphasiology: Disorders and clinical practice.* New York: Pearson.
Davis, G. A., & Wilcox, M. J. (1985). *Adult aphasia rehabilitation: Applied pragmatics.* San Diego, CA: Singular.
Davis, M., Guyker, W., & Persky, I. (2012). Uniting veterans across distance through a telephone-based reminiscence group therapy intervention. *Psychological Services, 9*(2), 206–208.
Davis, R. (1994). *My journey in Alzheimer's disease.* Carol Stream, IL: Tyndale House.
Dawson, D., Gaya, A., Hunt, A., Levine, B., Lemsky, C., & Polatajik, H. (2009). Using the Cognitive Orientation to Occupational Performance (CO-OP) with adults with executive dysfunction following traumatic brain injury. *Canadian Journal of Occupational Therapy, 76*(2), 115–127.
Dearden, N. M. (1998). Mechanisms and prevention of secondary brain damage during intensive care. *Clinical Neuropathology, 17,* 221–228.
De Bleser, R., & Kauschke, C. (2003). Acquisition and loss of nouns and verbs: Parallel or divergent patterns? *Journal of Neurolinguistics, 16,* 213–229.
de Boissezon, X., Marie, N., Castel-Lacanal, E., Marque, P., Bezy, C., Gros, H., . . . Demonet, I. (2009). Good recovery from aphasia is also supported by right basal ganglia: A longitudinal controlled PET study. *European Journal of Physical Rehabilitation and Medicine, 45,* 547–558.
de Boissezon, X., Peran, P., de Boysson, C., & Demonet, J. (2007). Pharmacotherapy of aphasia: Myth or reality? *Brain and Language, 102,* 114–125.
de Carvalho, I. A., & Mansur, L. L. (2008). Validation of ASHA FACS-functional assessment of communication skills for Alzheimer's disease population. *Alzheimer's Disease and Associated Disorders, 22*(4), 375–381.
Dechamps, A., Fasotti, L., Jungheim, J., Leone, E., Dood, E., Allioux, A., . . . Kessels, R. (2011). Effects of different learning methods for instrumental activities of daily living in patients with Alzheimer's dementia: A pilot study. *American Journal of Alzheimer's Disease and Other Dementias, 26*(4), 273–281.
DeDe, G., Parris, D., & Waters, G. (2003). Teaching self-cues: A treatment approach for verbal naming. *Aphasiology, 17,* 465–480.
De Deyn, P., De Reuck, J., Orgogozo, J. M., Vlietinck, R., & Deberdt, W. (1997). Treatment of acute ischemic stroke with piracetam. *Stroke, 28,* 2347–2352.
DeFilippis, N. A., & McCampbell, E. (1997). *Booklet category test* (2nd ed.). Lutz, FL: Psychological Assessment Resources.
DeFrances, C. J., Lucas, C. A., Buie, V. C., & Golosinskiy, A. (2008). 2006 National Hospital Discharge Survey. *National Health Status Report, 5,* 1–20.

de Haan, E., Nys, G., & van Zandvoort, M. (2006). Cognitive function following stroke and vascular cognitive impairment. *Current Opinion in Neurology, 19*(6), 559–564.

de Jong-Hagelstein, M., van de Sandt-Koenderman, W., Prins, N., Dippel, D., Koudstaal, P., & Visch-Brink, E. (2011). Efficacy of early cognitive linguistic treatment and communicative treatment in aphasia after stroke: A randomised controlled trial (RATS-2). *Journal of Neurology, Neurosurgery, and Psychiatry, 82*, 399–404.

Delano-Wood, L., Bondi, M., Sacco, J., Abeles, N., Jak, A., Libon, D., & Bozoki, A. (2009). Heterogeneity in mild cognitive impairment: Differences in neuropsychological profile and associated white matter lesion pathology. *Journal of the International Neuropsychological Society, 15*, 906–914.

DeLeo, G., Brivio, E., & Sautter, S. W. (2011). Supporting autobiographical memory in patients with Alzheimer's disease using smart phones. *Applied Neuropsychology, 18*, 69–76.

D'Elia, L. F., Satz, P., Uchiyama, C. L., & White, T. (1996). *Color trails test.* Lutz, FL: Psychological Assessment Resources.

Delis, D. C., Kaplan, E., & Kramer, J. H. (2001). *Delis-Kaplan executive function system—Examiner's manual.* San Antonio, TX: Psychological Corporation.

Delis, D. C., Kramer, J. H., Kaplan, E., & Ober, B. A. (2000). *California verbal learning test* (2nd ed.). San Antonio, TX: Psychological Corporation.

Delis, D. C., Squire, L. R., Bihrle, A., & Massman, P. (1992). Componential analysis of problem-solving ability: Performance of patients with frontal lobe damage and amnesic patients on a new sorting test. *Neuropsychologia, 30*, 683–697.

Della Barba, G., Frasson, E., Mantovan, M. C., Gallo, A., & Denes, G. (1996). Semantic and episodic memory in aphasia. *Neuropsychologia, 34*, 361–367.

Della Sala, S., Gray, C., Baddeley, A., & Wilson, L. (1997). *Visual patterns test.* Bury St. Edmunds, Suffolk, England: Thames Valley Test Company.

del Rio-Espinola, A., Mendioroz, M., Domingues-Montanari, S., Pozo-Rosich, P., Sole, E., Fernanadez-Morales, J., . . . Montaner, J. (2009). CADASIL management or what to do when there is little one can do. *Experimental Reviews of Neurotherapies, 9*(2), 197–210.

Del Toro, C., Bislick, L., Comer, M., Valozo, C., Romero, S., Gonzalez Rothi, L., & Kendall, D. (2011). Development of a short form of the Boston Naming Test for individuals with aphasia. *Journal of Speech, Language, and Hearing Research, 54*, 1089–1100.

Demir, S. O., Gorgulu, G., & Koseoglu, F. (2006). Comparison of rehabilitation outcome in patients with aphasic and non-aphasic traumatic brain injury. *Journal of Rehabilitation Medicine, 38*, 68–71.

Demonet, J. F., Thierry, G., & Cardebat, D. (2005). Renewal of the neurophysiology of language: Functional neuroimaging. *Physiological Revue, 85*(1), 49–95.

Denney, D. R., Hughes, A. J., Owens, E. M., & Lynch, S. G. (2012). Deficits in planning time but not performance in patients with multiple sclerosis. *Archives of Clinical Neuropsychology, 27*, 148–158.

Denti, L., Agosti, M., & Franceschini, M. (2008). Outcome predictors of rehabilitation for first stroke in the elderly. *European Journal of Physical Rehabilitation and Medicine, 44*, 3–11.

de Partz, M. P. (1986). Re-education of a deep dyslexic patient: Rationale of the method and results. *Cognitive Neuropsychology, 3*, 149–177.

de Partz, M. P., Seron, X., & Van der Linden, M. (1992). Re-education of a surface dysgraphia with a visual imagery strategy. *Cognitive Neuropsychology, 9*, 369–401.

DePompei, R., Gillette, Y., Goetz, E., Xenopoulos-Oddsson, A., Bryen, D., & Dowds, M. (2008). Practical applications for use of PDAs and smartphones with children and adolescents who have traumatic brain injury. *NeuroRehabilitation, 23*(6), 487–499.

DeRenzi, E., & Ferrari, C. (1978). The reporters test: A sensitive test to detect expressive disturbances in aphasics. *Cortex, 4*, 279–293.

de Riesthal, M. (2007). *Changes in written and spoken naming with a modified CART programme.* Paper presented at the annual convention of the American Speech-Language-Hearing Association, Boston, MA.

de Riesthal, M., & Wertz, R. T. (2004). Prognosis for aphasia: Relationship between selected biographical and behavioral variables and outcome and improvement. *Aphasiology, 18*, 899–915.

Derogatis, L. R. (2001). *Brief symptom inventory 18.* San Antonio, TX: Pearson.

Devine, J. M., & Zafonte, R. D. (2009). Physical exercise and cognitive recovery in acquired brain injury: A review of the literature. *PMR, 1*(6), 560–575.

De Witte, L., Engelborghs, S., De Deyn, P. & Marien, P. (2008). Crossed aphasia and visuo-spatial neglect following a right thalamic stroke: A case study and review of the literature. *Behavioural Neurology, 19*, 177–194.

De Witte, L., Brouns, R., Kavadias, D., Engelborghs, S., De Deyn, P., & Marien, P. (2011). Cognitive, affective and behavioural disturbances following vascular thalamic lesions: A review. *Cortex, 47*(3), 273–319.

Dickey, M. W., & Yoo, H. (2010). Predicting outcomes for linguistically specific sentence treatment protocols. *Aphasiology, 24*(6–8), 787–801.

Diener, E., Emmons, R. A., Larsen, R. J., Griffin, S. (1985). The Satisfaction with Life Scale. *Journal of Personality Assessment, 49*, 71–75.

Dietz, A., Ball, A., & Griffith, J. (2011). Reading and writing with aphasia in the 21st century: Technological applications of supported reading comprehension and written expression. *Topics in Stroke Rehabilitation, 18*(6), 758–769.

Dijkers, M. P. (2010). Issues in the conceptualization and measurement of participation: An overview. *Archives of Physical Medicine and Rehabilitation, 91*(Suppl. 9), S5–S16.

Ding, Q., Vaynman, S., Souda, P., Whitelegge, J. P., & Gomez-Pinilla, F. (2006). Exercise affects energy metabolism and neural plasticity-related proteins in the hippocampus as revealed by proteomic analysis. *The European Journal of Neuroscience, 24*(5), 1265–1276.

DiSimoni, F. G. (1989). *Comprehensive apraxia test*. Dalton, PA: Praxis House.

Dobie, D. J. (2002). Depression, dementia, and pseudodementia. *Seminars in Clinical Neuropsychiatry, 7*, 170–186.

Doesborgh, S. J., Mieke, van de Sandt-Koenderman, M., Dippel, D. W., van Harskamp, F., Koudstaal, P. J., & Visch-Brink, E. G. (2004). Effects of semantic treatment on verbal communication and linguistic processing in aphasia after stroke: A randomized controlled trial. *Stroke, 35*, 141–146.

Doesborgh, S., Van de Sandt-Koenderman, W., Dippel, D., Van Harskamp, F., Koudstaal, P., & Visch-Brink, E. (2003). Linguistic deficits in the acute phase of stroke. *Journal of Neurology, 250*, 977–982.

Dogil, G., Frese, I., Haider, H., Rohm, D., & Wokurek, W. (2004). Where and how does grammatically geared processing take place-and why is Broca's area often involved. A coordinated fMRI/ERBP study of language processing. *Brain and Language, 89*, 337–345.

Donkervoort, M., Dekker, J., van den Ende, E., Stehmann-Saris, J. C., & Deelman, B. G. (2000). Prevalence of apraxia among patients with a first left hemisphere stroke in rehabilitation centers and nursing homes. *Clinical Rehabilitation, 14*, 130–136.

Dore, J. (1974). A pragmatic description of early language development. *Journal of Psycholinguistic Research, 3*, 343–350.

Douglas, J. (2010). Relation of executive functioning to pragmatic outcome following severe traumatic brain injury. *Journal of Speech, Language and Hearing Research, 53*, 365–382.

Douglas, J. M., Bracy, C. A., & Snow, P. C. (2007). Measuring perceived communicative ability after traumatic brain injury: Reliability and validity of the La Trobe Communication Questionnaire. *Journal of Head Trauma Rehabilitation, 22*(1), 31–38.

Douglas, J., O'Flaherty, C., & Snow, P. (2000). Measuring perception of communicative ability: The development and evaluation of the La Trobe communication questionnaire. *Aphasiology, 14*, 251-268.

Douglas, K. (2003). *My stroke of luck*. New York: Harper Collins.

Dowden, P. A., Marshall, R. C., & Tompkins, C. A. (1981). Amer-Ind sign as a communicative facilitator for aphasic and apraxic patients. *Clinical Aphasiology, 10*, 133–140.

Downey, D., & Hurtig, R. (2006). Re-thinking AAC in acute care settings. *ASHA DAAC Perspectives on Augmentative and Alternative Communication, 15*, 3–8.

Downs, M., & Bowers, B. (2008). *Excellence in dementia care: Research into practice*. Maidenhead, UK: Open University Press.

Doyle, P. J., Goldstein, H., & Bourgeois, M. (1987). Experimental analysis of syntax training in Broca's aphasia: A generalization and social validation study. *Journal of Speech and Hearing Disorders, 52*, 143–155.

Doyle, P. J., McNeil, M. R., Mikolic, J. M., Prieto, L., Hula, W. D., Lustig, A. P., . . . Elman R. J. (2004). The Burden of Stroke Scale (BOSS) provides valid and reliable score estimates of functioning and well-being in stroke survivors with and without communication disorders. *Journal of Clinical Epidemiology, 57*, 997–1007.

Doyle, P. J., Tsironas, D., Goda, A. J., & Kalinyak, M. (1996). The relationship between objective measures and listeners' judgments of the communicative informativeness of the connected discourse of adults with aphasia. *American Journal of Speech-Language Pathology, 5*, 53–60.

Dreher, J. C., & Grafman, J. (2003). Dissociating the roles of the rostral anterior cingulated and the lateral prefrontal cortices in performing two tasks simultaneously or successively. *Cerebral Cortex, 13*, 329–339.

Dressel, K., Huber, W., Frings, L., Kummerer, D., Saur, D., Mader, I., . . . Abel, S. (2010). Model-oriented naming therapy in semantic dementia: A single-case fMRI study. *Aphasiology, 24*(12), 1537–1558.

Dronkers, N. N. (1996). A new brain region for coordinating speech articulation. *Nature, 384,* 159–161.

Drummond, S. S. (1993). *Dysarthria examination battery.* San Antonio, TX: Psychological Corporation.

D'Souza, C., Kay-Raining Bird, E., & Deacon, H. (2012). Survey of Canadian speech-language pathology service delivery to linguistically diverse clients. *Canadian Journal of Speech-Language Pathology and Audiology, 36*(1), 18-39.

Dubois, B., Slachevsky, A., Litvan, I., & Pillon, B. (2000). The FAB: A frontal assessment battery at bedside. *Neurology, 55,* 1621–1626.

Duering, M., Zieren, N., Hervé, D., Jouvent, E., Reyes, S., Peters, N., . . . Dichgans, M. (2011). Strategic role of frontal white matter tracts in vascular cognitive impairment: A voxel-based lesion-symptom mapping study in CADASIL. *Brain, 134*(Part 8), 2366–2375.

Duff, M., Proctor, A., & Haley, K. (2002). Mild traumatic brain injury: Assessment and treatment procedures used by speech-language pathologists. *Brain Injury, 16,* 773–787.

Duffy, J. (2013). *Motor speech disorders: Substrates, differential diagnosis, and management* (3rd ed.). St. Louis, MO: Elsevier Mosby.

Duffy, J., Fossett, T. R., & Thomas, J. E. (2011). Clinical practice in acute care hospital settings. In L. L. La Pointe (Ed.), *Aphasia and related neurogenic language disorders* (pp. 38–58). New York: Thieme.

Duffy, J. R., & Watkins, L. B. (1984). The effect of response choice relatedness on pantomime and verbal recognition ability in aphasic patients. *Brain and Language, 21,* 291–306.

Duffy, R. J., & Duffy, J. R. (1984). *Assessment of nonverbal communication.* Austin, TX: PRO-ED.

Duncan, P. W., Bode, R. K., Min Lai, S., & Perera, S. (2003). Rasch analysis of a new stroke-specific outcome scale: The Stroke Impact Scale. *Archives of Physical Medicine and Rehabilitation, 84*(7), 950–963.

Dunn, J., & Clare, L. (2007). Learning face–name associations in early-stage dementia: Comparing the effects of errorless learning and effortful processing. *Neuropsychological Rehabilitation, 17,* 735–754.

Dunn, L. M., & Dunn, E. S. (2007). *Peabody picture vocabulary test* (4th ed.) San Antonio, TX: Pearson.

Duval, J., Coyette, F., & Seron, X. (2008). Rehabilitation of the central executive component of working memory: A re-organisation approach applied to a single case. *Neuropsychological Rehabilitation, 18*(4), 430–460.

Eadie, T. L., Yorkston, K. M., Klasner, E. R., Dudgeon, B. J., Deitz, J. C., Baylor, C. R., . . . Amtmann, D. (2006). Measuring communicative participation: A review of self-report instruments in speech-language pathology. *American Journal of Speech-Language Pathology, 15*(4), 307–320.

Easton, J., Saver, J., Albers, G., Alberts, M., Chaturvedi, S., Feldmann, E., . . . Sacco, R. (2009). Definition and evaluation of transient ischemic attack. *Stroke, 40,* 2276–2293.

Edgeworth, J., Robertson, I. H., & MacMillan, T. (1998). *The balloons test.* Bury St. Edmunds, Suffolk, England: Thames Valley Test Company.

Edmonds, L., & Babb, M. (2011). Effect of Verb Network Strengthening treatment in moderate-to-severe aphasia. *American Journal of Speech-Language Pathology, 20,* 131–145.

Edmonds, L., & Donovan, N. (2012). Item-level psychometrics and predictors of performance for Spanish/English bilingual speakers on an object and action naming battery. *Journal of Speech, Language, and Hearing Research, 55,* 359–381.

Edmonds, L., Nadeau, S., & Kiran, S. (2009). Effect of Verb Network Strengthening Treatment (VNeST) on lexical retrieval of content words in sentences in persons with aphasia. *Aphasiology, 23,* 402–424.

Edwards, S. (1995). Profiling fluent aphasic spontaneous speech: A comparison of two methodologies. *European Journal of Disorders of Communication, 30,* 333–345.

Edwards, S., & Tucker, K. (2006). Verbal retrieval in fluent aphasia: A clinical study. *Aphasiology, 20*(7), 644–675.

Ehlardt, L., Sohlberg, M. M., Kennedy, M. R. T., Coelho, C., Turkstra, L., Ylvisaker, M., & Yorkston, K. (2008). Evidence-based practice guidelines for instructing individuals with acquired memory impairments: What have we learned in the past 20 years? *Neuropsychological Rehabilitation, 18*(3), 300–342.

Ehrlich, A., & Schroeder, C. (2009). *Medical terminology for health professions.* Clifton Park, NY: Delmar Cengage Learning.

Ellis, C. (2009). Does race/ethnicity really matter in adult neurogenics? *American Journal of Speech-Language Pathology, 18*, 310–314.

Ellis, C., Rosenbek, J., Rittman, M., & Boylstein, C. (2005). Recovery of cohesion in narrative discourse after left-hemisphere stroke. *Journal of Rehabilitation Research and Development, 42*(6), 737–746.

Ellis, H. C., & Hunt, R. R. (1993). *Fundamentals of human memory and cognition.* Dubuque, IA: William C. Brown.

Elman, R. (Ed.). (2007). *Group treatment of neurogenic communication disorders: The expert clinician's approach* (2nd ed.). San Diego, CA: Plural.

Enderby, P., Broeckx, J., Hospers, W., Schildermans, F., & Deberdt, W. (1994). Effect of piracetam on recovery and rehabilitation after stroke: A double-blind, placebo-controlled study. *Clinical Neuropharmacology, 17*, 320–331.

Enderby, P., & Palmer, R. (2008). *Frenchay dysarthria assessment* (2nd ed.). Austin, TX: PRO-ED.

Enderby, P., Wood, V., Wade, D., & Langton Hewer, R. (1997). *The Frenchay aphasia screening test.* Philadelphia: Taylor and Francis.

Engelter, S. T., Gostynski, M., Papa, S., Frein, M., Born, C,. Ajadacic-Gross, V., . . . Lyrer, P. A. (2006). Epidemiology of aphasia attributable to first ischemic stroke: Incidence, severity, fluency, etiology, and thrombolysis. *Stroke, 37*(6), 1379–1384.

Engle, R. W. (2002). Working memory capacity as executive attention. *Current Directions in Psychological Science, 11*, 19–23.

Ennis, M. R. (2001). Comprehension approaches for word retrieval training in aphasia. *Neurophysiology and Neurogenic Speech and Language Disorders, 11*, 18–23.

Eramudugolla, R., & Mattingley, J. B. (2008). Spatial gradient for unique-feature detection in patients with unilateral neglect: evidence from auditory and visual search. *Neurocase, 15*(1), 24–31.

Erkulwater, S., & Pillai, R. (1989). Amantadine and the end stage dementia of Alzheimer's type. *Southern Medical Journal, 82*, 550–554.

Eslinger, P. J., Moore, P., Anderson, C. & Grossman, M. (2011). Social cognition, executive functioning, and neuroimaging correlates of empathic deficits in frontotemporal dementia. *Journal of Neuropsychiatry and Clinical Neurosciences, 23*, 74–82.

Eslinger, P. J., Moore, P., Antani, S., Anderson, C., & Grossman, M. (2012). Apathy in frontotemporal dementia: Behavioral and neuroimaging correlates. *Behavioral Neurology, 25*(2), 127–136.

Evanofski, M. (1997). *Attention workbook volume 1* (2nd ed.). Dedham, MA: AliMed.

Evans, J. J., Emslie, H. C., & Wilson, B. A. (1998). External cueing systems in the rehabilitation of executive impairments of action. *Journal of the International Neuropsychology Society, 4*, 399–408.

Evans, J. J., Greenfield, E., & Wilson, B. (2009). Walking and talking therapy: Improving cognitive-motor dual tasking in neurological illness. *Journal of the International Neuropsychological Society, 15*, 112–120.

Evans, J. J., Wilson, B. A., Needham, P., & Brentnall, S. (2003). Who makes good use of memory aids? Results of a survey of people with acquired brain injury. *Journal of the International Neuropsychological Society, 9*, 925–935.

Evans, J. J., Wilson, B. A., Schuri, U., Andrade, J., Baddeley, A. D., Bruna, O., . . . Taussik, I. (2000). A comparison of "errorless" and "trial-and-error" learning methods for teaching individuals with acquired memory deficits. *Neuropsychological Rehabilitation, 10*, 67–101.

Ewing, S. E. A. (2007). Group process, group dynamics, and group techniques with neurogenic communication disorders. In R. J. Elman (Ed.), *Group treatment of neurogenic communication disorders: The expert clinician's approach* (2nd ed., pp. 11–23). San Diego, CA: Plural.

Ewing, S. A., & Pfalzgraf, B. (1991). *Pathways: Moving beyond stroke and aphasia.* Detroit, MI: Wayne State University Press.

Falconer, C., & Antonucci, S. M. (2012). Use of semantic feature analysis in group discourse treatment for aphasia: Extension and expansion. *Aphasiology, 26*(1), 64–82.

Falluji, N., Abou-Chebl, A., Rodriguez Castro, C. E., & Mukherjee, D. (2011). Reperfusion strategies for acute ischemic stroke. *Angiology*, doi: 10.1177/0003319711414269

Fan, J.-T., & Chen, K.-M. (2011). Using silver yoga exercises to promote physical and mental health of elders with dementia in long-term care facilities. *International Psychogeriatrics, 23*(8), 1222–1230.

Farias, D., Davis, C., & Harrington, G. (2006). Drawing: Its contribution to naming in aphasia. *Brain and Language, 97*(1), 53–63.

Farley, B. G., Derosa, S., Koshland, G. F., Fox, C. M., & Van Gemmert, A. W. (2006). *Training generalized amplitude across motor systems (training BIG and LOUD) transfers to an untrained handwriting task in early Parkinson disease* [Abstract]. Program no. 655.13, Society for Neuroscience, Atlanta, GA.

Farlow, M., Gracon, S. I., Hershey, L. A., Lewis, K. W., Sadowsky, C. H., & Dolan-Reno, J. (1992). A controlled trial of tacrine in Alzheimer's disease. *Journal of the American Medical Association, 268*, 2523–2529.

Faroqi-Shah, Y., Frymark, T., Mullen, R., & Wang, B. (2010). Effect of treatment for bilingual individuals with aphasia: A systematic review of the evidence. *Journal of Neurolinguistics, 23*, 319–341.

Fasotti, L., Kovacs, F., Eling, P., & Brouwer, W. H. (2000). Time pressure management as a compensatory strategy training after closed head injury. *Neuropsychological Rehabilitation, 10*, 47–65.

Fassbinder, W., & Tompkins, C. A. (2001). Slowed lexical-semantic activation in individuals with right hemisphere brain damage? *Aphasiology, 15*, 1079–1090.

Fatemi, Y., Boeve, B., Duffy, J., Petersen, R., Knopman, D., Cejka, . . . Geda, Y. (2011). Neuropsychiatric aspects of primary progressive aphasia. *Journal of Neuropsychiatry and Clinical Neuroscience, 23*, 168–172.

Faul, M., Xu, L., Wald, M. M., & Coronado, V. G. (2010). *Traumatic brain injury in the United States: Emergency department visits, hospitalizations and deaths 2002–2006*. Atlanta, GA: Centers for Disease Control and Prevention, National Center for Injury Prevention and Control.

Fausti, S., Wilmington, D., Gallun, F., Myers, P., & Henry, J. (2009). Auditory and vestibular dysfunction associated with blast-related traumatic brain injury. *Journal of Rehabilitation Research and Development, 46*(6), 797–810.

Federal Interagency Forum on Aging-Related Statistics. (2010). *Older Americans 2010: Key indicators of well-being*. Washington, DC: Author.

Feinberg, T., & Goodman, B. (1984). Affective illness, dementia, and pseudodementia. *Journal of Clinical Psychiatry, 45*, 99–103.

Ferguson, A., & Harper, A. (2010). Contributions to the talk of individuals with aphasia in multiparty interactions. *Aphasiology, 24*, 1605–1620.

Ferguson, N., Evans, K., & Raymer, A. (2012). A comparison of intention and pantomime gesture treatment for noun retrieval in people with aphasia. *American Journal of Speech-Language Pathology, 21*, S126–S139.

Fernando, M. S., & Ince, P. G. (2004). Vascular pathologies and cognition in a population-based cohort of elderly people. *Journal of the Neurological Sciences, 226*, 13–17.

Ferre, P., Ska, B., Lajoie, C., Bleau, A., & Joanette, Y. (2011). Clinical focus on prosodic, discursive, and pragmatic treatment for right hemisphere damaged adults: What's right? *Rehabilitation Research and Practice*, doi: 10.1155/2011/131820

Ferro, J. M., Mariano, G., & Madureira, S. (1999). Recovery from aphasia and neglect. *Cerebrovascular Disease, 9*(Suppl. 5), 6–22.

Fierce, D. W. (2002). *Surviving black ice: A survivor's insight to life after head injury*. Killingworth, CT: Writer's Block Press.

Filley, C. M. (2002). The neuroanatomy of attention. *Seminars in Speech and Language, 23*, 89–98.

Fillingham, J., Sage, K., & Lambon Ralph, A. (2005). Further explorations and an overview of errorless and errorful therapy for aphasic word-finding difficulties: The number of naming attempts during therapy affects outcome. *Aphasiology, 19*, 597–614.

Fillingham, J. K., Sage, K., & Lambon Ralph, M. A. (2006). The treatment of anomia using errorless learning. *Neuropsychological Rehabilitation, 16*, 129–154.

Fink, R. B, Bartlett, M. R., Lowery, J. S., Linebarger, M., & Schwartz, M. (2008). Aphasic speech with and without SentenceShaper: Two methods for assessing informativeness. *Aphasiology, 22*, 679–690.

Fink, R. B., Brecher, A., Schwartz, M. F., & Robey, R. R. (2002). A computer-implemented protocol for treatment of naming disorders: Evaluation of clinician-guided and partially self-guided instruction. *Aphasiology, 16*, 1061–1086.

Fink, R. B., Schwartz, M. F., & Myers, J. L. (1998). Investigations of the sentence-query approach to mapping therapy. *Brain and Language, 65*, 203–207.

Fink, R. B., Schwartz, M. F., Rochon, E., Myers, J. L., Socolof, G. S., & Bluestone, R. (1995). Syntax stimulation revisited: An analysis of generalization treatment effects. *American Journal of Speech-Language Pathology, 4*, 99–104.

Fischer, S., Trexler, L. E., & Gauggel, S. (2004). Awareness of activity limitations and prediction of performance in patients with brain injuries and orthopedic disorders. *Journal of the International Neuropsychological Society, 10*, 190–199.

Fish, J., Manly, T., Emslie, H., Evans, J. J., & Wilson, B. A. (2009). Compensatory strategies for acquired disorders of memory and planning: Differential effects of a paging system of patients with brain injury of traumatic versus cerebrovascular aetiology. *Journal of Neurology, Neurosurgery, & Psychiatry, 79*, 930–935.

Fish, J., Wilson, B. A., & Manly, T. (2010). The assessment and rehabilitation of prospective memory problems in people with neurological disorders: A review. *Neuropsychological Rehabilitation, 20*(2), 161–179.

Fisher, M. (2003). Recommendations for advancing development of acute stroke therapies: Stroke therapy academic industry roundtable 3. *Stroke, 34*, 1539–1546.

Fisher, M. (2011). New approaches to neuroprotective drug development. *Stroke, 42*(Suppl. 1), S24–S27.

Flamand-Roze, C., Falssard, B., Roze, E., Maintigneux, L., Beziz, J., Chacon, A., . . . Denier, C. (2011). Validation of a new language screening tool for patients with acute stroke: The Language Screening Test. *Stroke, 42*, 1224–1229.

Fleming, J. M., Strong, J., & Ashton, R. (1996). Self-awareness of deficits in adults with traumatic brain injury: How best to measure? *Brain Injury, 10*, 1–15.

Floel, A., Meinzer, M., Kirstein, R., Nijhof, S., Deppe, M., Knecht, S., & Breitenstein, C. (2011). Short-term anomia training and electrical brain stimulation. *Stroke, 42*, 2065–2067.

Floel, A., Poeppel, D., Buffalo, E. A., Braun, A., Wu, C. W., Seo, H. J., . . . Cohen, L. G. (2004). Prefrontal cortex asymmetry for memory encoding of words and abstract shapes. *Cerebral Cortex, 14*, 404–409.

Foldi, N. S., LoBosco, J. J., & Schaefer, L. A. (2002). The effect of attentional dysfunction in Alzheimer's disease: Theoretical and practical implications. *Seminars in Speech and Language, 23*, 139–150.

Folstein, M., & Folstein, S. (2010). *Mini-mental state examination* (2nd ed.) Lutz, FL: PAR.

Folstein, M. F., Folstein, S. E., & McHugh, P. R. (2001). *Mini-mental state examination*. Lutz, FL: Psychological Assessment Resources.

Formisano, R., Carlesimo, G. A., Sabbadini, M., Loasses, A., Penta, F., Vinicola, V., & Caltagirone, C. (2004). Clinical predictors and neuropsychological outcome in severe traumatic brain injury patients. *Acta Neurochirurgica, 146*, 457–462.

Forrester, G., & Geffen, G. (1995). *Julia Farr services post-traumatic amnesia scale*. Unley, Australia: Julia Farr Foundation.

Fotopoulou, A., Rudd, A., Holmes, P., & Kopelman, M. (2009). Self-observation reinstates motor awareness in anosognosia for hemiplegia. *Neuropsychologia, 47*, 1256–1260.

Fouladbakhsh, J. (2012). Complementary and alternative modalities to relieve osteoarthritis symptoms. *American Journal of Nursing, 112*(3 Suppl. 1), S44–S51.

Fox, B. D., Cheung, V. J., Patel, A. J., Suki, D., & Rao, G. (2011). Epidemiology of metastatic brain tumors. *Neurosurgery Clinics of North America, 22*, 1–6.

Fraas, M. (2006). Interactive multimedia training of names and faces following acquired brain injury. *International Journal of Cognition and Technology, 11*, 10–16.

Fraas, M., & Calvert, M. (2009). The use of narratives to identify characteristics leading to a productive life following acquired brain injury. *American Journal of Speech-Language Pathology, 18*(4), 315–328.

Francis, D. R., Clark, N., & Humphreys, G. W. (2003). The treatment of an auditory working memory deficit and the implications for sentence comprehension abilities in mild receptive aphasia. *Aphasiology, 17*, 723–750.

Frank, E. M., & Barrineau, S. (1996). Current speech-language protocols for adults with traumatic brain injury. *Journal of Medical Speech-Language Pathology, 4*, 81–101.

Frankel, T., & Penn C. (2007). Perseveration and conversation in TBI: Response to pharmacological intervention. *Aphasiology, 21*(10–11), 1039–1078.

Franklin, S., Buerk, F., & Howard, D. (2002). Generalised improvement in speech production for a subject with reproduction conduction aphasia. *Aphasiology, 16*(10/11), 1087–1114.

Fraser, S., Glass, J. N., Leathem, J. M. (1999). Everyday memory in an elderly New Zealand population: Performance on the Rivermead Behavioral Memory Test. *New Zealand Journal of Psychology, 28*, 118–123.

Frassinetti, F., Angeli, V., Menghello, F., Avanzi, S., & Ladavas, E. (2002). Long-lasting amelioration of visuospatial neglect by prism adaptation. *Brain, 125*, 608–623.

Fratiglioni, L., & Rocca, W. A. (2001). Epidemiology of dementia. In F. Bolla & S. F. Cappa (Eds.), *Handbook of neuropsychology* (Vol. 6, pp. 193–215). New York: Elsevier Science.

Frattali, C. M. (1994). Functional assessment. In R. Lubinski and C. Frattali (Eds.). *Professional issues in speech-language pathology and audiology* (pp. 306–320). San Diego, CA: Singular.

Frattali, C., Thompson, C., Holland, A., Wohl, A., & Ferketic, M. (1995). *American Speech-Language-Hearing Association Functional Assessment of Communication Skills for Adults*. Rockville, MD: ASHA.

Freed, D. (2004). Two case studies of family influence on treatment outcome after stroke. *Special Interest Division 2: Neurophysiology and Neurogenic Speech and Language Disorders Newsletter, 14*(4), 16–19.

Freed, D. (2012). *Motor speech disorders: Diagnosis and treatment* (2nd ed.). Clifton Park, NY: Delmar.

Freed, D., Celery, K., & Marshall, R. C. (2004). Effectiveness of personalized and phonological cueing on long-term naming performance by aphasic subjects: A clinical investigation. *Aphasiology, 18*, 743–757.

Freed, D. B., Marshall, R. C., & Chuhlantseff, E. A. (1996). Picture naming variability: A methodological consideration of inconsistent naming responses in fluent and nonfluent aphasia. *Clinical Aphasiology, 24*, 193–205.

Freedman, M., Alexander, M. P., & Naeser, M. A. (1984). Anatomic basis of transcortical motor aphasia. *Neurology, 34*, 409–417.

Freedman, M., Leach, L., Kaplan, E., Winocur, G., Shulman, K. I., & Delis, D. C. (1994). *Clock drawing: A neuropsychological analysis*. New York: Oxford Press.

Fridriksson, J., Baker, J. M., Whiteside, J., Eoute, D., Moser, D., Vesselinov, R., & Rorden, C. (2009). Treating visual speech perception to improve speech production in non-fluent aphasia. *Stroke, 40*(3), 853–858.

Fridriksson, J., Holland, A. L., Beeson, P., & Morrow, L. (2005). Spaced retrieval treatment of anomia. *Aphasiology, 19*, 99–109.

Fridriksson, J., Richardson, J. D., Baker, J. M., & Rorden, C. (2011). Transcranial direct current stimulation improves naming reaction time in fluent aphasia: A double-blind, sham-controlled study. *Stroke, 42*, 819–821.

Friederici, A. D. (2011). The brain basis of language processing: From structure to function. *Physiology Review, 91*(4), 1357–1392.

Friederici, A., & Frazier, L. (1992). Thematic analysis in agrammatic comprehension: Syntactic structure and task demands. *Brain and Language, 42*, 1–29.

Friedman, R. B., & Lott, S. N. (2000). Rapid word identification in pure alexia is lexical but not semantic. *Brain and Language, 72*, 219–237.

Fried-Oken, M. (2008). Augmentative and alternative communication treatment for persons with primary progressive aphasia. *Perspectives on Augmentative and Alternative Communication, 17*(3), 99–104.

Fromm, D., & Holland, A. (1989). Functional communication in Alzheimer's disease. *Journal of Speech and Hearing Disorders, 54*, 535–540.

Fucetola, R., Connor, L. T., Perry, J., Leo, P., Tucker, F. M., & Corbetta, M. (2006). Aphasia severity, semantics, and depression predict functional communication in acquired aphasia. *Aphasiology, 20*(5), 449–461.

Fucetola, R., Connor, L. T., Strube, M., & Corbetta, M. (2009). Unraveling nonverbal cognitive performance in acquired aphasia. *Aphasiology, 23*(12), 1418–1426.

Fujioka, M., Okuchi, K., Hiramatsu, K. L., Sakaki, T., Sakaguchi, S., & Ishii, Y. (1997). Specific changes in human brain after hypoglycemic injury. *Stroke, 28*, 584–587.

Fukui, T., & Lee, E. (2009). Visuospatial function is a significant contributor to functional status in patients with Alzheimer's disease. *American Journal of Alzheimer's Disease and Other Dementias, 24*(4), 313–321.

Fyffe, D., Mukherjee, S., Barnes, L., Manly, J., Bennett, D., & Crane, P. (2011). Explaining differences in episodic memory performance among older African Americans and Whites: The roles of factors related to cognitive reserve and test bias. *Journal of the International Neuropsychological Society, 17,* 625–638.

Gaber, T., Parsons, F., & Gautam, V. (2011). Validation of the language component of the Addenbrooke's Cognitive Examination–Revised (ACE-R) as a screening tool for aphasia in stroke patients. *Australasian Journal of Ageing, 30*(3), 156–158.

Gaddie, A., Kearns, K. P., & Yedor, K. (1991). A qualitative analysis of response elaboration training effects. *Clinical Aphasiology, 19,* 171–183.

Gainotti, G., Azzoni, A., Razzano, C., Lanzillotta M., Marra C., & Gasparini F. (1997). The post-stroke depression rating scale: A test specifically devised to investigate affective disorders of stroke patients. *Journal of Clinical and Experimental Neuropsychology, 19,* 340–356.

Galante, E., Gazzi, L., & Caffarra, S. (2011). Psychological activities in neurorehabilitation: From research to clinical practice. *Giornale Italiano di Medicina del Lavoro ed Ergonomia, 33*(1), A19–A28.

Galbiati, S., Recla, M., Pastore, V., Liscio, M., Bardoni, A., Castelli, E., & Strazzer, S. (2009). Attention remediation following traumatic brain injury in childhood and adolescence. *Neuropsychology, 23*(1), 40–49.

Gallo, J. J., Rabins, P. V., & Anthony, J. C. (1999). Sadness in older persons: 13-year follow-up of a community sample in Baltimore, Maryland. *Psychological Medicine, 29,* 341–350.

Galvin, J., Roe, C., Coats, M., & Morris, J. (2007). Patient's rating of cognitive ability: Using the AD8, a brief informant interview, as a self-rating tool to detect dementia. *Archives of Neurology, 64*(5), 725–730.

Gamino, J., Chapman, S., & Cook, L. (2009). Strategic learning in youth with traumatic brain injury: Evidence for stall in higher-order cognition. *Topics in Language Disorders, 29*(3), 224–235.

Garcin, B., Lillo, P., Hornberger, M., Piguet, O., Dawson, K., Nestor, P. J., & Hodges, J. R. (2009). Determinants of survival in behavioral variant frontotemporal dementia. *Neurology, 73*(20), 1656–1661.

Garrett, K. L. (1999). Measuring outcomes of group therapy. In R. J. Elman (Ed.), *Group treatment of neurogenic communication disorders: The expert clinician's approach* (pp. 17–29). Boston: Butterworth-Heinemann.

Garrett, K. L., & Lasker, J. P. (2005). *The multimodal communication screening test for persons with aphasia (MCST-A)*. Retrieved June 12, 2012, from http://aac.unl.edu/screen/screen.html

Garrett, K. L., Staltari, C. F., & Moir, L. J. (2007). Contextual group communication therapy for persons with aphasia: A scaffolded discourse approach. In R. J. Elman (Ed.), *Group treatment of neurogenic communication disorders: The expert clinician's approach* (2nd ed.; pp. 159–191). San Diego: Plural.

Garrett, M. F. (1988). Processes in language production. In F. J. Newmeyer (Ed.), *Linguistics: The Cambridge survey: III. Language: Psychological and biological aspects* (pp. 69–96). Cambridge: Cambridge University Press.

Geary, E. K., Kraus, M. F., Rubin, L., Pliskin, N., & Little, D. (2010). Verbal learning strategy following mild brain injury. *Journal of International Neuropsychological Society, 17,* 709–719.

Gentry, T., Wallace, J., Kvarfordt, C., & Lynch, K. B. (2008). Personal digital assistants as cognitive aids for individuals with severe traumatic brain injury: A community-based trial. *Brain Injury, 22*(1), 19–24.

George, M., Mercer, J., Walker, R., & Manly, T. (2008). A demonstration of endogenous modulation of unilateral spatial neglect: The impact of apparent time-pressure on spatial bias. *Journal of the International Neuropsychological Society, 14,* 33–41.

German, D. J. (1990). *The test of adolescent and adult word-finding.* Austin, TX: PRO-ED.

Gerritsen, M. J. J., Berg, I. J., Deelman, B. G., Visser-Keizer, A. C., & Meyboom-de Jong, B. (2003). Speed of information processing after unilateral stroke. *Journal of Clinical and Experimental Neuropsychology, 25,* 1–13.

Geyh, S., Cieza, A., Kollerits, B., Grimby, G., & Stucki, G. (2007). Content comparison of health-related quality of life measures used in stroke based on the international classification of functioning, disability and health (ICF): A systematic review. *Quality of Life Research, 16*(5), 833–851.

Giacino, J., & Malone, R. (2008). The vegetative and minimally conscious states. *Handbook of Clinical Neurology, 90,* 99–111.

Giacino, J., & Whyte, J. (2005). The vegetative and minimally conscious states: Current knowledge and remaining questions. *Journal of Head Trauma Rehabilitation, 20*(1), 30–50.

Gialanella, B. (2011). Aphasia assessment and functional outcome prediction in patients with aphasia after stroke. *Journal of Neurology, 258,* 343–349.

Gialanella, B., & Ferlucci, C. (2010). Functional outcome after stroke in patients with aphasia and neglect: Assessment by the Motor and Cognitive Functional Independence Measure instrument. *Cerebrovascular Disorders, 30,* 440–447.

Gialanella B., Monguzzi V., Santoro R., & Rocchi S. (2005). Functional recovery after hemiplegia in patients with neglect: The rehabilitative role of anosognosia. *Stroke, 36,* 2687–2690.

Gierut, J. A. (2007). Phonological complexity and language learnability. *American Journal of Speech Language Pathology, 16*(1), 6–17.

Giffords, G., & Kelly, M. (2011). *Gabby: A story of courage and hope.* New York: Scribner.

Gil, M., Cohen, M., Korn, C., & Groswasser, Z. (1996). Vocational outcome of aphasic patients following severe traumatic brain injury. *Brain Injury, 10,* 39–45.

Gilleard, C. J. (1997). Education and Alzheimer's disease: A review of recent international epidemiological studies. *Aging and Mental Health, 1,* 33–46.

Gillis, R. J. (2007). Traumatic brain injury: early intervention. In R. J. Elman (Ed.), *Group treatment of neurogenic communication disorders: The expert clinician's approach* (2nd ed., pp. 297–316). San Diego, CA: Plural.

Ginsberg, M. D. (2008). Neuroprotection for ischemic stroke: Past, present and future. *Neuropharmacology, 55,* 363–389.

Ginstfeldt, T., & Emanuelson, I. (2010). An overview of attention deficits after paediatric traumatic brain injury. *Brain Injury, 24*(10), 1123–1134.

Gitlin, L. N., Liebman, J., & Winter, L. (2003). Are environmental interventions effective in the management of Alzheimer's disease and related disorders?: A synthesis of evidence. *Alzheimer's Care Quarterly, 4,* 85–107.

Gitlin, L. N., Winter, L., Dennis, M. P., Hodgson, N., & Hauck, W. W. (2010). Targeting and managing behavioral symptoms in individuals with dementia: A randomized trial of a nonpharmacological intervention. *Journal of the American Geriatrics Society, 58*(8), 1465–1474.

Gitterman, M., Goral, M., & Obler, L. (2012). *Aspects of multilingual aphasia.* Bristol, UK: Multilingual Matters.

Gleason, J. B., Goodglass, H., Green, E., Ackerman, N., & Hyde, M. R. (1975). The retrieval of syntax in Broca's aphasia. *Brain and Language, 2,* 451–471.

Glisky, E. L. (1992). Computer-assisted instruction for patients with traumatic brain injury: Teaching of domain-specific knowledge. *Journal of Head Trauma Rehabilitation, 7,* 1–12.

Glisky, E. L., & Schacter, D. L. (1989). Extending the limits of complex learning in organic amnesia: Computer training in a vocational domain. *Neuropsychologia, 27,* 107–120.

Glisky, E. L., Schacter, D. L., & Tulving, E. (1989). Learning and retention of computer-related vocabulary in amnesic patients: Method of vanishing cues. *Journal of Clinical and Experimental Neuropsychology, 8,* 292–312.

Glosser, G., Baker, K. M., de Vries, J. J., Alavi, A., Grossman, M., & Clark, C. M. (2002). Disturbed visual processing contributes to impaired reading in Alzheimer's disease. *Neuropsychologia, 40,* 902–909.

Glosser, G., & Deser, T. (1990). Patterns of discourse production among neurological patients with fluent language disorders. *Brain and Language, 40,* 67–88.

Godefroy, O., Azouvi, P., Robert, P., Roussel, M., LeGall, D., & Meulemans, T. (2010). Dysexecutive syndrome: Diagnostic criteria and validation study. *Annals of Neurology, 68,* 855–864.

Godefroy, O., Fickl, A., Roussel, M., Auribault, C., Bugnicourt, J., Lamy, C., . . . Petitnicolas, G. (2011). Is the Montreal Cognitive Assessment superior to the Mini-Mental State Examination to detect poststroke cognitive impairment? A study with neuropsychological evaluation. *Stroke, 42,* 1712–1716.

Goff, R. A., Hinckley, J. J., & Wingo, B. E. (2011, May/June). *Examining Treatment Components: Interviews about Group Aphasia Therapy.* Paper presented at the Clinical Aphasiology Conference, Fort Lauderdale, FL.

Gold, M., VanDam, D., & Silliman, E. R. (2000). An open-label trial of bromocriptine in nonfluent aphasia: A qualitative analysis of word storage and retrieval. *Brain and Language, 74*, 141–156.

Goldberg, E., Podell, K., Bilder, R., & Jaeger, J. (2000). *Executive control battery*. Lutz, FL: Psychological Assessment Resources.

Golden, C. (2002). *Stroop color and word test*. Lutz, FL: Psychological Assessment Resources.

Goldenberg, G., & Spatt, J. (1994). Influence of size and site of cerebral lesions on spontaneous recovery of aphasia and on success of language therapy. *Brain and Language, 47*, 684–698.

Goldfarb, R., & Bader, E. (1979). Espousing melodic intonation therapy in aphasia rehabilitation: A case study. *International Journal of Rehabilitation Research, 2*, 333–342.

Golding, E. (1989). *Middlesex elderly assessment of mental state*. Bury St. Edmunds, Suffolk, England: Thames Valley Test Company.

Golding, H., Bass, E., Percy, A., & Goldberg, M. (2009). Understanding recent estimates of PTSD and TBI from Operations Iraqi Freedom and Enduring Freedom. *Journal of Rehabilitation Research and Development, 46*(5), vii–xiii.

Goldrick, M., Folk, J. R., & Rapp, B. (2010). Mrs. Malaprop's neighborhood: Using word errors to reveal neighborhood structure. *Journal of Memory and Language, 62*(2), 113–134.

Goldstein, K., & Scheerer, M. (1948). Abstract and concrete behavior in experimental study with special tests. *Psychological Monograph, 53*, 1–151.

Goldstein, K. H., & Scheerer, M. (1953). Tests of abstract and concrete behavior. In A. Weider (Ed.), *Contributions toward medical psychology: Theory and psychodiagnostic methods* (pp. 702–730). New York: Ronald Press.

Goldstein, L. B., Bushnell, C., Adams, R., Appel, L., Braun, L., Chaturvedi, S., . . . Pearson, T. A. (2010). Guidelines for the primary prevention of stroke: A guideline for healthcare professionals from the American Heart Association/American Stroke Association. *Stroke*, doi: 10.1161/STR.0b013e3181fcb238

Golisz, K. M. (1998). Dynamic assessment and multicontext treatment of unilateral neglect. *Topics in Stroke Rehabilitation, 5*, 11–28.

Goll, J., Crutch, S., Loo, J., Rohrer, J., Frost, C., Bamiou, D., & Warren, J. (2010). Non-verbal sound processing in the primary progressive aphasias. *Brain, 133*, 272–285.

Golper, L. C. (1996). Language assessment. In G. L. Wallace (Ed.), *Adult aphasia rehabilitation* (pp. 57–86). Boston: Butterworth-Heinemann.

Golper, L. C., Rau, M. T., Erskins, B., Langhans, J. J., & Houlihan, J. (1987). Aphasic patients' performance on a Mental Status Examination. *Clinical Aphasiology, 16*, 124–135.

Gonzalez Rothi, L., Fuller, R., Leon, S., Kendall, D., Moore, A., Wu, S., . . . Nadeau, S. E. (2009). Errorless practice as a possible adjuvant to donepezil in Alzheimer's disease. *Journal of the International Neuropsychological Society, 15*(1), 311–322.

Goodglass, H. (1981). The syndromes of aphasia: Similarities and differences in neurolinguistic features. *Topics in Language Disorders, 1*, 1–14.

Goodglass, H. (1993). *Understanding aphasia*. New York: Academic Press.

Goodglass, H. (1998). Stages of lexical retrieval. *Aphasiology, 4-5*, 287–298.

Goodglass, H., & Kaplan, E. (1983). *The assessment of aphasia and related disorders* (2nd ed.). Philadelphia: Lea & Febiger.

Goodglass, H., Kaplan, E., & Barresi, B. (2001). *Boston diagnostic aphasia examination* (3rd ed.). New York: Lippincott Williams & Wilkins.

Goodman, R. A., & Caramazza, A. (1986a). *The Johns Hopkins University dysgraphia battery*. Baltimore: Johns Hopkins University.

Goodman, R. A., & Caramazza, A. (1986b). *The Johns Hopkins University dyslexia battery*. Baltimore: Johns Hopkins University.

Gordon, J. K. (1998). The fluency dimension in aphasia. *Aphasiology, 12*, 673–688.

Gordon, W. P. (1983). Memory disorders in aphasia: I. Auditory immediate recall. *Neuropsychologia, 21*, 325–339.

Gordon, W., Cantor, J., Ashman, T., & Brown, M. (2006). Treatment of post-TBI executive dysfunction: Application of theory to clinical practice. *Journal of Head Trauma Rehabilitation, 21*(2), 156–167.

Gorno-Tempini, M., Hillis, A., Weintraub, S., Kertesz, A., Mendez, M., Cappa, S., . . . Grossman, M. (2011). Classification of primary progressive aphasia and its variants. *Neurology, 76*, 1006–1014.

Gotts, S. J., Incisa della Rocchetta, A., & Cipolotti, L. (2002). Mechanisms underlying perseveration in aphasia: Evidence from a single case study. *Neuropsychologia, 40,* 1930–1947.

Grace, J., & Malloy, P. (2001). *Frontal systems behavior scale.* Odessa, FL: PAR.

Graham, D. I. (1999). Pathophysiological aspects of injury and mechanisms of recovery. In M. Rosenthal, J. S. Kreutzer, E. R. Griffith, & B. Pentland (Eds.), *Rehabilitation of the adult and child with traumatic brain injury* (3rd ed., pp. 19–41). Philadelphia: F. A. Davis.

Graham, D., I., Adams, J. H., Nicoll, J. A. R., Maxwell, W. L., & Gennarelli, T. A. (1995). The nature, distribution, and causes of traumatic brain injury. *Brain Pathology, 4,* 397–406.

Grant, D. A., & Berg, E. A. (1993). *Wisconsin card sorting test.* Tampa, FL: Psychological Assessment Resources.

Grayson, E., Hilton, R., & Franklin, S. (1997). Early intervention in a case of jargon aphasia: Efficacy of language comprehension therapy. *European Journal of Disorders of Communication, 32,* 257–276.

Grealy, M. A., Johnson, D. A., & Rushton, S. K. (1999). Improving cognitive function after brain injury: The use of exercise and virtual reality. *Archives of Physical Medicine and Rehabilitation, 80,* 661–667.

Greenberg, D., & Veraellie, M. (2010). Interdependence of episodic and semantic memory: Evidence from neuropsychology. *Journal of the International Neuropsychological Society, 16,* 748–753.

Greenberg, L. (2011). *Test of variables of attention, Version 8.* Los Alamitos, CA: TOVA.

Greenwald, B., Kapoor, N., & Singh, A. (2012). Visual impairments in the first year after traumatic brain injury. *Brain Injury, 26*(11), 1338–1359.

Greenwald, M. (2004). "Blocking" lexical competitors in severe global agraphia: A treatment of reading and spelling. *Neurocase, 10*(2), 156–174.

Greenwald, M. L., & Gonzalez Rothi, L. J. (1998). Lexical access via letter naming in a profoundly alexic and anomic patient: A treatment study. *Journal of the International Neuropsychological Society, 4,* 595–607.

Grice, H. P. (1975). Logic and conversation. In P. Cole & J. Morgan (Eds.), *Studies in syntax and semantics: Vol. 3. Speech acts* (pp. 41–58). New York: Academic Press.

Griffin, R., Friedman, O., Ween, J., Winner, E., Happé, F., & Brownell, H. (2006). Theory of mind and the right cerebral hemisphere: Refining the scope of impairment. *Laterality: Asymmetries of Body, Brain and Cognition, 11,* 195–225.

Griffin, S. L., van Reekum, R., & Masanic, C. (2003). A review of cholinergic agents in the treatment of neurobehavioral deficits following traumatic brain injury. *Journal of Neuropsychiatry and Clinical Neuroscience, 15,* 17–26.

Grilli, M., & McFarland, C. (2011). Imagine that: Self-imagination improves prospective memory in memory-impaired individuals with neurological damage. *Neuropsychological Rehabilitation, 21*(6), 847–859.

Grodzinsky, Y. (1984). The syntactic characterization of agrammatism. *Cognition, 16,* 99–120.

Guilford, J. (1967). *The nature of human intelligence.* New York: McGraw-Hill.

Gronwall, D. (1977). Paced Auditory Serial Addition Test: A measure of recovery from concussion. *Perceptual and Motor Skills, 44,* 367–373.

Grossi, D., Lepore, M., Napolitano, A., & Trojano, L. (2001). On selective left neglect during walking in a child. *Brain and Cognition, 47,* 539–544.

Grossman, M., Libon, D., Forman, M., Massimo, L., Wood, E., Moore, P., . . . Trojanowski, J. Q. (2007). Distinct neuropsychological profiles in pathologically defined patients with frontotemporal lobe dementia. *Archives of Neurology, 64,* 1601–1609.

Grossman, M., Xie, S., Libon, D., Wang, X., Massimo, L., Moore, P., . . . Trojanowski, J. Q. (2008). Longitudinal decline in autopsy-defined frontotemporal lobar degeneration. *Neurology, 70,* 2036–2045.

Groves-Wright, K., Neils-Strunjas, J., Burnett, R., & O'Neill, M. J. (2004). A comparison of verbal and written language in Alzheimer's disease. *Journal of Communication Disorders, 37,* 109–130.

Guétin, S., Portet, F., Picot, M. C., Pommié, C., Messaoudi, M., Djabelkir, L., . . . Touchon, J. (2009). Effect of music therapy on anxiety and depression in patients with Alzheimer's type dementia: Randomised, controlled study. *Dementia and Geriatric Cognitive Disorders, 28*(1), 36–46.

Guilford, J. P., & Hoepfner, R. (1971). *The analysis of intelligence.* New York: McGraw-Hill.

Guitton, D., Buchtel, H. A., & Douglas, R. M. (1985). Frontal lobe lesions in man cause difficulties in suppressing reflexive glances and in generating goal-directed saccades. *Experimental Brain Research, 58,* 455–472.

Güngör, L., Terzi, M., & Onar, M. K. (2011). Does long term use of piracetam improve speech disturbances due to ischemic cerebrovascular diseases? *Brain and Language, 117*, 23–27.

Gupta, S. R., & Mlcoch, A. G. (1992). Bromocriptine treatment of nonfluent aphasia. *Archives of Physical Medicine and Rehabilitation, 73*, 373–376.

Gurland, G. B., Chwat, S. E., & Wollner, S. G. (1982). Establishing a communication profile in adult aphasia: Analysis of communicative acts and conversation consequences. *Clinical Aphasiology, 12*, 97–112.

Gustafson, M. (2006). *No-glamour sentence structure interactive software.* East Moline, IL: Linguisystems.

Guyatt, G., Haynes, B., Jaeschke, R., Meade, M., Wilson, M., Montori, V., & Richardson, S. (2008). The philosophy of evidence-based medicine. In G. Guyatt, D. Rennie, M. Meade, & D. Cook (Eds.), *Users' guides to the medical literature: A manual for evidence-based clinical practice* (2nd ed., pp. 9–16). Chicago: American Medical Association Press.

Guyatt, G. H., Sinclair, J., Cook, D. J., & Glasziou, P. (1999). Users' guides to the medical literature: XVI. How to use a treatment recommendation. *Journal of the American Medical Association, 281*, 1836–1843.

Haaland, K. Y., Vranes, L. F., Goodwin, J. S., & Garry, P. J. (1987). Wisconsin Card Sort Test in a healthy elderly population. *Journal of Gerontology, 42*, 345–346.

Hadjiev, D. I., & Mineva, P. P. (2007). A reappraisal of the definition and pathophysiology of the transient ischemic attack. *Medical Science Monitor, 13*(3), RA50–53.

Hagen, C. (1981). Language disorders secondary to closed head injury. *Topics in Language Disorders, 1*, 73–87.

Hall, K. M., Bushnik, T., Lakisic-Kazazic, B., Wright, J., & Cantagallo, A. (2001). Assessing traumatic brain injury outcome measures for long-term follow-up of community-based individuals. *Archives of Physical Medicine and Rehabilitation, 82*(3), 367–374.

Hall, K. S, Ogunniyi, A. O, Hendrie, H. C., & Brittain, H. M. (1996). A cross cultural community based study of dementias: Methods and performance of the survey instrument Indianapolis, U.S.A., and Ibadan, Nigeria. *International Journal of Methods in Psychiatric Research, 6*, 1–14.

Halliday, M. A. K. (1994). *An introduction to functional grammar* (2nd ed.). London: Edward Arnold.

Hallowell, B., & Chapey, R. (2008). Introduction to language intervention strategies in adult aphasia. In R. Chapey (Ed.), *Language intervention strategies in aphasia and related neurogenic communication disorders* (5th ed., pp. 3–19). New York: Lippincott, Williams, and Wilkins.

Halper, A. S., Cherney, L. R., Burns, M. S., & Mogil, S. I. (1996). *Clinical management of right hemisphere dysfunction* (2nd ed.). Rockville, MD: Aspen.

Halper, A. S., Cherney, L. R., Drimmer, D. P., & Chang, O. (1996). Right hemisphere stroke: Performance trends on word list recall and recognition. *Archives of Physical Medicine and Rehabilitation, 77*, 837.

Hama, S., Yamashita, H., Shigenobu, M., Watanabe, A., Hiramoto, K., Kurisu, K., . . . Kitaoka, T. (2007). Depression or apathy and functional recovery after stroke. *International Journal of Geriatric Psychiatry, 22*(10), 1046–1051.

Hamberger, M. J., & Seidel, W. T. (2003). Auditory and visual naming tests: Normative and patient data for accuracy, response time, and tip-of-the-tongue. *Journal of the International Neuropsychological Society, 9*, 479–489.

Hamer, M., & Chida, Y. (2009). Physical activity and risk of neurodegenerative disease: A systematic review of prospective evidence. *Psychological Medicine, 39*(01), 3–11.

Hamilton, M. (1959). The assessment of anxiety states by rating. *British Journal of Medical Psychology, 32*, 50–55.

Hamilton, M. (1960). A rating scale for depression. *Journal of Neurology, Neurosurgery, and Psychiatry, 23*, 56–62.

Hamilton, R. H., Coslett, H. B., Buxbaum, L. J., Whyte, J., Farne, A., Frassinetti, F., & Ferraro, M. K. (2008). Inconsistency of performance on neglect subtype tests following acute right hemisphere stroke. *Journal of the International Neuropsychological Society. 14*, 23–32.

Hamilton, R. H., Sanders, L., Benson, J., Faseyitan, O., Norise, C., Naeser M., . . . Coslett, H. B. (2010). Stimulating conversation: Enhancement of elicited propositional speech in a patient with chronic nonfluent aphasia following transcranial magnetic stimulation. *Brain and Language, 113*, 45–50.

Hammill, D. D., Brown, V. L., Larsen, S. C., & Wiederholt, J. L. (2007). *Test of adolescent and adult language* (4th ed.). Austin, TX: PRO-ED.

Hammill, D. D., & Larsen, S. C. (2009). *Test of written language* (4th ed.). Austin, TX: PRO-ED.

Hammill, D. D., Pearson, N. A., & Weiderholt, J. L. (2009). *Comprehensive test of nonverbal intelligence* (2nd ed.). Austin, TX: PRO-ED.

Hanlon, R. E., Brown, J. W., & Gerstman, L. J. (1990). Enhancement of naming in nonfluent aphasia through gesture. *Brain and Language, 38*, 298–314.

Hansen, A., & McNeil, M. (1986). Differences between writing with the dominant and nondominant hand by normal geriatric subjects on a spontaneous writing task: Twenty perceptual and computerized measures. *Clinical Aphasiology, 16*, 116–122.

Happé, F., Brownell, H., & Winner, E. (1999). Acquired "theory of mind" impairments following stroke. *Cognition, 70*, 211–240.

Harbeck-Seu, A., Brunk, I., Platz, T., Vajkoczy, P., Endres, M., & Spies, C. (2011). A speedy recovery: Amphetamines and other therapeutics that might impact the recovery from brain injury. *Current Opinion in Anesthesiology, 24*, 144–153.

Harciarek, M., Beidunkiewica, B., Lichodziejewska-Niemierko, M., Debska-Slizien, A., & Rutkowski, B. (2009). Cognitive performance before and after kidney transplantation: A prospective controlled study of adequately dialyzed patients with end-stage renal disease. *Journal of the International Neuropsychological Society, 15*, 684–694.

Harris, L., Olson, A., & Humphreys, G. (2012). Rehabilitation of past tense verb production and non-canonical sentence production in left inferior frontal non-fluent aphasia. *Aphasiology, 26*(2), 143–161.

Hart, T., Whyte, J., Polansky, M., Millis, S., Hammond, F. M., Sherer, M., . . . Kreutzer, J. (2003). Concordance of patient and family report of neurobehavioral symptoms at 1 year after traumatic brain injury. *Archives of Physical Medicine & Rehabilitation, 84*, 204–213.

Hartley, L. L., (1995). *Cognitive-communicative abilities following brain injury*. San Diego, CA: Singular.

Hartmann, A., Hupp, T., Koch, H. C., Dollinger, P., Stapf, C., Schmidt, R., . . . Mast, H. (1999). Prospective study on the complication rate of carotid surgery. *Cerebrovascular Diseases, 9*, 152–156.

Harvan, J., & Cotter, V. (2006). An evaluation of dementia screening in the primary care setting. *Journal of the American Academy of Nurse Practitioners, 18*(8), 351–360.

Haslam, C., Gilroy, D., Black, S., & Beesley, T. (2006). How successful is errorless learning in supporting memory for high and low-level knowledge in dementia? *Neuropsychological Rehabilitation, 16*(5), 505–536.

Haslam, C., Hodder, K., & Yates, P. (2011). Errorless learning and spaced retrieval: How do these methods fare in healthy and clinical populations? *Journal of Clinical and Experimental Neuropsychology, 33*(4), 432–447.

Haslam, C., Holme, A, Haslam, S., Iyer, A., Jetten, J., & Williams, W. (2008). Maintaining group memberships: Social idenitify continuity predicts well-being after stroke. *Neuropsychological Rehabilitation, 18*(5–6), 671–691.

Hawkins, K. A., & Bender, S. (2002). Norms and the relationship of Boston Naming Test performance to vocabulary and education: A review. *Aphasiology, 16*, 1143–1153.

Hawley, L., & Newman, J. (2010). Group Interactive Structured Treatment (GIST): A social competence intervention for individuals with brain injury. *Brain Injury, 24*(11), 1292–1297

Health Insurance Portability and Accountability Act of 1996 (HIPAA), 42 U.S.C. § 300gg *et seq.* (1996)

Heaton, R. K., Franklin, D., Ellis, R., McCutchan, J. A., Letendre, S., LeBlanc, S., . . . Grant, I. (2011). HIV-associated neurocognitive disorders before and during the era of combination antiretroviral therapy: Differences in rates, nature, and predictors. *Journal of Neurovirology, 17*, 3–16.

Hebert, L. E., Scherr, P. A., Bienias, J. L., Bennett, D. A., & Evans, D. A. (2003). Alzheimer's disease in the U.S. population: Prevalence estimates using the 2000 Census. *Archives of Neurology, 60*(8), 1119–1122.

Heeschen, C., & Kolk, H. (1988). Agrammatism and paragrammatism. *Aphasiology, 2*, 299–302.

Heilman, K. M., Rothi, L., Campanella, D., & Wolfson, S. (1979). Wernicke's and global aphasia without alexia. *Archives of Neurology, 36*, 129–133.

Heisters, D. (2011). Parkinson's: Symptoms, treatments and research. *British Journal of Nursing, 20*(9), 548–554.

Hellstrom, I., Nolan, M., Nordenfelt, L., & Lundh, U. (2007). Ethical and methodological issues in interviewing persons with dementia. *Nursing Ethics, 14*(5), 608–619.

Helm, N. A., & Barresi, B. (1980). Voluntary control of involuntary utterances: A treatment approach for severe aphasia. *Clinical Aphasiology, 10*, 308–315.

Helm-Estabrooks, N. (1981). *Helm elicited language program for syntax stimulation.* Austin, TX: PRO-ED.

Helm-Estabrooks, N. (1991). *Test of oral and limb apraxia.* Austin, TX: PRO-ED.

Helm-Estabrooks, N. (2001). *Cognitive linguistic quick test.* San Antonio, TX: Psychological Corporation.

Helm-Estabrooks, N. (2002). Cognition and aphasia: A discussion and a study. *Journal of Communication Disorders, 35,* 171–186.

Helm-Estabrooks, N., & Albert, M. L. (1991). *Manual of aphasia therapy.* Austin, TX: PRO-ED.

Helm-Estabrooks, N., & Albert, M. L. (2004). *Manual of aphasia and aphasia therapy* (2nd ed.). Austin, TX: PRO-ED.

Helm-Estabrooks, N., Albert, M., & Nicholas, M. (in press). *Manual of aphasia and aphasia therapy* (3rd ed.) Austin, TX: PRO-ED.

Helm-Estabrooks, N., Emery, P., & Albert, M. L. (1987). Treatment of Aphasic Perseveration (TAP) program: A new approach to aphasia therapy. *Archives of Neurology, 44,* 1253–1255.

Helm-Estabrooks, N., Fitzpatrick, P. M., & Barresi, B. (1981). Response of an agrammatic patient to a syntax stimulation program for aphasia. *Journal of Speech and Hearing Disorders, 46,* 422–427.

Helm-Estabrooks, N., Fitzpatrick, R., & Barresi, B. (1982). Visual Action Therapy for global aphasia. *Journal of Speech and Hearing Disorders, 44,* 385–389.

Helm-Estabrooks, N., & Hotz, G. (1991). *Brief test of head injury.* Austin, TX: PRO-ED.

Helm-Estabrooks, N., & Nicholas, M. (2000). *Sentence production program for aphasia.* Austin, TX: PRO-ED.

Helm-Estabrooks, N., & Nicholas, M. (2003). *Narrative story cards.* Austin, TX: PRO-ED.

Helm-Estabrooks, N., Nicholas, M., & Morgan, A. (1989). *Melodic intonation therapy program.* Austin, TX: PRO-ED.

Helm-Estabrooks, N., & Ramsberger, G. (1986a). Aphasia treatment delivered by telephone. *Archives of Physical Medicine and Rehabilitation, 67,* 51–53.

Helm-Estabrooks, N., & Ramsberger, G. (1986b). Treatment of agrammatism in long-term Broca's aphasia. *British Journal of Disorders of Communication, 21,* 39–45.

Helm-Estabrooks, N., Ramsberger, G., Morgan, A. R., & Nicholas, M. (1989). *Boston assessment of severe aphasia.* Austin, TX: PRO-ED.

Henderson, L. W., Frank, E. M., Pigatt, T., Abramson, R. K., & Houston, M. (1998). Race, gender, and educational level effects on Boston Naming Test scores. *Aphasiology, 12,* 901–911.

Hengst, J. A., Frame, S. R., Neuman-Stritzel. T., & Gannaway, R. (2005). Using others' words: Conversational use of reported speech by individuals with aphasia and their communication partners. *Journal of Speech, Language, and Hearing Research, 48,* 137–156.

Henke, K. (2010). A model for memory systems based on processing modes rather than consciousness. *Nature Reviews: Neuroscience, 11,* 523–532.

Henry, M. L., Beeson, P. M., & Rapcsak, S. Z. (2008). Treatment for lexical retrieval in progressive aphasia. *Aphasiology, 22*(7/8), 826–838.

Herbert, R., Hickin, J., Howard, D., Osborne, F., & Best, W. (2008). Do picture-naming tests provide a valid assessment of lexical retrieval in conversation in aphasia. *Aphasiology, 22*(2), 184–204.

Herrera, C., Chambon, C., Michel, B., Paban, V., & Alescio-Lautier, B. (2012). Positive effects of computer-based cognitive training in adults with mild cognitive impairment. *Neuropsychologia.* Retrieved from http://dx.doi.org/10.1016/j.neuropsychologia.2012.04.012

Herz, E., Hearne, J., Stone-Axelrad, J., Tritz, K., Baumrucker, E., Scott, C., . . . Rimkunas, R. (2005). *How Medicaid works: Program basics* (RL32277). Washington, DC: Congressional Research Service.

Heuer, S., & Hallowell, B. (2007). An evaluation of multiple-choice test images for comprehension assessment in aphasia. *Aphasiology, 21,* 883–900.

Hewitt, J., Evans, J. J., & Dritschel, B. (2006). Theory driven rehabilitation of executive functioning: Improving planning skills in people with traumatic brain injury through the use of an autobiographical episodic memory cueing procedure. *Neuropsychologia, 44*(8), 1468–1474.

Hickey, E. M., & Bourgeois, M. S. (2003). Beyond swallowing: Communication intervention in nursing homes. *Special Interest Division 2: Neurophysiology and Neurogenic Speech and Language Disorders Newsletter, 13,* 5–9.

Hickey, E. M., & Saunders, J. (2010). Group intervention for adolescents with chronic acquired brain injury: The Future Zone. *Perspectives on Neurophysiological and Neurogenic Speech and Language Disorders, 20*(4), 47–57.

Hickey, E. M., Bourgeois, M. S., & Olswang, L. B. (2004). Effects of training volunteers to converse with nursing home residents with aphasia. *Aphasiology, 5–7*, 625–637.

Hier, D. B., Mondlock, J., & Caplan, L. R. (1983). Recovery of behavioural abnormalities after right hemisphere stroke. *Neurology, 33*, 345–350.

Highnman, C. L., & Bleile, K. (2011). Language in the cerebellum. *American Journal of Speech-Language Pathology, 20*, 337–347.

Hilari, K., Byng, S., Lamping, D. L., & Smith, S. C. (2003). Stroke and Aphasia Quality of Life Scale–39 (SAQLS-39): Evaluation of acceptability, reliability, and validity. *Stroke, 34*, 1944–1950.

Hilari, K., Needle, J. J., & Harrison, K. L. (2012). What are the important factors in health-related quality of life for people with aphasia? A aystematic review. *Archives of Physical Medicine and Rehabilitation, 93*(1), S86–S95.

Hilari, K., Owen, S., & Farrelly, S. J. (2007). Proxy and self-report agreement on the Stroke and Aphasia Quality of Life Scale–39. *Journal of Neurology, Neurosurgery, and Psychiatry, 78*(10), 1072–1075.

Hillis, A. E. (1991). Effects of separate treatments for distinct impairments within the naming process. *Clinical Aphasiology, 19*, 255–265.

Hillis, A. E. (1993). The role of models of language processing in rehabilitation of language impairments. *Aphasiology, 7*, 5–26.

Hillis, A. E. (2008). Cognitive processes underlying reading and writing and their neural substrates. *Handbook of Clinical Neurology, 88*, 311–322.

Hillis, A. E., Barker, P. B., Wityk, R. J., Aldrich, E. M., Restrepo, L., Breese, E. L., . . . Work, M. (2004). Variability in subcortical aphasia is due to variable sites of cortical hypoperfusion. *Brain and Language, 89*, 524–530.

Hillis, A. E., & Caramazza, A. (1994). Theories of lexical processing and rehabilitation of lexical deficits. In M. Riddoch & G. W. Humphreys (Eds.), *Cognitive neuropsychology and cognitive rehabilitation* (pp. 449–484). Hillsdale, NJ: Erlbaum.

Hinckley, J. J. (1998). Investigating the predictors of lifestyle satisfaction among younger adults with chronic aphasia. *Aphasiology, 12*, 509–518.

Hinckley, J. J. (2000). Effective tools for family education. *Advance for Speech-Language Pathologists & Audiologists, 16*.

Hird, K., & Kirsner, K. (2003). The effect of right cerebral hemisphere damage on collaborative planning in conversation: An analysis of intentional structure. *Clinical Linguistics and Phonetics, 17*(4–5), 309–315.

Hirsch, F. M., & Holland, A. L. (1999). *How can we assess the quality of life of aphasic individuals? A study of five available measures.* Poster presented at the 1999 Clinical Aphasiology Conference, Key West, FL.

Hirsch, F. M., & Holland, A. L. (2000). Beyond activity: Measuring participation in society and quality of life. In L. E. Worrall & C. M. Frattali (Eds.), *Neurogenic communication disorders: A functional approach* (pp. 35–54). New York: Thieme.

Hochstadt, J., Nakano, H., Lieberman, P., & Friedman, J. (2006). The roles of sequencing and verbal working memory in sentence comprehension deficits in Parkinson's disease. *Brain and Language, 97*, 243–257.

Hodgson, C., & Lambon Ralph, M. (2008). Mimicking aphasic semantic errors in normal speech production: Evidence from a novel experimental paradigm. *Brain and Language, 104*, 89–101.

Hoerster, L., Hickey, E., & Bourgeois, M. (2001). Effects of memory aids on conversations between nursing home residents with dementia and nursing assistants. *Neuropsychological Rehabilitation, 11*, 399–427.

Hoffer, M. E., Balaban, C., Gottschall, K., Balough, B., Maddox, M., & Penta, J. (2010). Blast exposure vestibular consequences and associated characteristics. *Otology and Neurotology, 31*, 232–236.

Hoffman, P., Rogers, T., & Lambon Ralph, M. (2011). Semantic diversity accounts for the "missing" word frequency effect in stroke aphasia: Insights using a novel method to quantify contextual variability in meaning. *Journal of Cognitive Neuroscience, 23*(9), 2432–2446.

Holdsworth, S., & Bammer, R. (2008). Magnetic resonance imaging techniques: fMRI, DWI, and PWI. *Seminars in Neurology, 28*, 395–406.

Holland, A. L. (1980). *Communicative abilities in daily living.* Austin, TX: PRO-ED.

Holland, A. L. (1991). Pragmatic aspects of intervention in aphasia. *Journal of Neurolinguistics, 6*(2), 197–211.

Holland, A. L. (1996). Pragmatic assessment and treatment for aphasia. In G. L. Wallace (Ed.), *Adult aphasia rehabilitation* (pp. 161–173). Boston: Butterworth-Heinemann.

Holland, A. L. (2007). *Counseling in communication disorders: A wellness perspective.* San Diego, CA: Plural.

Holland, A. L., & Beeson, P. M. (1999). Aphasia groups: The Arizona experience. In R. J. Elman (Ed.), *Group treatment of neurogenic communication disorders: The expert clinician's approach* (pp. 77–83). Boston: Butterworth-Heinemann.

Holland, A. L., Fratalli, C. M., & Fromm, D. (1999). *Communication activities of daily living* (2nd ed.). Austin, TX: PRO-ED.

Holland, A. L., & Fridriksson, J. (2001). Aphasia management during the early phases of recovery following stroke. *American Journal of Speech-Language Pathology, 10,* 19–28.

Holland, A. L., Greenhouse, J., Fromm, D., & Swindell, C. S. (1989). Predictors of language restitution following stroke: A multivariate analysis. *Journal of Speech and Hearing Research, 32,* 232–238.

Holland, A. L., & Hinckley, J. J. (2002). Assessment and treatment of pragmatic aspects of communication in aphasia. In A. E. Hillis (Ed.), *The handbook of adult language disorders: Integrating cognitive neuropsychology, neurology, and rehabilitation* (pp. 413–427). New York: Psychology Press.

Holland, D., Witty, T., Lawler, J., & Lanzisera, D. (1999). Biofeedback-assisted relaxation training with brain injured patients in acute stages of recovery. *Brain Injury, 13,* 53–57.

Holtzapple, P., Pohlman, K., LaPointe, L. L., & Graham, L. F. (1989). Does SPICA mean PICA? *Clinical Aphasiology, 18,* 131–144.

Holtzer, R., Burright, R. G., & Donovick, P. J. (2004). The sensitivity of dual-task performance to cognitive status in aging. *Journal of the International Neuropsychology Society, 10,* 230–238.

Hoofien, D., Gilboa, A., Vakil, E., & Barak, O. (2004). Unawareness of cognitive deficits and daily functioning among persons with traumatic brain injuries. *Journal of Clinical and Experimental Neuropsychology, 26,* 278–290.

Hooper, H. E. (1983). *Hooper visual organization test.* Los Angeles: Western Psychological Services.

Hoppe, C., & Elger, C. (2011). Depression in epilepsy: A critical review from a clinical perspective. *Nature Reviews: Neurology, 7*(8), 462–472.

Hopper, T. (2007). The ICF and dementia. *Seminars in Speech and Language, 28*(4), 273–282.

Hopper, T., Bayles, K. A., Harris, F., & Holland, A. (2001). The relationship between Minimum Data Set ratings and scores on measures of communication and hearing among nursing home residents with dementia. *American Journal of Speech-Language Pathology, 10,* 370–381.

Hopper, T., Drefs, S., Bayles, K., Tomoeda, C., & Dinu, I. (2010). The effects of modified spaced-retrieval training on learning and retention of face-name associations by individuals with dementia. *Neuropsychological Rehabilitation, 20*(1), 81–102.

Horn, S., Gassaway, J., Pentz, L., & James, R. (2010). Practice-based evidence for clinical practice improvement: An alternative study design for evidence-based medicine. *Studies in Health Technology & Informatics, 151,* 446–460.

Hotz, G. A., Helm-Estabrooks, N., Nelson, N. W., & Plante, E. (2010). *The pediatric test of brain injury.* Baltimore: Brookes.

Hough, M. S. (1993). Treatment of Wernicke's aphasia with jargon: A case study. *Journal of Communication Disorders, 26,* 101–111.

Hough, M. S. (2010). Melodic Intonation Therapy and aphasia: Another variation on a theme. *Aphasiology, 24*(6–8), 775–786.

Hough, M. S., DeMarco, S., & Schmitzer, A. B. (1997). *Episodes of word retrieval failures after right hemisphere brain-damage.* Paper presented at the annual conference of the American Speech-Language-Hearing Association, Boston, MA.

Hough, M. S., & Johnson, R. K. (2009). Use of AAC to enhance linguistic communication skills in an adult with chronic severe aphasia. *Aphasiology, 23*(7–8), 965–976.

Howard, D., & Patterson, K. E. (1992). *Pyramids and palm trees.* Bury St. Edmunds, Suffolk, England: Thames Valley Test Company.

Howard, R. S. (2008). Coma and stupor. *Handbook of Clinical Neurology, 90,* 57–78.

Howe, T. J., Worrall, L. E., & Hickson, L. M. H. (2008). Interviews with people with aphasia: Environmental factors that influence their community participation. *Aphasiology, 22*(10), 1092–1120.

Howland, R. (2011). Alternative drug therapies for dementia. *Journal of Psychosocial Nursing, 49*(5), 17–20.

Hua, M., Chang, S., & Chen, S. (1997). Factor structure and age effects with an aphasia test battery in normal Taiwanese adults. *Neuropsychology, 11*, 156–162.

Huber, W., Poeck, K., Weniger, D., & Willmes, K. (1983). *Der aachener aphasie test*. Gottingen, Germany: Hogrefe.

Huber, W., Poeck, K., & Willmes, K. (1984). The Aachen Aphasia Test. In F. C. Rose (Ed.), *Progress in aphasiology*. New York: Raven Press.

Huber, W., Willmes, K., Poeck, K., Van Vleymen, B., & Deberdt, W. (1997). Piracetam in aphasia: A double-blind study. *Archives of Physical Medicine and Rehabilitation, 72*, 245–250.

Huckans, M., Pavawalla, S., Demadura, T., Kolessar, M., Seelye, A., Roost, N., . . . Storzbach, D. (2010). A pilot study examining effects of group-based Cognitive Strategy Training treatment on self-reported cognitive problems, psychiatric symptoms, functioning, and compensatory strategy use in OIF/OEF combat veterans with persistent mild cognitive disorder and history of traumatic brain injury. *Journal of Rehabilitation Research and Development, 47*(1), 43–60.

Huff, C. (2011). Does your patient really understand? *Hospital Health Network, 85*(10), 34–35, 37–38.

Hughes, J. D., Jacobs, D. H., & Heilman, K. M. (2000). Neuropharmacology and linguistic neuroplasticity. *Brain and Language, 71*, 96–101.

Hula, W. D., Donovan, N., Kendall, D., & Gonzalez Rothi, L. (2010). Item response theory analysis of the Western Aphasia Battery. *Aphasiology, 24*, 1326–1341.

Hula, W. D., Doyle, P. J., & Austermann Hula, S. N. (2010). Patient-reported cognitive and communicative functioning: 1 construct or 2? *Archives of Physical Medicine and Rehabilitation, 91*(3), 400–406.

Hula, W. D., Doyle, P. J., McNeil, M. R., & Mikolic, J. (2006). Rasch modeling of Revised Token Test performance: Validity and sensitivity to change. *Journal of Speech, Language & Hearing Research, 49*(1), 27–46.

Hula, W. D., McNeil, M. R., & Sung, J. E. (2007). Is there an impairment of language-specific attention processing in aphasia? *Brain and Language, 103*, 240–241.

Humphreys, G., Bickerton, W., Samson, D., & Riddoch, M. J. (2012). *Birmingham cognitive screen (BCoS)*. Hove, East Sussex, England: Psychology Press.

Hunkin, N. M., Squires, E. J., Aldrich, F. K., & Parkin, A. J. (1998). Errorless learning and the acquisition of word processing skills. *Neuropsychological Rehabilitation, 8*, 433–449.

Hunter, C. E., Ward, L., & Camp, C. (2012). Transitioning spaced retrieval training to care staff in an Australian residential aged care setting for older adults with dementia: A case study approach. *Clinical Gerontologist, 35*(1), 1–14.

Hurford, P., Stringer, A. Y., & Jann, B. (1998). Neuropharmacologic treatment of hemineglect: A case report comparing bromocriptine and methylphenidate. *Archives of Physical Medicine and Rehabilitation, 79*, 346–349.

Hurkmans, J., de Bruijn, M., Boonstra, A., Jonkers, R., Bastiaanse, R., . . . Reinders-Messelink, H. (2012). Music in the treatment of neurological language and speech disorders: A systematic review. *Aphasiology, 26*(1), 1–19.

Hurtig, R., & Downey, D. (2009). *Augmentative and alternative communication in acute and critical care settings*. San Diego, CA: Plural.

Hutchinson, N., & Oakes, P. (2011). Further evaluation of the criterion validity of the Severe Impairment Battery for the assessment of cognitive functioning in adults with Down Syndrome. *Journal of Applied Research in Intellectual Disabilities, 24*(2), 172–180.

Iliffe, S., Wilcock, J., & Haworth, D. (2006). Obstacles to shared care for patients with dementia: A qualitative study. *Family Practice, 23*, 353–362.

Ince, L. P. (1968). Desensitization with an aphasic patient. *Behavioral Research & Therapy, 6*, 235–237.

Irvine, A. B., Ary, D. V., & Bourgeois, M. S. (2003). An interactive multimedia program to train professional caregivers. *Journal of Applied Gerontology, 22*(2), 269–288.

Irwin, W., Wertz, R., & Avent, J. (2002). Relationships among language impairment, functional communication, and pragmatic performance in aphasia. *Aphasiology, 16*, 823–835.

Isaacson, J. E., & Rubin, A. M. (1999). Otolaryngologic management of dizziness in the older patient. *Clinics in Geriatric Medicine, 15*, 179–191.

Ishiai, S., Koyama, Y., Seki, K., Orimo, S., Sodeyama, N., Ozawa, E., . . . Hiroki, M. (2000). Unilateral spatial neglect in AD: Significance of line bisection performance. *Neurology, 55*, 364–370.

Isquith, P. D., Roth, R. M., & Gioia, G. A. (2010). *Tasks of executive control*. Lutz, FL: Psychological Assessment Resources.

Jackson, H. H. (1878). On affectations of speech from disease of the brain. *Brain, 1,* 304–330.

Jackson, W. T., Novack, T. A., & Dowler, R. N. (1998). Effective serial measurement of cognitive orientation in rehabilitation: The orientation log. *Archives of Physical Medicine and Rehabilitation, 79,* 718–720.

Jacobs, B. J. (2001). Social validity of changes in informativeness and efficiency of aphasic discourse following Linguistic Specific Treatment (LST). *Brain and Language, 78,* 115–127.

Jacobs, B. J., & Thompson, C. K. (1992, November). *Effects of semantically based training on lexical processing in severe aphasia*. Poster presentation at the annual ASHA Convention, San Antonio, TX.

Jacobs, B. J., & Thompson, C. K. (2000). Cross-modal generalization effects of training noncanonical sentence comprehension and production in agrammatic aphasia. *Journal of Speech, Language, and Hearing Research, 43,* 5–20.

Jacobs, D. H., Adair, J. C., Gold, M., Shuren, J., Williamson, D. J., Gonzalez Rothi, L., & Heilman, K. M. (1994). Physostigmine improves confrontation naming in two patients with anomic aphasia in an open-label, dose-escalating study. *Brain and Language, 47,* 532–535.

James, B., Wilson, R., Barnes, L., & Bennett, D. (2011). Late-life social activity and cognitive decline in old age. *Journal of the International Neuropsychological Society, 17,* 998–1005.

Jefferies, E., Patterson, K., Jones, R. W., & Lambon Ralph, M. A. (2009). Comprehension of concrete and abstract words in semantic dementia. *Neuropsychology, 23*(4), 492–499.

Jehkonen, M., Ahonen, J. P., Dastidar, P., Koivisto, A. M., Laippala, P., Vilkki, J., & Molnár, G. (2000). Visual neglect as a predictor of functional outcome one year after stroke. *Acta Neurologica Scandinavica, 101,* 195–201.

Jehkonen, M., Laihosalo, M., & Kettunen, J. (2006). Anosognosia after stroke: Assessment, occurrence, subtypes and impact on functional outcome reviewed. *Acta Neurologica Scandinavica, 114,* 293–306.

Jenicek, M., Croskerry, P., & Hitchcock, D. L. (2011). Evidence and its uses in health care and research: The role of critical thinking. *Medical Science Monitor, 17*(1), RA12–17. doi: 881321 [pii]

Joanette, Y., Goulet, P., & Hannequin, D. (1990). *Right hemisphere and verbal communication*. New York: Springer-Verlag.

Jodzio, K., Gasecki, D., Drumm, D. A., Lass, P., & Nyka, W. (2003). Neuroanatomical correlates of the post-stroke aphasias studied with cerebral blood flow SPECT scanning. *Medical Science Monitor, 9,* MT32–MT41.

Johns, J. S., Cifu, D. X., Keyser-Marcus, L., Jolles, P. R., & Fratkin, M. J. (1999). Impact of clinically significant heterotopic ossification on functional outcome after traumatic brain injury. *Journal of Head Trauma Rehabilitation, 14,* 269–276.

Johnson, A. F., Valachovic, A. M., & George, K. P. (2006). Speech-language pathology practice in the acute care setting: A consultative approach. In A. F. Johnson & B. H. Jacobson (Eds.), *Medical speech-language pathology: A practitioner's guide* (2nd ed., pp. 284–298). New York: Thieme.

Johnson, D., & Cannizzaro, M. (2009). Sentence comprehension in agrammatic aphasia: History and variability to clinical implications. *Clinical Linguistics and Phonetics, 23*(1), 15–37.

Johnson, F. (1990). *Right hemisphere stroke: A victim reflects on rehabilitative medicine*. Detroit, MI: Wayne State University Press.

Johnson, K., & Bourgeois, M. (1998). Language intervention for patients with dementia attending a respite program. *Special Interest Division 2: Neurophysiology and Neurogenic Speech and Language Disorders Newsletter, 8,* 11–16.

Johnson, N., Rademaker, A., Weintraub, S., Gitelman, D., Wienecke, C., & Mesulam, M. (2010). Pilot trial of memantine in primary progressive aphasia. *Alzheimer Disease and Associated Disorders, 24*(3), 308.

Johnson, P., & LoGiudice, C. (2011). *Spotlight on social skills adolescent* [Computer software]. East Moline, IL: Linguisystems.

Johnston, S. C. (2007). Transient ischemic attack: An update. *Stroke Clinical Updates, 17*(2). Retrieved July 20, 2011 from http://www.stroke.org

Johnstone, B., Childers, M. K., & Hoerner, J. (1998). The effects of normal ageing on neuropsychological functioning following traumatic brain injury. *Brain Injury, 12,* 569–576.

Joint Commission. (2010). *Advancing effective communication, cultural competence, and patient- and family-centered care: A roadmap for hospitals.* Oakbrook Terrace, IL: Author.

Jokel, R., & Anderson, N. D. (2012). Quest for the best: Effects of errorless and active encoding on word re-learning in semantic dementia. *Neuropsychological Rehabilitation, 22*(2), 187–214.

Jokel, R., De Nil, L., & Sharpe, A. (2007). Speech disfluencies in adults with neurogenic stuttering associated with stroke and traumatic brain injury. *Journal of Medical Speech-Language Pathology, 14,* 243–261.

Jokel, R., Rochon, E., & Anderson, N. D. (2010). Errorless learning of computer-generated words in a patient with semantic dementia. *Neuropsychological Rehabilitation, 20*(1), 81–102.

Jordan, L., Bell, L., Bryan, K., Maxim, J., & Axelrod, L. (2000). *Communicate: Evaluation of a training package for carers of older people with communication impairments.* Middlesex: University College London/Middlesex University.

Jorge, R., Starkstein, S., & Robinson, R. (2010). Apathy following stroke. *Canadian Journal of Psychiatry, 55*(6), 350–354.

Jorm, A. F., Christensen, J., Griffiths, K. M., & Rodgers, B. (2002). Effectiveness of complementary and self-help treatments for depression. *Medical Journal of Australia, 176,* S84–S96.

Josephs, A. (1992). *The invaluable guide to life after stroke: An owner's manual.* Milwaukee, WI: Amadeus Press.

Julian, L. J. (2011). Cognitive functioning in multiple sclerosis. *Neurology Clinics, 29,* 507–525.

Kabasawa, H., Matsubara, M., Kamimoto, K., Hibino, H., Banno, T., & Nagia, H. (1994). Effects of bi-femelane hydrochloride on cerebral circulation and metabolism in patients with aphasia. *Clinical Therapeutics, 16,* 471–482.

Kafer, K. L., & Hunter, M. (1997). On testing the face validity of planning/problem-solving tasks in a normal population. *Journal of the International Neuropsychology Society, 3,* 108–119.

Kaga, K., Nakamura, M., Takayama, Y., & Momose, H. (2004). A case of cortical deafness and anarthria. *Acta Oto-Laryngologica, 124,* 202–205.

Kagan, A., Black, S. E., Duchan, J. F., Simmons-Mackie, N., & Square, P. (2001). Training volunteers as conversation partners using "Supported Conversation for Adults with Aphasia" (SCA): A controlled trial. *Journal of Speech, Language, and Hearing Research, 44,* 624–638.

Kagan, A., Simmons-Mackie, N., Rowland, A., Huijbregts, M., Shumway, E., McEwan, S., . . . Sharp, S. (2008). Counting what counts: A framework for capturing real-life outcomes of aphasia intervention. *Aphasiology, 22*(3), 258–280.

Kagan, A., Simmons-MacKie, N., Victor, J. C., Carling-Rowland, A., Hoch, J., Huijbregts, D. Streiner, M., & Mok, A. (2010). *Assessment for living with aphasia.* Toronto, Ontario, Canada: Aphasia Institute.

Kahneman, D. (1973). *Attention and effort.* Englewood Cliffs, NJ: Prentice-Hall.

Kajs-Wyllie, M. (2002). Ritalin revisited: Does it really help in neurological injury? *Journal of Neuroscience Nursing, 34,* 303–313.

Kakuda, W., Abo, M., Kaito, N., Watanabe, M., & Senoo, A. (2010). Functional MRI-based therapeutic rTMS strategy for aphasic stroke patients: A case series pilot study. *International Journal of Neuroscience, 120*(1), 60–66.

Kalbe, E., Reinhold, N., Brand, M., Markowitsch, J. J., & Kessler, J. (2005). A new test battery to assess aphasic disturbances and associated cognitive dysfunctions—German normative data on the Aphasia Check List. *Journal of Clinical and Experimental Neuropsychology, 27,* 779–794.

Kalinyak-Fliszar, M., Kohen, F., & Martin, N. (2011). Remediation of language processing in aphasia: Improving activation and maintenance of linguistic representations in (verbal) short-term memory. *Aphasiology, 25*(10), 1095–1131.

Kalla, T., Downes, J. J., & van den Broek, M. (2001). The pre-exposure technique: Enhancing the effects of errorless learning in the acquisition of face-name associations. *Neuropsychological Rehabilitation, 11,* 1–16.

Kane, M. J., Bleckley, M. K., Conway, A. R. A., & Engle, R. W. (2001). A controlled-attention view of working-memory capacity. *Journal of Experimental Psychology: General, 130,* 169–183.

Kang, E. K., Sohn, H. M., Han, M., Kim, W., Han, T. R., & Paik, N. (2010). Severity of post-stroke aphasia according according to aphasia type and lesion location in Koreans. *Journal of Korean Medical Sciences, 25,* 123–127.

Kaplan, E., Goodglass, H., & Weintraub, S. (1983). *Boston naming test.* Philadelphia: Lea & Febiger.

Kaplan, E., Goodglass, H., & Weintraub, S. (2001). *Boston naming test* (2nd ed.). Philadelphia: Lippincott Williams & Wilkins.

Kaplan, E., Leach, L., Rewilak, D., Richards, B., & Proulx, G. (2000). *Kaplan Baycrest neurocognitive assessment*. San Antonio, TX: Psychological Corporation.

Karnath, H. O. (1994). Subjective body orientation in neglect and the interactive contribution of neck muscle proprioception and vestibular stimulation. *Brain, 117,* 1001–1012.

Kaschel, R., Della Sala, S., Cantagallo, A., Fahlbock, A., Laaksonen, R., & Kazen, M. (2002). Imagery mnemonics for the rehabilitation of memory: A randomized group controlled trial. *Neuropsychological Rehabilitation, 12,* 127–153.

Katz, D. I., Polyak, M., Coughlan, D., Nichols, M., & Roche, A. (2009). Natural history of recovery from brain injury after prolonged disorders of consciousness: Outcome of patients admitted to inpatient rehabilitation with 1–4 year follow-up. *Progress in Brain Research, 177,* 73–88.

Katz, R. C. (2000). The role of computers in the treatment of people with aphasia: Reflections on the past 20 years. *Special Interest Division 2: Neurophysiology and Neurogenic Speech and Language Disorders Newsletter, 10,* 6–10.

Katz, R. C., Hallowell, B., Code, C., Armstrong, E., Roberts, P., Pound, C., & Katz, L. (2000). A multinational comparison of aphasia management practices. *International Journal of Language and Communication Disorders, 35,* 303–314.

Katz, R. C., & Wertz, R. T. (1997). The efficacy of computer-provided reading treatment for chronic aphasic adults. *Journal of Speech, Language, and Hearing Research, 40,* 493–507.

Katzan, I. L., Furlan, A. J., Lloyd, L. E., Frank, J. I., Harper, D. L., Hinchey, J. A., . . . Sila, C. A. (2000). Use of tissue-type plasminogen activator for acute ischemic stroke: The Cleveland area experience. *Journal of the American Medical Association, 283,* 1151–1158.

Kaufer, D. I., Cummings, J. L., Ketchel, P., Smith, V., MacMillan, A., Shelley, T., . . . DeKosky, S. T. (2000). Validation of the NPI-Q, a brief clinical form of The Neuropsychiatric Inventory. *Journal of Neuropsychiatry and Clinical Neuroscience, 12,* 233–239.

Kaufman, A., & Kaufman, N. (2004). *Kaufman brief intelligence test* (2nd ed.). San Antonio, TX: Pearson.

Kauhanen, M.-L., Korpelainen, J. T., Hiltunen, P., Brusin, E., Mononen, H., Maatta, R., . . . Myllylä, V. V. (2000). Aphasia, depression, and non-verbal cognitive impairment in ischaemic stroke. *Cerebrovascular Disease, 10,* 455–461.

Kawano, N., Umegaki, H., Suzuki, Y., Yamamoto, S., Mogi, N., & Iguchi, A. (2010). Effects of educational background on verbal fluency task performance in older adults with Alzheimer's disease and mild cognitive impairment. *International Psychogeriatrics, 22*(6), 995–1002.

Kay, J., Lesser, R., & Coltheart, M. (1996). Psycholinguistic Assessments of Language Processing in Aphasia (PALPA): An introduction. *Aphasiology, 10,* 159–215.

Kay, J., Lesser, R., & Coltheart, M. (1997). *Psycholinguistic assessments of language processing in aphasia.* Hove, East Sussex: Psychology Press.

Kearns, K. P. (1985). Response elaboration training for patient initiated utterances. *Clinical Aphasiology, 14,* 196–204.

Kearns, K., & Elman, R. (2008). Group therapy for aphasia: Theoretical and practical considerations. In R. Chapey (Ed.), *Language intervention strategies in aphasia and related neurogenic communication disorders* (5th ed., pp. 376–400). Philadelphia: Lippincott Williams & Wilkins.

Kearns, K. P., & Scher, G. P. (1989). The generalization of response elaboration training effects. *Clinical Aphasiology, 18,* 223–245.

Keeley, S. P. (2003). *The source for executive function disorders.* East Moline, IL: Linguisystems.

Keenan, J. S., & Brassell, E. G. (1974). A study of factors related to prognosis for individual aphasic patients. *Journal of Speech and Hearing Disorders, 39,* 257–269.

Keil, K.., & Kaszniak, A. W. (2002). Examining executive function in individuals with brain injury: A review. *Aphasiology, 16,* 305–335.

Keith, R. W. (2009). *SCAN-3 tests for auditory processing disorders in adolescents and adults.* San Antonio, TX: Pearson.

Kellogg, C. E., & Morton, N. W. (1999). *Beta III.* San Antonio, TX: Psychological Corporation.

Kemper, S., & Harden, T. (1999). Experimentally disentangling what's beneficial about elderspeak from what's not. *Psychological Aging, 14,* 656–670.

Kempler, D., & Goral, M. (2008). Language and dementia: Neuropsychological aspects. *Annual Review of Applied Linguistics, 28,* 73–90.

Kempler, D., & Goral, M. (2011). A comparison of drill- and communication-based treatment for aphasia. *Aphasiology, 25*(11), 1327–1346.

Kempler, D., Teng, E. L., Taussig, M., & Dick, M. B. (2010). The Common Objects Memory Test (COMT): A simple test with cross-cultural applicability. *Journal of the International Neuropsychology Society, 16*(3), 537–545.

Kendall, D. L., Conway, T. W., Rosenbek, J., & Gonzalez Rothi, L. J. (2003). Phonological rehabilitation of acquired phonologic alexia. *Aphasiology, 17*(11), 1073–1096.

Kendall, D. L., Nadeau, S., Conway, T. W., Fuller, R., Riestra, A., & Gonzalez Rothi, L. J. (2006). Treatability of different components of aphasia: Insights from a case study. *Journal of Rehabilitation Research and Development, 43*(3), 323–336.

Kendall, D. L., Rosenbek, J. C., Heilman, K. M., Conway, T., Klenberg, K., Gonzalez Rothi, L. J., & Nadeau, S. (2008). Phoneme-based rehabilitation of anomia in aphasia. *Brain and Language, 105,* 1–17.

Kennedy, M. R. T. (2000). Topic scenes in conversations with adults with right-hemisphere brain damage. *American Journal of Speech-Language Pathology, 9,* 72–86.

Kennedy, M., Coelho, C., Turkstra, L., Ylvisaker, M., Sohlberg, M. M., Yorkston, K., . . . Kan, P. (2008). Intervention for executive functions after traumatic brain injury: A systematic review, meta-analysis, and clinical recommendations. *Neuropsychological Rehabilitation, 18,* 257–299.

Kennepohl, S., Shore, D., Nabors, N., & Hanks, R. (2004). African American acculturation and neuropsychological test performance following traumatic brain injury. *Journal of the International Neuropsychological Society, 10,* 566–577.

Kent, R. D., Kent, J. F., Duffy, J., & Weismer, G. (1998). The dysarthrias: Speech-voice profiles, related dysfunctions, and neuropathology. *Journal of Medical Speech-Language Pathology, 4,* 165–211.

Kent, R., Weismer, B., Kent, J., & Rosenbek, J. (1989). Toward phonetic intelligibility testing in dysarthria. *Journal of Speech and Hearing Disorders, 54,* 482–499.

Keogh, J. W. L., & MacLeod, R. D. (2012). Body composition, physical fitness, functional performance, quality of life, and fatigue benefits of exercise for prostate cancer patients: A systematic review. *Journal of Pain and Symptom Management, 43*(1), 96–110.

Kerkhoff, G. (2000). Multiple perceptual distortions and their modulation in patients with left visual neglect. *Neuropsychologia, 38,* 1073–1086.

Kerkhoff, G., Keller, I., Artinger, F., Hildebrandt, H., Marquardt, C., Reinhart, S., & Ziegler, W. (2012). Recovery from auditory and visual neglect after optokinetic stimulation with pursuit eye movements: Transient modulation and enduring treatment effects. *Neuropsychologia, 50,* 1164–1177.

Kertesz, A. (1979). *Aphasia and associated disorders: Taxonomy, localization, and recovery.* New York: Grune and Stratton.

Kertesz, A. (1982). *Western aphasia battery.* New York: Grune and Stratton.

Kertesz, A. (2006). *Western aphasia battery–Revised.* San Antonio, TX: Psychological Corporation.

Kertesz, A. (2010). Frontotemporal dementia, Pick's disease. *Ideggyo Gya Szati Szemle, 63*(1–2), 4–12.

Kertesz, A., Davidson, W., & Fox, H. (1997). Frontal behavioral inventory: Diagnostic criteria for frontal lobe dementia. *Canadian Journal of Neurological Sciences, 24,* 29–36.

Kertesz, A., Hillis, A., & Munoz, D. G. (2003). Frontotemporal degeneration, Pick's disease, Pick complex, and Ravel. *Annals of Neurology, 54,* S1–S2.

Kertesz, A., & McCabe, P. (1975). Intelligence and aphasia: Performance of aphasics on Raven's Coloured Progressive Matrices (RCPM). *Brain and Language, 2,* 387–395.

Kertesz, A., Morlog, D., Light, M., Blair, M., Davidson, W., Jesso, S., & Brashear R. (2008). Galantamine in frontotemporal dementia and primary progressive aphasia. *Dementia and Geriatric Cognitive Disorders, 25,* 178–185.

Kessels, R., & de Haan, E. (2003). Implicit learning in memory rehabilitation: A meta-analysis on errorless learning and vanishing cues methods. *Journal of Clinical and Experimental Neuropsychology, 25,* 805–814.

Kessels, R., Nys, G., Brands, A., van den Berg, E., & Van Zandvoort, M., (2006). The modified Location Learning Test: Norms for the assessment of spatial memory function in neuropsychological patients. *Archives of Clinical Neuropsychology, 21,* 841–846.

Kessler, J., Thiel, A., Karbe, H., & Heiss, W. D. (2000). Piracetam improves activated blood flow and facilitates rehabilitation of poststroke aphasic patients. *Stroke, 31*, 2112–2116.

Khan, F., & Curtice, M. (2011). Non-pharmacological management of behavioural symptoms of dementia. *British Journal of Community Nursing, 16*(9), 441–449.

Kiernan, R. J., Mueller, J., & Langston, J. W. (2011). *Cognistat and Cognistat assessment system manual.* Fairfax, CA: Cognistat.

Kim, E., Cleary, S., Hopper, T., Bayles, K., Mahendra, N., Azuma, T., & Rackley, A. (2006). Evidence-based practice recommendations for working with individuals with dementia: Group reminiscence therapy. *Journal of Medical Speech-Language Pathology, 14*(3), xxiii–xxxiv.

Kim, E., Rapcsak, S., Anderson, S., & Beeson, P. (2011). Multimodal alexia: Neuropsychological mechanisms and implications for treatment. *Neuropsychologia, 49*, 3551–3562.

Kim, H., & Na, D. L. (2004). Normative data on the Korean version of the Western Aphasia Battery. *Journal of Clinical and Experimental Neuropsychology, 26*(8), 1011–1020.

Kim, M., & Thompson, C. K. (2004). Verb deficits in Alzheimer's disease and agrammatism: Implications for lexical organization. *Brain & Language, 88*, 1–20.

King, N., & Kirwilliam, S. (2011). Permanent post-concussion symptoms after mild head injury. *Brain Injury, 25*(5), 462–470.

Kinsella, G. J. (1998). Assessment of attention following traumatic brain injury: A review. *Neuropsychological Rehabilitation, 8*, 351–375.

Kiran, S. (2008). Typicality of inanimate category exemplars in aphasia treatment: Further evidence for semantic complexity. *Journal of Speech, Language, and Hearing Research, 51*, 1550–1568.

Kiran, S., Caplan, D., Sandberg, C., Levy, J., Berardino, A., Ascenso, E., . . . Tripodis, Y. (2012). Development of a theoretically based treatment for sentence comprehension deficits in individuals with aphasia. *American Journal of Speech-Language Pathology, 21*, S88–S102.

Kiran, S., & Johnson, L. (2008). Semantic complexity in treatment of naming deficits in aphasia: Evidence from well-defined categories. *American Journal of Speech-Language Pathology, 17*, 389–400.

Kiran, S., Ntourou, K., & Eubank, M. (2007). The effect of typicality on online category verification of inanimate category exemplars in aphasia. *Aphasiology, 21*(9), 844–866.

Kiran, S., Sandberg, C., & Sebastian, R. (2011). Treatment of category generation and retrieval in aphasia: Effect of typicality of category items. *Journal of Speech, Language, and Hearing Research, 54*, 1101–1117.

Kiran, S., & Thompson, C. K. (2003). Effect of typicality on online category verification of animate category exemplars in aphasia. *Brain and Language, 85*(3), 441–450.

Klassman, L. (2011). Therapeutic hypothermia in acute stroke. *Journal of Neuroscience Nursing, 43*(2), 94–103.

Klein, E., & Hahn, S. (2007). *Focus on function: Gaining essential communication skills* (2nd ed.). Austin, TX: PRO-ED.

Klein, L., & Buchanan, J. (2009). Psychometric properties of the Pyramids and Palm Trees Test. *Journal of Clinical and Experimental Neuropsychology, 31*(7), 803–808.

Kleindorfer, D., Xu, Y., & Moomaw, T. (2009). U.S. geographic distribution of rt-PA utilization by hospital for acute ischemic stroke. *Stroke, 40*, 3580–3584.

Knapp, M., Thorgrimsen, L., Patel, A., Spector, A., Hallam, A., Woods, B., & Orrell, M. (2006). Cognitive stimulation therapy for people with dementia: Cost-effectiveness analysis. *British Journal of Psychiatry, 188*, 574–580.

Knauss, D. S. (1998). *Left visual inattention workbook.* San Antonio, TX: Communication Skill Builders.

Knight, J., & Kaplan, E. (Eds.) (2003). *The handbook of Rey-Osterrieth Complex Figure usage: Clinical and research applications.* Lutz, FL: PAR.

Knight, R. G., Titov, N., & Crawford, M. (2006). The effects of distraction on prospective remembering following traumatic brain injury assessed in a simulated naturalistic environment. *Journal of the International Neuropsychological Society, 12*, 8–16.

Knopman, D. S., Knudson, D., Yoes, M. E., & Weiss, D. J. (2000). Development and standardization of a new telephonic cognitive screening test: The Minnesota Cognitive Acuity Screen (MCAS). *Neuropsychiatry, Neuropsychology, & Behavioral Neurology, 13*, 286–296.

Knopman, D. S., & Rubens, A. B. (1986). The validity of computed tomography scan findings for the localization of cerebral functions. *Archives of Neurology, 43*, 328–332.

Knowlton, B., & Foerde, K. (2008). Neural representations of nondeclarative memories. *Current Directions in Psychological Science, 17*(2), 107–111.

Ko, M., Han, S., Park, S., Seo, J., & Kim, Y. (2008). Improvement of visual scanning after DC brain polarization of parietal cortex in stroke patients with spatial neglect. *Neuroscience Letters, 448*, 171–174.

Kocsis, J., & Tessler, A. (2009). Pathology of blast-related brain injury. *Journal of Rehabilitation Research and Development, 46*(6), 667–672.

Koenig-Bruhin, M., & Struder-Eichenberger, F. (2007). Therapy of short-term memory disorders in fluent aphasia: A single case study. *Aphasiology, 21*(5), 448–458.

Kohnert, K. (2004). Cognitive and cognate-based treatments for bilingual aphasia: A case study. *Brain and Language, 91*, 294–302.

Kohnert K. (2009) Cross-language generalization following treatment in bilingual speakers with aphasia: A review. *Seminars in Speech and Language, 30*, 174–186.

Koike, K. J. M., & Asp, C. W. (1981). Tennessee Test of Rhythm and Intonation Patterns. *Journal of Speech and Hearing Disorders, 46*, 81–87.

Kong, A. (2011). The main concept analysis in Cantonese aphasic oral discourse: External validation and monitoring chronic aphasia. *Journal of Speech, Language, and Hearing Research, 54*, 148–159.

Kong, E.-H., Evans, L. K., & Guevara, J. P. (2009). Nonpharmacological intervention for agitation in dementia: A systematic review and meta-analysis. *Aging & Mental Health, 13*(4), 512–520.

Kopelman, M., Thomson, A., Guerrini, I., & Marshall, E. (2009). The Korsakoff sydrome: Clinical aspects, psychology, and treatment. *Alcohol and Alcoholism, 44*(2), 148–154.

Kortte, K., & Hillis, A. E. (2009). Recent advances in the understanding of neglect and anosognosia following right hemisphere stroke. *Current Neurology and Neuroscience Report, 9*(6), 459–465.

Kortte, K., & Hillis, A. E. (2011). Recent trends in rehabilitation interventions for visual neglect and anosognosia for hemiplegia following right hemisphere stroke. *Future Neurology, 6*(1), 33–44.

Kostalova, M., Bartkova, E., Sajgalikova, K., Dolenska, A., Dusek, L., & Benarik, J. (2008). A standardization study of the Czech version of the Mississippi Aphasia Screening Test (MASTcz) in stroke patients and control subjects. *Brain Injury, 22*(10), 793–801.

Koul, R. (2011). *Augmentative and alternative communication for adults with aphasia.* Bingley, UK: Emerald Group.

Koul, R., Corwin, M., & Hayes, S. (2005). Production of graphic symbol sentences by individuals with aphasia: Efficacy of a computer-based augmentative and alternative communication intervention. *Brain and Language, 92*(1), 58–77.

Koul, R., & Van Sickle, A. J. (2010). There is a critical need for controlled data to support evidence based communication interventions in individuals with acquired brain injury, *Evidence-Based Communication Assessment and Intervention, 4*(4), 169–172.

Kounti, F., Tsolaki, M., & Kiosseoglou, G. (2006). Functional Cognitive Assessment Scale (FUCAS): A new scale to assess executive cognitive function in daily life activities in patients with dementia and mild cognitive impairment. *Human Psychopharmacology, 21,* 305–311.

Kovach, C. R. (2000). Sensoristasis and imbalance in persons with dementia. *Journal of Nursing Scholarship, 32,* 379–384.

Krackenfels Jones, D., Pierce, R., Mahoney, M., & Smeach, K. (2007). Effect of familiar content on paragraph comprehension in aphasia. *Aphasiology, 21*(2), 1218–1229.

Kramer, A. M., & Coleman, E. A. (1999). Stroke rehabilitation in nursing homes: How do we measure quality? *Clinics in Geriatric Medicine, 15,* 869–884.

Kramer, M., Chiu, C., Walz, N., Holland, S., Yuan, W., Karunanayaka, P., & Wade, S. (2008). Long-term neural processing of attention following early childhood traumatic brain injury: fMRI and neurobehavioral outcomes. *Journal of the International Neuropsychological Society, 14*(3), 424–435.

Krarup, L. H., Truelsen, T., Gluud, C., Andersen, G., Zeng, X., Kõrv, J., . . . Boysen, G. (2008). Prestroke physical activity is associated with severity and long-term outcome from first-ever stroke. *Neurology, 71*(17), 1313–1318.

Krasuski, J., Horwitz, B., & Rumsey, J. M. (1996). A survey of functional and anatomical neuroimaging techniques. In G. R. Lyon & J. M. Rumsey (Eds.), *Neuroimaging: A window to the neurological foundations of learning and behavior and children* (pp. 25–52). Baltimore: Brookes.

Kraus, J. F., & McArther, D. L. (1996). Epidemiologic aspects of brain injury. *Neurologic Clinics, 14,* 435–450.

Kraus, J. F., & McArthur, D. L. (1999). Incidence and prevalence of, and cost associated with, traumatic brain injury. In M. Rosenthal, J. S. Kreutzer, E. R. Griffith, & B. Pentland (Eds.), *Rehabilitation of the adult and child with traumatic brain injury* (3rd ed., pp. 3–18). Philadelphia: F. A. Davis Company.

Krauss, J. K., & Jankovic, J. (2002). Head injury and post-traumatic movement disorders. *Neurosurgery, 50*, 927–948.

Kremin, H., Perrier, D., De Wilde, M., Dordain, M., Le Bayon, A., Gatignol, P., . . . Arabia, C. (2001). Factors predicting success in picture naming in Alzheimer's disease and primary progressive aphasia. *Brain and Cognition, 46*, 180–183.

Kreutzer, J. S., Seel, R. T., & Marwitz, J. H. (1999*). Neurobehavioral functioning inventory.* San Antonio, TX: Psychological Corporation.

Krishnamoorthy, A., & Craufurd, D. (2011). Treatment of apathy in Huntington's disease and other movement disorders. *Current Treatment Options in Neurology, 13*, 508–519.

Kroenke, K., Spitzer, R., & Williams, J. (2001). The PHQ-9: Validity of a brief depression severity measure. *Journal of General Internal Medicine, 16*(9), 606–613.

Kubat-Silman, A. K., Dagenbach, D., & Absher, J. R. (2002). Patterns of impaired verbal, spatial and object working memory after thalamic lesions. *Brain and Cognition, 50*, 178–193.

Kumar, V. P., & Humphreys, G. W. (2008). The role of semantic knowledge in relearning spellings: Evidence from deep dysgraphia. *Aphasiolgy, 22*(5), 489–504.

Kurland, J., Baldwin, K., & Tauer, C. (2010). Treatment-induced neuroplasticity following intensive naming therapy in a case of chronic Wernicke's aphasia. *Aphasiology, 24*(6–8), 737–751.

Kurland, J., Pulvermuller, F., Silva, N., Burke, K., & Andrianopoulos, M. (2012). Constrained versus unconstrained intensive language therapy in two individuals with chronic, moderate-to-severe aphasia and apraxia of speech: Behavioral and fMRI outcomes. *American Journal of Speech-Language Pathology, 21*, S65-S87.

Laiacona, M., Luzzatti, C., Zonca, G., Guarnaschelli, C., & Capitani, E. (2001). Lexical and semantic factors influencing picture naming in aphasia. *Brain and Cognition, 46*, 184–187.

Lam, L. C. W., Chau, R. C. M., Wong, B. M. L., Fung, A. W. T., Lui, V. W. C., Tam, C. C. W., . . . Chan, W. M. (2011). Interim follow-up of a randomized controlled trial comparing Chinese style mind body (tai chi) and stretching exercises on cognitive function in subjects at risk of progressive cognitive decline. *International Journal of Geriatric Psychiatry, 26*(7), 733–740.

Lambon Ralph, M., Snell, C., Fillengham, J., Conroy, P., & Sage, K. (2010). Predicting the outcome of anomia therapy for people with aphasia post CVA: Both language and cognitive status are key predictors. *Neuropsychological Rehabilitation, 20*(2), 289–305.

Lancioni, G. E., Cuvo, A. J., & O'Reilly, M. F. (2002). Snoezelen: An overview of research with people with developmental disabilities and dementia. *Disability and Rehabilitation, 24*, 175–184.

Landesman, S., & Cooper, P. R. (1982). Infectious complications of head injury. In P. R. Cooper (Ed.), *Head injury* (pp. 343–362). Baltimore: Williams and Wilkins.

Langdon, H. W., & Cheng, L. L. (2002). *Collaborating with interpreters and translators: A guide for communication disorders professionals.* Austin, TX: PRO-ED.

Langenbahn, D., Rath, J., Hradil, A., Litke, D., Tucker, J., & Diller, L. (2008). Poster 8: A new approach to remediating problem-solving deficits in outpatients with moderate-to-severe cognitive impairments. *Archives of Physical Medicine and Rehabilitation, 89*, 1849–2040.

Langhorne, P., & Duncan, P. (2001). Does the organization of postacute stroke care really matter? *Stroke, 32*, 268–274.

Langlois, J. A., Ruthland-Brown, W., & Tomas, K. E. (2004). *Traumatic brain injury in the United States: Emergency department visits, hospitalizations, and deaths.* Atlanta, GA: Centers for Diseases Control and Prevention, National Center of Injury Prevention and Control.

LaPointe, L., & Eisenson, J. (2008). *Examining for aphasia* (4th ed.). Austin, TX: PRO-ED.

LaPointe, L. L., & Horner, J. (1998). *Reading comprehension battery for aphasia* (2nd ed.). Austin, TX: PRO-ED.

Larkins, B. (2007). The application of the ICF in cognitive-communication disorders following traumatic brain injury. *Seminars in Speech and Language, 28*(4), 334–342.

Larner, A. J. (2010). Cholinesterase inhibitors: Beyond Alzheimer's disease. *Expert Review of Neurotherapeutics, 10*, 1699–1706.

Laroi, F. (2003). The family systems approach to treating families of persons with brain injury: A potential collaboration between family therapist and brain injury professional. *Brain Injury, 17*, 175–187.

Laska, A., Bartfai, A., Hellblom, A., Murray, V., & Kahan, T. (2007). Clinical and prognostic properties of standardized and functional aphasia assessments. *Journal of Rehabilitation Medicine, 39*, 387–392.

Laska, A., Kahan, T., Hellblom, A., Murray, V., & von Arbin, M. (2011). A randomized controlled trial on very early speech and language therapy in acute stroke patients with aphasia. *Cerebrovascular Diseases, 1*, 66–74.

Lasker, J. P. (2008). AAC language assessment: Considerations for adults with aphasia. *Perspectives on Augmentative and Alternative Communication, 17*(3), 105–112.

Lasker, J. P., & Garrett, K. L. (2006). Using the Multimodal Communication Screening Test for Persons with Aphasia (MCST-A) to guide the selection of alternative communication strategies for people with aphasia. *Aphasiology, 20*, 217–232.

Lata-Caneda, M. C., Pineiro-Temprano, M., Garcia-Fraga, I., Garcia-Armesto, I., Barrueco-Egido, J., & Meijide-Failde, R. (2009). Spanish adaptation of the Stroke and Aphasia Quality of Life Scale–39 (SAQLS-39). *European Journal of Physical and Rehabilitation Medicine, 45*, 379–384.

Laures, J. S. (2005). Reaction time and accuracy in individuals with aphasia during auditory vigilance tasks. *Brain and Language, 95*(2), 353–357.

Lavin, J. H. (1985). *Stroke: From crisis to victory—A family guide*. New York: Franklin Watts.

Lavretsky, H., Epel, E. S., Siddarth, P., Nazarian, N., Cyr, N. S., Khalsa, D. S., . . . Irwin, M. R. (2012). A pilot study of yogic meditation for family dementia caregivers with depressive symptoms: Effects on mental health, cognition, and telomerase activity. *International Journal of Geriatric Psychiatry*. doi: 10.1002/gps.3790

Lazar, R., & Antoniello, D. (2008). Variability in recovery from aphasia. *Current Neurology and Neuroscience Reports, 8*, 497–502.

Le, K., Coelho, C., Mozeiko, J., & Grafman, J. (2011). Measuring goodness of story narratives. *Journal of Speech, Language, and Hearing Research, 54*, 118–126.

Leblanc, G. G., Meschia, J.F., Stuss, D. T., & Hachinski, V. (2006). Genetics of vascular cognitive impairment: The opportunity and the challenges. *Stroke, 37*, 248–255.

Le Dorze, G., & Brassard, C. (1995). A description of the consequences of aphasia on aphasic persons and their relatives and friends, based on the WHO model of chronic diseases. *Aphasiology, 9*, 239–255.

Lee, A. Y. (2011). Vascular dementia. *Chonnara Medical Journal, 47*, 66–71.

Lee, A., Harris, J., Atkinson, E., & Fowler, M. (2001). Evidence from a line bisection task for visuospatial neglect in left hemiparkinson's disease. *Vision Research, 41*, 2677–2686.

Lee, J. B., Kaye C., & Cherney, L. R. (2009). Conversational script performance in adults with non-fluent aphasia: Treatment intensity and aphasia severity. *Aphasiology, 23*(7–8), 885–897.

Lee, L. (1971). *Northwestern syntax screening test*. Evanston, IL: Northwestern University Press.

Lee, Y.-R., Sung, K.-T., & Kim, Y.-E. (2012). Effects of home-based stress management training on primary caregivers of elderly people with dementia in South Korea. *Dementia, 11*(2), 171–179.

Leemann, B., Laganaro, M., Chetelat-Mabillard, D., & Schnider, A. (2011). Crossover trial of subacute computerized aphasia therapy for anomia with the addition of either levodopa or placebo. *Neurorehabilitation and Neural Repair, 25*(1), 43–47.

Lehman, M. T., & Tompkins, C. A. (1998). Reliability and validity of an auditory working memory measure: Data from elderly and right-hemisphere damaged adults. *Aphasiology, 12*, 771–785.

Lehman Blake, M. (2003). Affective language and humor appreciation after right hemisphere brain damage. *Seminars in Speech and Language, 24*, 107–119.

Lehman Blake, M. L. (2007). Perspectives on treatment for communication deficits associated with right hemisphere brain damage. *American Journal of Speech-Language Pathology, 16*(4), 331–342.

Lehman Blake, M., Duffy, J. R., Myers, P. S., & Tompkins, C. A. (2002). Prevalence and patterns of right hemisphere cognitive/communicative deficits: Retrospective data from an inpatient rehabilitation unit. *Aphasiology, 16*, 537–547.

Leischner, A. (1996). Word class effects upon the intrahemispheric graphic disconnection syndrome. *Aphasiology, 10*, 443–451.

Leng, T. R., Woodward, M. J., Stokes, M. J., Swan, A. V., Wareing, L., & Baker, R. (2003). Effects of multisensory stimulation in people with Huntington's disease: A randomized controlled pilot study. *Clinical Rehabilitation, 17*, 30–41.

Leon, S. A., Rosenbek, J. C., Crucian, G. P., Hieber, B., Holiway, B., Rodriguez, A. D., . . . Gonzalez Rothi, L. (2005). Active treatments for aprosodia secondary to right hemisphere stroke. *Journal of Rehabilitation Research and Development, 41*(1), 93–102.

Leritz, E. C., McGlinchey, R. E., Lundgren, K., Grande, L. J., & Milberg, W. P. (2008). Using lexical familiarity judgments to assess verbally mediated intelligence in aphasia. *Neuropsychology, 22*(6), 687–696.

Lesniak, M., Bak, T., Czepiel, W., Seniow, J., & Czlonkowska, A. (2008). Frequency and prognostic values of cognitive disorders in stroke patients. *Dementia and Geriatric Cognitive Disorders, 26*, 356–363.

Lesser, R. (1990). Superior oral to written spelling: Evidence for separate buffers? *Cognitive Neuropsychology, 7*, 347–366.

Levin, H. S., O'Donnell, V. M., & Grossman, R. G. (1979). The Galveston Orientation and Amnesia Test: A practical scale to assess cognition after head injury. *Journal of Nervous and Mental Disease, 167*, 675–684.

Levine, B., Robertson, I. H., Clare, L., Carter, G., Hong, J., Wilson, B. A., . . . Stuss, D. (2000). Rehabilitation of executive functioning: An experimental-clinical validation of Goal Management Training. *Journal of the International Neuropsychological Society, 6*, 299–312.

Levine, D., & Langa, K. (2011). Vascular cognitive impairment: Disease mechanisms and therapeutic implications. *Neurotherapeutics, 8*, 361–373.

Lew, H. L., Poole, J. H., Guillory, S. B., Salerno, R. M., Leskin, G., & Sigford, B. (2006). Persistent problems after traumatic brain injury: The need for long-term follow-up and coordinated care. *Journal of Rehabilitation Research and Development, 43*(2), vii–x.

Lewis, M. S., Lilly, D. J., Hutter, M., Bourdette, D. N., Saunders, J., & Fausti, S. A. (2006). Some effects of multiple sclerosis on speech perception in noise: Preliminary findings. *Journal of Rehabilitation Research and Development, 43*(1), 91–98.

Lezak, M. D., Howieson, D., & Loring, D. (2004). *Neuropsychological assessment* (4th ed.). New York: Oxford University Press.

Li, E. C., Kitselman, K., Dusatko, D., & Spinelli, C. (1988). The efficacy of PACE in remediation of naming deficits. *Journal of Communication Disorders, 21*, 491–503.

Libin, A., & Cohen-Mansfield, J. (2004). Therapeutic robocat for nursing home residents with dementia: Preliminary inquiry. *American Journal of Alzheimer's Disease and Other Dementias, 19*, 111–116.

Libon, D., Rascovsky, K., Gross, R., White, M., Xie, S., Dreyfuss, M., . . . Grossman, M. (2011). The Philadelphia Brief Assessment of Cognition (PBAC): A validated screening measure for dementia. *Clinical Neuropsychology, 25*(8), 1314–1330.

Libon, D., Xie, S., Eppig, J., Wicas, G., Lamar, M., Lippa, C., . . . Wambach, D. M. (2010). The heterogeneity of mild cognitive impairment: A neuropsychological analysis. *Journal of the International Neuropsychological Society, 16*, 84–93.

Lichtheim, L. (1885). On aphasia. *Brain, 7*, 433–484.

Liddell, M. B., Lovestone, S., & Owen, M. J. (2001). Genetic risk of Alzheimer's disease: Advising relatives. *The British Journal of Psychiatry, 178*, 7–11.

Lieberman, J. D., Pasquale, M., Garcia, R., Cipolle, M., Li, M., & Wasser, T. (2003). Use of admission Glasgow Coma score, pupil size, and pupil reactivity to determine outcome for traumatic patients. *The Journal of Trauma Injury, Infection and Critical Care, 55*, 437–443.

Liman, T. G., Heuschmann, P. U., Endres, M., Flöel, A., Schwab, S., & Kolominsky-Rabas, P. L. (2011). Changes in cognitive function over 3 years after first-ever stroke and predictors of cognitive impairment and long-term cognitive stability: The Erlangen Stroke Project. *Dementia and Geriatric Cognitive Disorders, 31*(4), 291–299.

Lin, Y. C., Dai, Y. T., & Huang, S. L. (2003). The effect of reminiscence on the elderly population: A systematic review. *Public Health Nursing, 20*, 297–306.

Lindamood, C. H., & Lindamood, P. C. (1975). *Auditory discrimination in depth*. Austin, TX: PRO-ED.

Lindamood, P., & Lindamoood, P. D. (2011). *LiPS: The Lindamood phoneme sequencing program for reading, spelling, and speech* (4th ed.) Austin, TX: PRO-ED.

Lindell, A.K. (2006). In your right mind: Right hemisphere contributions to language processing and production. *Neuropsychology Review, 16*, 131–148.

Linebarger, M. C., & Schwartz, M. F. (2005). AAC for hypothesis-testing and treatment of aphasic language production: Lessons from a processing prosthesis. *Aphasiology, 19*, 930–942.

LinguiSystems. (2009). *Generations trivia: Interactive game shows for recall and deductive reasoning*. East Moline, IL: Author.

Little, A., & Doherty, B. (1996). Going beyond cognitive assessment: Assessment of adjustment, behavior, and the environment. In R. T. Woods (Ed.), *Handbook of the clinical psychology of ageing* (pp. 475–506). New York: John Wiley and Sons.

Liu, C. J., McDowd, J., & Lin, K. C. (2004). Visuospatial inattention and daily life performance in people with Alzheimer's disease. *American Journal of Occupational Therapy, 58*, 202–210.

Llanque, S. M., & Enriquez, M. (2012). Interventions for Hispanic caregivers of patients with dementia. *American Journal of Alzheimer's Disease and Other Dementias, 27*(1), 23–32.

Lloyd, J., Riley, G., & Powell, T. (2009). Errorless learning of novel routes through a virtual town in people with acquired brain injury. *Neuropsychological Rehabilitation, 19*(1), 98–109.

Lloyd, L., & Cuvo, A. (1994). Maintenance and generalization of behaviors after treatment of persons with traumatic brain injury. *Brain Injury, 8*, 529–540.

Lo, Y. L., & Cui, S. L. (2003). Acupuncture and the modulation of cortical excitability. *Neuroreport, 14*, 1229–1231.

Lock, S., Wilkinson, R., & Bryan, K., (2008). *SPPARC (Supporting partners of people with aphasia in relationships and conversation): A resource pack*. Bicester, England: Speechmark.

Logsdon, R. G., Gibbons, L. E., McCurry, S. M., & Teri, L. (1999). Quality of life in Alzheimer's disease: Patient and caregiver reports. *Journal of Mental Health and Aging, 5*(1), 21–32.

Logsdon, R. G., Gibbons, L. E., McCurry, S. M., & Teri, L. (2002). Assessing quality of life in older adults with cognitive impairment. *Psychosomatic Medicine, 64*(3), 510–519.

Lokk, J., Salman Roghani, R., & Delbari, A. (2011). Effect of methlphenidate and/or levodopa coupled with physiotherapy on functional and motor recovery after stroke: A randomized, double-blind, placebo-controlled trial. *Acta Neurologia Scandaniva, 123*(4), 266–273.

Lomas, J., Pickard, L., Bester, S., Elbard, H., Finlayson, A., & Zoghaib, C. (1989). The Communicative Effectiveness Index: Development and psychometric evaluation of functional communication measure for adult aphasia. *Journal of Speech and Hearing Disorders, 54*, 113–124.

Lombardi, F., Taricco, M., De Tanti, A., Telaro, E., & Liberati, A. (2002). Sensory stimulation of brain-injured individuals in coma or vegetative state: Results of a Cochrane systematic review. *Clinical Rehabilitation, 16*, 464–472.

Loonstra, A., Tarlow, A., & Sellars, A. (2001). COWAT metanorms across age, education, and gender. *Applied Neuropsychology, 8*(3), 161–166.

Lopez, O. (2011). The growing burden of Alzheimer's disease. *American Journal of Managed Care, 17*, S339–S345.

LoPresti, E., Simpson, R., Kirsch, N., Schreckenghost, D., & Hayashi, S. (2008). Distributed cognitive aid with scheduling and interactive task guidance. *Journal of Rehabilitation Research and Development, 45*(4), 505–522.

Lorenzen, B., & Murray, L. L. (2008a). Benefits of physical fitness training in healthy aging and neurogenic patient populations. *Perspectives on Neurophysiology and Neurogenic Speech and Language Disorders, 18*(3), 99–106.

Lorenzen, B., & Murray, L. L. (2008b). Bilingual aphasia: A theoretical and clinical review. *American Journal of Speech-Language Pathology, 17*, 1–19.

Lorenzen, B., & Murray, L. L. (2011, September). *Do aphasic symptoms benefit from physical fitness training?* Biennial International Conference of the British Aphasiology Society, Reading, England.

Lott, S. N., Carney, A. S., Glezer, L. S., & Friedman, R. B. (2010). Overt use of tactile/kinaesthetic strategy shifts to covert processing in rehabilitation of letter-by-letter reading. *Aphasiology, 24*(11), 1424–1442.

Lott, S. N., & Friedman, R. B. (1999). Can treatment for pure alexia improve letter-by-letter reading speed without sacrificing accuracy? *Brain and Language, 67*, 188–201.

Lubinski, R. (1991). Dysarthria: A breakdown in interpersonal communication. In D. Vogel & M. P. Cannito (Eds.), *Treating disordered speech motor control: For clinicians by clinicians* (pp. 153–181). Austin, TX: PRO-ED.

Lubinski, R. (2001). Environmental systems approach to adult aphasia. In R. Chapey (Ed.), *Language intervention strategies in aphasia and related neurogenic communication disorders* (4th ed., pp. 269–296). Philadelphia: Lippincott Williams and Wilkins.

Lucas, E. (1980). *Semantic and pragmatic language disorders: Assessment and remediation*. Rockville, MD: Aspen.

Luck, A., & Rose, M. (2007). Interviewing people with aphasia: Insights into method adjustments from a pilot study. *Aphasiology, 21*(2), 208–224.

Ludwig, B. (1993). Post-traumatic seizures. *Physical Medicine and Rehabilitation: State of the Art Reviews, 7*, 461–467.

Lukovits, T., Mazzone, T., & Gorelick, P. (1999). Diabetes mellitus and cerebrovascular disease. *Neuroepidemiology, 18*, 1–14.

Lumosity [online software program]. (2010). San Francisco, CA: Lumos Labs.

Lumos Labs. (2013). *About Lumosity*. Retrieved December 14, 2013, from www.lumosity.com/about

Lundgren, K., Brownell, H., Cayer-Meade, C., Milione, J., & Kearns, K. (2011). Treating metaphor interpretation deficits subsequent to right hemisphere brain damage: Preliminary results. *Aphasiology, 25*(4), 456–474.

Lundgren, K., Helm-Estabrooks, N., & Klein, R. (2010). Stuttering following acquired brain damage: A review of the literature. *Journal of Neurolinguistics, 23*, 447–454.

Lundqvist, A., Linnros, H., Orlenius, H., & Samuelsson, K. (2010). Improved self-awareness and coping strategies for patients with acquired brain injury—A group therapy programme. *Brain Injury, 24*(6), 823–832.

Luterman, D. M. (2008). *Counseling persons with communication disorders and their families*. Austin, TX: PRO-ED.

Luukinen, H., Viramo, P., Koski, K., Laippala, P., & Kivela, S. L. (1999). Head injuries and cognitive decline among older adults: A population-based study. *Neurology, 52*, 557–562.

Luukkainen-Markkula, R., Tarkka, I. M., Pitkanen, K., Sivenius, J., & Hamalainen, H. (2009). Rehabilitation of hemispatial neglect: A randomized study using either arm activation or visual scanning training. *Restorative Neurology and Neuroscience, 27*(6), 663–672.

Luzzatti, C., Colombo, C., Frustaci, M., & Vitolo, F. (2000). Rehabilitation of spelling along the sub-word-level routine. *Neuropsychological Rehabilitation, 10*(3), 249–278.

Luzzi, S., & Piccirilli, M. (2003). Slowly progressive pure dysgraphia with late apraxia of speech: A further variant of the focal cerebral degeneration. *Brain and Language, 87*, 355–360.

Lyon, J. G. (1998). *Coping with aphasia*. San Diego, CA: Singular.

Lyon, J. G., Cariski, D., Keisler, L., Rosenbek, J., Levine, R., Kumpula, J., . . . Blanc, M. (1997). Communication partners: Enhancing participation in life and communication for adults with aphasia in natural settings. *Aphasiology, 11*, 693–708.

Lyon, J. G., & Helm-Estabrooks, N. (1987). Drawing: Its communicative significance for expressively restricted aphasic adults. *Topics in Language Disorders, 8*, 61–71.

Maas, M. B., Lev, M. H., Ay, H., Singhal, A. B., Greer, D. M., Smith, W. S., . . . Furie, K. L. (2012). The prognosis for aphasia in stroke. *Journal of Stroke and Cerebrovascular Diseases, 21*(5), 350–357.

MacDonald, S. (2005). *Functional assessment of verbal reasoning and executive strategies*. Guelph, Ontario, Canada: CCD.

MacDonald, S. (2010). *Functional assessment of verbal reasoning and executive strategies–Adolescent edition*. Guelph, Ontario, Canada: CCD.

Mackay, L. E., Chapman, P. E., & Morgan, A. S. (1997). *Maximizing brain injury recovery*. Gaithersburg, MD: Aspen.

MacKenzie, C. (2000). The relevance of education and age in the assessment of discourse comprehension. *Clinical Linguistics and Phonetics, 14*, 151–161.

MacNeill Horton, A., Soper, H., & Reynolds, C. (2010). Executive functions in children with traumatic brain injury. *Applied Neuropsychology, 17*, 99–103.

Maddicks, R., Marzillier, S. L., & Parker, G. (2003). Rehabilitation of unilateral neglect in the acute recovery stage: The efficacy of limb activation therapy. *Neuropsychological Rehabilitation, 13*, 391–408.

Mahendra, N., & Arkin, S. (2003). Effects of four years of exercise, language, and social interventions on Alzheimer discourse. *Journal of Communication Disorders, 36*, 395–422.

Mahendra, N., & Arkin, S. (2004). Exercise and volunteer work: Contexts for AD language and memory interventions. *Seminars in Speech and Language, 25*, 151–165.

Mahendra, N., & Engineer, N. (2009). Effects of vascular dementia on cognition and linguistic communication: A case study. *Perspectives on Neurophysiology and Neurogenic Speech and Language Disorders, 19*(4), 107–116.

Mahendra, N., Scullion, A., & Hamerschlag, C. (2011). Cognitive-linguistic interventions for persons with dementia: A practitioner's guide to 3 evidence-based techniques. *Topics in Geriatric Rehabilitation, 27*(4), 278–288.

Maher, L. M., Clayton, M. C., Barrett, A. M., Schober-Peterson, D., & Rothi, L. J. G. (1998). Rehabilitation of a case of pure alexia: Exploiting residual abilities. *Journal of the International Neuropsychological Society, 4*, 636–647.

Maher, L. M., Kendall, D., Swearengin, J. A., Rodriguez, A., Leon, S. A., Pingel, K., . . . Gonzalez Rothi, L. J. (2006). A pilot study of use-dependent learning in the context of Constraint Induced Language Therapy. *Journal of the International Neuropsychological Society, 12*(6), 843–852.

Mailles, A., De Broucker, T., Costanzo, P., Martinez-Almoyna, L., Vaillant, V., & Stahl, J. P. (2012). Long-term outcome of patients presenting with acute infectious encephalitis of various causes in France. *Clinical Infectious Diseases, 54*(10), 1455–1464.

Malia, K. B., Bewick, K. C., Raymond, M. J., & Bennet, T. L. (2002). *Brainwave–Revised: Cognitive strategies and techniques for brain injury rehabilitation*. Austin, TX: PRO-ED.

Malone, M., Skrajner, M., Camp, C., Neundorfer, M., & Gorzelle, G. (2007). Research in practice II: Spaced retrieval. A memory intervention. *Alzheimer's Care Quarterly, 8*, 65–74.

Man, D. W., & Li, R. (2001). Assessing Chinese adults' memory abilities: Validation of the Chinese version of the Rivermead Behavioral Memory Test. *Clinical Gerontologist, 24*, 27–36.

Man, D., Soong, W., Tam, S., & Hui-Chan, C. (2006). A randomized clinical trial study on the effectiveness of a tele-analogy-based problem-solving programme for people with acquired brain injury (ABI). *NeuroRehabilitation, 21*, 205–217.

Manchikanti, L., Singh, V., Smith, H. S., & Hirsch, J. A. (2009). Evidence-based medicine, systematic reviews, and guidelines in interventional pain management: Part 4: Observational studies. *Pain Physician, 12*(1), 73–108.

Manheim, L. M., Halper, A. S., & Cherney, L. R. (2009). Patient-reported changes in communication after computer-based script training for aphasia. *Archives of Physical Medicine and Rehabilitation, 90*(4), 623–627.

Manly, T. (2002). Cognitive rehabilitation for unilateral neglect: Review. *Neuropsychological Rehabilitation, 12*, 289–310.

Manly, T., Hawkins, K., Evans, J., Woldt, K., & Robertson, I. H. (2002). Rehabilitation of executive function: Facilitation of effective goal management on complex tasks using periodic auditory alerts. *Neuropsychologia, 40*, 271–281.

Manly, T., Joost, H., Davison, B., Gaynord, B., Greenfield, E., Parr, A., . . . Robertson, R. H. (2004). An electronic knot in the handkerchief: "Content free cueing" and the maintenance of attentive control. *Neuropsychological Rehabilitation, 14*, 89–117.

Manning, K., Gordon, B., Pearlson, G., & Schretlen, D. (2007). The relationship of recency discriminaton to explicit memory and executive functioning. *Journal of International Neuropsychological Society, 13*(4), 710–715.

Manochiopinig, S., Reed, V. A., Sheard, C., & Choo, P. (1997). Significant others' perceptions of speech pathology services for Thai aphasic speakers. *Aphasiology, 11*, 210–217.

Mapou, R. L., Kramer, J. H., & Blusewicz, M. J. (1989). Performance on the California Discourse Memory Test following closed head injury. *Journal of Clinical and Experimental Neuropsychology, 11*, 58.

Marchina, S., Zhu, L., Norton, A., Zipse, L., Wan, C., & Schlaug, G. (2011). Impairment of speech production predicted by lesion load of the left arcuate fasciculus. *Stroke, 42*, 2251–2256.

Marien, P., Paghera, B., De Deyn, P., & Vignolo, L. (2004). Adult crossed aphasia in dextrals revisited. *Cortex, 40*, 41–74.

Marini, A., Caltagirone, C., Paqualetti, P., & Carlomagno, S. (2007). Patterns of language improvement in adults with non-chronic non-fluent aphasia after specific therapies. *Aphasiology, 21*(2), 164–186.

Marini, A., Carlomagno, S., Caltagirone, C., & Nocentini, U. (2005). The role played by the right hemisphere in the organization of complex textual structures. *Brain and Language, 93*, 46–54.

Markova, I., & Berrios, G. (2006). Approaches to the assessment of awareness: Conceptual issues. *Neuropsychological Rehabilitation, 16*(4), 439–455.

Markowitsch, H. (1998). Cognitive neuroscience of memory. *Neurocase, 4*, 429–435.

Markwardt, F. C. (1997). *Peabody individual achievement test* (Rev. ed.). Circle Pines, MN: American Guidance Service.

Marquez de la Plata, C., Arango-Lasprilla, J. C., Alegret, M., Moreno, A., Tarraga, L., Lara, M., . . . Cullum, C. M. (2009). Item analysis of three Spanish naming tests: A cross-cultural investigation. *NeuroRehabilitation, 24*, 75–85.

Marsh, E., & Hillis, A. (2006). Recovery from aphasia following brain injury: The role of reorganization. *Progress in Brain Research, 157,* 143–156.

Marsh, N. V., Kersel, D. A., Havill, J. H., & Sleigh, J. W. (2002). Caregiver burden during the year following severe traumatic brain injury. *Journal of Clinical and Experimental Neuropsychology, 24,* 434–447.

Marshall, J. (2010). Classification of aphasia: Are there benefits for practice? *Aphasiology, 24*(3), 408–412.

Marshall, J., Best, W., Cocks, N., Cruice, M., Pring, T., Bulcock, G., . . . Caute, A. (2012). Gesture and naming therapy for people with severe aphasia: A group study. *Journal of Speech, Language, and Hearing Research, 55*(3), 726–738.

Marshall, J. C., & Halligan, P. W. (1988). Blindsight and insight in visuo-spatial neglect. *Nature, 336,* 766–767.

Marshall, R. C. (1997). Aphasia treatment in the early postonset period: Managing our resources effectively. *American Journal of Speech-Language Pathology, 6,* 5–11.

Marshall, R. C. (2001). Management of Wernicke's aphasia: Context-based approach. In R. Chapey (Ed.), *Language intervention strategies in aphasia and related neurogenic communication disorders* (4th ed., pp. 435–456). Philadelphia: Lippincott Williams and Wilkins.

Marshall, R. C. (2007). A problem-focused group treatment program for clients with mild aphasia. In R. J. Elman (Ed.), *Group treatment of neurogenic communication disorders: The expert clinician's approach* (2nd ed., pp. 95–109). San Diego, CA: Plural.

Marshall, R., & Karow, C. (2008). Update on a clinical measure for the assessment of problem solving. *American Journal of Speech-Language Pathology, 17,* 377–388.

Marshall, R. C., Karow, C. M., Freed, D., & Babcock, P. (2002). Effects of personalized cue form on the learning of subordinate category names by aphasic and non-brain-damaged subjects. *Aphasiology, 16,* 763–771.

Marshall, R. C., Karow, C. M., Morelli, C. A., Iden, K. K., & Dixon, J. (2003). A clinical measure for the assessment of problem solving in brain-injured adults. *American Journal of Speech-Language Pathology, 12,* 333–348.

Marshall, R. C., & Neuburger, S. (1984). Extended comprehension training reconsidered. *Clinical Aphasiology, 14,* 181–187.

Marshall, R. C., & Watts, M. T. (1976). Relaxation training: Effects of communicative ability of aphasic adults. *Archives of Physical Medicine and Rehabilitation, 57,* 464–467.

Martelli, M. (1999, December). Protocol for increasing initiation, decreasing adynamia. *HeadsUp: RSS Newsletter,* 2 & 9.

Martin, I., & McDonald, S. (2003). Weak coherence, no theory of mind, or executive dysfunction? Solving the puzzle of pragmatic language disorders. *Brain and Language, 85,* 451–466.

Martin, N. (2006). *Test of visual perceptual skills* (3rd ed.). Novato, CA: Academic Therapy.

Martin, N., & Brownell, R. (2011a). *Expressive one-word picture vocabulary test* (4th ed.). Ann Arbor, MI: Academic Therapy.

Martin, N., & Brownell, R. (2011b). *Receptive one-word picture vocabulary test* (4th ed.). Ann Arbor, MI: Academic Therapy.

Martin, N., & Reilly, J. (2012). Short-term/working memory impairments in aphasia: Data, models, and their application to aphasia rehabilitation. *Aphasiology, 26*(3–4), 253–257.

Martin, N., Schwartz, M. F., & Kohen, F. P. (2006). Assessment of the ability to process semantic and phonological aspects of words in aphasia: A multi-measurement approach. *Aphasiology, 20,* 154–166.

Martin, P., Naeser, M., Ho, M., Doron, K., Kurland, J., Kaplan, J., . . . Pascual-Leone, A. (2009). Overt naming fMRI pre-and post-TMS: Two nonfluent aphasia patients, with and without improved naming post-TMS. *Brain and Language, 111*(1), 20–35.

Martin, R. C. (2003). Language processing: Functional organization and neuroanatomical basis. *Annual Review of Psychology, 54,* 55–89.

Martin, R. C., & Allen, C. (2008). A disorder of executive function and its role in language processing. *Seminars in Speech and Language, 29,* 201–210.

Martinaud, O., Opolczynski, G., Gaillard, M., & Hannequin, D. (2009). Relevant category-specific effect on naming in Alzheimer's disease. *Dementia and Geriatric Cognitive Disorders, 28,* 413–418.

Martin-Saez, M., Deakins, J., Winson, R., Watson, P., & Wilson, B. (2011). A 10-year follow up of a paging service for people with memory and planning problems within a healthcare system: How do recent users differ from the original users? *Neuropsychological Rehabilitation, 21*(6), 769–783.

Massaro, M. E., & Tompkins, C. A. (1992). Feature analysis for treatment of communication disorders in traumatically brain injured patients: An efficacy study. *Clinical Aphasiology, 22*, 245–256.

Mateer, C. A. (1999). Executive function disorders: Rehabilitation challenges and strategies. *Seminars in Clinical Neuropsychiatry, 4*, 50–59.

Mateer, C. A. (2009). Neuropsychological interventions for memory impairment and the role of single-case design methodologies. *Journal of the International Neuropsychological Society, 15*, 623–628.

Mateer, C. A., Kerns, K. A., & Eso, K. L. (1999). Management of attention and memory disorders following traumatic brain injury. *Journal of Learning Disabilities, 29*, 618–632.

Mateer, C. A., Polen, S. B., Ojemann, G. A., & Wyler, A. R. (1982). Cortical localization of finger spelling and oral language: A case study. *Brain and Language, 17*, 46–57.

Mateer, C. A., Rapport, R. L., & Kettrick, C. (1984). Cerebral organization of oral and signed language responses: Case study evidence from amytal and cortical stimulation studies. *Brain and Language, 21*, 123–135.

Matesich, J., & Dressler, R. (2006). *Language activity resource kit* (2nd ed.) [CD-ROM]. Austin, TX: PRO-ED.

Mathias, J. L., Beall, J., & Bigler, E. D. (2004). Neuropsychological and information processing deficits following mild traumatic brain injury. *Journal of the International Neuropsychological Society, 10*, 286–297.

Matthews, C. G., Harley, J. P., & Malec, J. F. (1992). Guidelines for computer-assisted neuropsychological rehabilitation and cognitive remediation. In K. M. Adams & B. P. Rouke (Eds.), *The TCN guide to professional practice in clinical neuropsychology* (pp. 120–136). Amsterdam, Netherlands: Swets & Zeitlinger.

Mattis, S. (2001). *Dementia rating scale* (2nd ed.). Lutz, FL: Psychological Assessment Resources.

Mätzig, S., Druks, J., Masterson, J., & Vigliocco, G. (2009). Noun and verb differences in picture naming: Past studies and new evidence. *Cortex, 45*(6), 738–758.

Maxim, J., Bryan, K., Axelrod, L., Jordan, L., & Bell, L. (2001). Speech and language therapists as trainers: Enabling care staff working with older people. *International Journal of Language and Communication, 33*, 194–199.

Maxwell, W. L., Watt, C., Graham, D. I., & Gennarelli, T. A. (1993). Ultrastructural evidence of axonal shearing as a result of lateral acceleration of the head in non-human primates. *Acta Neuropathologica, 86*, 136–144.

Mayer, J. F., & Murray, L. L. (2002). Approaches to the treatment of alexia in chronic aphasia. *Aphasiology, 16*, 727–744.

Mayer, J. F., & Murray, L. L. (2003). Functional measures of naming in aphasia: Word-retrieval in confrontation naming versus connected speech. *Aphasiology, 17*, 481–498.

Mayer, J. F., & Murray, L. L. (2013). The nature of working memory deficits in aphasia. *Journal of Communication Disorders, 45*(5), 325–339.

Mayer, J. F., Murray, L. L., & Bishop, L. (2012). Applying a structured cognitive training protocol to address progressive cognitive decline in vascular dementia. *American Journal of Speech-Language Pathology, 21*, 167–179.

Mayer, J. F., Murray, L. L., & Karcher, L. A. (2004). *Treatment of anomia in severe aphasia*. Clinical Aphasiology Conference, Park City, UT.

Maynard, C. K. (2003). Differentiate depression from dementia. *The Nurse Practitioner, 28*(3), 18–27.

Mazaux, J. M., & Orgozo, J. M. (1981). *Boston diagnostic aphasia examination: Échelle française*. Paris, France: Éditions scientifiques et psychologiques.

McCall, D., Virata, T., Linebarger, M., & Berndt, R. (2009). Integrating technology and targeted treatment to improve narrative production in aphasia: A case study. *Aphasiology, 23*(4), 438–461.

McCarty, J. P., & White, S. C. (2012). *Health plan coding and claims guide*. Rockville, MD: American Speech-Language-Hearing Association.

McCooey, R., Toffolo, D., & Code, C. (2000). A socioenvironmental approach to functional communication in hospital in-patients. In L. Worrall & C. M. Frattali (Eds.), *Neurogenic communication disorders: A functional approach* (pp. 295–311). New York: Thieme.

McCurry, S., Pike, K., Vitiello, M., Logsdon, R., Larson, E., & Teri, L. (2011). Increasing walking and bright light exposure to improve sleep in community dwelling persons with Alzheimer's disease: Results of a randomized, controlled trial. *Journal of the American Geriatric Society, 59*, 1393–1402.

McDonald, S. (2000). Exploring the cognitive basis of right-hemisphere pragmatic language disorders. *Brain and Language, 75*, 82–107.

McDonald, S. (2012). New frontiers in neuropsychological assessment: Assessing social perception using a standardised instrument, The Awareness of Social Inference Test. *Australian Psychologist, 47*, 39–48.

McDonald, S., Bornhofen, C., Togher, L., Flanagan, S., Gertler, P., & Bowen, R. (2009). *Improving first impressions: A step-by-step socials skills program*. Australasian Society for the Study of Brain Impairment. Available from http://www.assbi.com.au/assbi%20products.html

McDonald, S., & Flanagan, S. (2004). Social perception deficits after traumatic brain injury: Interaction between emotion recognition, mentalizing ability, and social communication. *Neuropsychology, 18*, 572–579.

McDonald, S., Flanagan, S., & Rollins, J. (2011). *The awareness of social inference test* (Rev. ed.). Sydney, Australia: Pearson Assessment.

McDonald, S., Tate, R., Togher, L., Bornhofen, C., Long, E., Gertler, P., & Bowen, R. (2008). Social skills treatment for people with severe, chronic acquired brain injuries: A multicenter trial. *Archives of Physical Medicine and Rehabilitation, 89*, 1648–1659.

McDonald, S., Togher, L., & Code, C. (Eds.). (1999). *Communication disorders following traumatic brain injury*. East Sussex, UK: Psychology Press.

McDonnell, M. N., Smith, A. E., & Mackintosh, S. F. (2011). Aerobic exercise to improve cognitive function in adults with neurological disorders: A systematic review. *Archives of Physical Medicine and Rehabilitation, 92*(7), 1044–1052.

McFarlane, L. (2012). Motivational interviewing: Practical strategies for speech-language pathologists and audiologists. *Canadian Journal of Speech-Language Pathology and Audiology, 36*(1), 1–16.

McGann, W., & Werven, G. (1999). *Social communication skills for children: A workbook for principle-centered communication*. Austin, TX: PRO-ED.

McGowin, D. (1994). *Living in the labyrinth: A personal journey through the maze of Alzheimer's*. New York: Dell.

McGuire, L. M., Burright, R. G., Williams, R., & Donovick, P. J. (1998). Prevalence of traumatic brain injury in psychiatric and non-psychiatric subjects. *Brain Injury, 12*, 207–214.

McIntosh, R.D., Brodie, E. E., Beschin, N., & Robertson, I. H. (2000). Improving the clinical diagnosis of personal neglect: A reformulated comb and razor test. *Cortex, 36*(2), 289–292.

McKelvey, M., Hux, K., Dietz, A., & Beukelman, D. (2010). Impact of personal relevance and contextualization on word-picture matching by people with aphasia. *American Journal of Speech-Language Pathology, 19*, 22–33.

McKerracher, G., Powell, T., & Oyebode, J. (2005). A single case experimental design comparing two memory notebook formats for a man with memory problems caused by traumatic brain injury. *Neuropsychological Rehabilitation, 15*(2), 115–118.

McKhann, G. M., Knopman, D. S., Chertkow, H., Hyman, B. T., Jack, C. R., Kawas, D. H., . . . Phelps, C. H. (2011). The diagnosis of dementia due to Alzheimer's disease: Recommendations from the National Institute on Aging–Alzheimer's Association workgroups on diagnostic guidelines for Alzheimer's disease. *Alzheimer's and Dementia, 7*, 263–269.

McKinlay, A., Dalrymple-Alford, J., Grace, R., & Roger, D. (2009). The effect of attentional set-shifting, working memory, and processing speed on pragmatic language functioning in Parkinson's disease. *European Journal of Cognitive Psychology, 21*(2–3), 330–346.

McKinlay, A., Grace, R. C., Horwood, L. J., Fergusson, D. M., Ridder, E. M., & MacFarlene, M. (2008). Prevalence of traumatic brain injury among children, adolescents and young adults: Prospective evidence from a birth cohort. *Brain Injury, 22*(2), 175–181.

McKitrick, L. A., & Camp, C. J. (1993). Relearning the names of things: The spaced-retrieval intervention implemented by caregivers. *Clinical Gerontologist, 14*, 60–62.

McNeil, M. R., Odell, K., & Tseng, C. (1991). Toward the integration of resource allocation into and general theory of aphasia. *Clinical Aphasiology, 20*, 21–36.

McNeil, M. R., & Prescott, T. E. (1978). *Revised token test*. Baltimore: University Park Press.

McNeil, M. R., Small, S. L., Masterson, R. J., & Fossett, T. R. (1995). Behavioral and pharmacological treatment of lexical-semantic deficits in a single patient with primary progressive aphasia. *American Journal of Speech-Language Pathology, 4*, 76–87.

McNeil, M., Sung, J., Yang, D., Pratt, S., Fossett, T., & Doyle, P. (2007). Comparing connected language elicitation procedures in persons with aphasia: Concurrent validation of the Story Retell Procedure. *Aphasiology, 216*(8), 775–790.

McVicker, S., Parr, S., Pound, C., & Duchan, J. (2009). The Communication Partner Scheme: A project to develop long-term, low-cost access to conversation for people living with aphasia. *Aphasiology, 23*(1), 52–71.

Medina, J., Norise, C., Faseyitan, O., Coslett, H. B., Turkeltaub, P., & Hamilton, R. (2012). Finding the right words: Transcranial magnetic stimulation improves discourse productivity in non-fluent aphasia after stroke. *Aphasiology, 26*(9), 1153–1168.

Meiland, F., Bouman, A., Savenstedt, S., Bentvelzen, S., Davies, R., Mulvenna, M., . . . Droes, R. (2012). Usability of a new electronic assistive device for community-dwelling persons with mild dementia. *Aging and Mental Health, 16*(5), 584–591.

Meinzer, M., Obleser, J., Flaisch, T., Eulitz, C., & Rockstroh, B. (2007). Recovery from aphasia as a function of language therapy in an early bilingual patient demonstrated by fMRI. *Neuropsychologia, 45*, 1247–1256.

Meinzer, M., Streiftau, S., & Rockstroh, B. (2007). Intensive language training in the rehabilitation of chronic aphasia: Efficient training by laypersons. *Journal of the International Neuropsychological Society, 13*, 846–853.

Melamed, L. E. (2000). *Kent visual perceptual test*. Odessa, FL: Psychological Assessment Resources.

Melton, A., & Bourgeois, M. (2005). Training compensatory memory strategies via the telephone for persons with TBI. *Aphasiology, 19*, 353–364.

Menn, L., Ramsberger, G., & Helm-Estabrooks, N. (1994). A linguistic communication measure for aphasic narratives. *Aphasiology, 8*, 343–359.

Mentis, M., & Prutting, C. (1991). Analysis of topic as illustrated in a head-injured and normal adult. *Journal of Speech and Hearing Research, 34*, 583–595.

Merritta, C., Cherian, B., Macaden, A. S., & John, J. A. (2010). Measurement of physical performance and objective fatigability in people with mild-to-moderate traumatic brain injury. *International Journal of Rehabilitation Research, 33*(2), 109–114.

Messenger, B., & Ziarnek, N. (2004). *Functional rehabilitation activity manuals*. Wake Forest, NC: Lash & Associates.

Messinis, L., Malegiannaki, A., Christodoulou, T., Panagiotopoulos, V., & Papthanasopoulos, P. (2011). Color Trails Test: Normative data and criterion validity for the Greek adult population. *Archives of Clinical Neuropsychology, 26*(4), 322–330.

Mesulam, M. M. (1981). A cortical network for directed attention and unilateral neglect. *Annals of Neurology, 10*, 309–325.

Metter, E. J., Kempler, D., Jackson, C., Hanson, W. R., Mazziotta, J. C., & Phelps, M. E. (1989). Cerebral glucose metabolism in Wernicke's, Broca's, and conduction aphasia. *Archives Neurology, 46*, 27–34.

Metter, E. J., Riege, W. H., Hanson, W. R., Kuhl, D. E., Phelps, M. E., Squire, L. R., . . . Benson, D. F. (1983). Comparison of metabolic rates, language, and memory in subcortical aphasias. *Brain and Language, 19*, 33–47.

Metzler-Baddeley, C., & Jones, R. W. (2010). Cognitive rehabilitation of executive functioning in a case of craniopharyngioma. *Applied Neuropsychology, 17*, 299–304.

Meyer, M. J., Megyesi, J., Meythaler, J., Murie-Fernandez, M., Aubut, J.-A., Foley, N., . . . Teasell, R. (2010). Acute management of acquired brain injury Part III: An evidence-based review of interventions used to promote arousal from coma. *Brain Injury, 24*(5), 722–729.

Meyers, J. E., & Meyers, K. R. (1995). *Rey complex figure test and recognition trial*. Odessa, FL: Psychological Assessment Resources.

Meyers, J. E., Volkert, K., & Diep, A. (2000). Sentence Repetition test: Updated norms and clinical utility. *Applied Neuropsychology, 7*(3), 154–159.

Meythaler, J. M., Depalma, L., Devivo, M. J., Guin-Renfroe, S., & Novack, T. A. (2001). Sertraline to improve arousal and alertness in severe traumatic brain injury secondary to motor vehicle crashes. *Brain Injury, 15*, 321–331.

Middleton, E., & Schwartz, M. (2010). Density pervades: An analysis of phonological neighborhood density effects in aphasic speakers with different types of naming impairment. *Cognitive Neuropsychology, 27*(5), 401–427.

Middleton, E., & Schwartz, M. (2012). Errorless learning in cognitive rehabilitation: A critical review. *Neuropsychological Rehabilitation, 22*(2), 138–168.

Miertsch, B., Meisel, J., & Isel, F. (2009). Non-treated languages in aphasia therapy of polyglots benefit from improvement in the treated language. *Journal of Neurolinguistics, 22,* 135–150.

Milev, R. V., Kellar, T., McLean, M., Mileva, V., Luthra, V., Thompson, S., & Peever, L. (2008). Multisensory stimulation for elderly with dementia: A 24-week single-blind randomized controlled pilot study. *American Journal of Alzheimer's Disease and Other Dementias, 23*(4), 372–376.

Miller, E., Murray, L., Richards, L., Zorowitz, R., Bakas, T., Clark, P., & Sullivan, K. (2010). Comprehensive overview of nursing and interdisciplinary rehabilitation care of the stroke patient. *Stroke, 41*(10), 2402–2448.

Miller, N. (2002). The neurological bases of apraxia of speech. *Seminars in Speech and Language, 23*(4), 223–230.

Mills, H. (2004). *A mind of my own: Memoir of recovery from aphasia.* Bloomington, IN: Authorhouse.

Milman, L., & Holland, A. (2012). *Scales of cognitive and communicative ability for neurorehabilitation.* Austin, TX: PRO-ED.

Mioshi, E., Dawson, K., Mitchell, J., Arnold, R., & Hodges, J. (2006). Addenbrooke's Cognitive Examination–Revised (ACE-R): A brief cognitive test battery for dementia screening. *International Journal of Geriatric Psychiatry, 21,* 1078–1085.

Miotto, E., Cinalli, F., Serrao, V., Benute, G., Lucia, M., & Scaff, M. (2010). Cognitive deficits in patients with mild to moderate traumatic brain injury. *Arquives Neuropsiquiatria, 68*(8), 862–868.

Mirman, D. (2011). Effects of near and distant semantic neighbors on word production. *Cognitive, Affective, & Behavioral Neuroscience, 11*(1), 32–43.

Mirman, D., & Magnuson, J. S. (2008). Attractor dynamics and semantic neighborhood density: Processing is slowed by near neighbors and speeded by distant neighbors. *Journal of Experimental Psychology. Learning, Memory, and Cognition, 34*(1), 65–79.

Mitchell, J. P. (2008). Contributions of functional neuroimaging to the study of social cognition. *Current Directions in Psychological Science, 17*(2), 142–146.

Mitchum, C. C., & Berndt, R. S. (1991). Diagnosis and treatment of the non-lexical route in acquired dyslexia: An illustration of the cognitive neuropsychological approach. *Journal of Neurolinguistics, 6,* 103–137.

Mitrushina, M., Boone, J. B., Razani, J., & D'Elia, L. F. (2005). *Handbook of normative data for neuropsychological assessment* (2nd ed.). New York: Oxford University Press.

Mittelman, M. S., Haley, W. E., Clay, O. J., & Roth, D. L. (2006). Improving caregiver well-being delays nursing home placement of patients with Alzheimer disease. *Neurology, 67,* 1592–1599.

Miyake, A., Emerson, M. J., & Friedman, N. P. (2000). Assessment of executive functions in clinical settings: Problems and recommendations. *Seminars in Speech and Language, 21,* 169–183.

Miyake, A., Friedman, N. P., Emerson, M. J., Witzki, A. H., Howerter, A., & Wager, T. D. (2000). The unity and diversity of executive functions and their contributions to complex "frontal lobe" tasks: A latent variable analysis. *Cognitive Psychology, 41*(1), 49–100.

Mizuno, E., Hosaka, T., Ogihara, R., Higano, H., & Mano, Y. (1999). Effectiveness of a stress management program for family caregivers of the elderly at home. *Journal of Medical and Dental Sciences, 46,* 145–153.

Molina, C. A. (2011). Reperfusion therapies for acute ischemic stroke: Current pharmacological and mechanical approaches. *Stroke, 42*(Suppl. 1), S16–S19.

Molrine, C. J., & Pierce, R. S. (2002). Black and white adults' expressive language performance on three tests of aphasia. *American Journal of Speech-Language Pathology, 11,* 139–150.

Montgomery, M. (2010). *Alzheimer diary: A wife's journal.* Scotts Valley, CA: CreateSpace.

Monti, A., Cogiamanian, F., Marceglia, S., Ferrucci, R., & Mameli, F. (2008). Improved naming after transcranial direct current stimulation in aphasia. *Journal of Neurology, Neurosurgery, and Psychiatry, 79,* 451–453.

Montoya, A., Price, B., Menear, M., & Lepage, M. (2006). Brain imaging and cognitive dysfunctions in Huntington's disease. *Journal of Psychiatry Neuroscience, 31*(1), 21–29.

Moran, A. J. (1976). Six cases of severe head injury treated by exercise in addition to other therapies. *Medical Journal of Australia, 1,* 396–397.

Moran, C., & Gillon, G. (2004). Language and memory profiles of adolescents with traumatic brain injury. *Brain Injury, 18*, 273–288.

Morgan, A. L. R., & Helm-Estabrooks, N. (1987). Back to the drawing board: A treatment program for nonverbal aphasic patients. *Clinical Aphasiology, 19*, 64–72.

Moriarty Mystery Dinner [computer software]. (2005). Blacksburg, VA: Bungalow Software.

Morris, J., Franklin, S., Ellis, A. W., Turner, J. E., & Bailey, P. J. (1996). Remediating a speech perception deficit in an aphasic patient. *Aphasiology, 10*, 137–158.

Morris, R. G., Worsley, C., & Matthews, D. (2000). Neuropsychological assessment in older people: Old principles and new directions. *Advances in Psychiatric Treatment, 6*, 362–372.

Morrow, K. L., & Fridriksson, J. (2006). Comparing fixed- and randomized-interval spaced retrieval in anomia treatment. *Journal of Communication Disorders, 39*, 2–11.

Morton, N., & Barker, L. (2010). The contribution of injury severity, executive and implicit functions to awareness of deficits after traumatic brain injury (TBI). *Journal of International Neuropsychological Society, 16*, 1089–1098.

Mosch, S. C., Max, J. E., & Tranel, D. (2005). A matched lesion analysis of childhood versus adult-onset brain injury due to unilateral stroke: Another perspective on neural plasticity and recovery of social functioning. *Cognitive and Behavioral Neurology, 18*(1), 5–17.

Moses, M. S., Nickels, L. A., & Sheard, C. (2004). "I'm sitting here feeling aphasic!" A study of recurrent perseverative errors elicited in unimpaired speakers. *Brain and Language, 89*, 157–173.

Moss, A., & Nicholas, M. (2006). Language rehabilitation in chronic aphasia and time postonset. *Stroke, 37*, 3043–3051.

Mount, J., Pierce, S., Parker, J., DiEgidio, R., Woessner, R., & Spiegel, L. (2007). Trial and error versus errorless learning of functional skills in patients with acute stroke. *NeuroRehabilitation, 22*, 123–132.

Moyle, W., Gracia, N., Murfield, J. E., Griffiths, S. G., & Venturato, L. (2011). Assessing quality of life of older people with dementia in long-term care: A comparison of two self-report measures. *Journal of Clinical Nursing*. doi: 10.1111/j.1365-2702.2011.03688.x

Murphy, J., Gray, C. M., & Cox, S. (2007). Talking mats: The effectiveness of a low technology communication framework to help people with dementia express their views. *Journal of Assistive Technologies, 1*(2), 30–34.

Murphy, J., Tester, S., Hubbard, G., Downs, M., & MacDonald, C. (2005). Enabling frail older people with a communication difficulty to express their views: The use of Talking Mats as an interview tool. *Health and Social Care in the Community, 13*(2), 95–107.

Murray, H., Maslany, G., & Jeffery, B. (2006). Assessment of family needs following acquired brain injury in Saskatchewan. *Brain Injury, 20*(6), 575–585.

Murray, L. L. (1998). Longitudinal treatment of primary progressive aphasia: A case study. *Aphasiology, 12*, 651–672.

Murray, L. L. (1999). Attention and aphasia: Theory, research and clinical implications. *Aphasiology, 13*, 91–112.

Murray, L. L. (2000a). The effects of varying attentional demands on the word-retrieval skills of adults with aphasia, right hemisphere brain-damage or no brain-damage. *Brain and Language, 72*, 40–72.

Murray, L. L. (2000b). Spoken language production in Huntington's and Parkinson's diseases. *Journal of Speech, Language and Hearing Research, 43*, 1350–1366.

Murray, L. L. (2002a). Attention deficits in aphasia: Presence, nature, assessment and treatment. *Seminars in Speech and Language, 23*, 107–116.

Murray, L. L. (2002b). Cognitive distinctions between depression and early Alzheimer's disease in the elderly. *Aphasiology, 16*, 573–586.

Murray, L. L. (2004a). Cognitive treatments for aphasia: Should we and can we help attention and working memory problems? *Medical Journal of Speech-Language Pathology, 12*, xxi–xxxviii.

Murray, L. L. (2004b). *Semantic processing in aphasia and right hemisphere brain damage: The effects of increased attention demands.* Paper presented at the Clinical Aphasiology Conference, Park City, UT.

Murray, L. L. (2008a). The application of relaxation training approaches to patients with neurogenic disorders and their caregivers. *Perspectives on Neurophysiology and Neurogenic Speech and Language Disorders, 18*(3), 90–98.

Murray, L. L. (2008b). Language and Parkinson's disease. *Annual Review of Applied Linguistics, 28,* 1–15.

Murray, L. L. (2010). Distinguishing clinical depression from early Alzheimer's disease in the elderly: Can narrative analysis help? *Aphasiology, 24*(6), 928–939.

Murray, L. L. (2012a). Assessing cognitive functioning in older patients: The why, who, what, and how. *Perspectives on Gerontology, 17* (1), 17–26.

Murray, L. L. (2012b). Attention and other cognitive deficits in aphasia: Presence and relation to language and communication measures. *American Journal of Speech-Language Pathology, 21,* 167–179.

Murray, L. L. (2012c). Direct and indirect treatment approaches for addressing short-term or working memory deficits in aphasia. *Aphasiology, 26*(3-4), 317–337.

Murray, L. L., Ballard, K., & Karcher, L. (2004). Linguistic specific treatment: Just for Broca's aphasia? *Aphasiology, 18,* 785–809.

Murray, L. L., & Chapey, R. (2001). Assessment of language disorders in adults. In R. Chapey (Ed.), *Language intervention strategies in adult aphasia* (4th ed., pp. 55–126). New York: Lippincott Williams & Wilkins.

Murray, L. L., & Coppens, P. (2011). Formal and informal assessment of aphasia. In I. Papathanasiou, P. Coppens, & C. Potagas (Eds.), *Aphasia and related neurogenic communication disorders* (pp. 67–92). Sudbury, MA: Jones & Bartlett.

Murray, L. L., Dickerson, S., Lichtenberger, B., & Cox, C. (2003). Effects of toy stimulation on the cognitive, communicative, and emotional functioning of adults in the middle stages of Alzheimer's disease. *Journal of Communication Disorders, 36,* 101–127.

Murray, L. L., Holland, A. L., & Beeson, P. M. (1998). Spoken language of individuals with mild fluent aphasia under focused and divided attention conditions. *Journal of Speech, Language, and Hearing Research, 41,* 213–227.

Murray, L. L., & Karcher, L. (2000). Treating written verb retrieval and sentence construction skills: A case study. *Aphasiology, 14,* 585–602.

Murray, L. L., & Kean, J. (2004). Resource theory and aphasia: Time to abandon or time to revise? *Aphasiology, 18,* 830–835.

Murray, L. L., Keeton, R. J., & Karcher, L. (2006). Treating attention in mild aphasia: Evaluation of Attention Process Training-II. *Journal of Communication Disorders, 39,* 37–61.

Murray, L. L., & Kim, H. Y. (2004). A review of select alternative treatment approaches for acquired neurogenic disorders: Relaxation therapy and acupuncture. *Seminars in Speech and Language, 25,* 133–149.

Murray, L. L., & Ramage, A. E. (2000). Assessing the executive function abilities of adults with neurogenic communication disorders. *Seminars in Speech and Language, 21,* 153–168.

Murray, L. L., & Ray, A. H. (2001). A comparison of relaxation training and syntax stimulation for chronic nonfluent aphasia. *Journal of Communication Disorders, 34,* 87–113.

Murray, L. L., & Stout, J. C. (1999). Discourse comprehension in Huntington's and Parkinson's Diseases. *American Journal of Speech-Language Pathology, 8,* 137–148.

Murray, L. L., Timberlake, A., & Eberle, R. (2007). Treatment of underlying forms in a discourse context. *Aphasiology, 21,* 139–163.

Murray Law, B. (2012, June 05). Giffords comes home to aphasia treatment. *The ASHA Leader.* Retrieved from http://www.asha.org/Publications/leader/2012/120605/Giffords-Comes-Home-to-Aphasia-Treatment.htm

Musicco, M., Salamone, G., Caltagirone, C., Cravello, L., Fadda, L., Lupo, F., . . . Palmer, K. (2010). Neuropsychological predictors of rapidly progressing patients with Alzheimer's disease. *Dementia and Geriatric Cognitive Disorders, 30*(3), 219–228.

Muslimovic, D., Post, B., Speelman, J., De Haan, R., & Schmand, B. (2009). Cognitive decline in Parkinson's disease: A prospective longitudinal study. *Journal of the International Neuropsychological Society, 15,* 426–437.

Myers, P. (1999). *Right hemisphere damage: Disorders of communication and cognition.* San Diego, CA: Singular-Thomson Learning.

Myers, P., & Blake, M. L. (2008). Communication disorders associated with right-hemisphere damage. In R. Chapey (Ed.), *Language intervention strategies in aphasia and related neurogenic communication disorders* (5th ed., pp. 963–987). New York: Lippincott Williams & Wilkins.

Naeser, M. A., Baker, E. H., Palumbo, C. L., Nicholas, M., Alexander, M. P., Samaraweera, R., . . . Weissman, T. (1998). Lesion site patterns in severe, nonverbal aphasia to predict outcome with a computer-assisted treatment program. *Archives of Neurology, 55*, 1438–1448.

Naeser, M., Martin, P., Lundgren, K., Klein, R., Kaplan, J., Treglia, E., . . . Pascual-Leone, A. (2010). Improved language in a chronic nonfluent aphasia patient following treatment with CPAP and TMS. *Cognitive and Behavioral Neurology, 23*(1), 29–38.

Naeser, M., Martin, P., Nicholas, M., Baker, E., Seekins, H., Kobayashi, M., . . . Pascual-Leone, A. (2005). Improved picture naming in chronic aphasia after TMS to part of right Broca's area: An open-protocol study. *Brain and Language, 93*(1), 95–105.

Naeser, M., & Helm-Estabrooks, N. (1985). CT scan lesion localization and response to Melodic Intonation Therapy with nonfluent aphasia cases. *Cortex, 21*, 203–223.

Naeser, M., & Paulumbo, C. L. (1994). Neuroimaging and language recovery in stroke. *Journal of Clinical Neurophysiology, 11*, 150–174.

Nagaratnam, N., Phan, T. A., Barnett, C., & Ibrahim, N. (2002). Angular gyrus syndrome mimicking depressive pseudodementia. *Journal of Psychiatry and Neuroscience, 27*, 364–368.

Nair, A. K., Gavett, B. E., Damman, M., Dekker, W., Green, R. C., Mandel, A., . . . Stern, R. A. (2010). Clock drawing test ratings by dementia specialists: Interrater reliability and diagnostic accuracy. *Journal of Neuropsychiatry and Clinical Neuroscience, 22*(1), 85–92.

Nakase-Thompson, R. (2004). *The Mississippi aphasia screening test*. The Center for Outcome Measurement in Brain Injury. Accessed March 23, 2012, at http://www.tbims.org/combi/mast

Nakase-Thompson, R., Manning, E., Sherer, M., Yablon, S., Gontkovsky, S., & Vickery, C. (2005). Brief assessment of severe language impairments: Initial validation of the Mississippi Aphasia Screening Test. *Brain Injury, 29*(9), 685–691.

Nanda, U., McLendon, P., Andresen, E., & Armbrecht, E. (2003). The SIP68: An abbreviated sickness impact profile for disability outcomes research. *Quality of Life Research, 12*, 583–595.

Nasreddine, Z. S., Phillips, N. A., Bedirian, V., Charbonneau, S., Whitehead, V., Collin, I., . . . Chertkow, H. (2005). The Montreal Cognitive Assessment, MoCA: A brief screening tool for mild cognitive impairment. *Journal of the American Geriatric Society, 53*, 695–699.

National Center for Complementary and Alternative Medicine. (2013). *Complementary, alternative, or integrative health: What's in a name?* Publication No. D347. Betheseda, MD: Author.

National Head Injury Foundation (NHIF) Task Force on Special Education. (1989). *An educator's manual: What educators need to know about students with traumatic brain injury*. Southborough, MA: Author.

National Institute for Health and Clinical Excellence. (2006). *Dementia: Supporting people with dementia and their carers in health and social care. NICE clinical guideline*. London, England: Author.

National Institute of Neurological Disorders and Stroke. (2007). *NINDS Wernicke-Korsakoff syndrome information page*. Available from http://www.ninds.nih.gov/disorders/wernicke_korsakoff/wernicke-korsakoff.htm

National Institute of Neurological Disorders and Stroke. (2009). *NINDS paraneoplastic syndromes information page*. Available from http://www.ninds.nih.gov/disorders/paraneoplastic/paraneoplastic.htm

National Institute of Neurological Disorders and Stroke. (2010). *Huntington's disease: Hope through research*. Available from http://www.ninds.nih.gov/disorders/huntington/detail_huntington.htm

National Institute of Neurological Disorders and Stroke. (2011a). *Multiple sclerosis: Hope through research*. Available from http://www.ninds.nih.gov/disorders/multiple_sclerosis/detail_multiple_sclerosis.htm

National Institute of Neurological Disorders and Stroke. (2011b). *Traumatic brain injury: Hope through research*. Retrieved July 22, 2011, from http://www.ninds.nih.gov/disorders/tbi/detail_tbi.htm

National Institutes of Health. (2011). *Estimates of funding for various research, condition, and disease categories*. Retrieved August 2, 2011, from http://report.nih.gov/rcdc/categories/

Neils-Strunjas, J., Groves-Wright, K., Mashima, P., & Harnish, S. (2006). Dysgraphia in Alzheimer's disease: A review for clinical and research purposes. *Journal of Speech-Language, and Hearing Research, 49*, 1313–1330.

Neimeier, J. P., Cifu, D. X., & Kishore, R. (2001). The lighthouse strategy: Improving the functional status of patients with unilateral neglect after stroke and brain injury using a visual imagery intervention. *Topics in Stroke Rehabilitation, 8*(2), 10–18.

Neisser, U. (1967). *Cognitive psychology*. New York: Appleton-Century-Crofts.

Nelson, A., Fogel, B. S., & Faust, D. (1986). Bedside cognitive screening instruments: A critical assessment. *Journal of Nervous and Mental Disorders, 174*, 73–83.

Nelson, E. C., Wasson, J., Kirk, J., Keller, A., Clark, D., Dietrich, A., . . . Zubkoff, M. (1987). Assessment of function in routine clinical practice: Description of the COOP Chart method and preliminary findings. *Journal of Chronic Diseases, 40*, 55S–69S.

Neugroschl, J., & Wang, S. (2011). Alzheimer's disease: Diagnosis and treatment across the spectrum of disease severity. *Mount Sinai Journal of Medicine, 78*, 596–612.

Newberg, A. B., Wintering, N., Khalsa, D. S., Roggenkamp, H., & Waldman, M. R. (2010). Meditation effects on cognitive function and cerebral blood flow in subjects with memory loss: A preliminary study. *Journal of Alzheimer's disease, 20*(2), 517–526.

Newborn, B. (1997). *Return to Ithaca*. Rockport, MA: Element.

Newman, G. C., Bang, H., Hussain, S. I., & Toole, J. F. (2007). Association of diabetes, homocysteine, and HDL with cognition and disability after stroke. *Neurology, 69*(22), 2054–2062.

Ni, W., Constable, R. T., Mencl, W. E., Pugh, K. R., Fulbright, R. K., Shaywitz, S. E., . . . Shankweiler, D. (2000). An event-related neuroimaging study distinguishing form and content in sentence processing. *Journal of Cognitive Neuroscience, 12*, 120–133.

Nicholas, L. E., & Brookshire, R. H. (1993). A system for quantifying the informativeness and efficiency of the connected speech of adults with aphasia. *Journal of Speech and Hearing Research, 36*, 338–350.

Nicholas, L. E., & Brookshire, R. H. (1995a). Comprehension of spoken narrative discourse by adults with aphasia, right-hemisphere brain damage, or traumatic brain injury. *American Journal of Speech-Language Pathology, 4*, 69–81.

Nicholas, L. E., & Brookshire, R. H. (1995b). Presence, completeness, and accuracy of main concepts in the connected speech of non-brain-damaged adults and adults with aphasia. *Journal of Speech and Hearing Research, 38*, 145–156.

Nicholas, L. E., MacLennan, D. L., & Brookshire, R. H. (1986). Validity of multiple-sentence reading comprehension tests for aphasic adults. *Journal of Speech and Hearing Disorders, 51*, 82–87.

Nicholas, M., & Elliott, S. (1999). *C-Speak Aphasia: A communication system for adults with aphasia*. Solana Beach, CA: Mayer-Johnson.

Nicholas, M., Sinotte, M., & Helm-Estabrooks, N. (2011). C-Speak Aphasia alternative communication program for people with severe aphasia: Importance of executive functioning and semantic knowledge. *Neuropsychological Rehabilitation, 21*(3), 322–366.

Nicholson, K. G., Baum, S., Kilgour, A., Koh, C. K., Munhall, K. G., & Cuddy, L. L. (2003). Impaired processing of prosodic and musical patterns after right hemisphere damage. *Brain and Cognition, 52*, 382–389.

Nickels, L. A. (1995). Getting it right? Using aphasic naming errors to evaluate theoretical models of spoken word production. *Language and Cognitive Processes, 10*, 13–45.

Nickels, L., & Best, W. (1996). Therapy for naming disorders (Part I): Principles, puzzles, and progress. *Aphasiology, 10*, 21–47.

Nickels, L. A., & Cole-Virtue, J. (2004). Reading tasks from PALPA: How do controls perform on visual lexical decision, homophony, rhyme, and synonym judgements? *Aphasiology, 18*, 103–126.

Nickels, L. A., & Howard, D. (1995). Aphasic naming: What matters? *Neuropsychologia, 33*, 1281–1303.

Nielsen, N., & Wiig, E. (2006). Alzheimer's Quick Test cognitive screening criteria for West African Speakers of Krio. *Age and Ageing, 35*(5), 503–507.

Niemann, H., Ruff, R. M., & Baser, C. A. (1990). Computer-assisted attention retraining in head-injured individuals: A controlled efficacy study of an outpatient program. *Journal of Consulting and Clinical Psychology, 58*, 811–817.

Niemeier, J. P. (1998). The lighthouse strategy: Use of a visual imagery technique to treat visual inattention in stroke patients. *Brain Injury, 12*, 399–406.

Niemeier, J. P., Cifu, D., & Kishore, R. (2001). The lighthouse strategy: Improving the functional status of patients with unilateral neglect after stroke and brain injury using a visual imagery intervention. *Topics in Stroke Rehabilitation, 8*(2), 10–18.

Niemeier, J. P., Kreutzer, J. S., & Taylor, L. A. (2005). Acute cognitive and neurobehavioural intervention for individuals with acquired brain injury: Preliminary outcome data. *Neuropsychological Rehabilitation, 15*(2), 129–146.

Nitsche, M., & Paulus, W. (2011). Transcranial direct current stimulation–Update 2011. *Restorative Neurology ad Neuroscience, 29*, 463–492.

Nobis-Bosch, R., Springer, L., Radermacher, I., & Huber, W. (2011). Supervised home training of dialogue skills in chronic aphasia: A randomized parallel group study. *Journal of Speech, Language, and Hearing, 54*, 1118–1136.

Noda, R., Maeda, Y., & Yoshino, A. (2004). Therapeutic time window for musicokinetic therapy in a persistent vegetative state after severe brain damage. *Brain Injury, 18*(5), 509–515.

Nolin, P., Villemure, R., & Heroux, L. (2006). Determining long-term symptoms following mild traumatic brain injury: Method of interview affects self-report. *Brain Injury, 20*(11), 1147–1154.

Noonan, V. K., Kopec, J. A., Singer, J., & Dvorak, M. F. (2009). A review of participation instruments based on the International Classification of Functioning, Disability, and Health. *Disability and Rehabilitation, 31*(23), 1883–1901.

Norman, D. A., & Shallice, T. (1986). Attention to action: Willed and automatic control of behavior. In R. J. Davidson, G. E. Schwartz, & D. Shapiro (Eds.), *Consciousness and self-regulation* (pp. 1–18). New York: Plenum Press.

Norman, M. A., Moore, D. J., Taylor, M., Franklin, D., Cysique, L., Ake, C., . . . Heaton, R. K. (2011). Demographically corrected norms for African Americans and Caucasians on the Hopkins Verbal Learning Test–Revised, Brief Visuospatial Memory Test–Revised, Stroop Color and Word Test, and Wisconsin Card Sorting Test 64-Card Version. *Journal of Clinical and Experimental Neuropsychology, 33*(7), 793–804.

North Carolina Board of Examiners. (1999). *Speech-language pathology assistants. North Carolina Board of Examiners Directory* (1999 ed.). Greensboro, NC: North Carolina Board of Examiners.

Nurmi, L., Kettunen, J., Laihosalo, M., Ruuskanen, E., Koivisto, A., & Jehkonen, M. (2010). Right hemisphere infarct patients and halthy controls: Evaluation of starting points in cancellation tasks. *Journal of the International Neuropsychology Society, 16*(5), 902–909.

Nussbaum, P. D. (1994). Pseudodementia: A slow death. *Neuropsychology Review, 4*, 71–90.

Nussbaum, P. D. (1998). Neuropsychological assessment of the elderly. In G. Goldstein, P. D., Nussbaum, & S. R. Beers (Eds.), *Neuropsychology* (pp. 83–105). New York: Plenum Press.

Nyberg, L. (2002). Levels of processing: A view from functional brain imaging. *Memory, 10*(5–6), 345–348.

Nys, G. M., Van Zandvoort, M., De Kort, P., Jansen, B., Kappelle, L., & De Haan, E. (2005a). Restrictions of the Mini-Mental State Examination in acute stroke. *Archives of Clinical Neuropsychology, 20*(5), 623–629.

Oberg, L. W., & Turkstra, L. S. (1998). The use of elaborative encoding to facilitate vocabulary learning after adolescent traumatic brain injury: Two case illustrations. *Journal of Head Trauma Rehabilitation, 3*, 44–62.

O'Brien, J. T., Erkinjuntti, T., Reisberg, B., Roman, G., Sawada, T., Pantoni, L., . . . DeKosky, S. T. (2003). Vascular cognitive impairment. *The Lancet: Neurology, 2*, 89–98.

OCEBM Levels of Evidence Working Group. (2011). *The Oxford 2011 levels of evidence.* Available from http://www.cebm.net/index.aspx?o=5653

O'Connell, M., Mateer, C., & Kerns, K. (2003). Prosthetic systems for addressing problems with initiation: Guidelines for selection, training, and measuring efficacy. *NeuroRehabilitation, 18*, 9–20.

Oda, H., Ohkawa, S., & Maeda, K. (2008). Hemispatial visual defect in Alzheimer's disease. *Neurocase, 14*(2), 141–146.

Odell, K. H., Wollack, J. A., & Flynn, M. (2005). Functional outcomes in patients with right hemisphere brain damage. *Aphasiology, 19*(9), 807–830.

Oelschlaeger, M. L., & Thorne, J. C. (1999). Application of the correct information unit analysis to the naturally occurring conversation of a person with aphasia. *Journal of Speech, Language and Hearing Research, 42*, 636–648.

Office of Technology Assessment. (1978). *Assessing the safety and efficacy of medical technologies.* Washington, DC: Author.

Ogar, J. M. (2010). Primary progressive aphasia and its three variants. *Perspectives on Neurophysiology and Neurogenic Speech and Language Disorders, 20*(1), 5–12.

Ogrezeanu, V., Voinescu, I., Mihailescu, L., & Jipescu, I. (1994). "Spontaneous" recovery in aphasics after single ischaemic stroke. *Romanian Journal of Neurology and Psychiatry, 32*, 77–90.

Oh, H., & Seo, W. (2003). Sensory stimulation programme to improve recovery in comatose patients. *Journal of Clinical Nursing, 12*, 394–404.

Ojemann, G. A., & Mateer, C. (1979). Human language cortex: Localization of memory, syntax, and sequential motor-phoneme identification systems. *Science, 205*, 1401–1403.

Ojemann, G. A., & Whitaker, H. A. (1978). Language localization and variability. *Brain and Language, 6*, 239–260.

O'Keeffe, F., Dockree, P., Moloney, P., Carton, S., & Robertson, I. H. (2007). Awareness of deficits in traumatic brain injury: A multidimensional approach to assessing metacognitive knowledge and online-awareness. *Journal of the International Neuropsychological Society, 13*, 38–49.

Oken, B. S., Flegal, K., Zajdel, D., Kishiyama, S. S., Lovera, J., Bagert, B., & Bourdette, D. N. (2006). Cognition and fatigue in multiple sclerosis: Potential effects of medications with central nervous system activity. *Journal of Rehabilitation Research and Development, 43*(1), 83–90.

Okie, S. (2005). Traumatic brain injury in the war zone. *The New England Journal of Medicine, 352*(20), 2043–2047.

Oleksiak, M., Smith, B., St. Andre, J., Caughlan, C., & Steiner, M. (2012). Audiological issues and hearing loss among veterans with mild traumatic brain injury. *Journal of Rehabilitation Research and Development, 49*(7), 995–1004.

Oliveira, F., & Damasceno, B. (2011). Global aphasia as a predictor of mortality in the acute phase of a first stroke. *Arquivos de Neuro-Psiquiatria, 69*(2-B), 277–282.

Oliveira, R. M., Gurd, J. M., Nixon, P., Marshall, J. C., & Passingham, R. E. (1997). Micrographia in Parkinson's disease: The effect of providing external cues. *Journal of Neurology, Neurosurgery, and Psychiatry, 63*, 429–433.

Olsen, E., Freed, D., & Marshall, R. (2012). Generalization of personalized cueing to enhance word finding in natural settings. *Aphasiology, 26*(5), 618–631.

One, K., Yalçinkaya, E. Y., Toklu, B. C., & Cağlar, N. (2009). Effects of age, gender, and cognitive, functional and motor status on functional outcomes of stroke rehabilitation. *NeuroRehabilitation, 25*(4), 241–249.

O'Neil-Pirozzi, T., Stangman, G., Goldstein, R., Katz, D., Savage, D., Kelkar, K., . . . Glenn, M. (2010). A controlled treatment study of internal memory strategies following traumatic brain injury. *Journal of Head Trauma Rehabilitation, 25*(1), 43–51.

Orange, J. B., & Colton-Hudson, A. (1998). A case study of a spousal communication education and training program for Alzheimer's disease. *Special Interest Division 2: Neurophysiology and Neurogenic Speech and Language Disorders Newsletter, 8*, 22–29.

Orenstein, E., & Shisler, R. (2009, May 26–30). *Effects of mindfulness meditation on three individuals with aphasia*. Paper presented at the Clinical Aphasiology Conference, Keystone, CO.

Osaka, N., Osaka, M., Kondo, H., Morishita, M., Fukuyama, H., & Shibasaki, H. (2004). The neural basis of executive function in working memory: An fMRI study based on individual differences. *Neuroimage, 21*, 623–631.

Osborn, C. (2000). *Over my head*. Kansas City, MO: Andrews McMeel.

Osher, J. E., Wicklund, A. H., Rademaker, A., Johnson, N., & Weintraub, S. (2008). The mini-mental state examination in behavioral variant frontotemporal dementia and primary progressive aphasia. *American Journal of Alzheimer's Disease and Other Dementias, 22*(6), 468–473.

O'Sullivan, T., & Fagan, S. C. (1998). Drug-induced communication and swallowing disorders. In A. F. Johnson & B. H. Jacobson (Eds.), *Medical speech-language pathology: A practitioner's guide* (pp. 176–191). New York: Thieme.

Owens, R. E. (2012). *Language development: An introduction* (8th ed). Columbus, OH: Allyn & Bacon.

Owens, R. E., Metz, D. E., & Haas, A. (2007). *Introduction to communication disorders: A life span perspective*. Boston: Allyn & Bacon.

Ownsworth, T., Fleming, J., Desbois, J., Strong, J., & Kuipers, P. (2006). A metacognitive contextual intervention to enhance error awareness and functional outcome following traumatic brain injury: A single-case experimental design. *Journal of the International Neuropsychological Society, 12*(1), 54–63.

Ownsworth, T., & McFarland, K. (1999). Memory remediation in long-term acquired brain injury: Two approaches in diary training. *Brain Injury, 13*, 605–626.

Ownsworth, T., Turpin, M., Andrew, B., & Fleming, J. (2008). Participant perspectives on an individualised self-awareness intervention following stroke: A qualitative case study. *Neuropsychological Rehabilitation, 18*(5–6), 692–712.

Ozeren, A., Sarica, Y., Mavi, Y., & Demirkiran, M. (1995). Bromocriptine is ineffective in the treatment of chronic nonfluent aphasia. *Acta Neurologica Belgium, 95*, 235–238.

Pagni, C., Frosini, D., Ceravolo, R, Giunti, G., Unti, E., Poletti, M., . . . Tognoni, G. (2011). Event-based prospective memory in newly diagnosed, drug-naïve Parkinson's disease patients. *Journal of the International Neuropsychological Society, 17*, 1158–1162.

Pagonabarraga, J., Kulisevsky, J., Llebaria, G., Garcia-Sanchez, C., Pascual-Sedano, B., & Gironell, A. (2008). Parkinson's disease–cognitive rating scale (PD-CRS): A new cognitive scale specific for Parkinson's disease. *Movement Disorders, 23*, 998–1005.

Pakhomov, S., Smith, G., Marino, S., Birnbaum, A., Graff-Radford, N., Caselli, R., . . . Knopman, D. (2010). A computerized technique to assess language use patterns in patients with frontotemporal dementia. *Journal of Neurolinguistics, 23*(2), 127–144.

Palmese, C. A., & Raskin, S. A. (2000). The rehabilitation of attention in individuals with mild traumatic brain injury using the APT-II programme. *Brain Injury, 14*, 535–548.

Pang, D. (1985). Pathophysiologic correlates of neurobehavioral syndromes following closed head injury. In M. Ylvisaker (Ed.), *Head injury rehabilitation: Children and adolescents* (pp. 3–70). San Diego, CA: College-Hill Press.

Pang, Y., Wu, L. B., & Liu, D. H. (2010). Acupuncture therapy for apoplectic aphasia: A systematic review. *Zhongguo Zhen Jiu, 30*(7), 612–616.

Pantiga, C., Rodrigo, L., Cuesta, M., Lopez, L., & Arias, J. (2003). Cognitive deficits in patients with hepatic cirrhosis and in liver transplant recipients. *Journal of Neuropsychiatry and Clinical Neurosciences, 15*, 84–89.

Paolucci, S., Antonucci, G., Guariglia, C., Magnotti, L., Pizzamiglio, L., & Zoccolotti, P. (1996). Facilitory effect of neglect rehabilitation on the recovery of left hemiplegic stroke patients: A cross-over study. *Journal of Neurology, 243*, 308–314.

Papathanassiou, I., Filipovic, S., Whurr, R., & Jahnashahi, M. (2003). Plasticity of motor cortex excitability induced by rehabilitation therapy for writing. *Neurology, 61*, 977–980.

Paradis, M. (2004). *A neurolinguistic theory of bilingualism*. The Netherlands: John Benjamins.

Paradis, M. (2011). Principles underlying the Bilingual Aphasia Test (BAT) and its uses. *Clinical Linguistics and Phonetics, 25*(6–7), 427–443.

Paradis, M., & Libben, G. (1987). *The assessment of bilingual aphasia*. Hillsdale, NJ: Erlbaum.

Paradis, M., & Libben, G. (1993). *Evaluacion de la afasia en los bilingues*. Barcelona, Spain: Masson.

Paradise, M., Cooper, C., & Livingston, G. (2009). Systematic review of the effect of education on survival in Alzheimer's disease. *International Psychogeriatrics, 21*(1), 25–32.

Parenté, R., & Herrmann, D. (2010). *Retraining cognition: Techniques and applications* (3rd ed.). Austin, TX: PRO-ED.

Park, K. W., Kim, H. S., Cheon, S., Cha, J., Kim, S., & Kim, J. W. (2011). Dementia with Lewy bodies versus Alzheimer's disease and Parkinson's disease dementia: A comparison of cognitive profiles. *Journal of Clinical Neurology, 7*, 19–24.

Park, N. W., & Ingles, J. L. (2001). Effectiveness of attention rehabilitation after an acquired brain injury: A meta-analysis. *Neuropsychology, 15*, 199–210.

Park, N. W., Proulx, G. B., & Towers, W. M. (1999). Evaluation of the Attention Process Training programme. *Neuropsychological Rehabilitation, 9*, 135–154.

Parr, S. (2007). Living with severe aphasia: Tracking social exclusion. *Aphasiology, 21*(1), 98–123.

Parron, T., Requena, M., Hernandez, A., & Alarcon, R. (2011). Association between environmental exposure to pesticides and neurodegenerative diseases. *Toxicology and Applied Pharmacology, 256*(3), 379–385.

Pashek, G. V., & Bachman, D. L. (2003). Cognitive, linguistic, and motor speech effects of donepezil hydrocholoride in a patient with stroke-related aphasia and apraxia of speech. *Brain and Language, 87*, 179–180.

Pashler, H. (1994a). Dual-task interference in simple tasks: Data and theory. *Psychological Bulletin, 116*, 220–244.

Pashler, H. (1994b). Graded capacity-sharing in dual-task interference? *Journal of Experimental Psychology: Human Perception and Performance, 20,* 330–342.

Patient Protection and Affordable Care Act of 2010, 42 U.S.C. § 18001 *et seq.* (2010)

Patricacou, A., Psallida, E., Pring, T., & Dipper, L. (2007). The Boston Naming Test in Greek: Normative data and the effects of age and education on naming. *Aphasiology, 21*(12), 1157–1170.

Patrick, P. D., Buck, M. L., Conaway, M. R., & Blackman, J. A. (2003). The use of dopamine enhancing medications with children in low response states following brain injury. *Brain Injury, 17,* 497–506.

Pattee, C., Von Berg, S., & Ghezzi, P. (2006). Effects of alternative communication on the communicative effectiveness of an individual with a progressive language disorder. *International Journal of Rehabilitation Research, 29*(2), 151–153.

Paul, N. A., & Sanders, G. F. (2010). Applying an ecological framework to education needs of communication partners of individuals with aphasia. *Aphasiology, 24*(9), 1095–1112.

Paul-Brown, D., Frattali, C. M., Holland, A. L., Thompson, C. K., Caperton, C. J., & Slater, S. C. (2004). *Quality of communication life scale.* Rockville, MD: American Speech-Language-Hearing Association.

Pavlik, V. N., Doody, R. S., Massman, P. J., & Chan, W. (2006). Influence of premorbid IQ and education on progression of Alzheimer's disease. *Dementia and Geriatric Cognitive Disorders, 22,* 367–377.

Payne, J. C. (1994). *Communication profile: A functional skills survey.* San Antonio, TX: Communication Skill Builders.

Peach, R. K. (2001). Further thoughts regarding management of acute aphasia following stroke. *American Journal of Speech-Language Pathology, 10,* 29–36.

Peach, R. K., & Wong, P. C. M. (2004). Integrating the message level into treatment for agrammatism using story retelling. *Aphasiology, 18,* 429–441.

Pedersen, P. M., Vinter, K., & Olsen, T. S. (2004). Aphasia after stroke: Type, severity and prognosis. The Copenhagen aphasia study. *Cerebrovascular Disorders, 17,* 35–43.

Pedraza, O., & Mungas, D. (2008). Measurement in cross-cultural neuropsychology. *Neuropsychology Review, 18,* 184–193.

Pelosof, L. C., & Gerber, D. E. (2010). Paraneoplastic syndromes: An approach to diagnosis and treatment. *Mayo Clinic Proceedings, 85*(9), 838–854.

Peña-Casanova, J., Quiñones-Ubeda, S., Quintana-Aparicio, M., Aguilar, M., Badenes, D., Molinuevo, J. L., . . . Blesa, R. (2009). Spanish Multicenter Normative Studies (NEURONORMA Project): Norms for verbal span, visuospatial span, letter and number sequencing, trail making test, and symbol digit modalities test. *Archives of Clinical Neuropsychology, 24*(4), 321–341.

Penfield, W., & Roberts, L. (1959). *Speech and brain mechanisms.* Princeton, NJ: Princeton University Press.

Penn, C. (1988). The profiling of syntax and pragmatics in aphasia. *Clinical Linguistics and Phonetics, 2,* 179–207.

Penn, C., Jones, D., & Joffe, V. (1997). Hierarchial discourse therapy: A method for the mild patient. *Aphasiology, 11,* 601–632.

Pentland, B., Hutton, L., MacMillan, A., & Mayer, V. (2003). Training in brain injury rehabilitation. *Disability and Rehabilitation, 25,* 544–548.

Pentland, B., & Whittle, I. R. (1999). Acute management of brain injury. In M. Rosenthal, J. S. Kreutzer, E. R. Griffith, & Pentland, B. (Eds.), *Rehabilitation of the adult and child with traumatic brain injury* (3rd ed., pp. 42–52). Philadelphia: F. A. Davis.

Peper, M., & Irle, E. (1997). Categorical and dimensional coding of emotional intonations in patients with focal brain lesions. *Brain and Language, 58,* 233–264.

Perenboom, R. J., & Chorus, A. M. (2003). Measuring participation according to the International Classification of Functioning, Disability, and Health (ICF). *Disability and Rehabilitation, 25*(11–12), 577–587.

Perkins, L., Whitworth, A., & Lesser, R. (1997). *Conversation analysis profile for people with cognitive impairment.* Philadelphia: Taylor & Francis.

Pero, S., Incoccia, C., Caracciolo, B., Zoccolotti, P., & Formisano, R. (2006). Rehabilitation of attention in two patients with traumatic brain injury by means of "attention process training." *Brain Injury, 20,* 1207–1219.

Phelps-Terasaki, D., & Phelps-Gunn, T. (2007). *Test of pragmatic language* (2nd ed.). Austin, TX: PRO-ED.

Pickens, S., Ostwald, S., Murphy-Pace, K., & Bergstrom, N. (2010). Systematic review of current executive function measures in adults with and without cognitive impairments. *International Journal of Evidence Based Heatlhcare, 8,* 110–125.

Pimental, P. A., & Kingsbury, N. A. (1989). *Mini inventory of right brain injury.* Austin, TX: PRO-ED.

Pimental, P. A., & Knight, J. A. (2000). *Mini inventory of right brain injury* (2nd ed.). Austin, TX: PRO-ED.

Pinto, E., & Peters, R. (2009). Literature review of the Clock Drawing Test as a tool for cognitive screening. *Dementia and Geriatric Cognitive Disorders, 27*(3), 201–213.

Piolino, P., Desgranges, B., Manning, L., North, P., Jokic, C., & Eustache, F. (2007). Autobiographical memory, the sense of recollection and executive functions after severe traumatic brain injury. *Cortex, 43,* 176–195.

Piras, F., Borella, E., Incoccia, C., & Carlesimo, G. (2011). Evidence-based practice recommendations for memory rehabilitation. *European Journal of Physical Rehabilitation and Medicine, 47,* 149–175.

Pitel, A., Beaunieux, H., Lebaron, N., Joyeaux, F., Desgranges, B., & Eustache, F. (2006). Two case studies in the application of errorless learning techniques in memory impaired patients with additional executive deficits. *Brain Injury, 20,* 1099–1110.

Pizzamiglio, I., Mammucari, A., & Razzano, C. (1985). Evidence for sex differences in brain organization in recovery in aphasia. *Brain and Language, 25,* 213–223.

Plass, B. (2005). *Functional vocabularly for adolescents and adults.* East Moline, IL: Linguisystems.

Plassman, B. L., Langa, K. M., Fisher, G. G., Heeringa, S. G., Weir, D. R., Ofstedal, M. B., . . . Wallace, R. B. (2007). Prevalence of dementia in the United States: The aging, demographics, and memory study. *Neuroepidemiology, 29*(1–2), 125–132.

Plowman, E., Hentz, B., & Ellis, C. (2011). Post-stroke aphasia prognosis: A review of patient-related and stroke-related factors. *Journal of Evaluation in Clinical Practice, 18,* 689–694.

Polanowska, K., Seniów, J., Paprot, E., Lešniak, M., & Członkowska, A. (2009). Left-hand somatosensory stimulation combined with visual scanning training in rehabilitation for post-stroke hemineglect: A randomised, double-blind study. *Neuropsychological Rehabilitation, 19*(3), 364–382.

Polster, M. R., & Rose, S. B. (1998). Disorders of auditory processing: Evidence for modularity in audition. *Cortex, 34,* 47–65.

Popovici, M., Mihailescu, L., & Voinescu, I. (1992). Melodic Intonation Therapy in the rehabilitation of Romanian aphasics with buccolingual apraxia. *Review of Romanian Neurology and Psychiatry, 30,* 99–113.

Porch, B. E. (2001). *Porch index of communicative ability* (Rev. ed.). Albuquerque, NM: PICA Programs.

Porter, K. R., McCarthy, B. J., Freels, S., Kim, Y., & Davis, F. G. (2010). Prevalence estimates for primary brain tumors in the U.S. by age, gender, behavior, and histology. *Neuro-Oncology, 12*(6), 520–527.

Porteus, S. D. (1965). *Porteus maze test. Fifty years application.* Palo Alto, CA: Pacific.

Portugal, M., Marinho, V., & Laks, J. (2011). Pharmacological treatment of frontotemporal lobar degeneration: Systematic review. *Revista Brasileira de Psiquiatria, 33*(1), 81–90.

Posteraro, L., Formis, A., Grassi, E., Bighi, M., Nati, P., Proietti Bocchini, C., . . . Franceschini, M. (2006). Quality of life and aphasia. Multicentric standardization of a questionnaire. *Europa Medicophysica, 42*(3), 227–230.

Potter, J., Deighton, T., Patel, M., Fairhurst, M., Guest, R., & Donnelly, N. (2000). Computer recording of standard tests of visual neglect in stroke patients. *Clinical Rehabilitation, 14,* 441–446.

Poulin, V., Korner-Bitensky, N., Dawson, D., & Bherer, L. (2012). Efficacy of executive function interventions after stroke: A systematic review. *Topics in Stroke Rehabilitation, 19*(2), 158–171.

Pound, C. (1996). Writing remediation using preserved oral spelling: A case for separate output buffers. *Aphasiology, 10,* 283–296.

Prins, R., & Bastiaanse, R. (2004). Analysing the spontaneous speech of aphasic speakers. *Aphasiology, 18,* 1075–1091.

Proto, D., Pella, R. D., Hill, B. D., & Gouvier, W. D. (2009). Assessment and rehabilitation of acquired visuospatial and proprioceptive deficits associated with visuospatial neglect. *NeuroRehabilitation, 24*(2), 145–157.

Prutting, C. (1979). The action of moving forward progressively from one point to another on the way to completion. *Journal of Speech and Hearing Research, 14,* 776–792.

Prutting, C. A., & Kirchner, D. M. (1987). A clinical appraisal of the pragmatic aspects of language. *Journal of Speech and Hearing Disorders, 52*, 105–119.

Pryor, J. (2004). What environmental factors irritate people with acquired brain injury? *Disability and Rehabilitation, 26*(16), 974–980.

PSSCogRehab [computer software]. (2012). Indianapolis, IN: Psychological Software Service.

Psycholinguistic Technologies. (2012). *SentenceShaper 2.* Jenkintown, PA: Author.

Psychological Corporation. (1996). *Vigil continuous performance test.* San Antonio, TX: Author.

Ptak, R., der Linden, M. V., & Schnider, A. (2010). Cognitive rehabilitation of episodic memory disorders: From theory to practice. *Frontiers in Human Neuroscience, 4.* doi: 10.3389/fnhum.2010.00057

Purdy, M. (2002). Executive function ability in persons with aphasia. *Aphasiology, 16*, 549–557.

Purdy, M., & Dietz, A. (2010). Factors influencing AAC usage by individuals with aphasia. *Perspectives on Augmentative and Alternative Communication, 19*(3), 70–78.

Purdy, M., & Koch, A. (2006). Prediction of strategy usage by adults with aphasia. *Aphasiology, 20*(2–4), 337–348.

Pylyshyn, Z. (1999). Is vision continuous with cognition? The case for cognitive impenetrability of visual perception. *Behavioral and Brain Sciences, 22*, 341–423.

Rabins, P. V. (1983). Reversible dementia and the misdiagnosis of dementia: A review. *Hospital Community Psychiatry, 9*, 830–835.

Rabinstein, A. A., & Shulman, L. (2003). Acupuncture in clinical neurology. *Neurology, 9*, 137–148.

Rabuffetti, M., Farina, E., Alberoni, M., Pellegatta, D., Appollonio, I., Affanni, P., . . . Ferrarin, M. (2012). Spatio-temporal features of visual exploration in unilaterally brain-damaged subjects with or without neglect: Results from a touchscreen test. *PLoS One, 7*(2), e31511. doi: 10.1371/journal.pone.0031511

Radanovic, M., & Scaff, M. (2003). Speech and language disturbances due to subcortical lesions. *Brain and Language, 84*, 337–352.

Radford, K., Lah, S., Thayer, Z., Say, M., & Miller, L. (2012). Improving memory in outpatients with neurological disorders using a group-based training program. *Journal of the International Neuropsychological Society, 18*, 1–11.

Radice-Neumann, D., Zupan, B., Tomita, M., & Willer, B. (2009). Training emotional processing in persons with brain injury. *Journal of Head Trauma Rehabilitation, 24*, 313–323.

Radloff, L. W., & Teri, L. (1986). Assessing depression in older adults: The CES-D scale. *Clinical Gerontologist, 5*, 119–137.

Raglio, A., Bellelli, G., Traficante, D., Gianotti, M., Ubezio, M. C., Villani, D., & Trabucchi, M. (2008). Efficacy of music therapy in the treatment of behavioral and psychiatric symptoms of dementia. *Alzheimer Disease & Associated Disorders, 22*(2), 158–162.

Ramage, A., Beeson, P., & Rapcsak, S. Z. (1998). *Dissociation between oral and written spelling: Clinical characteristics and possible mechanisms.* Presentation at the Clinical Aphasiology Conference, Asheville, NC.

Rami, L., Serradell, M., Bosch, B., Caprile, C., Sekler, A., Villar, A., . . . Molinuevo, J. (2008). Normative data for the Boston Naming Test and the Pyramids and Palm Trees Test in the elderly Spanish population. *Journal of Clinical and Experimental Neuropsychology, 30*(1), 1–6.

Ramsberger, G. (2005). Achieving conversational success in aphasia by focusing on nonlinguistic cognitive skills: A potentially promising new approach. *Aphasiology, 19*(10/11), 1066–1073.

Ramsberger, G., & Helm-Estabrooks, N. (1989). Visual Action Therapy for bucco-facial apraxia. *Clinical Aphasiology, 20*, 395–400.

Ramsing, S., Blomstrand, C., & Sullivan, M. (1991). Prognostic factors for return to work in stroke patients with aphasia. *Aphasiology, 5*, 583–588.

Rand, D., Weiss, P., & Katz, N. (2009). Training multitasking in a virtual supermarket: A novel intervention after stroke. *American Journal of Occupational Therapy, 63*, 535–542.

Randolph, C. (2012). *Repeatable battery for the assessment of neuropsychological status update.* San Antonio, TX: Pearson.

Rankin, K., Salazar, A., Gorno-Tempini, M., Sollberger, M., Wilson, S., Pavlic, D., . . . Miller, B. L. (2009). Detecting sarcasm from paralinguistic cues: Anatomic and cognitive correlates in neurodegenerative disease. *Neuroimage, 47*(4), 2005–2015.

Rao, P. R. (1995). Drawing and gesture as communication options in a person with severe aphasia. *Topics in Stroke Rehabilitation, 2*, 49–56.

Rao, P. (2001). Use of Amer-Ind code by persons with severe aphasia. In R. Chapey (Ed.), *Language intervention strategies in adult aphasia* (4th ed., pp. 688–701). Baltimore: Williams & Wilkins.

Rapp, B., & Caramazza, A. (1998). A case of selective difficulty in writing verbs. *Neurocase, 4*(2), 127–140.

Rapp, S., Brenes, G., & Marsh, A. P. (2002). Memory enhancement training for older adults with mild cognitive impairment: A preliminary study. *Aging and Mental Health, 6*, 5–11.

Raskin, D., & Buckheit, C. (2010). *Memory for intentions test.* Lutz, FL: PAR.

Raskin, S. A., & Sohlberg, M. M. (1996). The efficacy of prospective memory training in two adults with brain injury. *Journal of Head Trauma Rehabilitation, 11*, 32–51.

Raskin, D., & Sohlberg, M. (2009). Prospective memory intervention: A review and evaluation of a pilot restorative intervention. *Brain Impairment, 10*(1), 76–86.

Rath, J. F., Langebahn, D. M., Simon, D., Sherr, R., Fletcher, J., & Diller, L. (2004). The construct of problem solving in higher level neuropsychological assessment and rehabilitation. *Archives of Clinical Neuropsychology, 19*, 613–635.

Rath, J. F., Simon, D., Langenbahn, D. M., Sherr, R. L., & Diller, L. (2003). Group treatment of problem solving deficits in outpatients with traumatic brain injury: A randomised outcome study. *Neuropsychological Rehabilitation, 13*(4), 461–488.

Rathore, S. S., Hinn, A. R., Cooper, L. S., Tyroler, H. A., & Rosamond, W. D. (2002). Characterization of incident stroke signs and symptoms: Findings from the atherosclerosis risk in communities study. *Stroke, 33*, 2718–2721.

Raven, J. C. (2003). *Raven's progressive matrices.* San Antonio, TX: Pearson.

Ravizza, S., McCormick, C., Schlerf, J., Justus, T., Ivry, R., & Fiez, J. (2006). Cerebellar damage produces selective deficits in verbal working memory. *Brain, 129*, 306–320.

Raymer, A. M. (2003). Treatment of adynamia in aphasia. *Frontiers in Bioscience, 8*, S845–S851.

Raymer, A. M., Bandy, D., & Adair, J. C. (2001). Effects of bromocriptine in a patient with crossed nonfluent aphasia: A case report. *Archives of Physical Medicine and Rehabilitation, 82*, 139–144.

Raymer, A. M., McHose, B., Smith, K., Iman, L., Ambrose, A., & Casselton, C. (2012). Contrasting effects of errorless naming treatment and gestural facilitation for word retrieval in aphasia, *Neuropsychological Rehabilitation, 22*(2), 235–266.

Raymer, A. M., & Rothi, L. J. G. (2001). Cognitive approaches to impairments of word comprehension and production. In R. Chapey (Ed.), *Language intervention strategies in adult aphasia* (4th ed., pp. 524–550). New York: Lippincott Williams & Wilkins.

Raymer, A. M., Singletary, F., Rodriguez, A., Ciampitti, M., Heilman, K. M., & Gonzalez Rothi, L. J. (2006). Effects of gesture + verbal treatment for noun and verb retrieval in aphasia. *Journal of the International Neuropsychological Society, 12*, 867–882.

Raymer, A. M., Thompson, C. K., Jacobs, B., Le Grand, H. R. (1993). Phonological treatment of naming deficits in aphasia: Model-based generalization analysis. *Aphasiology, 7*, 27–53.

Rayner, H., & Marshall, J. (2003). Training volunteers as conversation partners for people with aphasia. *International Journal of Language and Communication Disorders, 38*, 149–164.

Raz, A. (2006). Individual differences and attentional varieties. *Europa Medicophysica, 42*(1), 53–58.

Records, N. L. (1994). A measure of the contribution of a gesture to the perception of speech in listeners with aphasia. *Journal of Speech and Hearing Research, 37*, 1086–1099.

Records, N. L., Tomblin, J. B., & Freese, P. R. (1992). The quality of life of young adults with histories of specific language impairment. *American Journal of Speech-Language Pathology, 1*, 44–53.

Reed, D., Johnson, N., Thompson, C., Weintraub, S., & Mesulam, M. (2004). A clinical trial of bromocriptine for treatment of primary progressive aphasia. *Annals of Neurology, 56*(5), 750.

Rehabilitation Act of 1973, 29 U.S.C. 70 § 701 *et seq.* (1973)

Reilly, J., Rodriguez, A., Lamy, M., & Neils-Strunjas, J. (2010). Cognition, language, and clinical pathological features of non-Alzheimer's dementias: An overview. *Journal of Communication Disorders, 43*(5), 438–452.

Reilly, S. (2004). The challenges in making speech pathology evidence based. *Advances in Speech-Language Pathology, 6*, 113–124.

Reinmuth, O. M. (1997). Stroke: Mechanisms and effects. *Special Interest Division 2: Neurophysiology and Neurogenic Speech and Language Disorders Newsletter, 7,* 16–19.

Reitan, R. M., & Wolfson, D. (1993). *The Halstead-Reitan neuropsychological test battery: Theory and clinical interpretation* (2nd ed). Tucson, AZ: Neuropsychology Press.

Reiter, E., & Costanzo, R. (2010). Chemosensory impairment after traumatic brain injury: Assessment and management. *International Brain Injury Association Newsletter, 5.* Available at: http://www.internationalbrain.org/?q=node/149

Rende, B. (2000). Cognitive flexibility: Theory, assessment and treatment. *Seminars in Speech and Language, 21,* 121–134.

Renison, B., Ponsford, J., Testa, R., Richardson, B., & Brownfield, K. (2008). *Virtual library task.* Melbourne, Australia: Monash University.

Renison, B., Ponsford, J., Testa, R., Richardson, B., & Brownfield, K. (2012). The ecological and construct validity of a newly developed measure of executive function: The Virtual Library Task. *Journal of the International Neuropsychological Society, 18,* 1–11.

Renner, C., Hummelsheim, H., Kopczak, A., Steube, D., Schneider, H., Schneider, M., . . . Stalla, G. (2012). The influence of gender on the injury severity, course and outcome of traumatic brain injury. *Brain Injury, 26*(11), 1360–1371.

Rey, G. J., Sivan, A. B., & Benton, A. L. (1991). *Multilingual aphasia examination–Spanish version.* Lutz, FL: Psychological Assessment Resources.

Reynolds, C. R. (2002). *Comprehensive trail-making test.* Lutz, FL: Psychological Assessment Resources.

Reynolds, C., & Horton, A. M. (2007). *Test of verbal conceptualization and fluency.* Austin, TX: PRO-ED.

Reynolds, C., & Voress, J. (2007). *Test of memory and learning* (2nd ed.). Austin, TX: PRO-ED.

Reynolds, C., & Voress, J. (2012). *Test of memory and learning* (Senior ed.). Austin, TX: PRO-ED.

Reynolds, W. (1999). *Multidimensional anxiety questionnaire.* Odessa, FL: PAR.

Reynolds, W., & Kobak, K. (1998). *Reynolds depression screening inventory.* Lutz, FL: PAR.

Rhodes-Kropf, J., Cheng, H., Castillo, E., & Fulton, A. (2011). Managing the patient with dementia in long-term care. *Clinics in Geriatric Medicine, 27,* 135–152.

Richards, K., Singletary F., Gonzalez Rothi, L. J., Koehler, S., & Crosson, B. (2002). Activation of intentional mechanisms through utilization of nonsymbolic movements in aphasia rehabilitation. *Journal of Rehabilitation Research and Development, 39,* 445–454.

Richardson, J. T., & Barry, C. (1985). The effects of minor closed head injury upon human memory: Further evidence on the role of mental imagery. *Cognitive Neuropsychology, 2,* 149–168.

Richeson, N. E. (2003). Effects of animal-assisted therapy on agitated behaviors and social interactions of older adults with dementia. *American Journal of Alzheimer's Disease and Other Dementias, 18,* 353–358.

Rider, J., Wright, H., Marshall, R., & Page, J. (2008). Using semantic feature analysis to improve contextual discourse in adults with aphasia. *American Journal of Speech-Language Pathology, 17*(2), 161–172.

Riederer, P., & Sian-Hülsmann, J. (2012). The significance of neuronal lateralisation in Parkinson's disease. *Journal of Neural Transmission.* doi: 10.1007/s00702-012-0775-1

Rinere O'Brien, S. (2010). Trends in inpatient rehabilitation stroke outcomes before and after advent of the prospective payment system: A systematic review. *Journal of Neurology and Physical Therapy, 34*(1), 17–23.

Rinne, J. O., Portin, R., Ruottinen, H., Nurmi, I., Bergman, J., Haaparanta, M., . . . Solin, O. (2000). Cognitive impairment and the brain dopaminergic system in Parkinson's disease. *Archives of Neurology, 57,* 470–475.

Rios, M., Perianez, J. A., & Munoz-Cespedes, J. M. (2004). Attentional control and slowness of information processing after severe traumatic brain injury. *Brain Injury, 18,* 257–272.

Ripich, D. N. (1996). *Alzheimer's disease communication guide: The FOCUSED program for caregivers.* San Antonio, TX: Psychological Corporation.

Ritchie, K., & Lovestone, S. (2002). The dementias. *The Lancet, 360,* 1759–1766.

Roach, E., Golomb, M., Adams, R., Biller, J., Daniels, S., deVeber, G., . . . Smith, E. R. (2008). Management of stroke in infants and children: A scientific statement from a special writing group of the American Heart Association Stroke Council and the Council on Cardiovascular Disease in the Young. *Stroke, 39.* doi: 10.1161/CIR.0b013e31823ac046

Roberts, C. B., Rafal, R., & Coetzer, B. R. (2006). Feedback of brain-imaging findings: Effect on impaired awareness and mood in acquired brain injury. *Brain Injury, 20*(5), 485–497.

Roberts, P. (2008). Issues in assessment and treatment for bilingual and culturally diverse patients. In R. Chapey (Ed.), *Language intervention strategies in aphasia and related neurogenic communication disorders* (5th ed., pp. 245–275). New York: Lippincott Williams & Wilkins.

Roberts, P., & Doucet, N. (2011). Performance of French-speaking Quebec adults on the Boston Naming Test. *Canadian Journal of Speech-Language Pathology and Audiology, 35*(3), 254–264.

Robertson, I. H. (1996). *Goal management training: A clinical manual.* Cambridge, UK: PsyConsult.

Robertson, I. H., & Halligan, P. W. (1999). *Spatial neglect: A clinical handbook for diagnosis and treatment.* Hove, UK: Psychology Press.

Robertson, I. H., Hogg, K., & McMillan, T. M. (1998). Rehabilitation of unilateral neglect: Improving function by contralesional limb activation. *Neuropsychological Rehabilitation, 8,* 19–29.

Robertson, I. H., & Murre, J. M. (1999). Rehabilitation of brain damage: Brain plasticity and principles of guided recovery. *Psychological Bulletin, 25,* 544–575.

Robertson, I. H., North, N., & Geggie, C. (1992). Spatio-motor cueing in unilateral neglect: Three single case studies of its therapeutic effectiveness. *Journal of Neurology, Neurosurgery, and Psychiatry, 55,* 799–805.

Robertson, I. H., Ward, T., Ridgeway, V., & Nimmo-Smith, I. (1994). *The test of everyday attention.* Gaylord, MI: Northern Speech Services.

Robertson, I. H., Ward, T., Ridgeway, V., & Nimmo-Smith, I. (1996). The structure of normal human attention: The Test of Everyday Attention. *Journal of the International Neuropsychological Society, 2,* 525–534.

Robey, R. R. (2004). A five-phase model for clinical-outcome research. *Journal of Communication Disorders, 37,* 401–411.

Robey, R. R., & Schultz, M. C. (1998). A model for conducting clinical-outcome research: An adaptation of the standard protocol for use in aphasiology. *Aphasiology, 12,* 787–810.

Robinson, R., & Spalletta, G. (2010). Poststroke depression: A review. *Canadian Journal of Psychiatry, 55*(6), 341–349.

Robson, J., Marshall, J., Chiat, S., & Pring, T. (2001). Enhancing communication in jargon aphasia: A small group study of writing therapy. *International Journal of Language and Communication Disorders, 36,* 471–488.

Robson, J., Pring, T., Marshall, J., Morrison, S., & Chiat, S. (1998). Written communication in undifferentiated jargon aphasia: A therapy study. *International Journal of Language and Communication Disorders, 33,* 305–328.

Rochon, E., Laird, L., Bose, A., & Scofield, J. (2005). Mapping therapy for sentence production impairments in nonfluent aphasia. *Neuropsychological Rehabilitation, 15*(1), 1–36.

Rochon, E., & Reichman, S. (2003). A modular treatment for sentence processing impairment in aphasia: Sentence production. *Journal of Speech-Language Pathology and Audiology, 27,* 202–210.

Rochon, E., & Reichman, S. (2004). A modular treatment for sentence processing impairment in aphasia: Sentence comprehension. *Journal of Speech-Language Pathology and Audiology, 28,* 25–33.

Rochon, E., Saffran, E. M., Berndt, R. S., & Schwartz, M. F. (2000). Quantitative analysis on aphasic sentence production: Further development and new data. *Brain and Language, 72,* 193–218.

Rode, G., Tilikete, C., Luaute, J., Rossetti, Y., Vighetto, A., & Boisson, D. (2002). Bilateral vestibular stimulation does not improve visual hemineglect. *Neuropsychologia, 40,* 1104–1106.

Rodriguez, A. (2009). Aprosodia secondary to right hemisphere damage. *Perspectives on Neurophysiology and Neurogenic Speech and Language Disorders, 19*(3), 71–76.

Roger, V. L., Go, A. S., Lloyd-Jones, D., Benjamin, E., Berry, J., Borden, W., . . . Turner, M. B. (2011). Heart disease and stroke statistics–2012 update. A report from the American Heart Association writing group members. *Circulation.* doi: 10.1161/CIR.0b013e3182009701

Rogers, H. B., Schroeder, T., Secher, N. H., & Mitchell, J. (1990). Cerebral blood flow during static exercise in humans. *Journal of Applied Physiology, 68,* 2358–2361.

Romero, M., Sanchez, A., Marin, C., Navarro, M., Ferri, J., & Noe, E. (2011). Clinical usefulness of the Spanish version of the Mississippi Aphasia Screening Test (MASTsp): Validation in stroke patients. *Neurologia, 27*(4), 216–224.

Rorden, C., & Karnath, H. (2004). Using human brain lesions to infer function: A relic from a past era in the fMRI age? *Nature Reviews Neuroscience, 5*(10), 813–819.

Rose, M. (2006). The utility of arm and hand gestures in the treatment of aphasia. *Advances in Speech-Language Pathology, 8,* 92–109.

Rose, M., & Douglas, J. (2002). The comparative effectiveness of gesture and verbal treatments for a specific phonologic naming impairment. *Aphasiology, 16*(10–11), 1001–1030.

Rose, M., & Douglas, J. (2006). A comparison of verbal and gesture treatments for a word production deficit resulting from acquired apraxia of speech. *Aphasiology, 20*(12), 1186–1209.

Rose, M., & Sussmilch, G. (2008). The effects of semantic and gesture treatments on verb retrieval and verb use in aphasia. *Aphasiology, 22,* 691–706.

Rosen, H. J., & Viskontas, I. V. (2008). Cortical neuroanatomy and cognition. *Handbook of Clinical Neurology, 88,* 41–60.

Rosenbek, J. C., LaPointe, L. L., & Wertz, R. T. (1989). *Aphasia: A clinical approach.* Austin, TX: PRO-ED.

Rosenbek, J. C., Rodriguez, A. D., Hieber, B., Leon, S. A., Crucian, G. P., Kettersonm, T. U., . . . Gonzalez Rothi, L. J. (2006). Effects of two treatments for aprosodia secondary to acquired brain injury. *Journal of Rehabilitation Research and Development, 43*(3), 379–390.

Rosenthal, W. S. (2004). Group therapy is better than individual therapy: With special attention to stuttering. *Special Interest Division 2: Neurophysiology and Neurogenic Speech and Language Disorders Newsletter, 14,* 3–8.

Rosetta Stone language learning programs [Computer software]. (2001). Harrisonburg, VA: Fairfield Language Technologies.

Ross, A., Winslow, I., & Marchant, P. (2006). Evaluation of communication, life participation and psychological well-being in chronic aphasia: The influence of group intervention. *Aphasiology, 20*(5), 427–448.

Ross, C. A., & Tabrizi, S. (2011). Huntington's disease: From molecular pathogenesis to clinical treatment. *Lancet Neurology, 10,* 83–98.

Ross, D. (1986). *Ross information processing assessment.* Austin, TX: PRO-ED.

Ross, E. D., Thompson, R. D., & Yenkosky, J. (1997). Lateralization of affective prosody in brain and the callosal integration of hemispheric language functions. *Brain and Language, 56,* 27–54.

Ross, K. B., & Wertz, R. T. (1999). Comparison of impairment and disability measures for assessing severity of, and improvement in, aphasia. *Aphasiology, 13,* 113–124.

Ross, K. B., & Wertz, R. T. (2001). Possible demographic influences on differentiating normal from aphasic performance. *Journal of Communication Disorders, 34,* 115–130.

Ross, K. B., & Wertz, R. T. (2002). Relationships between language-based disability and quality of life in chronically aphasic adults. *Aphasiology, 16,* 791–800.

Ross, K. B., & Wertz, R. T. (2003). Discriminative validity of selected measures for differentiating normal from aphasic performance. *American Journal of Speech-Language Pathology, 12,* 312–319.

Ross, K. B., & Wertz, R. T. (2004). Accuracy of formal tests for diagnosing mild aphasia: An application of evidence-based medicine. *Aphasiology, 18,* 337–355.

Rossi, S., Hallett, M., Rossini, P. M., Pascual-Leone, A., & the Safety of TMS Consensus Group. (2009). Safety, ethical considerations, and application guidelines for the use of transcranial magnetic stimulation in clinical practice and research. *Clinical Neurophysiology, 120,* 2008–2039.

Rossor, M. N. (2001). Pick's disease: A clinical overview. *Neurology, 56*(Suppl. 4), S3–S5.

Ross-Swain, D. (1996). *Ross information processing assessment* (2nd ed.). Austin, TX: PRO-ED.

Ross-Swain, D., & Fogle, P. (2012). *Ross information processing assessment–Geriatric: 2.* Austin, TX: PRO-ED.

Roth, C. (2007). Mechanisms and sequelae of blast injuries. *Perspectives on Neurophysiological and Neurogenic Speech and Language Disorders, 17*(3), 20–24.

Roth, E. J., & Lovell, L. (2003). Seven year trends in stroke rehabilitation: Patient characteristics, medical complications, and functional outcomes. *Topics in Stroke Rehabilitation, 9,* 1–9.

Roth, H., & Heilman, K. M. (2000). Aphasia: A historical perspective. In S. Nadeau, L. J. Gonzales Rothi, & B. Crosson (Eds.), *Aphasia and language: Theory to practice* (pp. 3–28). New York: Guilford Press.

Roth, R., Isquith, P., & Gioia, G. (2005). *Behavior rating inventory of executive function–Adult version.* Odessa, FL: PAR.

Rothi, L. J. G., & Moss, S. (1992). Alexia without agraphia: Potential for model assisted therapy. *Clinics in Communication Disorders, 2,* 11–18.

Rothi, L. J. G., Raymer, A. M., & Heilman, K. M. (1997). Limb praxis assessment. In L. J. G. Rothi & K. M. Heilman (Eds.), *Apraxia: The neuropsychology of action* (pp. 61–73). East Sussex, UK: Psychology Press.

Rountree, S., Chan, W., Pavlik, V., Darby, E., & Doody, R. (2012). Factors that influence survival in a probable Alzheimer disease cohort. *Alzheimer's Research and Therapy, 4*(3). doi:10.1186/alzrt119

Rousseaux, M., Daveluy, W., & Koslowski, O. (2010). Communication in conversation in stroke patients. *Journal of Neurology, 257,* 1099–1107.

Rousseaux, M., Delacourt, A., Wyrzykowski, N., & Lefeuvre, M. (2001). *TLC: Test Lillois de Communication. Ortho e´dition,* Isbergues.

Rousseaux, M., Seve, A., Vallet, M., Pasquier, F., & Mackowiak-Cordoliani, M. (2010). An analysis of communication in conversation in patients with dementia. *Neuropsychologia, 48,* 3884–3890.

Roux, F. E., Lubrano, V., Lauwers-Cances, V., Tremoulet, M., Mascott, C. R., & Demonet, J. F. (2004). Intra-operative mapping of cortical areas involved in reading in mono- and bilingual patients. *Brain, 127,* 1796–1810.

Rowe, F., & VIS Group UK. (2009). Visual perceptual consequences of stroke. *Strabismus, 17,* 24–28.

Rowe, F., Wright, D., Brand, D., Jackson, C., Price, A., Walker, L., . . . Freeman, C. (2011). Reading difficulty after stroke: Ocular and non-ocular causes. *Journal of Stroke, 6*(5), 404–411.

Royall, D. R., Cordes, J. A., & Polk, M. (1998). CLOX: An executive clock drawing task. *Journal of Neurology, Neurosurgery, and Psychiatry, 64,* 588–594.

Royall, D. R., Espino, D. V., Polk, M. J., Verdeja, R., Vale, S., Gonzales, H., . . . Markides, K. P. (2003). Validation of a Spanish translation of the CLOX for use in Hispanic samples: The Hispanic EPESE study. *International Journal of Geriatric Psychiatry, 18,* 135–141.

Royall, D. R., Mahurin, R. K., & Gray, K. F. (1992). Bedside assessment of executive dyscontrol: The Executive Interview (EXIT). *Journal of the American Geriatrics Society, 40,* 1221–1226.

Ruff, R. (1996). *Ruff figural fluency test.* Lutz, FL: Psychological Assessment Resources.

Ryan, L. M., & Warden, D. (2003). Post concussion syndrome. *International Review of Psychiatry, 15*(4), 310–316.

Ryff, C. D. (1989). Happiness is everything, or is it? Explorations on the meaning of psychological well-being. *Journal of Personality and Social Psychology, 57,* 1069–1081.

Rymer, S., Salloway, S., Norton, L., Malloy, P., Correia, S., & Monast, D. (2002). Impaired awareness, behavior disturbance, and caregiver burden in Alzheimer disease. *Alzheimer Disease and Associated Disorders, 16,* 248–253.

Sabbagh, M. N., Silverberg, N., Majeed, B., Samant, S., Sparks, D. L., Seward, J., & Connor, D. J. (2003). Length of stay in skilled nursing facilities is longer for patients with dementia. *Journal of Alzheimer's Disease, 5*(1), 57–63.

Sacchett, C., & Black, M. (2011). Drawing as a window to event conceptualisation: Evidence from two people with aphasia. *Aphasiology, 25*(1), 3–26.

Sacchett, C., Byng, S., Marshall, J., & Pound, C. (1999). Drawing together: Evaluation of a therapy programme for severe aphasia. *International Journal of Language and Communication disorders, 34*(3), 265–289.

Sacco, K., Angeleri, R., Bosco, F. M., Colle, L., Mate, D., & Bara, B. G. (2008). Assessment battery for communication – AbaCo: A new instrument for the evaluation of pragmatic abilities. *Journal of Cognitive Science, 9,* 111–157.

Sackett, D. L., Richardson, W. S., Rosenberg, W., & Haynes, R. B. (1997). *Evidence-based medicine: How to practice and teach EBM.* London: Churchill-Livingstone.

Sackett, D. L., Rosenberg, W. M., Gray, J. A., Haynes, B., & Richardson, W. S. (1996). Evidence based medicine: What it is and what it isn't. *British Medical Journal 312,* 71–72.

Sackett, D. L., Strauss, S. E., Richardson, W. S., Rosenberg, W., & Haynes, R. B. (2000). *Evidence-based medicine: How to practice and teach EBM* (2nd ed.). London: Churchill Livingstone.

Saez-Fonseca, J. A., Lee, L., & Walker, Z. (2007). Long-term outcome of depressive pseudodementia in the elderly. *Journal of Affective Disorders, 101,* 123–129.

Safaz, I., Alaca, R., Yasar, E., Tok, F., & Yilmaz, B. (2008). Medical complications, physical function and communication skills in patients with traumatic brain injury: A single centre 5-year experience. *Brain Injury, 22*(10), 733–739.

Sage, K., Hesketh, A., & Lambon Ralph, M. A. (2005). Using errorless learning to treat letter-by-letter reading: Contrasting word versus letter-based therapy. *Neuropsychological Rehabilitation, 15*, 619–642.

Sahin, H. A., Gurvit, I. H., Bilgic, B., Hanagasi, H., & Emre, M. (2002). Therapeutic effects of an acetylcholinesterase inhibitor (donepezil) on memory in Wernicke-Korsakoff's disease. *Clinical Neuropharmacology, 25*(1), 16–20.

Sakurai, Y., Asami, M., & Mannen, T. (2010). Alexia and agraphia with lesions of the angular and supramarginal gyri: Evidence for the disruption of sequential processing. *Journal of the Neurological Sciences, 288*, 1–2.

Salis, C. (2012). Short-term memory treatment: Patterns of learning and generalisation to sentence comprehension in a person with aphasia. *Neuropsychological Rehabiliation, 22*(3), 428–448.

Salter, K., Jutai, J., Foley, N., Hellings, C., & Teasell, R. (2006). Identification of aphasia post stroke: A review of screening assessment tools. *Brain Injury, 20*(6), 559–568.

Samsa, G. P., & Matchar, D. B. (2004). How strong is the relationship between functional status and quality of life among persons with stroke. *Journal of Rehabilitation Research and Development, 41*, 279–282.

Samuel, C., Louis-Dreyfus, A., Kaschel, R., Makiela, E., Troubat, M., Anselmi, N., . . . Azouvi, P. (2000). Rehabilitation of very severe unilateral neglect by visuospatiomotor cueing: Two single case studies. *Neuropsychological Rehabilitation, 10*, 385–399.

Sansoni, J., Marosszeky, N., Jeon, Y.-H., Chenoweth, L., Hawthorne, G., King, M., . . . Low, L. (2007). *Final report: Dementia outcomes measurement suite project*. Centre for Health Service Development, University of Wollongong.

Santo Pietro, M. J., & Boczko, F. (1998). The Breakfast Club: Results of a study examining the effectiveness of a multi-modality group communication treatment. *American Journal of Alzheimer's Disease, 13*, 146–158.

Sardina, A. (2010). *A recreation therapy twist to sign language: An intervention for primary progressive aphasia* (Master's thesis). University of North Carolina Greensboro.

Sarno, M. T. (1969). *The functional communication profile*. New York: NYU Medical Center Monograph Department.

Sarno, M. T. (1997). Quality of life in aphasia in the first post-stroke year. *Aphasiology, 11*(7), 665–679.

Sarno, M. T., Buonaguro, A., & Levin, E. (1986). Characteristics of verbal impairment in closed head injured patients. *Archives of Physical Medicine and Rehabilitation, 67*, 400–405.

Sarno, J. E., Sarno, M. T., & Levita, E. (1973). The functional life scale. *Archives of Physical and Medical Rehabilitation, 54*, 214–220.

Saunders, N. L., & Summers, M. J. (2011). Longitudinal deficits to attention, executive, and working memory in subtypes of mild cognitive impairment. *Neuropsychology, 25*(2), 237–248.

Savundranayagam, M., & Orange, J. B. (2011). Relationships between appraisals of caregiver communication strategies and burden among spouses and adult children. *International Psychogeriatrics*. doi: 10.1017/S1041610211000408

Sawyer, E., Mauro, L. S., & Ohlinger, M. J. (2008). Amantadine enhancement of arousal and cognition after traumatic brain injury. *The Annals of Pharmacotherapy, 42*, 247–252.

Saxton, J., Swihart, A. A., & Boller, F. (1993). *Severe impairment battery*. Bury St. Edmunds, Suffolk, England: Thames Valley Test Company.

Saygin, A. P., Dick, F., Wilson, S. M., Dronkers, N. F., & Bates, E. (2003). Neural resources for processing language and environmental sounds: Evidence from aphasia. *Brain, 126*, 928–945.

Sbordone, R. J., Seyranian, G. D., & Ruff, R. M. (1998). Are the subjective complaints of traumatically brain injured patients reliable? *Brain Injury, 12*, 505–515.

Schacter, D. L. (1992). Understanding implicit memory. *American Psychologist, 47*, 559–569.

Schacter, D., & Buckner, R. L. (1998). On the relations among priming, conscious recollection, and intentional retrieval: Evidence from neuroimaging research. *Neurobiology of Learning and Memory, 70*, 284–303.

Schapira, A. (2009). Neurobiology and treatment of Parkinson's disease. *Trends in Pharmacological Sciences, 30*(1), 41–47.

Scherder, E. J., Bouma, A., & Steen, L. (1992). Influence of transcutaneous electrical nerve stimulation on memory in dementia of the Alzheimer's type. *Journal of Clinical and Experimental Neuropsychology, 14*, 951–960.

Scherder, E. J., Bouma, A., & Steen, L. (1995). Effects of short-term transcutaneous electrical nerve stimulation on memory and affective behavior in patients with probable Alzheimer's disease. *Behavioral Brain Research, 67*, 211–219.

Scherder, E. J., Vuijk, P. J., Swaab, D. F., & van Someren, E. J. (2007). Estimating the effects of right median nerve stimulation on memory in Alzheimer's disease: A randomized controlled pilot study. *Experimental Aging Research, 33*(2), 177–186.

Schindler, I., Kerkhoff, G., Karnath, H. O., Keller, I., & Goldenberg, G. (2002). Neck muscle vibration induces lasting recovery in spatial neglect. *Journal of Neurology, Neurosurgery, and Psychiatry, 73*, 412–419.

Schinka, J., Raj, A., Loewenstein, D., Small, B., Duara, R., & Potter, H. (2010). The cognitive change checklist (3CL): Cross-validation of a measure of change in everday cognition. *International Journal of Geriatric Psychiatry, 25*, 266–274.

Schlaug, G., Marchina, S., & Norton, A. (2008). From singing to speaking: Why singing may lead to recovery of expressive language function in patients with Broca's aphasia. *Music Perception, 25*(5), 315–323.

Schlund, M. W. (1999). Self awareness: Effects of feedback and review on verbal self reports and remembering following brain injury. *Brain Injury, 13*, 375–380.

Schmidt, G., Kranjec, A., Cardillo, E., & Chatterjee, R. (2010). Beyond laterality: A critical assessment of research on the neural basis of metaphor. *Journal of the International Neuropsychological Society, 11*, 795–806.

Schmidt, J., Fleming, J., Ownsworth, T., Lannin, N., & Khan, A. (2012). Feedback interventions for improving self-awareness after brain injury: A protocol for a pragmatic randomized controlled trial. *Australian Occupational Therapy Journal, 59*, 138–146.

Schmitter-Edgecombe, M., Howard, J., Pavawalla, S., Howell, L., & Rueda, A. (2008). Multidyad memory notebook intervention for very mild dementia: A pilot study. *American Journal of Alzheimer's Disease and Other Dementias, 23*(5), 477–487.

Schmitter-Edgecombe, M., Parsey, C., & Cook, D. (2011). Cognitive correlates of functional performance in older adults: Comparison of self-report, direct observation, and performance-based measures. *Journal of the International Neuropsychological Society, 17*, 1–12.

Schmitter-Edgecombe, M., & Wright, M. J. (2004). Event-based prospective memory following severe closed head injury. *Neuropsychology, 18*, 353–361.

Schneider, L. S., Olin, J. T., Doody, R., Clark, C., Morris, J., Reisberg, B., ... Thomas, R. G. (1997). Validity and reliability of the Alzheimer's Disease Cooperative Study–Clinical Global Impression of Change. *Alzheimer's Disease and Associated Disorders, 11*(Suppl. 2), S22–S32.

Schneider, S., Haack, L., Owens, J., Herrington, D., & Zelek, A. (2009). An interdisciplinary treatment approach for soldiers with TBI/PTSD: Issues and outcomes. *Perspectives on Neurophysiological and Neurogenic Speech and Language Disorders, 19*(2), 36–46.

Schneider, S. L., Thompson, C. K., & Luring, B. (1996). Effects of verbal plus gestural matrix training on sentence production in a patient with primary progressive aphasia. *Aphasiology, 10*, 297–317.

Schouten, J., Cinque, P., Gisslen, M., Reiss, P., & Portegies, P. (2011). HIV-1 infection and cognitive impairment in the cart era: A review. *AIDS, 25*, 561–575.

Schretlen, D. (1997). *Brief test of attention*. Lutz, FL: Psychological Assessment Resources.

Schretlen, D. (2011). *Modified Wisconsin card sorting test*. Lutz, FL: PAR.

Schretlen, D., & Vannorsdall, T. (2011). *Calibrated ideational fluency assessment*. Lutz, FL: PAR.

Schroder, A., Wist, E., & Homberg, V. (2008). TENS and optokinetic stimulation in neglect therapy after cerebrovascular accident: A randomized controlled study. *European Journal of Neurology, 15*, 922–927.

Schuell, H., & Jenkins, J. J. (1959). The nature of language deficit in aphasia. *Psychological Review, 66*, 45–67.

Schuell, H., Jenkins, J. J., & Jimenese-Pabon, E. (1964). *Aphasia in adults.* New York: Harper and Row.

Schultheis, M. T., Caplan, B., Ricker, J. H., & Woessner, R. (2000). Fractioning the Hooper: A multiple-choice response format. *Clinical Neuropsychologist, 14*, 196–201.

Schultz, C. (2010). *Crossing the void: My aphasic journey.* Scotts Valley, CA: CreateSpace.

Schwartz, M. F., Buxbaum, L. J., Veramonti, T., Ferraro, M., & Segal, M. (2002). *Naturalistic Action Test.* Bury St. Edmunds, Suffolk, England: Thames Valley Test Company.

Schwartz, M. F., Dell, G. S., Martin, N., Gahl, S., & Sobel, P. (2006). A case-series test of the interactive two-step model of lexical access: Evidence from picture naming. *Journal of Memory and Language, 54*, 228–264.

Schwartz, M. F., Saffran, E. M., Fink, R. B., Myers, J. L., & Martin, N. (1994). Mapping therapy: A treatment programme for agrammatism. *Aphasiology, 8*, 19–54.

Schwartz, R. (1989). Early rehabilitation in trauma centers: Have speech-language pathology services progressed? *American Speech-Language-Hearing Association, 31*, 91–94.

Schutz, L. (2005). Broad-perspective perceptual disorder of the right hemisphere. *Neuropsychology Review, 15*(1), 11–27.

Scott, S. G., Belanger, H. G., Vanderploeg, R. D., Massengale, J., & Scholten, J. (2006). Mechanism-of-injury approach to evaluating patients with blast-related polytrauma. *Journal of the American Osteopathology Association, 106*, 265–270.

Searl, J., & Gabel, R. (2003). Speech-language pathologists' attitudes toward aging and the elderly. *Contemporary Issues in Communication Science and Disorders, 30*, 146–155.

Searle, J. (1969). *Speech acts.* London: Cambridge University Press.

Seashore, C., Lewis, D., & Saetveit, J. (1960). *Seashore measures of musical talents.* New York: Psychological Corporation.

Semel, E., Wiig, E., & Secord, W. (2013). *Clinical evaluation of language fundamentals* (5th ed.). San Antonio, TX: Pearson.

Sendroy-Terrill, M., Whiteneck, G., & Brooks, C. (2010). Aging with traumatic brain injury: Cross-sectional follow-up of people receiving inpatient rehabilitation over more than 3 decades. *Archives of Physical Medicine and Rehabilitation, 91*, 489–497.

Seniow, J., Litwin, M., Litwin, T., Lesniak, M., & Członkowska, A. (2009). New approach to the rehabilitation of post-stroke focal cognitive syndrome: Effect of levodopa combined with speech and language therapy on functional recovery from aphasia. *Journal of Neurological Sciences, 283*, 214–218.

Shadden, B. (1998). Obtaining the discourse sample. In L. R. Cherney, B. Shadden, & C. A. Coelho (Eds.). *Analyzing discourse in communicatively impaired adults.* Gathersburg, MD: Aspen.

Shallice, T. (1988). *From neuropsychology to mental structure.* Cambridge, MA: Cambridge University Press.

Shames, J., Treger, I., Ring, H., & Giaquinto, S. (2007). Return to work following traumatic brain injury: Trends and challenges. *Disability and Rehabilitation, 29*(17), 1387–1395.

Shankar, K. K., Walker, M., Frost, D., & Orrell, M. W. (1999). The development of a valid and reliable scale for rating anxiety in dementia. *Aging and Mental Health, 3*, 39–49.

Shankweiler, D., Palumbo, L., Fulbright, R., Mencl, W., Van Dyke, J., Kollia, B., . . . Harris, K. (2010). Testing the limits of language production in long-term survivors of major stroke: A psycholinguistic and anatomic study. *Aphasiology, 24*(11), 1455–1485.

Shapiro, L. P. (1997). Tutorial: An introduction to syntax. *Journal of Speech, Language, and Hearing Research, 40*, 254–272.

Shaw, D., & May, H. (2001). Sharing knowledge with nursing home staff: An objective investigation. *International Journal of Language and Communication, 33*, 200–205.

Shelton, J. R., Weinrich, M., McCall, D., & Cox, D. M. (1996). Differentiating globally aphasic patients: Data from in-depth language assessments and production training using C-VIC. *Aphasiology, 10*, 319–342.

Sherratt, S., & Bryan, K. (2012). Discourse production after right brain damage: Gaining a comprehensive picture using a multi-level processing model. *Journal of Neurolinguistics, 25*, 213–239.

Sherratt, S. M., & Penn, C. (1990). Discourse in a right-hemisphere brain-damaged subject. *Aphasiology, 4*, 539–560.

Shewan, C. M. (1979). *Auditory comprehension test for sentences.* Chicago: Biolinguistics Clinical Institutes.

Shewan, C. M., & Kertesz, A. (1980). Reliability and validity characteristics of the Western Aphasia Battery. *Journal of Speech and Hearing Disorders, 45*, 308–324.

Shewan, C. M., & Kertesz, A. (1984). Effects of speech and language treatment on recovery from aphasia. *Brain and Language, 23*, 272–299.

Shiel, A., Wilson, B. A., McLellan, D. L., Horn, S., & Watson, M. (2000). *Wessex head injury matrix*. Bury St. Edmunds, Suffolk, England: Thames Valley Test Company.

Shiraishi, H., Yamakawa, Y., Itou, A., Muraki, T., & Asada, T. (2008). Long-term effects of prism adaptation on chronic neglect after stroke. *NeuroRehabilitation, 23*, 137–151.

Shum, D., Fleming, J., Gill, H., Gullo, M., & Strong, J. (2011). A randomized controlled trial of prospective memory rehabilitation in adults with traumatic brain injury. *Journal of Rehabilitation Medicine, 43*, 216–223.

Shuster, L. I. (2004). Resource theory and aphasia reconsidered: Why alternative theories can better guide our research. *Aphasiology, 18*, 811–830.

Sigurdardottir, S., Andelic, N., Roe, C., & Schanke, A. (2009). Cognitive recovery and predicators of functional outcome 1 year after traumatic brain injury. *Journal of the International Neuropsychological Society, 15*, 740–750.

Sieroff, E., Piquard, A., Auclair, L., Lacomblez, L., Derouesne, C., & Laberge, D. (2004). Deficit of preparatory attention in frontotemporal dementia. *Brain and Cognition, 55*, 444–451.

Sikkes, S., Knol, D., van den Berg, M., de Lange-de Klerk, E., Scheltens, P., Klein, M., . . . Uitdehaag, B. M. J. (2011). An informant questionnaire for detecting Alzheimer's disease: Are some items better than others? *Journal of the International Neuropsychological Society, 17*, 674–681.

Silbergleit, A. K., & Basha, M. A. (2007). Speech-language pathology in the intensive care unit. In A. F. Johnson & B. H. Jacobson (Eds.), *Medical speech-language pathology: A practitioner's guide* (pp. 260–283). New York: Thieme.

Silverberg, N. D., & Millis, S. R. (2009). Impairment versus deficiency in neuropsychological assessment: Implications for ecological validity. *Journal of the International Neuropsychological Society, 15*, 94–102.

Simmons-Mackie, N. N. (2008). Social approaches to aphasia intervention. In R. Chapey (Ed.), *Language intervention strategies in aphasia and related neurogenic communication disorders* (5th ed, pp. 290– 318). Philadelphia: Lippincott Williams & Wilkins.

Simmons-Mackie, N. N., & Damico, J. S. (1996). Accounting for handicaps in aphasia: Communicative assessment from an authentic social perspective. *Disability and Rehabilitation, 18*, 540–549.

Simmons-Mackie, N., & Damico, J. S. (2001). Intervention outcomes: A clinical application of qualitative methods. *Topics in Language Disorders, 21*(4), 21–36.

Simmons-Mackie, N., & Elman, R. J. (2011). Negotiation of identity in group therapy for aphasia: The Aphasia Café. *International Journal of Language & Communication Disorders, 46*(3), 312–323.

Simmons-Mackie, N., & Kagan, A. (1999). Communication strategies used by "good" versus "poor" speaking partners of individuals with aphasia. *Aphasiology, 13*, 807–820.

Simmons-Mackie, N., & Kagan, A. (2007). Application of the ICF in aphasia. *Seminars in Speech and Language, 28*(4), 244–253.

Simmons-Mackie, N., Kearns, K., & Potechin, G. (2005 [1987]). Treatment of aphasia through family member training. *Aphasiology, 19*, 583–593.

Simmons-Mackie, N., Kingston, D., & Schultz, M. (2004). Speaking for another: The management of participant frames in aphasia. *American Journal of Speech-Language Pathology, 13*, 114–127.

Simmons-Mackie, N., Raymer, A., Armstrong, E., Holland, A., & Cherney, L. R. (2010). Communication partner training in aphasia: A systematic review. *Archives of Physical Medicine and Rehabilitation, 91*(12), 1814–1837.

Simmons-Mackie, N., Threats, T. T., & Kagan, A. (2005). Outcome assessment in aphasia: A survey. *Journal of Communication Disorders, 38*, 1–27.

Simon, H. A. (1975). The functional equivalence of problem solving skill. *Cognitive Psychology, 7*, 268–288.

Sinanovic, O. (2010). Neuropsychology of acute stroke. *Psychiatria Danubina, 22*(2), 278–281.

Sinanovic, O., Mrkonjic, Z., Zukic, S., Vidovic, M., & Imamovic, K. (2011). Post-stroke language disorders. *Acta Clinic Croatia, 50*(1), 79–94.

Singer, B. D., & Bashir, A. S. (1999). What are executive functions and self-regulation and what do they have to do with language-learning disorders? *Language, Speech, and Hearing Services in Schools, 30*, 265–273.

Sinotte, M., & Coelho, C. (2007). Attention training for reading impairment in mild aphasia: A follow-up study. *NeuroRehabilitation, 22*, 303–310.

Sivan, A. B. (1991). *Benton visual retention test.* San Antonio, TX: Psychological Corporation.

Skelly, M. (1979). *Amer-Ind gestural code based on universal American Indian hand talk.* New York: Elsevier.

Skrine, R., & Brown, J. (2011). Home care rule will take effect on April 1. *The ASHA Leader.* http://www.asha.org/Publications/leader/2011/110315/Home-Care-Rule-Will-Take-Effect-on-April-1/

Slachevsky, A., Villalpando, J. M., Sarazin, M., Hahn-Barma, V., Pillon, B., & Dubois, B. (2004). Frontal assessment battery and differential diagnosis of frontotemporal dementia and Alzheimer disease. *Archives of Neurology, 61*, 1104–1107.

Slevc, L., Martin, R., Hamilton, A., & Joanisse, M. (2011). Speech perception, rapid temporal processing, and the left hemisphere: A case study of unilateral pure word deafness. *Neuropsychologia, 49*(2), 216–230.

Slovarp, L., Azuma, T., & LaPointe, L. (2012). The effect of traumatic brain injury on sustained attention and working memory. *Brain Injury, 26*(1) 48–57.

Small, J. A. (2012). A new frontier in spaced retrieval memory training for persons with Alzheimer's disease. *Neuropsychological Rehabilitation, 22*(3), 329–361.

Small, J. A., & Gutman, G. (2002). Recommended and reported use of communication strategies in Alzheimer caregiving. *Alzheimer Disease and Associated Disorders, 16*, 270–278.

Small, J. A., & Perry, J. (2005). Do you remember? How caregivers question their spouses who have Alzheimer's disease and the impact on communication. *Journal of Speech, Language, and Hearing Research, 48*, 125–136.

Small, J. A., Geldart, K., & Gutman, G. (2000). Communication between individuals with Alzheimer's disease and their caregivers during activities of daily living. *American Journal of Alzheimer's Disease, 15*, 291–302.

Small, J. A., Geldart, K., Gutman, G., & Clarke Scott, M. (1998). The discourse of self in dementia. *Ageing and Society, 18*, 291–316.

Small, S. L. (2002). Biological approaches to the treatment of aphasia. In A. E. Hillis (Ed.), *The handbook of adult language disorders: Integrating cognitive neuropsychology, neurology, and rehabilitation* (pp. 392–411). New York: Psychology Press.

Small, S. L. (2009). A biological basis for aphasia treatment: Mirror neurons and observation-execution matching. *Poznan Studies in Contemporary Linguistics, 45*(2), 313–326.

Smith, S. C., Lamping, D. L., Banerjee, S., Harwood, R. H., Foley, B., Smith, P., . . . Knapp, M. (2007). Development of a new measure of health-related quality of life for people with dementia: DEMQOL. *Psychological Medicine, 37*(5), 737–746.

Smollan, T., & Penn, C. (1997). The measurement of emotional reaction and depression in a South African stroke population. *Disability and Rehabilitation, 19*, 56–63.

Snow, P. C., & Douglas, J. M. (2000). Conceptual and methodological challenges in discourse assessment with TBI speakers: Towards an understanding. *Brain Injury, 14*, 397–415.

Sohlberg, M. M. (2000). Assessing and managing unawareness of self. *Seminars in Speech and Language, 21*, 135–152.

Sohlberg, M. M. (2002). An overview of approaches for managing attention impairments. *Perspectives on Neurophysiology and Neurogenic Speech and Language Disorders, 12*, 4–8.

Sohlberg, M. M. (2011). Assistive technology for cognition. *ASHA Leader, 16*(2), 14–17.

Sohlberg, M. M., Avery, J., Kennedy, M., Ylvisaker, M., Coelho, C., Turkstra, L., & Yorkston, K. (2003). Practice guidelines for direct attention training. *Journal of Medical Speech-Language Pathology, 11*, xix–xxxix.

Sohlberg, M. M., Johnson, L., Paule, L., Raskin, S. A., & Mateer, C. A. (2001). *Attention Process Training-II: A program to address attentional deficits for persons with mild cognitive dysfunction* (2nd ed.). Wake Forest, NC: Lash & Associates.

Sohlberg, M., Kennedy, M., Avery, J., Coelho, C., Turkstra, L., Ylvisaker M., & Yorkston, K. (2007). Evidence-based practice for the use of external aids as a memory rehabilitation technique. *Journal of Medical Speech-Language Pathology, 15*, xv–li.

Sohlberg, M. M., & Mateer, C. A. (1986). *Attention process training (APT).* Puyallup, WA: Association for Neuropsychological Research and Development.

Sohlberg, M. M., & Mateer, C. A. (2001). *Cognitive rehabilitation: An integrative neuropsychological approach.* New York: Guilford Press.

Sohlberg, M. M., & Mateer, C. (2010). *Attention process training–III.* Youngsville, NC: Lash & Associates.

Sohlberg, M. M., McLaughlin, K., Pavese, A., Heidrich, A., & Posner, M. I. (2000). Evaluation of attention process training and brain injury education in persons with acquired brain injury. *Journal of Clinical and Experimental Neuropsychology, 22,* 656–676.

Sohlberg, M. M., Sprunk, H., & Metzelaar, K. (1988). Efficacy of an external cuing system in an individual with severe frontal lobe damage. *Cognitive Rehabilitation, 6,* 36–41.

Sohlberg, M. M., & Turkstra, L. S. (2011). *Optimizing cognitive rehabilitation: Effective instructional methods.* New York: Guilford Press.

Sohlberg, M. M., White, O., Evans, E., & Mateer, C. A. (1992). Background and initial case studies into the effects of prospective memory training. *Brain Injury, 6,* 129–138.

Solomon, P. R. (2002). *Alzheimer's disease caregiver's questionnaire.* Lutz, FL: Psychological Assessment Resources.

Song, W., Du, B., Xu, Q., Hu, J., Wang, M., & Luo, Y. (2009). Low-frequency transcranial magnetic stimulation for visual spatial neglect: A pilot study. *Journal of Rehabilitation Medicine, 41,* 162–165.

Sorin-Peters, R. (2004). The evaluation of a learner-centred training programme for spouses of adults with chronic aphasia using qualitative case study methodology. *Aphasiology, 18,* 951–975.

Sparks, R. (2001). Melodic Intonation Therapy. In R. Chapey (Ed.), *Language intervention strategies in aphasia and related neurogenic communication disorders* (4th ed., pp. 703–717). New York: Lippincott Williams & Wilkins.

Sparks, R., Helm, N., & Albert, M. (1974). Aphasia rehabilitation resulting from Melodic Intonation Therapy. *Cortex, 10,* 303–316.

Speech, T. J., Rao, S. M., Osmon, D. C., & Sperry, L. T. (1993). A double-blind controlled study of methylphenidate treatment in closed head injury. *Brain Injury, 7,* 333–338.

Spikman, J., Boelen, D., Lamberts, K., Brouwer, W., & Fasotti, L. (2009). Effects of a multifaceted treatment program for executive dysfunction after acquired brain injury on indications of executive functioning in daily life. *Journal of the International Neuropsychological Society, 16,* 118–129.

Spreen, O., & Strauss, E. (2006). *A compendium of neuropsychological tests* (3rd ed.). New York: Oxford University Press.

Squire, L. R. (1987). *Memory and brain.* New York: Oxford University Press.

Squires, E. J., Hunkin, N. M., & Parkin, A. J. (1996). Memory notebook training in a case of severe amnesia: Generalizing from paired associate learning to real life. *Neuropsychological Rehabilitation, 6,* 55–65.

Stadie, N., Schröder, A., Postler, J., Lorenz, A., Swoboda-Moll, M., Burchert, F., & De Bleser, R. (2008). Unambiguous generalization effects after treatment of non-canonical sentence production in German agrammatism. *Brain and Language, 104*(3), 211–229.

Stanczak, D. E., Lynch, M. D., McNeil, C. K., & Brown, B. (1998). The Expanded Trail Making Test: Rationale, development, and psychometric properties. *Archives of Clinical Neuropsychology, 13,* 473–487.

Starkstein, S., Jorge, R., & Robinson, R. (2010). Frequency, clinical correlates, and mechanism of anosognosia after stroke. *Canadian Journal of Psychiatry, 55*(6), 355–361.

State University of New York at Buffalo Research Foundation. (1993). *Guide for the use of the uniform data set for medical rehabilitation: Functional independence measure.* Buffalo: State University of New York.

Steele, R. (2006). AAC use and communicative improvements in chronic aphasia: Evidence comparing global with severe Broca's aphasia. *Perspectives on Augmentative and Alternative Communication, 15*(4), 18–22.

Stein, N. L., & Glenn, C. G. (1979). An analysis of story comprehension in elementary school children. In R. O. Freedle (Ed.), *New directions in discourse processing* (pp. 53–120). Norwood, NJ: Ablex.

Stein, R. A., & Strickland, T. L. (1998). A review of the neuropsychological effects of commonly used prescription medications. *Archives of Clinical Neuropsychology, 13,* 259–284.

Steinberg, B., Bileiauskas, L., Smith, G., & Ivnik, R. (2005). Mayo's older Americans normative studies: Age- and IQ-adjusted norms for the Trail Making Test, the Stroop Test, and MAE Controlled Oral Word Association Test. *Clinical Neuropsychology, 19*(3–4), 329–377.

Stern, R. A. (1998). *Visual analog mood scales.* Odessa, FL: Psychological Assessment Resources.

Stern, R. A., Javorsky, D. J., Singer, E. A., Singer Harris, N. G., Somerville, J. A., Duke, L. M., . . . Kaplan, E. (1999). *The Boston qualitative scoring system for the Rey-Osterrieth complex figure*. Lutz, FL: Psychological Assessment Resources.

Stern, R. A., & White, T. (2003). *Neuropsychological assessment battery*. Lutz, FL: Psychological Assessment Resources.

Stern, R. A., & White, T. (2009a). *NAB mazes test*. Lutz, FL: Psychological Assessment Resources.

Stern, R. A., & White, T. (2009b). *NAB naming test*. Lutz, FL: Psychological Assessment Resources.

Stern, R. A., & White, T. (2009c). *NAB visual discrimination test*. Lutz, FL: Psychological Assessment Resources.

Stern, R. A., & White, T. (2010). *NAB writing test*. Lutz, FL: Psychological Assessment Resources.

Stone, A., Casadesus, G., Gustaw-Rothenberg, K., Siedlak, S., Wang, X., Zhu, X., . . . Smith, M. A. (2011). Frontiers in Alzheimer's disease therapeutics. *Therapeutic Advances in Chronic Diseases, 2*(1), 9–23.

Storey, J. E., Rowland, J. T. J., Conforti, D. A., & Dickson, H. G. (2004). The Rowland Universal Dementia Assessment Scale (RUDAS): A multicultural cognitive assessment scale. *International Psychogeriatrics, 16*, 13–31.

Strauss, E., Sherman, E. M. S., & Spreen, O. (2006). *A compendium of neuropsychological tests: Administration, norms, and commentary* (3rd ed.). New York: Oxford University Press.

Stringer, A. Y. (1996). Treatment of motor aprosodia with pitch biofeedback and expression modeling. *Brain Injury, 10*, 583–590.

Stroop, J. R. (1935). Studies of interference in serial verbal reactions. *Journal of Experimental Psychology, 18*, 643–662.

Struchen, M. A., Clark, A., Sander, A., Mills, M., Evans, G., & Kurtz, D. (2008a). Relation of executive functioning and social communication measures to functional outcomes following traumatic brain injury. *NeuroRehabilitation, 23*, 185–198.

Struchen, M. A., Pappadis, M., Mazzei, D., Clark, A., Davis, L., & Sander, A. (2008b). Perceptions of communication abilities for persons with traumatic brain injury: Validity of the La Trobe Communication Questionnaire. *Brain Injury, 22*(12), 940–951.

Sturm, W., Longoni, F., Weis, S., Specht, K., Herzog, H., Vohn, R., . . . Willmes, K. (2004). Functional reorganisation in patients with right hemisphere stroke after training of alertness: A longitudinal PET and fMRI study in eight cases. *Neuropsychologia, 42*, 434–450.

Sturm, W., Willmes, K., Orgass, B., & Hartje, W. (1997). Do specific attention deficits need specific training? *Neuropsychological Rehabilitation, 7*, 81–103.

Stuss, D. T. (2011). Functions of the frontal lobes: Relation to executive functions. *Journal of the International Neuropsychological Society, 17*, 759–765.

Suarez, J. I. (2000). Acute ischemic stroke: Current treatment and future direction. *Special Interest Division 2: Neurophysiology and Neurogenic Speech and Language Disorders Newsletter, 10*, 5–10.

Suhr, J. S., Anderson, S., & Tranel, D. (1999). Progressive muscle relaxation in the management of behavioral disturbance in Alzheimer's disease. *Neuropsychological Rehabilitation, 9*, 31–44.

Sullivan, E. V., Rose, J., Rohling, T., & Pfefferbaum, A. (2009). Postural sway reduction in aging men and women: Relation to brain structure, cognitive status, and stabilizing factors. *Neurobiology of Aging, 30*, 793–807.

Sunderland, T., Alterman, I. S., Yount, D., Hill, J. L., Tariot, P. N., Newhouse, P. A., . . . Cohen, R. M. (1988). A new scale for assessment of depressed mood in demented patients. *American Journal of Psychiatry, 145*, 955–959.

Sundin, K., Jansson, L., & Norberg, A. (2000). Communicating with people with stroke and aphasia: Understanding through sensation without words. *Journal of Clinical Nursing, 9*, 481–488.

Sung, J. E., McNeil, M. R., Pratt, S. R., Dickey, M. W., Hula, W. D., Szuminsky, N. J., & Doyle, P. J. (2009). Verbal working memory and its relationship to sentence-level reading and listening comprehension in persons with aphasia. *Aphasiology, 23*(7–8), 1040–1052.

Surian, L., & Siegal M. (2001). Sources of performance on theory of mind tasks in right hemisphere-damaged patients. *Brain and Language, 78*, 224–232.

Sutcliffe, L. M., & Lincoln, N. B. (1998). The assessment of depression in aphasic stroke patients: The development of the Stroke Aphasic Depression Questionnaire. *Clinical Rehabilitation, 12*, 506–513.

Sutherland, G., Andersen, M. B., & Morris, T. (2005). Relaxation and health-related quality of life in multiple sclerosis: The example of autogenic training. *Journal of Behavioral Medicine, 28*(3), 249–256.

Sutton-Brown, M., & Suchowersky, O. (2003). Clinical and research advances in Huntington's disease. *Canadian Journal of Neurological Sciences, 30*, S45–S52.

Svoboda, E., & Richards, B. (2009). Compensating for anterograde amnesia: A new training method that capitalizes on emerging smartphone technologies. *Journal of the International Neuropsychological Society, 15*, 629–638.

Svoboda, E., Richards, B., Polsinelli, A., & Guger, S. (2010). A theory-driven training programme in the use of emerging commercial technology: Application to an adolescent with severe memory impairment. *Neuropsychological Rehabilitation, 20*(4), 562–586.

Swanson, K. L., & Chrumka, M. (1999). *I'll carry the fork!: Recovering a life after brain injury*. Los Altos, CA: Rising Star Press.

Swartz, R., Miller, B. L., Darby, A., & Schuman, S. (1997). Frontotemporal dementia: Treatment response to serotonin selective reuptake inhibitors. *Journal of Clinical Psychiatry, 58*, 212–216.

Sweet, J., Nelson, N., & Moberg, P. (2006). The TCN/AACN 2005 "Salary Survey:" Professional practices, beliefs, and incomes of U.S. neuropsychologists. *Clinical Neuropsychology, 20*, 325–364.

Swigert, N. B. (1997). *The source for dysarthria*. East Moline, IL: Linguisystems.

Swinbourne, K., & Byng, S. (2006). *The communication disability profile*. London: Connect Press.

Swinburn, K., Porter, G., & Howard, D. (2004). *Comprehensive aphasia test*. Hove, England: Psychology Press.

Szaflarski, J., Ball, A. L., Grether, S., Al-fwaress, F., Griffith, N. M., Neils-Strunjas, J., . . . Reichhardt, R. (2008). Constraint-induced aphasia therapy stimulates language recovery in patients with chronic aphasia after ischemic stroke. *Medical Science Monitor, 14*(5), 243–250.

Szaflarski, J., Vannest, J., Wu, S., DeFrancesco, M., Banks, C., & Gilbert, D. (2011). Excitatory repetitive transcranial magnetic stimulation induces improvement in chronic post-stroke aphasia. *Medical Science Monitor, 25*(17), 132–139.

Tanaka, Y., Albert, M. L., Aketa, S., Hujita, K., Noda, E., Takashima, M., . . . Tanaka, M. (2004). Serotonergic therapy for fluent aphasia. *Neurology, 62*, A166.

Tanaka, Y., & Bachman, D. L. (2007). Pharmacotherapy of aphasia. In L. S. Connor & L. K. Obler (Eds.), *Neurobehavior of language and cognition studies of normal aging and brain damage* (pp. 159–162). Berlin, Germany: SpringerLink.

Tanaka, Y., Miyazaki, M., & Albert, M. L. (1997). Effects of increased cholinergic activity on naming in aphasia. *The Lancet, 350*, 116–117.

Tanner, D. C., & Culbertson, W. (1999a). *Caregiver-administered communication inventory*. Oceanside, CA: Academic Communication Associates.

Tanner, D. C., & Culbertson, W. (1999b). *Quick assessment for aphasia*. Oceanside, CA: Academic Communication Associates.

Tanner, D. C., & Culbertson, W. (1999c). *Quick assessment for apraxia of speech*. Oceanside, CA: Academic Communication Associates.

Tanner, D. C., & Culbertson, W. (1999d). *Quick assessment for dysarthria*. Oceanside, CA: Academic Communication Associates.

Tariot, P. N., Farlow, M. R., Grossberg, G. T., Graham, S. M., McDonald, S., & Gergel, I. (2004). Memantine treatment in patients with moderate-to-severe Alzheimer disease already receiving donepezil. *Journal of the American Medical Association, 291*, 317–324.

Tartaglia, M., Rosen, H., & Miller, B. (2011). Neuroimaging in dementia. *Neurotherapeutics, 8*, 82–92.

Tate, R. (2010). *A compendium of tests, scales, and questionnaires: The practitioner's guide to measuring outcomes after acquired brain impairment*. New York: Psychology Press.

Taylor, J. (2008). *My stroke of insight: A brain scientist's personal journey*. New York: Viking Press.

Taylor, R. (2006). *Alzheimer's from the inside out*. Baltimore: Health Professions Press.

Teasdale, G., & Jennett, B. (1976). Assessment and prognosis of coma after head injury. *Acta Neurochirurgica, 34*, 45–55.

Teasdale, T. W., Emslie, H., Quirk, K., Evans, J., Fish, J., & Wilson, B. A. (2009). Alleviation of carer strain during the use of the NeuroPage device by people with acquired brain injury. *Journal of Neurology, Neurosurgery, and Psychiatry, 80*(7), 781–783.

Tekur, P., Nagarathna, R., Chametcha, S., Hankey, A., & Nagendra, H. R. (2012). A comprehensive yoga programs improves pain, anxiety and depression in chronic low back pain patients more than exercise: An RCT. *Complementary Therapies in Medicine, 20*(3), 107–118.

Terrell, B., & Ripich, D. (1989). Discourse competence as a variable in intervention. *Seminars in Speech and Language, 10,* 282–297.

Tesar, N., Bandion, K., & Baumhackl, U. (2005). Efficacy of a neuropsychological training programme for patients with multiple sclerosis: A randomised controlled trial. *Wiener klinische Wochenschrift, 117*(21–22), 747–754.

Tessier, C., Weill-Chounlamountry, A., Michelot, N., & Pradat-Diehl, P. (2007). Rehabilitation of word deafness due to auditory analysis disorder. *Brain Injury, 21*(11), 1165–1174.

Testa, R., Bennett, P., & Ponsford, J. (2012). Factor analysis of nineteen executive function tests in a healthy adult population. *Archives of Clinical Neuropsychology, 27,* 213–224.

Theodoros, D. G., Murdoch, B. E., & Goozee, J. V. (2001). Dysarthria following traumatic brain injury: Incidence, recovery and perceptual features. In B. E. Murdoch & D. G. Theodoros (Eds.), *Traumatic brain injury: Associated speech, language, and swallowing disorders* (pp. 27–51). San Diego, CA: Singular.

Thickpenny-Davis, K., & Barker-Collo, S. (2007). Evaluation of a structured group format memory rehabilitation program for adults following brain injury. *Journal of Head Trauma Rehabiliation, 22,* 303–313.

Thiel, A., Habedank, B., Winhuisen, L., Herholz, K., Kessler, J., Haupt, W. F., & Heiss, W. D. (2005). Essential language function of the right hemisphere in brain tumor patients. *Annals of Neurology, 57,* 128–131.

Thiel, A., Herholz, K., Koyuncu, A., Ghaemi, M., Kracht, L. W., Habedank, B., & Heiss, W. D. (2001). Plasticity of language networks in patients with brain tumors: A positron emission tomography activation study. *Annals of Neurology, 50,* 620–629.

Thimm, M., Fink, G., Kust, J., Karbe, H., Willmes, K., & Sturm, W. (2009). Recovery from hemineglect: Differential neurobiological effects of optokinetic stimulation and alertness training. *Cortex, 45,* 850–862.

Thom, J., & Clare, L. (2011). Rationale for combined exercise and cognition-focused interventions to improve functional independence in people with dementia. *Gerontology, 57*(3), 265–275.

Thompson, C. K. (2008). Treatment of syntactic and morphologic deficits in agrammatic aphasia: Treatment of underlying forms. In R. Chapey (Ed.), *Language intervention strategies in adult aphasia and related neurogenic communication disorders* (5th ed., pp. 735–755). New York: Lippincott Williams & Wilkins.

Thompson, C. K., Ballard, K. J., & Shapiro, L. P. (1998). The role of syntactic complexity in training wh-movement structures in agrammatic aphasia: Optimal order for promoting generalization. *Journal of the International Neuropsychological Society, 4,* 661–674.

Thompson, C. K., Choy, J. J., Holland, A., & Cole, R. (2010). Sentactics: Computer-automated treatment of underlying forms. *Aphasiology, 24*(10), 1242–1266.

Thompson, C. K., & Shapiro, L. P. (2005). Treating agrammatic aphasia within a linguistic framework: Treatment of underlying forms. *Aphasiology, 19*(10–11), 1021–1036.

Thompson, C. K., & Shapiro, L. P. (2007). Complexity in treatment of syntactic deficits. *American Journal of Speech-Language Pathology, 16*(1), 30–42.

Thompson, C. K., Shapiro, L. P., Kiran, S., & Sobecks, J. (2003). The role of syntactic complexity in treatment of sentence deficits in agrammatic aphasia: The complexity account of treatment efficacy (CATE). *Journal of Speech, Language, and Hearing Research, 46,* 591–607.

Thompson, C. K., Shapiro, L. P., Tait, M. E., Jacobs, B. J., Schneider, S. L., & Ballard, K. J. (1995). A system for the linguistic analysis of agrammatic language production. *Brain and Language, 51,* 124–129.

Threats, T. (2009). Severe aphasia: Possible contributions of using the ICF in assessment. *Perspectives on Neurophysiology and Neurogenic Speech and Language Disorders, 19*(1), 7–14.

Thurstone, L. L., & Thurstone, T. G. (1962). *Primary mental abilities* (Rev. ed.). Chicago: Science Research Associates.

Tiberti, C., Sabe, L., Jason, L., Leiguarda, R., & Starkstein, S. (1998). A randomized, double-blind, placebo-controlled study of methylphenidate in patients with organic amnesia. *European Journal of Neurology, 5,* 297–299.

Tingley, S. J., Kyte, C. S., Johnson, C. J., & Beitchman, J. H. (2003). Single-word and conversational measures of word-finding proficiency. *American Journal of Speech-Language Pathology, 12*, 359–368.

Togher, L. (2001). Discourse sampling in the 21st century. *Journal of Communication Disorders, 34*, 131–150.

Togher, L. (2012). Challenges inherent in optimizing speech-language pathology outcomes: It's not just about counting the hours. *International Journal of Speech-Language Pathology.* doi:10.3109/17549507.2012.689334

Togher, L., McDonald, S., Tate, R., Power, E., & Rietdijk, R. (2009). Training communication partners of people with traumatic brain injury: Reporting the protocol for a clinical trial. *Brain Impairment, 10*(02), 188–204.

Toglia, J. P. (1993). *Contextual memory test.* San Antonio, TX: Psychological Corporation.

Toglia, J., Johnston, M. V., Goverover, Y., & Dain, B. (2010). A multicontext approach to promoting transfer of strategy use and self regulation after brain injury: An exploratory study. *Brain Injury, 24*(4), 664–677.

Tombaugh, T. N., & Hubley, A. M. (1997). The 60-item Boston Naming Test: Norms for cognitively intact adults aged 25 to 88 years. *Journal of Clinical and Experimental Neuropsychology, 19*, 922–932.

Tombaugh, T. N., & McIntyre, N. J. (1992). The Mini-Mental State Examination: A comprehensive review. *Journal of the American Geriatrics Society, 40*, 922–935.

Tomlin, K. J. (2007). *Workbook of activities for language and cognition–1: Aphasia rehab* (Spanish). East Moline, IL: Linguisystems.

Tompkins, C. A. (1995). *Right hemisphere communication disorders: Theory and management.* San Diego, CA: Singular.

Tompkins, C. A. (2008). Theoretical considerations for understanding "understanding" by adults with right hemisphere brain damage. *Perspectives on Neurophysiology and Neurogenic Speech and Language Disorders, 18*(2), 45–54.

Tompkins, C. A. (2012). Rehabilitation for cognitive-communication disorders in right hemisphere brain damage. *Archives of Physical Medicine and Rehabilitation, 93*(Suppl. 1), S61–S69.

Tompkins, C. A., Blake, M., Wambaugh, J., & Meigh, K. (2011). A novel, implicit treatment for language comprehension processes in right hemisphere brain damage: Phase I data. *Aphasiology, 25*(6–7), 789–799.

Tompkins, C. A., Bloise, C. G. R., Timko, M. L., & Baumgaertner, A. (1994). Working memory and inference revision in brain-damaged and normally aging adults. *Journal of Speech and Hearing Research, 37*, 896–912.

Tompkins, C. A., Fassbinder, W., Blake, M. L., Baumgaertner, A., & Jayaram, N. (2004). Inference generation during text comprehension by adults with right hemisphere brain damage: Activation failure versus multiple activation. *Journal of Speech, Language, and Hearing Research, 47*, 1380–1395.

Tompkins, C. A., Fassbinder, W., Scharp, V. L., & Meigh, K. (2008). Activation and maintenance of peripheral semantic features of unambiguous words after right hemisphere brain damage in adults. *Aphasiology, 22*(2), 119–138.

Tompkins, C. A., & Flowers, C. R. (1985). Perception of emotional intonation by brain-damaged adults: The influence of task processing levels. *Journal of Speech and Hearing Research, 28*, 527–538.

Tompkins, C. A., Jackson, S., & Schulz, R. (1990). On prognostic research in adult neurologic disorders. *Journal of Speech and Hearing Research, 33*, 398–401.

Tompkins, C. A., Klepousniotoou, E., & Gibbs Scott, A. (2011). Nature and assessment of right hemisphere disorders. In I. Papathanasiou, P. Coppens, & C. Potagas (Eds.), *Aphasia and related neurogenic communication disorders* (pp. 297–343). Sudbury, MA: Jones & Bartlett.

Tompkins, C. A., & Lehman, M. T. (1997). Outcomes measurement in cognitive communication disorders. Section 2: Right-hemisphere brain damage. In C. M. Frattali (Ed.), *Measuring outcomes in speech-language pathology* (pp. 281–292). New York: Thieme.

Tompkins, C. A., Lehman Blake, M., Baumgaertner, A., & Fassbinder, W. (2001). Mechanisms of discourse comprehension impairment after right hemisphere brain damage: Suppression in inferential ambiguity resolution. *Journal of Speech, Language and Hearing Research, 44*, 400–415.

Tompkins, C. A., Meigh, K., Scott, A., & Lederer, L. (2009). Can high-level inferencing be predicted by Discourse Comprehension Test performance in adults with right hemisphere brain damage? *Aphasiology, 23*(7–8), 1016–1027.

Tompkins, C. A., Scharp, V. L., Fassbinder, W., Meigh, K., & Armstrong, E. M. (2008). A different story on "Theory of Mind" deficit in adults with right hemisphere brain damage. *Aphasiology, 22*(1), 42–61.

Tompkins, C. A., Scharp, V. L., Meigh, K., Blake, M., & Wambaugh, J. (2012). Generalization of a novel implicit treatment for coarse coding deficit in right hemisphere brain damage: A single-participant experiment. *Aphasiology, 26*(5), 689–708.

Tompkins, C. A., Scharp, V. L., Meigh, K., & Fassbinder, W. (2008). Coarse coding and discourse comprehension in adults with right hemisphere brain damage. *Aphasiology, 22*(2), 204–223.

Torgesen, J. K., Wagner, R., & Rashotte, C. (2012). *Test of word reading efficiency* (2nd ed.). Austin, TX: PRO-ED.

Torti, F. M., Gwyther, L., Reed, S. D., Friedman, J., & Schulman, K. (2004). A multinational review of recent trends and reports in dementia caregiver burden. *Alzheimer Disease and Associated Disorders, 18*, 99–109.

Tosto, G., Gasparini, M., Lenzi, G., & Bruno, G. (2011). Prosodic impairment in Alzheimer's disease: Assessment and clinical relevance. *Journal of Neuropsychiatry and Clinical Neuroscience, 23*(2), E21–E23.

Trahan, D. E., & Larrabee, G. J. (1988). *Continuous visual memory test*. Lutz, FL: Psychological Assessment Resources.

Trenerry, M. R., Crosson, B., DeBoe, J., & Leber, W. R. (1989). *Stroop neuropsychological screening test*. Lutz, FL: Psychological Assessment Resources.

Trenerry, M. R., Crosson, B., DeBoe, J., & Leber, W. R. (1990). *Visual search and attention test*. Lutz, FL: Psychological Assessment Resources.

Troster, A. (2011). A précis of recent advances in the neuropsychology of mild cognitive impairment in Parkinson's disease and a proposal of preliminary research criteria. *Journal of the International Neuropsychological Society, 17*, 393–406.

True, G., Bartlett, M. R., Fink, R. B., Linebarger, M., & Schwartz, M. (2010). Perspectives of persons with aphasia towards SentenceShaper To Go: A qualitative study. *Aphasiology, 24*, 1032–1050.

Truelle, J. L., Koskinen, S., Hawthorne, G., Sarajuuri, J., Formisano, R., Von Wild, K., . . . Von Steinbuechel, N. (2010). Quality of life after traumatic brain injury: The clinical use of the QOLIBRI, a novel disease-specific instrument. *Brain Injury, 24*(11), 1272–1291.

Tsang, M. H., Sze, K. H., & Fong, K. N. (2009). Occupational therapy treatment with right half-field eye-patching for patients with subacute stroke and unilateral neglect: A randomised controlled trial. *Disability and Rehabilitation, 31*(8), 630–637.

Tsegaye, M., de Bleser, R., & Iribarren, C. (2011). The effect of literacy on oral language processing: Implication for aphasia tests. *Clinical Linguistics and Phonetics, 25*(6–7), 628–639.

Tsirlin, I., Dupierrix, E., Chokron, S., Coquillart, S., & Ohlmann, T. (2009). Uses of virtual reality for diagnosis, rehabilitation, and study of unilateral spatial neglect: Review and analysis. *Cyberpsychology and Behavior, 12*, 175–181.

Tu, L., Togher, L., & Power, E. (2011). The impact of communication partner and discourse task on a person with traumatic brain injury: The use of multiple perspectives. *Brain Injury, 25*(6), 560–580.

Tucker, J., & Reed, G. (2008). Evidentiary pluralism as a strategy for research and evidence-based practice in rehabilitation psychology. *Rehabilitation Psychology, 53*(3), 279–293.

Tuomiranta, L., Rautakoski, P., Rinne, J., Martin, N., & Laine, M. (2012). Long-term maintenance of novel vocabulary in persons with chronic aphasia. *Aphasiology, 26*(8), 1053–1073.

Turkstra, L. S. (2001). Treating memory problems in adults with neurogenic communication disorders. *Seminars in Speech and Language, 22*, 149–156.

Turkstra, L. S., & Bourgeois, M. S. (2005). Intervention for a modern day HM: Errorless learning of practical goals. *Journal of Medical Speech Language Pathology, 13*(3), 205–212.

Turkstra, L. S., & Flora, T. (2002). Compensation for executive function impairments after TBI: A single case study of functional intervention. *Journal of Communication Disorders, 35*, 167–182.

Turkstra, L. S., & Holland, A. L. (1998). Assessment of syntax after adolescent brain injury: Effects of memory on test performance. *Journal of Speech, Language and Hearing, 41*, 137–149.

Turkstra, L., Ylvisaker, M., Coelho, C., Kennedy, M., Sohlberg, M., Avery, J., & Yorkston, K. (2005). Practice guidelines for standardized assessment for person with traumatic brain injury. *Journal of Medical Speech-Language Pathology, 13*(2), ix–xxxviii.

Turton, A., Dewar, S., Lievesley, A., O'Leary, K., Gabb, J., & Gilchrist, I. D. (2009). Walking and wheelchair navigation in patients with left visual neglect. *Neuropsychological Rehabilitation, 19*, 274–290.

Uc, E. Y., Rizzo, M., Anderson, S. W., Sparks, J., Rodnitzky, R. L., & Dawson, J. D. (2006). Impaired visual search in drivers with Parkinson's disease. *Annals of Neurology, 60*(4), 407–413.

Ulatowska, H. K., Olness, G. S., Hill, C. L., Roberts, J. A., & Keebler, M. W. (2000). Repetition in narratives of African Americans: The effects of aphasia. *Discourse Processes, 30*, 265–283.

Ulatowska, H. R., & Richardson, S. M. (1974). A longitudinal study of an adult with aphasia: Considerations for research and therapy. *Brain and Language, 1*, 151–166.

Urban, P. P., Rolke, R., Wicht, S., Keilmann, A., Stoeter, P., Hopf, H. C., & Dieterich, M. (2006). Left-hemispheric dominance for articulation: A prospective study on acute ischaemic dysarthria at different localizations. *Brain, 129*, 767–777.

Urbenjaphol, P., Jitpanya, C., & Khaoropthum, S. (2009). Effects of the sensory stimulation program on recovery in unconscious patients with traumatic brain injury. *Journal of Neuroscience Nursing, 41*(3), E10–E16.

U.S. Department of Health and Human Services. (2012). *The healthcare law and you*. Accessed December 9, 2012, from http://www.healthcare.gov/law

Utz, K., Dimova, V., Oppelander, K., & Kerkhoff, G. (2010). Electrified minds: Transcranial direct current stimulation (tDCS) and galvanic vestibular stimulation (GVS) as methods of non-invasive brain stimulation in neuropsychology—A review of current data and future implications. *Neuropsychologia, 48*, 2789–2810.

Vakil, E. (2005). Effect of moderate to severe traumatic brain injury (TBI) on different aspects of memory: A selective review. *Journal of Clinical and Experimental Neuropsychology, 27*, 977–1021.

Vallar, G. (2007). Spatial neglect, Balint-Holmes' and Gerstmann's syndromes, and other spatial disorders. *CNS Spectrums, 12*(7), 527–536.

Vallar, G., Rusconi, M. L., & Bernardini, B. (1996). Modulation of neglect hemianesthesia by transcutaneous electrical stimulation. *Journal of the International Neuropsychology Society, 2*, 452–459.

Vallat, C., Azouvi, P., Hardisson, H., Meffert, R., Tessier, C., & Pradat-Diehl, P. (2005). Rehabilitation of verbal working memory after left hemisphere stroke. *Brain Injury, 19*(3), 1157–1164.

Vanbellingen, T., & Bohlhalter, S. (2011). Apraxia in neurorehabilitation: Classification, assessment and treatment. *NeuroRehabilitation, 28*, 91–98.

Vanbellingen, T., Kersten, B., Van Hemelrijk, B., Van de Winckel, A., Bertschl, M., Muri, R., . . . Bohlhalter, S. (2010). Comprehensive assessment of gesture production: A new test of upper limb apraxia (TULIA). *European Journal of Neurology, 17*, 59–66.

van der Meulen, I., van de Sandt-Koenderman, M. E., & Ribbers, G. (2012). Melodic Intonation Therapy: Present controversies and future opportunities. *Archives of Physical Medicine and Rehabilitation, 93*(Suppl. 1), S46–S52.

van de Sandt-Koenderman, M. W. M. (2004). High-tech AAC and aphasia: Widening horizons? *Aphasiology, 18*, 245–263.

van de Sandt-Koenderman, W. M. (2011). Aphasia rehabilitation and the role of computer technology: Can we keep up with modern times? *International Journal of Speech Language Pathology, 13*(1), 21–27.

van de Sandt-Koenderman, W. M., Wiegers, J., & Hardy, P. (2005). A computerised communication aid for people with aphasia. *Disability and Rehabilitation, 27*(9), 529–533.

van de Sandt-Koenderman, W. M., Wiegers, J., Wielaert, S. M., Duivenvoorden, H. J., & Ribbers, G. M. (2007). A computerised communication aid in severe aphasia: An exploratory study. *Disability and Rehabilitation, 29*(22), 1701–1709.

Van Dijk, K. R., Luijpen, M. W., Van Someren, E. J., Sergeant, J. A., Scheltens, P., & Scherder, E. J. (2006). Peripheral electrical nerve stimulation and rest-activity rhythm in Alzheimer's disease. *Journal of Sleep Research, 15*(4), 415–423.

Vangel, S., Rapport, L., & Hanks, R. (2011). Effects of family and caregiver psychosocial functioning on outcomes in persons with traumatic brain injury. *Journal of Head Trauma Rehabilitation, 26*(1), 20–29.

van Harskamp, F., & Visch-Brink, E. (1991). Goal recognition in aphasia therapy. *Aphasiology, 5*, 529–539.

van Kessel, K., Moss-Morris, R., Willoughby, E., Chalder, T., Johnson, M. H., & Robinson, E. (2008). A randomized controlled trial of cognitive behavior therapy for multiple sclerosis fatigue. *Psychosomatic Medicine, 70*(2), 205–213.

Van Zomeren, A. H., & Brouwer, W. H. (1994). *Clinical neuropsychology of attention*. New York: Oxford University Press.

Varley, R. (2011). Rethinking aphasia therapy: A neuroscience perspective. *International Journal of Speech-Language Pathology, 13*(1), 11–20.

Varney, N. R. (1998). Neuropsychological assessment of aphasia. In G. Goldstein, P. D. Nussbaum, & S. R. Beers (Eds.), *Neuropsychology* (pp. 357–378). New York: Plenum Press.

Vaynman, S., Ying, Z., & Gomez-Pinilla, F. (2003). Interplay between brain-derived neurotrophic factor and signal transduction modulators in the regulation of the effects of exercise on synaptic-plasticity. *Neuroscience, 122*(3), 647–657.

Verny, M., Hugonot-Diener, L., Saillon, A., Caputo, L., Dobigny-Roman, N., Dieudonne, B., . . . Poller, F. (1999). Evaluation de la démence sévère: Échelles cognitives et comportementales (groupe de travail du GRECO). *L'année Gérontologique Serdi, 13*, 156–168.

Vickers, C. (2004). Communicating in groups: One stop on the road to improved participation for persons with aphasia. *Perspectives on Neurophysiology and Neurogenic Speech and Language Disorders, 14*, 16–20.

Vickers, C. (2010). Social networks after the onset of aphasia: The impact of aphasia group attendance. *Aphasiology, 24*(6–8), 902–913.

Vigen, C., Mack, W., Keefe, R., Sano, M., Sultzer, D., Stroup, T., . . . Schneider, L. (2011). Cognitive effects of atypical antipsychotic medications in patients with Alzheimer's disease: Outcomes form CATIE-AD. *American Journal of Psychiatry, 168*(8), 831–839.

Vignolo, L. A. (2003). Music agnosia and auditory agnosia: Dissociations in stroke patients. *Annals of the New York Academy of Sciences, 999*, 50–57.

Vignolo, L. A., Boccardi, E., & Caverni, L. (1986). Unexpected CT-scan findings in global aphasia. *Cortex, 22*, 55–69.

Vines, B., Norton, A., & Schlaug, G. (2011). Non-invasive brain stimulation enhances the effects of melodic intonation therapy. *Frontiers in Psychology, 2*. doi: 10.3389/fpsyg.2011.00230

Vink, A. C., Bruinsma, M. S., & Scholten. R. (2011). There is no substantial evidence to support nor discourage the use of music therapy in the care of older people with dementia. *Cochrane Summaries*. Retreived from http://www.summaries.cochrane.org

Viola, L., Nunes, P., Yassuda, M., Aprahamian, I., Santos, F., Santos, G., . . . Forlenza, O. (2011). Effects of a multidisciplinary cognitive rehabilitation program for patients with mild Alzheimer's disease. *Clinics (San Paolo), 66*(8), 1395–1400.

Visser-Keizer, A. C., Meyboom-de Jong, B., Deelman, B. G., Berg, I. J., & Gerritsen, M. J. J. (2002). Subjective changes in emotion, cognition, and behavior after stroke: Factors affecting the perception of patients and partners. *Journal of Clinical and Experimental Neuropsychology, 24*, 1032–1045.

Vitali, P., Abutalebi, J., Tettamanti, M., Danna, M., Ansaldo, A., Perani, D., . . . Cappa, S. (2007). Training-induced brain remapping in chronic aphasia: A pilot study. *Neurorehabilation and Neural Repair, 21*, 152–160.

Vitali, P., Tettamanti, M., Abutalebi, J., Ansaldo, A., Perani, D., Cappa, S., & Joanette, Y. (2010). Generalization of the effects of phonological training for anomia using structural equation modeling: A multiple single-case study. *Neurocase, 16*(2), 93–105.

Vogel, D., Carter, J. E., & Carter, P. B. (2000). *The effects of drugs on communication disorders*. San Diego, CA: Singular.

von Cramon, D. Y., & Matthes-von Cramon, G. (1992). Reflections on the treatment of brain-injured patients suffering from problem-solving disorders. *Neuropsychological Rehabilitation, 2*, 207–230.

von Steinbuchel, N., Wilson, L., Gibbons, H., Hawthorne, G., Hofer, S., Schmidt, S., . . . Truelle, J. L. (2010). Quality of Life After Brain Injury (QOLIBRI): Scale validity and correlates of quality of life. *Journal of Neurotrauma, 27*(7), 1157–1165.

Vukovic, M., Vuksanovic, J., & Vukovic, I. (2008). Comparison of recovery patterns of language and cognitive functions in patients with post-traumatic language processing deficits and in patients with aphasia following stroke. *Journal of Communication Disorders, 41*, 531–552.

Wagner, A. K., Sasser, H. C., Hammond, F. M., Wierciseiwski, D., & Alexander, J. (2000). Intentional traumatic brain injury: Epidemiology, risk factors, and associations with injury severity and mortality. *The Journal of Trauma Injury, Infection, and Critical Care, 49*, 404–410.

Wagner, R., Torgesen, J., Rashotte, C., & Pearson, N. (2010). *Test of silent reading efficiency and comprehension*. Austin, TX: PRO-ED.

Waldron, H., Whitworth, A., & Howard, D. (2011). Comparing monitoring and production based approaches to the treatment of phonological assembly difficulties in aphasia. *Aphasiology, 25*(10), 1153–1173.

Walker, R., Young, A. W., & Lincoln, N. B. (1996). Eye patching and rehabilitation in unilateral neglect. *Neuropsychological Rehabilitation, 6*, 219–231.

Walker-Batson, D., Curtis, S., Natarajan, R., Ford, J., Dronkers, N., Salmeron, E., . . . Unwin, D. H. (2001). A double-blind, placebo-controlled study of the use of amphetamine in the treatment of aphasia. *Stroke, 32*, 2093–2098.

Walker-Batson, D., Curtis, S., Wolf, T., & Porch, B. (1996). Amphetamine treatment accelerates recovery from aphasia. *Brain and Language, 55*, 27–29.

Walker-Batson, D., Unwin, H., Curtis, S., Allen, E., Wood, M., Smith, P., . . . Greenlee, R. G. (1992). Use of amphetamine in the treatment of aphasia. *Restorative Neurology and Neuroscience, 4*, 47–50.

Wallace, G., & Hammill, D. D. (2013). *Comprehensive receptive and expressive vocabulary test* (3rd ed.). Austin, TX: PRO-ED.

Wallace, T., & Bradshaw, A. (2011). Technologies and strategies for people with communication problems following brain injury or stroke. *NeuroRehabilitation, 28*(3), 199–209.

Wambaugh, J. L. (2003). A comparison of the relative effects of phonologic and semantic cueing treatments. *Aphasiology, 17*, 433–441.

Wambaugh, J. L., Doyle, P. J., Martinez, A. L., & Kalinyak-Fliszar, M. (2002). Effects of two lexical retrieval cueing treatments on action naming in aphasia. *Journal of Rehabilitation Research and Development, 39*, 455–466.

Wambaugh, J. L., & Ferguson, M. (2007). Application of semantic feature analysis to retrieval of action names in aphasia. *Journal of Rehabilitation Research & Development, 44*(3), 381–394.

Wambaugh, J. L., & Martinez, A. L. (2000). Effects of modified response elaboration training with apraxia and aphasic speakers. *Aphasiology, 14*, 603–617.

Wambaugh, J. L., Martinez, A. L., & Alegre, M. N. (2001). Qualitative changes following application of modified response elaboration training with apraxic-aphasic speakers. *Aphasiology, 15*, 965–976.

Ward, H., Shum, D., Dick, B., McKinlay, L., & Baker-Tweney, S. (2004). Interview study of the effects of paediatric traumatic brain injury on memory. *Brain Injury, 18*, 471–495.

Ward-Lonergan, J., & Nicholas, M. (1995). Drawing to communicate: A case report of an adult with global aphasia. *European Journal of Disorders of Communication, 30*, 475–491.

Warner, T. T., & Schapira, A. H. V. (2003). Genetic and environmental factors in the cause of Parkinson's disease. *Annals of Neurology, 53*, S16–S25.

Warren, R. L. (1992). Functional outcome: An introduction. *Clinical Aphasiology, 21*, 59–65.

Warrington, E. K. (1999). *Recognition memory test*. Lutz, FL: Psychological Assessment Resources.

Warrington, E. K., & James, M. (1991). *Visual object and space perception battery*. Gaylord, MI: National Rehabilitation Services.

Watanabe, M., Martin, E., DeLeon, O., Gaviria, M., Pavel, D., & Trepashko, D. (1995). Successful methylphenidate treatment of apathy after subcortical infarcts. *Journal of Neuropsychiatry, 7*(4), 502–504.

Watanabe, S., & Amimoto, K. (2010). Generalization of prism adaptation for wheelchair driving task in patients with unilateral spatial neglect. *Archives of Physical Medicine and Rehabilitation, 91*, 443–447.

Webster, J., & Gordon, B. (2009). Contrasting therapy effects for verb and sentence processing difficulties: A discussion of what worked and why. *Aphasiology, 23*(10), 1231–1251.

Webster, J. S., McFarland, P. T., Rapport, L. J., Morrill, B., Roades, L. A., & Abadee, P. S. (2001). Computer-assisted training for improving wheelchair mobility in unilateral neglect patients. *Archives of Physical Medicine and Rehabilitation, 82*, 769–775.

Wechsler, D. (2001). *Wechsler test of adult reading*. San Antonio, TX: Psychological Corporation.

Wechsler, D. (2008). *Wechsler adult intelligence scale* (4th ed.) San Antonio, TX: Pearson.

Wechsler, D. (2009). *Wechsler memory scale* (4th ed.). San Antonio, TX: Pearson.

Wee, J., & Hopman, W. (2008). Comparing consequences of right and left unilateral neglect in a stroke rehabilitation population. *American Journal of Physical Medicine Rehabilitation, 87*(11), 910–920.

Wee, J., & Menard, M. R. (1999). "Pure word deafness:" Implications for assessment and management in communication disorder—A report of two cases. *Archives of Physical Medicine and Rehabilitation, 80*, 1106–1109.

Weigl, E. (1981). *Neuropsychology and neurolinguistics: Selected papers*. New York: Mouton.

Wertz, R. T., & Katz, R. C. (2004). Outcomes of computer-provided treatment for aphasia. *Aphasiology, 18,* 229–244.

Weiduschat, N., Thiel, A., Rubi-Fessen, I., Hartmann, A., Kessler, J., Merl, P., . . . Heiss, W. (2011). Effects of repetitive transcranial magnetic stimulation in aphasic stroke. *Stroke, 42,* 409–415.

Weintraub, S., & Mesulam, M. M. (1985). *Verbal and nonverbal cancellation test.* Philadelphia: FA Davis.

Weintraub, S., Rubin, N. P., & Mesulam, M. M. (1990). Primary progressive aphasia: Longitudinal course, neuropsychological profile, and language features. *Archives of Neurology, 47,* 1329–1335.

Weir, D. W., Sturrack, A., & Leavitt, B. R. (2011). Development of biomarkers for Huntington's disease. *Lancet Neurology, 10,* 573–590.

Weissling, K., & Prentice, C. (2010). The timing of remediation and compensation rehabilitation programs for individuals with acquired brain injuries: Opening the conversation. *Perspectives on Augmentative and Alternative Communication, 19*(3), 87–96.

Welden, S., & Yesavage, J. (1982). Behavioral improvement with relaxation training in senile dementia. *Clinical Gerontologist, 1,* 43–49.

Welland, R. J., Lubinski, R., & Higginbotham, D. J. (2002). Discourse comprehension test performance of elders with dementia of the Alzheimer's type. *Journal of Speech, Language and Hearing Research, 45,* 1175–1187.

Welsh, J., & Zhabo, G. (2011). Teaching nursing assistant students about aphasia and communication. *Seminars in Speech and Language, 32*(3), 243–255.

Wen, P. Y., Fine, H. A., Black, P. M., Shrieve, D. C., Alexander, E., & Loeffler, J. S. (1995). High-grade astrocytomas. *Neurologic Clinics, 13,* 875–900.

Wertz, R. T., & Irwin, W. H. (2001). Darley and the efficacy of language rehabilitation in aphasia. *Aphasiology, 15,* 231–247.

West, J., Sands, E., & Ross-Swain, D. (1998). *Bedside evaluation screening test of aphasia* (2nd ed.). Austin, TX: PRO-ED.

Wetherell, J. L. (1998). Treatment of anxiety in older adults. *Psychotherapy, 35,* 444–458.

Wharton, S. B., Brayne, C., Savva, G. M., Matthews, F. E., Forster, G., Simpson, J., . . . Ince, P. G. (2011). Epidemiological neuropathology: The MRC Cognitive Function and Aging Study Experience. *Journal of Alzheimer's Disease, 25*(2), 359–372.

Whiteneck, G. G., Charlifue, S. W., Gerhart, K. A., Overholser, J. D., & Richardson, G. N. (1992). Quantifying handicap: A new measure of long-term rehabilitation outcomes. *Archives of Physical and Medical Rehabilitation, 73,* 519–526.

Whiting, E., Chenery, H. J., Chalk, J., & Copland, D. A. (2008). Dexamphetamine boosts naming treatment effects in chronic aphasia. *Journal of International Neuropsychological Society, 13,* 972–979.

Whitworth, A., Perkins, L., & Lesser, R. (1997). *Conversation analysis profile for people with aphasia.* Philadelphia: Taylor & Francis.

Whitworth, A., Webster, J., & Howard, D. (2005). *A cognitive neuropsychological approach to assessment and intervention in aphasia.* Hove, England: Psychology Press.

Whurr, M., & Lorch, M. (1991). The use of a prosthesis to facilitate writing in aphasia and right hemiplegia. *Aphasiology, 5,* 411–418.

Whurr, R. (2011). *Aphasia screening test–Third edition.* Milton Keynes, United Kingdom: Speechmark.

Whyte, J., Gordon, W., Nash, J., & Gonzalez Rothi, L. (2009). A phased developmental approach to neurorehabilitation research: The science of knowledge building. *Archives of Medical Rehabilitation, 90*(Suppl. 1), S3–S10.

Whyte, J., Hart, T., Ellis, C., & Chervoneva, I. (2008). The Moss Attention Rating Scale for traumatic brain injury: Further explorations of reliability and sensitivity to change. *Archives of Physical Medicine and Rehabilitation, 89*(5), 966–973.

Wiederholt, J. L., & Blalock, G. (2001). *Gray silent reading test.* Austin, TX: PRO-ED.

Wiederholt, J. L., & Bryant, B. R. (2012). *Gray oral reading tests* (5th ed.). Austin, TX: PRO-ED.

Wierenga, C., Maher, L., Moore, A., White, K., McGregor, K., Soltysik, D., . . . Crosson, B. (2006). Neural substrates of syntactic mapping treatment: An fMRI study of two cases. *Journal of the International Neuropsychological Society, 12,* 132–146.

Wiig, E. H., Nielsen, N. P., Minthon, L., & Warkentin, S. (2002). *Alzheimer's quick test: Assessment of parietal function.* San Antonio, TX: Psychological Corporation.

Wiig, E. H., & Secord, W. (1989). *Test of language competence* (Expanded ed.). San Antonio, TX: Psychological Corporation.
Wiig, E. H., & Secord, W. A. (1992). *Test of word knowledge.* San Antonio, TX: Psychological Corporation.
Wilkinson, D., Roman, G., Salloway, S., Hecker, J., Boundy, K., Kumar, D., . . . Schindler, R. (2010). The long-term efficacy and tolerability of donepezil in patients with vascular dementia. *International Journal of Geriatric Psychiatry, 25,* 305–313.
Wilkinson, G. S., & Robertson, G. (2006). *Wide range achievement test* (4th ed.). Odessa, FL: PAR.
Wilkinson, R. (2010). Interaction-focused intervention: A conversation analytic approach to aphasia therapy. *Journal of Interactional Research in Communication Disorders, 1,* 45–68.
Wilkinson, R., Bryan, K., Lock, S., & Sage, K. (2010). Implementing and evaluating aphasia therapy targeted at couples' conversations: A single case study. *Aphasiology, 24,* 869–886.
Wilkinson, R., Lock, S., Bryan, K., & Sage, K. (2011). Interaction-focused intervention for acquired language disorders: Facilitating mutual adaptation in couples where one partner has aphasia. *International Journal of Speech-Language Pathology, 13*(1), 74–87.
Wilkinson, R., Bryan, K., Lock, S., Bayley, K., Maxim, J., Bruce, C., . . . Moir, D. (1998). Therapy using conversation analysis: Helping couples adapt to aphasia in conversation. *International Journal of Language and Communication Disorders, 33,* 144–149.
Willer, B., Rosenthal, M., Kreutzer, J. S., Gordon, W.A., & Rempel, R. (1993). Assessment of community integration following rehabilitation for traumatic brain injury. *Journal of Head Trauma Rehabilitation, 8,* 75–87.
Williams, K. N., Herman, R., Gajewski, B., & Wilson, K. (2009). Elderspeak communication: Impact on dementia care. *American Journal of Alzheimers Disease and Other Dementias, 24*(1), 11–20.
Williams, K., Kemper, S., & Hummert, M. L. (2005). Enhancing communication with older adults: Overcoming elderspeak. *Journal of Psychosocial Nursing and Mental Health Services, 43*(5), 12–16.
Williams, K. T. (2007). *Expressive vocabulary test* (2nd ed.). San Antonio, TX: Pearson.
Williams, L., Abdi, H., French, R., & Orange, J. B. (2010). A tutorial on Multiblock Discriminant Correspondence Analysis (MUDICA): A new method for analyzing discourse data from clinical populations. *Journal of Speech, Language, and Hearing Research, 53,* 1372–1393.
Williams, L. S., Weinberger, M., Harris, L. E., Clark, D. O., & Biller, H. (1999). Development of a stroke-specific quality of life scale. *Stroke, 30,* 1362–1369.
Williams, M. (1990). *Test of auditory perception.* Woodsboro, MD: Cool Spring Software.
Williams, M. (1994a). *The category test.* Marlton, NJ: Brainmetric Software.
Williams, M. (1994b). *Criterion-oriented test of attention.* Marlton, NJ: Brainmetric Software.
Williams, M. (1994c). *Test of visual field attention.* Marlton, NJ: Brainmetric Software.
Williams, M. (1994d). *Williams inhibition test.* Marlton, NJ: Brainmetric Software.
Williams, M. (1996). *The naming test.* Marlton, NJ: Brainmetric Software.
Williams, S. E., Ris, M. D., Ayyangar, R., Schefft, B. K., & Berch, D. (1998). Recovery in pediatric brain injury: Is psychostimulant medication beneficial? *Journal of Head Trauma Rehabilitation, 13*(3), 73–81.
Wilson, B. A. (1996). *Wilson reading system.* Milbury, MA: Wilson Language Training.
Wilson, B. A., Alderman, N., Burgess, P., Emslie, H., & Evans, J. J. (1996). *Behavioral Assessment of the Dysexecutive Syndrome.* Bury St. Edmunds, Suffolk, England: Thames Valley Test Company.
Wilson, B. A., Cockburn, J., & Halligan, P. (1987). *The behavioral inattention test.* Bury St. Edmunds, Suffolk, England: Thames Valley Test Company.
Wilson, B. A., Emslie, H. C., Quirk, K., & Evans, J. J. (2001). Reducing everyday memory and planning problems by means of a paging system: A randomized control crossover study. *Journal of Neurology, Neurosurgery, and Psychiatry, 70,* 477–482.
Wilson, B. A., & Evans, E. (1996). Error-free learning in the rehabilitation of people with memory impairments. *Journal of Head Trauma Rehabilitation, 11,* 54–64.
Wilson, B. A., Evans, J. J., Emslie, H., & Malinek, V. (1997). Evaluation of NeuroPage: A new memory aid. Journal of Neurology, *Neurosurgery and Psychiatry, 63,* 113–115.
Wilson, B. A., Greenfield, E., Clare, L., Baddeley, A., Cockburn, J., Watson, P., . . . Nannery, R. (2008). *The Rivermead behavioral memory test* (3rd ed.). Bury St. Edmunds, Suffolk, England: Thames Valley Test Company.
Wilson, B. A., Shiel, A., Foley, J., Emslie, H., Groot, Y., Hawkins, K., & Watson, P. (2005). *Cambridge prospective memory test.* Bury St. Edmunds, Suffolk, England: Thames Valley Test Company.

Wilson, B. A., Watson, P. C., Baddeley, A. D., Emslie, H., & Evans, J. J. (2000). Improvement or simply practice? The effects of twenty repeated assessments on people with and without brain injury. *Journal of the International Neuropsychological Society, 6*, 469–479.

Wilson, C., & Manly, T. (2003). Sustained attention training and errorless learning facilitates self-care functioning in chronic ipsilesional neglect following severe traumatic brain injury. *Neuropsychological Rehabilitation, 13*, 537–549.

Wilson, C., & Robertson, I. H. (1992). A home-based intervention for attentional slips during reading following head injury: A single case study. *Neuropsychological Rehabilitation, 2*, 193–205.

Wilson, K., Donders, J., & Nguyen, L. (2011). Self and parent ratings of executive functioning after adolescent traumatic brain injury. *Rehabilitation Psychology, 56*(2), 100–106.

Wilson, R., Rochon, E., Mihailidis, A., & Leonard, C. (2012). Examining success of communication strategies used by formal caregivers assisting individuals with Alzheimer's disease during an activity of daily living. *Journal of Speech, Language, and Hearing Research, 55*(2), 328–341.

Wilson, R. S., Rosenbaum, G., & Brown, B. (1979). The problem of premorbid intelligence in neuropsychological assessment. *Journal of Clinical Neuropsychology, 1*, 49–53.

Wilson, S. J., Parsons, K., & Reutens, D. C. (2006). Preserved singing in aphasia. *Music Perception, 24*(1), 23–36.

Wilson, S. L., Powell, G. E., Elliot, K., & Thwaites, H. (1993). Evaluation of sensory stimulation as a treatment for prolonged coma: Seven single experimental case studies. *Neuropsychological Rehabilitation, 3*, 191–201.

Winkens, I., Van Heugten, C., Fasotti, L., & Wade, D. (2009). Reliability and validity of two new instruments for measuring aspects of mental slowness in the daily lives of stroke patients. *Neuropsychological Rehabilitation, 19*(1), 64–85.

Winkens, I., Van Heugten, C., Wade, D., & Fasotti, L. (2009). Training patients in Time Pressure Management: A cognitive strategy for mental slowness. *Clinical Rehabilitation, 23*, 79–90.

Winnicka, K., Tomasiak, M., & Bielawska, A. (2005). Piracetam an old drug with novel properties. *Acta Poloniae Pharmaceutica, 62*(5), 405–409.

Winocur, G., & Moscovitch, M. (2011). Memory transformation and systems consolidation. *Journal of the International Neuropsychological Society, 17*, 766–780.

Winograd, P., & Hare, V. C. (1988). Direct instruction of reading comprehension strategies: The nature of teacher explanation. In C. Weinstein, E. Goetz, & P. Alexander (Eds.), *Learning and study strategies: Issues in assessment, instruction and evaluation* (pp. 121–138.). New York: Academic Press.

Wisely, J. (2010). Skilled nursing facility assessment tool focuses on patient communication. *ASHA Leader, 15*(6), 8–9.

Wiseman-Hakes, C., Stewart, M. L., Wasserman, R., & Schuller, R. (1998). Peer group training of pragmatic skills in adolescents with acquired brain injury. *Journal of Head Trauma Rehabilitation, 13*, 23–28.

Wolman, R. L., Cornall, C., Flucher, K. R., & Greenwood, R. (1994). Aerobic training in brain-injured patients. *Clinical Rehabilitation, 8*, 253–257.

Wong, M., Murdoch, B., & Whelan, B. (2010). Language disorders subsequent to mild traumatic brain injury (MTBI): Evidence from four cases. *Aphasiology, 24*(10), 1155–1169.

Wong, V., Cheuk, D. K., Lee, S., & Chu, V. (2011). Acupuncture for acute management and rehabilitation of traumatic brain injury. *Cochrane Database of Systematic Reviews, 5*. CD007700. doi: 10.1002/14651858.CD007700.pub2

Woodcock, R. W. (2011). *Woodcock reading mastery tests* (3rd ed.). San Antonio, TX: Pearson.

Woodruff, L., & Woodruff, B. (2007). *In an instant: A family's journey of love and healing*. New York: Random House.

Woolley, J., Khan, B., Murtthy, N., Miller, B., & Rankin, K. (2011). The diagnostic challenge of psychiatric symptoms in neurodegenerative disease: Rates of and risk factors for prior psychiatric diagnosis in patients with early neurodegenerative disease. *Journal of Clinical Psychiatry, 72*(2), 126–133.

World Health Organization. (1978). *Declaration of Alma-Ata*. Available at http://www.who.int/publications/almaata_declaration_en.pdf

World Health Organization. (1980). *International classification of impairments, disabilities, and handicaps: A manual relating to the consequences of disease*. Geneva, Switzerland: Author.

World Health Organization. (2001). *ICF: International classification of functioning, disability, and health*. Geneva, Switzerland: Author.

Wressle, E., Eeg-Olofsson, A., Marcusson, J., & Henriksson, C. (2002). Improved client participation in the rehabilitation process using a client-centred goal formulation structure. *Journal of Rehabilitation Medicine, 34*, 5–11.

Wright, H. H., & Fergadiotis, G. (2012). Conceptualising and measuring working memory and its relationship to aphasia. *Aphasiology, 26*(3–4), 258–278.

Wright, H. H., & Newhoff, M. (2005). Pragmatics. In L. L. La Pointe (Ed.), *Aphasia and related neurogenic language disorders* (3rd ed., pp. 237–248). New York: Thieme.

Wright, P., Rogers, N., Hall, C.,Wilson, B., Evans, J., Emslie, H., & Bartram C. (2001). Comparison of pocket-computer memory aids for people with brain injury. *Brain Injury, 15*, 787–800.

Wright, S., & Persad, C. (2007). Distinguishing between depression and dementia in older persons: Neuropsychological and neuropathological correlates. *Journal of Geriatric Psychiatry and Neurology, 20*, 189–198.

Wright Willis, A., Evanoff, B., Lian, M., Criswel, S., & Racette, B. (2010). Geographic and ethnic variation in Parkinson disease: A population-based study of U.S. Medicare beneficiaries. *Neuroepidemiology, 34*, 143–151.

Wu, T., & Garmel, G. (2005). Improved neurological function after Amantadine treatment in two patients with brain injury. *The Joural of Emergency Medicine, 28*, 289–292.

Wymer, J. H., Lindman, L. S., & Booksh, R. L. (2002). A neuropsychological perspective of aprosody: Features, function, assessment and treatment. *Applied Neuropsychology, 9*, 37–47.

Wynia, M., & Osborn, C. (2010). Health literacy and communication quality in health care organizations. *Journal of Health Communication, 15*(Suppl. 2), 102–115.

Xie, S., Libon, D., Wang, X., Massimo, L., Moore, P., Vesely, L., . . . Grossman, M. (2010). Longitudinal patterns of semantic and episodic memory in frontotemporal lobar degeneration and Alzheimer's disease. *Journal of the International Neuropsychological Society, 16*, 278–286.

Yamadera, H., Ito, T., Suzuki, H., Asayama, K., Ito, R., & Endo, S. (2000). Effects of bright light on cognitive and sleep-wake (circadian) rhythm disturbances in Alzheimer-type dementia. *Psychiatry and Clinical Neurosciences, 54*, 352–254.

Yampolsky, S., & Waters, G. (2002). Treatment of single word oral reading in an individual with deep dyslexia. *Aphasiology, 16*, 455–471.

Yang, C., Huang, S., Lin, W., Tsai, Y., & Hua, M. (2011). National Taiwan University Irritability Scale: Evaluating irritability in patients with traumatic brain injury. *Brain Impairment, 12*(3), 200–209.

Yang, Z., Zhao, X., Wang, C., Chen, H., & Zhang, Y. (2008). Neuroanatomic correlation of the post-stroke aphasias studied with imaging. *Neurological Research, 30*, 356–360.

Yantis, S. (2008). The neural basis of selective attention. *Current Directions in Psychological Science, 17*(2), 86–90.

Yasuda, K., Misu, T., Beckman, B., Watanabe, O., Ozawa, Y., & Nakamura, T. (2002). Use of an IC Recorder as a voice output memory aid for patients with prospective memory impairment. *Neuropsychological Rehabilitation, 12*, 155–166.

Yasuda, K., Nakamura, T., & Beckman, B. (2000). Comprehension and storage of four serially presented radio news stories by mild aphasic subjects. *Brain and Language, 75*, 399–415.

Yeates, K. O. (2010). Mild traumatic brain injury and postconcussive symptoms in children and adolescents. *Journal of International Neuropsychological Society, 16*, 953–960.

Yesavage, J. A., Brink, T. L., Rose, T. L., Lum, O., Huang, V., Adey, M., & Leirer, V. O. (1983). Development and validation of a geriatric depression screening scale: A preliminary report. *Journal of Psychiatric Research, 17*, 37–49.

Yeung, O., & Law, S.-P. (2010). Executive functions and aphasia treatment outcomes: Data from orthophonological cueing therapy for anomia in Chinese. *International Journal of Speech-Language Pathology, 12*(6), 529–544.

Ylvisaker, M., & Feeney, T. (1998). A Vygotskyan approach to rehabilitation after TBI: A case illustration. *Special Interest Division 2: Neurophysiology and Neurogenic Speech and Language Disorders Newsletter, 8*, 14–18.

Ylvisaker, M., Szekeres, S. F., & Feeney, T. J. (1998). Cognitive rehabilitation: Executive functions. In M. Ylvisaker (Ed.), *Traumatic brain injury rehabilitation: Children and adolescents* (2nd ed., pp. 221–269). Boston: Butterworth-Heinemann.

Ylvisaker, M., Szekeres, S., & Feeney, T. (2008). Communication disorders associated with traumatic brain injury. In R. Chapey (Ed.), *Language and intervention strategies in aphasia and related neurogenic communication disorders* (5th ed.). Philadelphia: Lippincott Williams & Wilkins.

Ylvisaker, M., Turkstra, L., Coehlo, C., Yorkston, K., Kennedy, M., Sohlberg, M. M., & Avery, J. (2007). Behavioral interventions for children and adults with behavior disorders after TBI: A systematic review of the evidence. *Brain Injury, 21*(8), 769–805.

Yokota, O., Tsuchiya, K., Arai, T., Yagishita, S., Matsubara, O., Mochizuki, A., . . . Akiyama, H. (2009). Clinicopathological characterization of Pick's versus frontotemporal lobar degeneration with ubiquitin/TDP-43-positive inclusions. *Acta Neuropathology, 117,* 429–444.

Yoo, E., Park, E., & Chung, B. (2001). Mental practice effect on line-tracing accuracy in persons with hemiparetic stroke: A preliminary study. *Archives of Physical Medicine and Rehabilitation, 82,* 1213–1218.

Yorkston, K., & Baylor, C. (2011). Measurement of communicative participation. In A. Lowit & R. Kent (Eds.), *Assessment of motor speech disorders* (pp. 123–157). San Diego, CA: Plural.

Yorkston, K. M., Baylor, C. R., Dietz, J., Dudgeon, B. J., Eadie, T., Miller, R. M., & Amtmann, D. (2008). Developing a scale of communicative participation: A cognitive interviewing study. *Disability and Rehabilitation, 30*(6), 425–433.

Yorkston, K., & Beukelman, D. (1980). An analysis of connected speech samples of aphasic and normal speakers. *Journal of Speech and Hearing Disorders, 45,* 27–36.

Yorkston, K. M., Beukelman, D. R., & Traynor, C. (1984). *Assessment of intelligibility of dysarthric speech*. Austin, TX: PRO-ED.

You, D. S., Dae-Yul, K., Chun, M., Jung, S. E., & Park, S. (2011). Cathodal transcranial direct current stimulation of the right Wernicke's area improves comprehension in subacute stroke patients. *Brain and Language, 119*(1), 1–5.

Youmans, G., Holland, A. L., Munoz, M., & Bourgeois, M. (2005). Script training and automaticity in two individuals with aphasia. *Aphasiology, 19*(3–5), 435–450.

Young, A., Perrett, D., Calder, A., Sprengelmeyer, R., & Elkman, P. (2002). *Facial expression stimuli and test*. Bury St. Edmunds, Suffolk, England: Thames Valley Test Company.

Young, J. A. (2011). Pharmacotherapy for traumatic brain injury: Focus on sympathomimetics. *Pharmacology and Therapeutics*. doi:10.1016/j.pharmthera.2011.08.003

Zammitt, N. N., Warren, R. E., Deary, I. J., & Frier, B. M. (2008). Delayed recovery of cognitive function following hypoglycemia in adults with type 1 diabetes: Effect of impaired awareness of hypoglycemia. *Diabetes, 57*(3), 732–736.

Zangwill, O. L. (1967). Speech and the minor hemisphere. *Acta Neurologica et Psychiatrica Belgica, 67,* 1013–1020.

Zeman, A. (1997). Persistent vegetative state. *Lancet, 350,* 795–799.

Zerwic, J., Hwang, S. Y., & Tucco, L. (2007). Interpretation of symptoms and delay in seeking treatment by patients who have had a stroke: Exploratory study. *Heart and Lung, 36,* 25–34.

Zgaljardic, D. J., Borod, J. C., Foldi, N. S., & Mattis, P. (2003). A review of the cognitive and behavioral sequelae of Parkinson's disease: Relationship to frontostriatal circuitry. *Cognitive and Behavioral Neurology, 16,* 193–210.

Zhang, L., Abreu, B., Gonzales, V., Seale, G., Masel, B., & Ottenbacher, K. (2002). Comparison of the Community Integration Questionnaire, the Craign Handicap Assessment and Reporting Technique, and the Disability Rating Scale in traumatic brain injury. *Journal of Head Trauma Rehabilitation, 17*(6), 497–509.

Zhang, Z. (1989). Efficacy of acupuncture in the treatment of post-stroke aphasia. *Journal of Traditional Chinese Medicine, 9,* 87–89.

Zhang, Z., & Zhao, C. (1990). Comparative observations on the curative results of the treatment of central aphasia by puncturing the yumen point versus conventional acupuncture methods. *Journal of Traditional Chinese Medicine, 10,* 260–263.

Zheng, X., Alsop, D. C., & Schlaug, G. (2011). Effects of transcranial direct current stimulation (tDCS) on human regional cerebral blood flow. *Neuroimage, 58,* 26–33.

Ziegler, W. (2002). Psycholinguistic and motor theories of apraxia of speech. *Seminars in Speech and Language, 23,* 231–244.

Zientz, J., Rackley, A., Bond-Chapman, S., Hopper, T., & Mahendra, N. (2007). Evidence-based practice recommendations: Caregiver-administered active cognitive stimulation for individuals with Alzheimer's disease. *Journal of Medical Speech-Language Pathology, 15*(3), xxvii–xxxiv.

Ziino, C., & Ponsford, J. (2006). Vigilance and fatigue following traumatic brain injury. *Journal of the International Neuropsychological Society, 12*, 100–110.

Zinn, S., Bosworth, H., Hoenig, H., & Swartzwelder, H. (2007). Executive function deficits in acute stroke. *Archives of Physical Medicine and Rehabilitation, 88*(2), 173–180.

Zoccolotti, P., Cantagallo, A., De Luca, M., Guariglia, C., Serion, A., & Trojano, L. (2011). Selective and integrated rehabilitation programs for disturbances of visual/spatial attention and executive function after brain damage: A neuropsychological evidence-based review. *European Journal of Physical Rehabilitation and Medicine, 47*, 123–147.

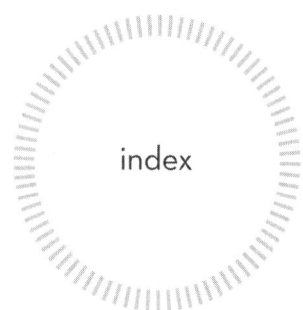

index

In this index, *f* denotes figure, *s* denotes sidebar, and *t* denotes table.

A

AAC. *See* Augmentative or alternative communication (AAC)
Abandoned utterances, 200
ABCD. *See Arizona Battery for Communication Disorders of Dementia* (ABCD)
ABS. *See Affect Balance Scale* (ABS)
Abstract letter identification, 16*f*, 17
Accommodations. *See also* Compensatory strategies; Interpreters; Modifications, 122, 129, 131–132, 149, 152
Accreditation agencies, 122, 279, 281, 283
Acetylcholine. *See also* Cholinergic system, 397*s*, 402
Achromatopsia, 55*t*, 73, 152
Acoustic environment, 448–449
Acoustic-phonological conversion, 15, 16*f*
Acquired dysgraphia, 41
Acquired dyslexia, 40–41
Acquired immune deficiency syndrome (AIDS), 93
Activity and participation. *See also* Assessments of activity, participation, and quality of life, 3–4, 5, 488
Activity-focused treatment. *See also* Participation-focused treatment, 412–425, 426*f*, 427–451
Acupuncture, 461–462
Acute-care settings
    assessment goals in, 117, 117*t*
    assessment restrictions in, 135, 136
    hidden deficits due to, 59–60
    observations in, 167
    overview of, 474–477
    patient interview and limitations from, 128
    process measures and, 279–280*s*
AD. *See* Alzheimer's disease (AD)
AD8 Dementia Screening Interview, 229
ADA. *See* Americans with Disabilities Act (1990)
Adaptive treatment. *See* Accommodations; Compensatory strategies; Modifications; Restorative versus adaptive treatment
ADD. *See Auditory Discrimination in Depth* (ADD)

601

Adolescents. *See also* Children, 150, 182–183, 198, 206, 209, 259, 262
Advocacy
    in assessment procedures, 116, 122
    for referrals and services, 123–124, 149, 299–300, 423s, 490
    for self, 379
    for treatment intensity, 355
    for use of AAC, 422–423
Affect Balance Scale (ABS), 290–291
Affordable Care Act (2010), 482
A-FROM. *See Living With Aphasia: Framework for Outcome Measurement* (A-FROM)
Age, as a testing confound, 214
Age, as prognostic factor, 216t, 217, 267–268
Ageism, 217
Aging population, differential diagnostic difficulties in, 112
Agitation. *See* Disruptive behaviors
Agonists, 397
Agrammatism, 37t, 38, 39f, 335, 337, 338
Agraphia, 41, 42t, 51
Agraphia treatment. *See* Orthographic treatment approaches
AIDS, 93
Akinetopsia, 152
ALA. *See Assessment for Living With Aphasia* (ALA)
Alcohol abuse, 110, 111
Alexia, 40–41, 42t, 51
Alexia treatment. *See* Orthographic treatment approaches
ALFA. *See Assessment of Language-Related Functional Activities* (ALFA)
Allesthesia, 57–58
Allographic conversion deficits, 309
AllTalk, 421
Alphabet search, 369
Alzheimer's disease (AD). *See also* Dementia
    angular gyrus syndrome versus, 111
    causes of, 103–105
    complicating conditions in, 152, 157, 159
    diagnosing, 103, 104t, 112
    lesion location for, 73s
    perceptual deficits in, 73
    Pick's disease versus, 105
    PPA and, 52
    prevalence of, 102
    prognostic factors in, 270
    pseudodementia versus, 112
    quality-of-life measures for, 293
    risk and protective factors for, 102, 103t
    symptoms of, 22, 74, 75–76, 219
Alzheimer's Disease Caregiver's Questionnaire, 232
Alzheimer's disease tests, 184, 206, 208, 212, 232
Alzheimer's disease treatment. *See also* Behavioral approaches for cognitive disorders
    CAM, 458, 460, 462, 463, 464
    memory treatment, 373, 374

pharmacotherapy approaches, 399–400t, 405, 406, 407, 408
taped autobiographical narratives, 368
Alzheimer's Quick Test, 232–233
Amantadine, 399t, 405
American Heart Association, 36
American Sign Language (ASL), 416
American Speech-Hearing Association (ASHA)
  on advocacy, 490
  on documentation, 488
  on EBP, 10–11s
  ICF and, 2
  on practice economics, 487
  on prevention activities, 470s
  program evaluations by, 281, 282t
  quality-of-life measures by, 293
  on SLPAs, 487
  support organization resources, 456
Americans With Disabilities Act (1990), 448, 482
Amer-Ind signs, 213, 416–417
Amnesia. *See* Post-traumatic amnesia (PTA)
Amphetamines, 399–400t, 401–402
Amusia, 150
Aneurysms, 88, 88f
Angular gyrus, 29
Angular gyrus syndrome, 111
Anomia, 38–40, 41, 71
Anomia treatment, 391
Anomic aphasia, 48t, 50, 51, 221
Anosodiaphoria, 59
Anosognosia
  assessments for, 264–265
  definition of, 59
  in frontotemporal dementia, 75
  functional outcomes of, 226
  as prognostic factor, 222, 270
  in TBI, 228
Antagonists, 397
Anterograde amnesia, 69–70
Anterograde memories, 22, 31
Anticipatory awareness deficit, 70
Antipsychotic medications, 400t, 407–408
Anxiety, 220
Aphasia
  A-FROM and, 275s
  apraxia of speech versus, 153–154
  classification systems for, 46–47, 48t, 49–52, 179
  complicating conditions after, 150, 153
  contextual variability of, 133
  definition and prevalence of, 36, 49, 50, 51
  explanations of, 45–46

frontotemporal dementia and, 63–64s
patient interview and limitations from, 128
prognostic factors in, 219, 220–221
psychiatric disorders screenings and, 160
symptoms of, 36–45
types of, 50–52, 53t
Aphasia groups, 437
Aphasia screenings, 172t, 173
Aphasia tests. *See also* Lexical–semantic processing tests; Morphosyntactic processing tests; Orthographic processing tests; Phonological processing tests; *specific tests*
    dementia patients and use of, 183–184
    overview of, 175–179, 185, 191, 198, 212
    RHD tests versus, 180
    TBI tests versus, 183
Aphasia treatment. *See also* Lexical–semantic treatment approaches; Morphosyntactic treatment approaches; Orthographic treatment approaches; Phonological treatment approaches
    AAC considerations in, 419–420, 421–422
    Amer-Ind signs, 417
    APT, 364, 390
    CAM, 458, 461–462, 464
    in groups, 437
    PACE, 432–434
    pharmacotherapy approaches, 399–400t, 401–403, 408
    SCA, 443–444
    sentence repetition tasks, 390
    variables for consideration in, 37
Applications (Apps). *See also* Software and applications, as treatment activities, 421–422
Apraxia Battery for Adults–Second Edition, 153, 157, 213
Apraxia of speech, 128, 153–154
APT. *See* Attention Process Training (APT)
Arcuate fasciculus, 29
Arizona Battery for Communication Disorders of Dementia (ABCD), 176t, 184
Arteriovenous malformation (AVM), 88–89
ASHA. *See* American Speech-Hearing Association (ASHA)
ASHA Functional Assessment of Communication Skills for Adults (ASHA FACS), 281, 283, 285
ASHA QCL. *See Quality of Communication Life Scale* (ASHA QCL)
ASL. *See* American Sign Language (ASL)
Assessment confounds. *See* Complicating conditions
Assessment for Living With Aphasia (ALA), 295, 296f
Assessment of Communicative Effectiveness in Severe Aphasia, 176t, 178
Assessment of Intelligibility of Dysarthric Speech, 154
Assessment of Language-Related Functional Activities (ALFA), 176t, 284–285
Assessment of Nonverbal Communication, 213
Assessment procedures, 124–144, 166, 171–174
Assessments. *See also* Cognitive disorders assessment of body structure and function; Linguistic disorders assessment of body structure and function; *specific tests*
    in acute care, 473, 475–476
    approach considerations for, 119–123
    goals of, 116, 117–119, 121s
    non-standardized procedures in, 476s

in outpatient settings, 480
  in rehabilitation phase, 478
  reimbursement issues with, 116s
  sharing results of, 144–145
Assessments of activity, participation, and quality of life
  approach considerations for, 278–279
  authentic assessment and ethnography, 295, 297–298
  environmental factors and, 448
  functional measures for, 279–286
  importance of, 273–274, 288–289
  list of measures by population, 276–277t
  participation measures, 286–288
  quality-of-life measures, 289–294
  relationship among measures, 294–295, 296f
  term definitions in, 274–275
Association areas and fibers, 29
Ataxia, 158
Attention, 19–20, 30–31
Attention deficits
  with aphasia, 43
  in dementia, 74
  in RHD, 54, 56–58, 60, 62
  in TBI, 68–69
Attention Process Training (APT), 363, 364
Attention Process Training–II (APT-II), 363, 364, 366, 390
Attention Process Training–III (APT-III), 363, 364, 364t, 366
Attention switching, 20, 20t, 31
Attention tests, 233, 239–240, 248–252
Attention treatment. *See also* Intention treatment
  attention training or retraining, 360, 363–365, 390
  cognitive strategies, 424
  combined approaches, 366–367
  for neglect, 358–363
  strategy training, 365
Audiologists, 148, 150, 449
Audiology, 120t
Audio recordings, 368, 378, 380
Auditory agnosias, 55t, 73–74, 150
Auditory Discrimination in Depth (ADD), 304t
Auditory perceptual deficits screenings, 150, 151t
Auditory phonological analysis, 15, 16f
Auditory sound agnosia, 150
Auditory-verbal working memory tests, 253–254
Auditory word-picture matching, 302
Augmentative or alternative communication (AAC). *See also* External devices, 418–422
Authentic assessment and ethnography, 295, 297–298
Authentic context, 454
Autobiographical memory. *See also* Episodic memory, 58
Autopagnosia, 152
AVM. *See* arteriovenous malformation (AVM)

Awareness training, 377–378, 379t, 380
Axonal shearing, 98, 99f

B

Back to the Drawing Board, 413
Backward chaining, 373
Bacterial meningitis, 92
BADS. *See Behavioral Assessment of Dysexecutive Syndrome* (BADS)
Balanced Budget Act of 1997, 484
Balloons Test, 250, 251
Barkley Deficits in Executive Functioning Scale (BDEFS), 243
Barotraumas. *See* Blast injuries
Barrier games, 345–346, 433
BASA. *See Boston Assessment of Severe Aphasia* (BASA)
Basal ganglia, 29, 30f, 31, 33, 83
Basement effect, 239
BAT. *See Bilingual Aphasia Test* (BAT)
BDAE. *See Boston Diagnostic Aphasia Examination* (BDAE)
BDAE-3. *See Boston Diagnostic Aphasia Examination–Third Edition* (BDAE-3)
BDEFS. *See Barkley Deficits in Executive Functioning Scale* (BDEFS)
BEAC. *See* Behavior, Emotion, Attitude, and Communication questionnaire (BEAC)
Bedside Evaluation Screening Test of Aphasia–Second Edition (BEST-2), 173
Behavior, Emotion, Attitude, and Communication questionnaire (BEAC), 291
Behavioral approaches for cognitive disorders, 357–392
Behavioral approaches for linguistic disorders, 299–355
Behavioral Assessment of Dysexecutive Syndrome (BADS), 229, 242
Behavioral Inattention Test (BIT), 251
Behavior Rating Inventory of Executive Function–Adult Version (BRIEF-A), 243
Benign brain tumors, 91
BEST-2. *See Bedside Evaluation Screening Test of Aphasia–Second Edition* (BEST-2)
Bifemelane hydrochloride, 399t, 402
Bilingual aphasia, 51–52
Bilingual Aphasia Test (BAT), 176t, 178
Bilingualism, 338–339s
Bilingual speakers. *See also specific types of speakers*, 125, 142–143s, 173, 178
Biofeedback, 458
Biographical factors, in prognosis, 217–218, 267–268
BIT. *See Behavioral Inattention Test* (BIT)
Blast injuries, 96–97, 100, 148, 152
Blood clots, 88, 97, 98t
Blood supply, in brain, 80–84
BNT. *See Boston Naming Test* (BNT)
Board games, 350
Body structure and body function, 2, 5
Booklet Category Test–Second Edition, 260
Books, 467t
BOSS. *See Burden of Stroke Scale* (BOSS)
Boston Assessment of Severe Aphasia (BASA), 176t, 178, 179
Boston Diagnostic Aphasia Examination (BDAE), 183, 381
Boston Diagnostic Aphasia Examination–Third Edition (BDAE-3), 47, 173, 176t, 177–178, 203
Boston Naming Test (BNT), 121s, 138, 197

Boston Naming Test–Second Edition, 178
Bradykinesia, 158
Brain. *See* Blood supply, in brain; Neuroanatomy
Brain abcesses, 92–93
Brain attacks. *See also* Strokes, 89
Brain-behavior relationships, 25–27s
Brain damage. *See* Primary brain damage; Secondary brain damage; *specific conditions*
Brain stimulation approaches, 331–332
Brain tumors, 90–92, 113, 219, 374
BRIEF-A. *See* Behavior Rating Inventory of Executive Function–Adult Version (BRIEF-A)
Brief Test of Head Injury (BTHI), 176t, 182
Broca's aphasia. *See also* Expressive aphasia, 48t, 49, 221, 338, 464
Broca's area, 28, 29s, 31, 83
Bromocriptine, 399t, 401
BTHI. *See* Brief Test of Head Injury (BTHI)
Bubble maps. *See* Metaphor Training Program (MTP)
Burden of Stroke Scale (BOSS), 292
Burns Brief Inventory of Communication and Cognition, 176t, 180–181

C

CADL-2. *See* Communicative Activities of Daily Living–Second Edition (CADL-2)
Calibrated Ideational Fluency Assessment (CIFA), 264
California Verbal Learning Test–Second Edition (CVLT-2). *See also Rey's Visual Design Learning Test* (RVDLT), 252–253
CAM. *See* Complementary and alternative medicine (CAM)
Cambridge Prospective Memory Test, 255
Cancellation tasks, 249, 251, 360, 362
Canonical word order, 18, 203
Cantonese speakers, 197
Capitation systems, 485
Caps or limits, 484, 486
Caregiver-Administered Communication Inventory, 167
Caregiver assessments, 143–144
Caregiver attitudes, 216t, 218, 460
Caregiver burden, 143, 226
Caregiver education. *See also* Counseling and education; Family education
    assessment results sharing and, 145
    communication partner training, 210, 415, 440–448, 454
    on environmental modifications, 448–451
    on external devices use, 427, 431–432
    in home health care, 480
    on memory books, 428–430
    prognosis and, 219
    relaxation therapy and, 459
    on spaced retrieval, 371
    on strategies, 431–432
    on topic coherence and cohesion treatment, 347
    on treatment purposes, 301s, 354
Caregivers. *See also* Families
    case history input of, 228
    functional measures and, 284

observations of interactions with, 167
quality-of-life measures for, 293
screening input of, 174, 229, 232
workbooks and software use as respite for, 352
Caregiver strategies, negative, 133, 144, 167
CARF. *See* Commission on Accreditation of Rehabilitation Facilities (CARF)
Carotid arterial system, 80–81, 82*f*, 83, 84
CART. *See* Copy and Recall Treatment (CART)
Case histories, 124–126, 167, 168–170*f*, 228–229
Case-mix adjustment, 486
Case rate systems, 485, 486
CATE. *See* Complexity Account of Treatment Efficacy (CATE)
Catecholamine system, 398, 401–402, 404–405
Category Test, 260
Caudate nucleus, 30*f*, 31, 33, 109
CC. *See* Coarse coding (CC)
CDP. *See* Communicative Drawing Program (CDP)
CELF-5. *See Clinical Evaluation of Language Fundamentals–Fifth Edition* (CELF-5)
Cell phones. *See* iPhones; Smartphones
Centers for Disease Control and Prevention (CDC), 94
Centers for Medicare and Medicaid Services (CMS), 283, 482, 486
Cerebellum, 31, 32*f*, 33
Cerebral arteries. *See* Cerebral vascular system
Cerebral hemispheres. *See also* Left hemisphere; Neuroanatomy; Right hemisphere, 81, 82*f*
Cerebral vascular system, 80–84
Cerebrovascular accidents. *See* Strokes
CETI. *See Communicative Effectiveness Index* (CETI)
Chaining techniques. *See also* Cueing hierarchies, 373–374, 375
CHART. *See Craig Handicap Assessment and Reporting Technique* (CHART)
Chemosensory impairments, 149–150
Children. *See also* Adolescents
    stroke incidence in, 85
    TBI incidence and, 94, 95
    tests for, 182–183, 208–209, 258, 262
    tumor incidence in, 91
Chinese speakers, 60, 178, 197, 265
Cholinergic system, 402–403, 406
CIAT. *See* Constraint-induced aphasia therapy (CIAT)
CIFA. *See Calibrated Ideational Fluency Assessment* (CIFA)
Cingulate gyrus, 31, 32*f*
Circle of Willis, 83–84, 89
Circumlocutions, 37*t*, 39, 40*t*, 200
CIUs. *See* Correct information units (CIUs)
Classical conditioning, 21*f*, 22
Clinical competency
    to advocate for referrals, 299–300
    on formal test utility, 135, 136, 138–139, 140–141, 175, 184, 190
    on range of communication, 349–350*s*
    on workbook and software use, 353
Clinical Evaluation of Language Fundamentals–Fifth Edition (CELF-5), 182

Clinical reasoning, 7, 11, 476
Clinician-developed probe tasks, 171–172, 208, 209, 210, 213–214
Clinician Interview-Based Impression of Change—Plus Caregiver Information (CIBIC+), 132
Clock Drawing, 233
Closed class words, 202
Closed head injuries. *See also* Traumatic brain injuries (TBI), 96, 97–98, 99*f*
CLQT. *See Cognitive Linguistic Quick Test* (CLQT)
CMS. *See* Centers for Medicare and Medicaid Services (CMS)
Coarse coding (CC). *See also* Contextual Constraint Treatment, 341
Cocaine abuse. *See* Substance abuse
Cognistat, 173
Cognitive Change Checklist, 232
Cognitive-communicative disorders. *See also* specific disorders, 53–54, 71, 227*s*
Cognitive-communicative disorders tests. *See also* specific tests, 140–141, 176–177*t*, 185
Cognitive disorders. *See also* specific disorders, 8*t*, 111–113
Cognitive disorders assessment of body structure and function. *See also* specific tests, 225–270
Cognitive disorders treatment. *See* Activity-focused treatment; Behavioral approaches for cognitive disorders; Participation-focused treatment; Pharmacotherapy approaches
Cognitive flexibility, 24, 32, 45
Cognitive flexibility tests, 258, 262
Cognitive functioning, general, tests for, 235, 236–237*t*, 238–239
Cognitive inflexibility, 75
Cognitive Linguistic Quick Test (CLQT), 258, 265
Cognitive neuropsychological approaches, 300–301, 322–330
Cognitive outcomes and prognosis, 221–222
Cognitive processing, 14, 18–24, 30–33, 42–45, 270
Cognitive stimulation general approaches, 386–387
Cognitive strategies, compensatory, 423–425
Cognitive treatment, 390–392
Cohesion analyses, 210–213
Color Trails Test, 248, 249
Coma, 65
Combine approaches, in attention remediation, 366
Combined semantic and phonological treatment approaches, 330–331
Commission on Accreditation of Rehabilitation Facilities (CARF), 122
Common Objects Memory Test, 265
Communication, 13–14
Communication approaches, multimodality, 413–418
Communication books. *See* Memory books
Communication partners. *See also* Caregivers; Families
    AAC and, 418
    in barrier games, 345–346
    discourse sampling and, 210
    memory books and, 430
    in topic coherence and cohesion treatment, 347
    training of, 415, 440–448, 454
Communication symptoms. *See also* Aphasia, 59–63, 75–76, 216*t*, 219–220
Communication systems, in ICUs, 473–474
Communicative Activities of Daily Living–Second Edition (CADL-2), 284–285
Communicative Drawing Program (CDP), 413–414

Communicative Effectiveness Index (CETI), 132, 284
Communicative Participation Item Bank, 287–288
Communicative Profiling System (CPS), 295, 297
Community-based teams, 123s
Community Integration Questionnaire (CIQ), 286–287
Community resources, 455–457
Compensatory strategies. *See also* Accommodations; Modifications
    for activity-focused treatment, 412–434
    for allographic conversion deficits, 309
    group treatment and, 438
    lighthouse imagery strategy, 361
    metacognitive training, 358
    mnemonic strategies, 368–369
    practice of, 430–434
    strategy training, 365, 368–370
    for writing deficits, 311t
Competency. *See* Clinical competency
Complementary and alternative medicine (CAM), 457–464
Complex Figure Test, 256
Complexity Account of Treatment Efficacy (CATE), 337
Complicating conditions
    observations of, 134
    overview of, 147–164
    as prognostic factors, 216t, 220, 222, 268–269
    sensitivity to, 229
Comprehension deficits
    in aphasia, 37–38, 46–47
    figurative language approaches for, 342–344
    linguistic stimulation approaches for, 310–313
    phonological treatment approaches for, 329
    semantic treatment approaches for, 323–324
    suprasegmental impairments treatment for, 304–305
Comprehensive Aphasia Test, 176t
Comprehensive Apraxia Test, 153
Comprehensive Receptive and Expressive Vocabulary Test–Third Edition (CREVT-III), 198, 204
Comprehensive Test of Nonverbal Intelligence–Second Edition (CTONI-2), 262, 265
Comprehensive Trail-Making Test, 248
Computer-Assisted Visual Communication system (C-VIC), 420
Computerized tomography (CT scans), 26s
Computers. *See* Software and applications, as treatment activities
Conduction aphasia, 48t, 50, 221
Confabulation, 61
Confidentiality, 482
Congruent overlap, 441
Conjunctive devices, 211
Connectionist classification systems, 47, 48t, 49–50
Conners' Continuous Performance Test III, 248
Consciousness disorders, 65–67
Constraint-induced aphasia therapy (CIAT), 355
Construct validity, 136t, 137
Content validity, 136–137

Contextual Constraint Treatment, 342, 343*f*
Contextual factors. *See also* Environmental factors
    aphasia and, 37, 45
    attention deficits and, 62
    definitions of, 4
    generalization and, 354
    in home health care, 480
    in LTC settings, 479
    pragmatics and discourse impairments treatment and, 348–349
    pragmatics and discourse processing and, 60–61, 340, 341
Continuous quality improvement. *See* Program evaluations
Continuous Visual Memory Test (CVMT), 257
Continuum of care, 470–481
Contrastive stress procedures, 305, 306*t*
Controlled Oral Word Association Test, 263
Conversation, CIUs and, 199
Conversational rules, 18
Conversational script training, 322, 454
Conversational skills treatment, 347–348
Conversation Analysis Profile for People With Aphasia, 167
Conversation Analysis Profile for People With Cognitive Impairment, 167
Conversation partners. *See* Communication partners
Cooking tasks, 242–243
Cooling therapy, 90
Coping style, as prognostic factor, 269
Coping With Aphasia, 466
Copy and Recall Treatment (CART), 313–314
Copying tasks, 309–310
Correct/incorrect judgments, 302
Correct information units (CIUs), 199
Cortical dementia. *See also* Dementia, 73*s*
Cortical stimulation, 26*s*
Cost effectiveness. *See* Health-care economics
Counseling and education. *See also* Caregiver education; Family education; Patient education, 464–465, 467*t*, 468
Coup and contrecoup injuries, 97–98, 99*f*
Craig Handicap Assessment and Reporting Technique (CHART), 286–287
CREVT-III. *See Comprehensive Receptive and Expressive Vocabulary Test–Third Edition* (CREVT-III)
Criterion-Oriented Test of Attention, 248
Criterion-related validity, 137
Critical appraisals, 9, 10, 11
Critical care units. *See* Intensive care units (ICUs)
Critical thinking. *See also* Clinical reasoning, 7, 11, 476
Crossed aphasia, 51
CTONI-2. *See Comprehensive Test of Nonverbal Intelligence–Second Edition* (CTONI-2)
CT scans. *See* Computerized tomography (CT scans)
Cueing approaches, in neglect treatment, 360–363
Cueing hierarchies. *See also* Chaining techniques, 314, 315*t*, 316–317
Cultural variables. *See* Ethnocultural variables
C-VIC. *See* Computer-Assisted Visual Communication system (C-VIC)

CVLT-2. *See California Verbal Learning Test–Second Edition* (CVLT-2)
CVMT. *See Continuous Visual Memory Test* (CVMT)
Czech speakers. *See also* Non-English speakers, 173

D
Daily Mishaps Test, 214
Dartmouth COOP Functional Assessment Charts, 290
Databases, 7, 8*t*
DCT. *See Discourse Comprehension Test* (DCT)
Deblocking activities. *See also* Speech perception tasks, 310–311
Declarative memory, 20, 21*f*, 22, 31
Delis-Kaplan Executive Function System (D-KEFS), 207, 239, 241–242
Dementia. *See also* Progressive neurological diseases; *specific conditions*
  AIDS and HIV and, 93
  chemosensory impairments and, 149–150
  complicating conditions in, 152, 154
  functional outcomes of, 74, 76
  inappropriate assessment of, 227*s*, 234*s*
  overview of, 72, 73*s*
  patient interview and limitations from, 128
  prognostic factors in, 219
  psychiatric disorders screenings an, 160
  quality-of-life measures for, 293
  symptoms of, 73–76
Dementia Outcomes Measurement Suite (DOMS), 293
Dementia Quality of Life Questionnaire (DQOL), 293
Dementia Rating Scale–Second Edition, 232, 262
Dementia tests, 176–177*t*, 183–185, 232, 233, 239, 262
Dementia treatment. *See also* Behavioral approaches for cognitive disorders
  CAM, 458, 460, 463–464
  communication partner training, 444–445
  general cognitive stimulation approaches, 386
  in groups, 438–439
  lack of referrals for, 299–300
  memory treatment, 371, 374
  pharmacotherapy approaches, 399*t*, 402, 408
  reality orientation to environment, 449–450
  social conventions treatment, 348
Dementia with Lewy bodies. *See also* Dementia, 74, 158, 212, 219, 399*t*, 406
DEMQOL, 293
Depression
  caregiving consequences and, 143
  as a complicating condition, 158–159
  as prognostic factor, 220
  pseudodementia and, 112
  SSRIs and, 408
  tests for, 206
Derivational morphemes, 18, 202
Diabetes, as prognostic factor, 268*t*, 269
Diagnosis-related groups (DRGs), 486
Diagnostic questions, 9*s*

Diagnostic reports, 144–145
Dichotomous classification systems, 46–47
Differential diagnosis, 472, 473, 475, 476
Disability, 3
Discharge recommendations, 476–477, 478
Discounted fee-for-service model, 484
Discourse Comprehension Test (DCT), 206
Discourse genres, 209–210, 212–213
Discourse informativeness, 61, 71, 199
Discourse interpretations, 62
Discourse macrostructure, 61, 71
Discourse processing. *See* Pragmatics and discourse processing
Discourse samples, 191, 199, 204–205, 209–213
Disinhibition, 75, 158, 382–383
Disjunct markers, 441
Disruptive behaviors. *See also* Complicating conditions, 440, 445, 450, 459, 460
Divided attention, 20, 249
Documentation. *See also* Diagnostic reports, 488
DOMS. *See* Dementia Outcomes Measurement Suite (DOMS)
Donepezil, 399t, 403, 406, 407
Dopamine. *See also* Catecholamine system, 397–398
DQOL. *See* Dementia Quality of Life Questionnaire (DQOL)
Drawings, 57f, 214, 233, 250, 413–416
DRGs. *See* Diagnosis-related groups (DRGs)
Drug treatments. *See* Pharmacotherapy approaches
Dual coding, 369
Dysarthria, 128, 154, 155t, 156, 156s
Dysarthria Examination Battery, 154
Dysphagia treatment. *See also* Swallowing function and services, 487, 490s

E
Ecological validity, 137, 392
Economics. *See* Health-care economics
Edema, in the brain, 100
Education. *See* Caregiver education; Counseling and education; Family education; Team education
Education, as a testing confound, 214–215, 229
Education, as prognostic factor, 268
EEG. *See* Electroencephalography (EEG)
Efficacy. *See* Treatment efficacy
Effortful learning, 374, 375
Egocentric output, 61
Elder Rehab program, 463
Electroencephalography (EEG), 27s
Electronic indexes, 7, 8t
Ellipsis, 211
Embolic stroke, 86–87
Embolus, 86
Emotion perception deficits and treatment, 349
"Empty speech," 38
Encoding, 21f, 23–24, 31

Encoding deficits, 58, 69–70
Endarterectomy, 87
Energent awareness deficit, 70
Environmental adaptation approaches, 376–377
Environmental agnosia, 152
Environmental factors. *See also* Contextual factors
    acoustics, 448–449
    definition of, 4
    formal tests and effects of, 134
    hidden deficits due to, 59–60, 123, 228, 266
    ICF assessment goals and, 118, 122
    modifications to, 448–451
    MS and, 109
    neglect syndrome and, 249
    observations and, 133, 285
    Parkinson's disease and, 107
    pragmatics and discourse processing and, 341, 348–349
    principles for organizing, 450–451
    psychiatric disorders and, 159
    screenings and, 174*s*
    TBI attention deficits and, 68
    variability in aphasia symptoms across, 133
Episodic memory, 21–22, 31, 69
Error analyses, 199–201, 204–205
Errorless learning, 373, 374–375, 391, 432
Ethics. *See also* Clinical reasoning, 116*s*
Ethnic differences. *See also* Ethnocultural variables; Racial differences, 85, 102
Ethnocultural variables. *See also* Authentic assessment and ethnography
    AAC and, 420
    in assessments, 139*s*, 142–143*s*
    generalization and, 354
    pragmatics and discourse processing and, 340
    as a testing confound, 215, 229
    in tests, 178
Event Drawing Task, 214
Evidence-based practice (EBP). *See also* Functional outcomes, 6–13, 490
Examining for Aphasia–Fourth Edition, 176*t*
Executive functioning, 24, 32–33, 222, 270, 369
Executive functioning deficits, 44–45, 59, 70–71, 75
Executive functioning screenings, 229
Executive functioning tests, 207, 233, 241–243, 257–265
Executive Function Route-Finding Task, 259
Executive function treatment, 376–378, 379*t*, 380–386
Exercise, 462–465
Expanded Trail Making Test, 248, 249
Expression deficits. *See* Production deficits
Expressive aphasia. *See also* Broca's aphasia, 46–47
Expressive Vocabulary Test–Second Edition, 198
External devices. *See also* Augmentative or alternative communication (AAC); Memory aids,
  413–418, 425, 426*t*, 427–432

F

Facebook, 443s
"Face-saving" repair strategies, 442–443
Falls, 95
False starts, 200, 200t
Families. *See also* Caregivers, 122, 164s, 210
Family attitudes. *See also* Caregiver attitudes, 216t, 218
Family education. *See also* Caregiver education; Counseling and education
    in acute care, 477
    HIPPA and, 482
    in ICUs, 474
    lighthouse imagery strategy, 361
    prognosis and, 219
    in SNFs, 478–479
FAS test, 263
FAVRES. *See Functional Assessment of Verbal Reasoning and Executive Strategies* (FAVRES)
FCMs. *See Functional Communication Measures* (FCMs)
FCP. *See Functional Communication Profile* (FCP)
FDA-2. *See Frenchay Dysarthria Assessment–Second Edition* (FDA-2)
Fee-for-service model, 483–484
Figurative language, 60, 71, 76, 446t
Figurative language and alternative meanings treatment, 341–345
Fillers, 200
FIM. *See Functional Independence Measure* (FIM)
FLCI. *See Functional Linguistic Communication Inventory* (FLCI)
Floor effect, 239
Florida Affect Battery, 192
FLS. *See Functional Life Scale* (FLS)
Fluency. *See* Speech fluency
Fluency tests, 263
Fluent aphasia, 46, 47
Fluvoxamine, 400t, 408
FMRI. *See* Functional magnetic resonance imaging (fMRI)
Focused attention, 20, 20t, 62
Focused attention tests, 248–249
Formal test procedures, 134–143
Fornix, 32f
Forward chaining, 373–374
Frenchay Dysarthria Assessment–Second Edition (FDA-2), 154
French speakers, 239, 243
Frontal Assessment Battery, 232
Frontal lobe lesions, tests for, 207
Frontal lobes
    blood supply for, 81, 82f
    Coup and contrecoup injuries in, 98
    dopamine and, 401
    functions of, 28f, 31, 32–33
    Korsakoff's disease and, 110
Frontotemporal dementia. *See also* Dementia
    aphasia and, 63–64s, 202

diagnosing, 106–107s
pharmacotherapy approaches for, 399t, 406, 408
prognostic factors in, 270
symptoms of, 73–74, 75, 76, 219
tests for, 208, 212
Frontotemporal lobar degeneration (FTLD)
complicating conditions in, 158, 159
definition and overview of, 105–107
PPA and, 52
screenings for, 173
tests for, 184, 232
Functional Assessment of Verbal Reasoning and Executive Strategies (FAVRES), 259
Functional communication. *See* Assessments of activity, participation, and quality of life
Functional Communication Measures (FCMs), 281, 282t, 283, 286
Functional Communication Profile (FCP), 283–284
Functional deficits, 488
Functional Independence Measure (FIM). *See also ASHA Functional Assessment of Communication Skills for Adults* (ASHA FACS), 280, 285
Functional Life Scale (FLS), 287
Functional Linguistic Communication Inventory (FLCI), 176t, 184
Functional magnetic resonance imaging (fMRI), 27s
Functional measures, 274–275, 279–286
Functional outcomes. *See also* Cognitive outcomes and prognosis; Linguistic outcomes and prognosis; *specific cognitive-communication disorder*
amnesia and, 67, 69
anosognosia and, 59, 226
blast injuries and, 97
CAM and, 460, 461–462, 463, 464
caregiver assessment and, 143
complicating conditions and, 134
external devices and, 427
group treatment and, 434
ICF assessment goals and, 118
limb apraxia and, 157
making assumptions about, 118–119
of memory books, 430
neglect and, 43, 56, 226
psychiatric disorders and, 159
thorough assessments and, 116
vegetative state and, 66
vocation and, 226
Functional tasks integration, for generalization, 366
Functional tests, 242–243, 252, 262–263
Funding agencies. *See also* Health-care funding models; Medicaid; Medicare; Private insurers; Third-party payers, 355

G
Galantamine, 400t, 402, 406
Gaming platforms, 388

GCS. *See* Glasgow Coma Scale (GCS)
Gender differences
    Alzheimer's disease and, 102
    FTLD and, 105
    meningiomas and, 91
    MS and, 109
    Parkinson's disease and, 107
    Pick's disease and, 105
    as prognostic factors, 216*t*, 217–218, 268
    strokes and, 85
    TBI and, 95
General cognitive functioning tests, 235, 236–237*t*, 238–239
Generalization
    of attention treatment, 364–365
    of computer-assisted therapy programs, 353
    external devices and, 427
    factors to encourage, 354–355, 392, 431–432
    of general cognitive stimulation approaches, 387
    of linguistic stimulation treatment, 317, 319, 321, 322
    of morphosyntactic treatment, 334, 336, 338, 342, 344
    of neglect treatment, 360, 361
    of phonological treatment, 307
    of semantic treatment, 323, 326, 328
Genres. *See* Discourse genres
Geographic differences, 85, 109, 123*s*
German speakers, 243
Gestures, 41, 213, 416–418
GI. *See* Guided imagery (GI)
GIST. *See* Group Interactive Structure Treatment (GIST)
Glasgow Coma Scale (GCS), 65
Glioblastomas, 91
Global aphasia, 48*t*, 49, 221
Goal Management Training (GMT), 384, 385*f*
Goal setting, planning, and problem-solving impairments treatment, 383–386
GORT-5. *See* Gray Oral Reading Tests–Fifth Edition (GORT-5)
Graphemes, 17
Graphemic processing. *See* Orthographic processing
Graphic displays. *See* Metaphor Training Program (MTP)
Gray Oral Reading Tests–Fifth Edition (GORT-5), 207
Greek speakers, 197, 292
Group Interactive Structure Treatment (GIST), 350
Group treatment
    awareness training, 380
    as compensatory strategy, 415*f*, 416
    conversational skills and, 347
    in LTC settings, 479
    overview of, 434–439
    social conventions treatment and, 348, 349, 350
Guided imagery (GI), 458

H

HAND (HIV-associated neurocognitive disorders), 93
Handicap, 3
HD. *See* Huntington's disease (HD)
Health-care delivery models. *See* Continuum of care
Health-care economics, 476, 483–490
Health-care funding models, 483–486
Health-care providers. *See also specific professionals*, 447–448, 449, 474, 477, 478–479, 489–490
Health-care reform. *See* Patient Protection and Affordable Care Act (2010)
Health-care settings. *See also specific levels of care*, 116, 116s, 117, 123
Health Insurance Portability and Accountability Act (HIPAA 1996), 482
Health literacy, 145, 160
Hearing loss. *See also* Acoustic environment, 148
Hearing screenings, 148
Helm Elicited Program for Syntax Stimulation (HELPSS), 333–335
HELPSS. *See Helm Elicited Program for Syntax Stimulation* (HELPSS)
Hematomas, 88, 97, 98t
Hemiakinesia, 57
Hemianesthesia, 149
Hemianopsia, 149
Hemi-inattention. *See also* Neglect syndrome, 56–57
Hemiparesis, 156
Hemiplegia, 156
Hemispatial neglect. *See also* Neglect syndrome, 56–57
Hemispatial patching or sunglasses, 359
Hemorrhagic strokes, 86f, 88–89
HHRGs. *See* Home health resource groups (HHRGs)
Hierarchy for cueing. *See* Cueing hierarchies
Hierarchy of evidence, 6
Hierarchy of pre-stimulation cues. *See* Contextual Constraint Treatment
Hierarchy of syntactic constructions. *See Helm Elicited Program for Syntax Stimulation* (HELPSS)
Higher-level language processes. *See also* Pragmatics and discourse processing, 180
HIPAA. *See* Health Insurance Portability and Accountability Act (HIPAA 1996)
Hippocampus, 31
HIV, 93
Holistic treatment. *See* Complementary and alternative medicine (CAM)
Home health care, 118, 479–480
Home health resource groups (HHRGs), 486
Homonymous hemianopsia, 149
Hopkins Verbal Learning Test–Revised, 252
Hospitals. *See* Health care settings; *specific levels of care*
Human immunodeficiency virus (HIV), 93
Humor appreciation, 60, 350
Huntington's disease (HD)
    complicating conditions in, 157, 158
    lesion location for, 73s
    overview of, 108–109, 219
    pharmacotherapy approaches for, 400t, 405, 406

sensory stimulation and, 460
tests for, 196, 206
Hypoxic-ischemic brain injuries, 100, 101

I

ICD-50. *See* Sony IC Recorder (ICD-50)
ICF. *See* International Classification of Functioning, Disability, and Health (ICF)
ICIDH. *See* International Classification of Impairment, Disability, and Handicap (ICIDH)
Iconic gestures, 213
ICUs. *See* Intensive care units (ICUs)
Ideational apraxia, 157
Identification cards, 422
Ideomotor apraxia, 157
Illogical verbal output, 54
Imagery. *See* Guided imagery (GI); Lighthouse imagery strategy; Visual imagery
Impairment, 3
Impulsivity. *See* Disinhibition
Incentives, therapy, 487
Indefinite substitutions, 39, 40*t*, 200
Infarcts, 86
Infections, 92–94, 100, 113
Inferencing, 61, 63, 347
Inflectional morphemes, 18, 202
Informativeness. *See* Discourse informativeness
Inhibition, 23, 24, 32, 45, 258, 261–262
Initiation, 32, 75
In-network providers, 484–485*s*
Inpatient rehabilitation, 477–478
Insurance agencies. *See* Private insurers
Intake form, 168–170*f*
Intellectual awareness deficit, 70
Intelligence. *See* Premorbid intelligence
Intensive care units (ICUs), 472–474
Intention treatment, 392
Interaction, 454
Internal capsule, 29, 30*f*, 83
International Classification of Functioning, Disability, and Health (ICF)
    assessment goals in, 117*t*, 118, 122, 133, 144
    assessments of activity, participation, and quality of life and, 274–275
    CAM and, 457
    EBP applied to, 11, 13
    overview of, 2–6
International Classification of Impairment, Disability, and Handicap (ICIDH), 2
Interpreters, 142–143*s*
Inter-rater reliability, 135, 136*t*
Intervention. *See specific approaches or treatments*
Interview formats, 132–133
Intracranial pressure, 100
iPads, 420, 421

iPhones, 421
Irreversible dementia. *See also* Vascular dementia, 107, 110, 112
Ischemic strokes. *See also* Strokes, 86–87, 89–90
Isolation aphasia. *See* Transcortical aphasia
Italian speakers, 292

J
Jargon, 37*t*, 39
Joint Commission of Accreditation of Healthcare Organizations (JCAHO), 122

K
Keywords, 308–309
Kindle Fires, 420
Knowledge base. *See* Declarative memory
Korean speakers, 243
Korsakoff's disease, 110, 373

L
Labeling behavior, 199
Lability, 67, 158
Lacunar stroke, 86
Language. *See also* Bilingualism; Bilingual speakers; Linguistic processing, 14, 28–29, 30*f*
Language disorders. *See also specific conditions*, 8*t*, 111–113
"Language neurotransmitter," 397–398*s*
Language sampling. *See also* Discourse samples, 198–201, 209–213
Language Screening Test, 172
La Trobe Communication Questionnaire, 167, 174, 286
Learning. *See* Encoding
Left frontal lobe, 28, 31
Left hemisphere, 28–29, 56, 401
Left hemisphere disorders. *See also* Aphasia; Right-sided neglect
    ASHA FACS and, 281
    assessment goals in, 117*t*, 119
    complicating conditions after, 150, 153, 156–157
    prognostic factors in, 269–270
Left parietal lobe, 29
Left prefrontal cortex, 31
Left-sided neglect. *See also* Neglect syndrome, 68
Legibility. *See also* Spelling deficits treatment, 41
Legislation, 481–482, 486–490
Lesion locations
    assessment goals and, 117*t*, 119, 165–166
    as prognostic factors, 216*t*, 218–219, 222, 269–270
Lesion method, 26*s*
Letter-to-sound rules, 16*f*, 17
Levels-of-evidence rating scales, 10
Levodopa, 399*t*, 401
Lewy body dementia. *See* Dementia with Lewy bodies
Lexical ambiguity resolution, 61
Lexical markers, 211

Lexical Orthographic Familiarity Test, 218
Lexical–semantic processing, 16*f*, 17, 41, 60, 76, 194–195*t*
Lexical–semantic processing tests, 193–201
Lexical–semantic treatment approaches. *See also* Combined semantic and phonological treatment approaches
    brain stimulation approaches, 331–332
    cognitive neuropsychological approaches, 322–331
    linguistic stimulation approach, 310–314, 315*t*, 316–319, 320*t*, 321–322
Life Participation Approach to Aphasia (LPAA). *See also* Social models, 452–453
Lighthouse imagery strategy, 361
Lighting, 449
Liles Communication Test, 212
Limb activation training, 361–362
Limb and head movements, as intention treatment, 392
Limb apraxia, 41, 156–157
Limbic system, 33
Lindamood Phoneme Sequencing Program for Reading, Spelling, and Speech (LiPS). *See also Auditory Discrimination in Depth* (ADD), 303
Line bisection tasks, 249, 251
Lingraphica system, 421
Linguistic ambiguity awareness, 341–342
Linguistic disorders assessment of body structure and function
    cognitive ability evaluation during, 266–267
    overview of, 166–174
    specific tests for, 185, 186–214
    test confounds, 214–215
Linguistic disorders treatment. *See* Activity-focused treatment; Behavioral approaches for linguistic disorders; Participation-focused treatment; Pharmacotherapy approaches
Linguistic outcomes and prognosis, 215, 216*t*, 217–221
Linguistic processing, 15, 16*f*, 17–18, 25, 40
Linguistic Specific Treatment. *See* Treatment of underlying forms (TUF)
Linguistic stimulation approaches, 300, 310–321, 333–335
Linguistic-theory-motivated approaches, 335–338
LiPS. *See Lindamood Phoneme Sequencing Program for Reading, Spelling, and Speech* (LiPS)
Literacy. *See* Health literacy; Reading
Literacy, as a testing confound, 215
Literacy problems. *See* Reading deficits treatment
Literal paraphasias. *See* Phonemic or literal paraphasias
Living With Aphasia: Framework for Outcome Measurement (A-FROM), 275*s*
Location Learning Test, 257
Logopenic progressive aphasia, 52, 53*t*
Long-term care (LTC) settings, 117, 117*t*, 282, 479
Long-term memory, 20–22, 23–24, 31–32, 44
LPAA. *See* Life Participation Approach to Aphasia (LPAA)
LTC. *See* Long-term care (LTC) settings

M

Magnetic resonance imaging (MRI), 26*s*, 332
Magnetoencephalography (MEG), 27*s*
Maintenance. *See* Generalization

Malignant brain tumors, 91, 92
Managed care models, 484–486
Mapping therapy, 335–336, 391
Marketing of services, 489–490
MAST. *See Mississippi Aphasia Screening Test* (MAST)
Maze completion tests, 258
MCST-A. *See Multimodal Communication Screening Task for Persons With Aphasia* (MCST-A)
MDS. *See* Minimum Data Set (MDS)
Medicaid. *See also* Centers for Medicare and Medicaid Services (CMS), 281, 439, 481–482, 484
Medical factors, in prognosis, 218–220
Medical professionals. *See also specific type of professional*, 447–448
Medical records review, 124–126
Medicare. *See also* Centers for Medicare and Medicaid Services (CMS)
  case rate system in, 486
  documentation and, 488
  fee-for-service model and, 484
  group treatment and, 436–437s, 439
  MDS and, 281
  overview of, 481
Medications. *See also* Pharmacotherapy approaches, 216t, 269
Meditation, 458
MEG. *See* Magnetoencephalography (MEG)
Melodic Intonation Therapy (MIT), 319–321
Mematine, 400t, 408
Memory, 20–24, 31–32
Memory aids. *See also* External devices, 375–376, 377
Memory books, 428–430
Memory deficits
  AAC and, 420
  anterograde amnesia and, 69
  with aphasia, 43–44
  in dementia, 74–75
  in RHD, 58
  in TBI, 69–70, 71
Memory for Intentions Test (MIST), 255–256
Memory retrieval, 21f, 23–24, 31
Memory tests, 233, 240–241, 252–257
Memory treatment, 367–376
Men. *See* Gender differences
Meningiomas, 91
Mental Slowness Questionnaire, 229
Mental-state inferencing, 32
Meta-cognitive abilities, 24
Metacognitive training, 358
Metalinguistic awareness. *See also* Linguistic ambiguity awareness; Topic coherence and cohesion, 340–341
Metalinguistic comments, 200t
Metaphor Training Program (MTP), 343–344
Metastatic brain tumors, 91
Methylphenidate, 399t, 404
Micrographia, 107, 108f

Mild cognitive impairment (MCI), 72, 364, 374, 458
Mild language impairments tests, 190
Mini Inventory of Right Brain Injury (MIRBI), 180
Mini Inventory of Right Brain Injury–Second Edition (MIRBI-II), 140, 176*t*, 180
Minimally conscious state, 66–67
Mini-Mental State Examination (MMSE), 231, 233, 234*s*
Mini-Mental State Examination–Second Edition (MMSE-2), 227*s*, 231, 265
Minimum Data Set (MDS), 281–283, 486
MIRBI. *See Mini Inventory of Right Brain Injury* (MIRBI)
MIRBI-II. *See Mini Inventory of Right Brain Injury–Second Edition* (MIRBI-II)
Mississippi Aphasia Screening Test (MAST), 173
MIST. *See Memory for Intentions Test* (MIST)
MIT. *See* Melodic Intonation Therapy (MIT)
MMSE. *See Mini-Mental State Examination* (MMSE)
MMSE-2. *See Mini-Mental State Examination–Second Edition* (MMSE-2)
Mnemonic strategies, 368–369
Modafinil, 400*t*, 408
Modifications. *See also* Accommodations; Compensatory strategies
    environmental adaptation approaches, 376–377
    of environment and task for neglect treatment, 358–360
    of physical environment, 448–451
    qualitative information from, 142
    to social environment, 440–448
    in stimulus and test administration, 142
    theoretical framework and treatment, 301*s*
    of treatment protocols, 319*s*
Modified Wisconsin Card Sorting Test (M-WCST), 260
Monocular eye patching, 359
MOR. *See* Multiple Oral Rereading (MOR)
Morphemes, 18
Morphosyntactic processing, 17–18, 38, 41, 76
Morphosyntactic processing tests, 202–205
Morphosyntactic treatment approaches, 333–338
Mosquitoes, 93–94*s*
Moss Attention Rating Scale, 229
Motivation, 32, 216*t*, 218
Motor extinction or neglect, 57
Motoric impairments screenings, 153–154, 156–158
MRI. *See* Magnetic resonance imaging (MRI)
MTP. *See* Metaphor Training Program (MTP)
Multicomponent Intervention Program, 387
Multidisciplinary involvement. *See also* Team approach, 5
Multilingual aphasia, 51–52
Multilingual Aphasia Examination, 178
Multilingualism. *See also* Bilingual speakers, 338–339*s*
Multimodal Communication Screening Task for Persons With Aphasia (MCST-A), 419
Multimodality communication approaches, 415*f*, 441–442
Multiple Oral Rereading (MOR), 324
Multiple sclerosis (MS)
    lesion location for, 73*s*
    meditation and, 458

pharmacotherapy approaches, 399t, 400t
prevalence of, 109
reversible dementia in, 112
symptoms of, 109–110
tests for, 206, 243
M-WCST. *See Modified Wisconsin Card Sorting Test* (M-WCST)

N

NAB. *See Neuropsychological Assessment Battery* (NAB)
NAB Mazes Test, 258
NAB Naming Test, 198
Naming. *See* Anomia
Naming errors, 54
Narrative rules, 18
National Aphasia Association, 422
National Center for Complementary and Alternative Medicine (NCCAM), 457
National Head Injury Foundation, 94
National Institutes of Health (NIH), 94s
National Outcomes Measurement System (NOMS), 281, 282t, 283
Native language, RHD and, 60
Naturalistic Action Test, 157
Naturalistic tests, 242–243, 252, 262–263
N-back tasks, 254, 255f
NCCAM. *See* National Center for Complementary and Alternative Medicine (NCCAM)
Neck stimulation, 363
Neglect-alert device, 361
Neglect dysgraphia, 58
Neglect dyslexia, 58
Neglect syndrome
    AAC and, 419
    dementia and, 74
    environmental factors and, 249
    overview of, 54, 56–58
    as prognostic factor, 222, 269, 270
    right-sided neglect, 43, 68
    TBI and, 68
    TENS and, 462
Neglect tests, 249–252
Neglect treatment, 358–363, 424
Neologisms, 37t, 39, 40t, 50, 200
Neoplasms. *See* Brain tumors
Neuroanatomy
    in aphasia, 47, 48t, 49, 50
    of cognition, 30–33
    functional outcomes and, 71–72
    of language, 28–29, 30f
Neurobehavioral Functioning Inventory, 167
Neurogenic stuttering, 156s
Neuroleptic medications, 400t, 407–408
Neurological examination procedures, 129t

Neurological incidences, xi
Neurologists, 472
Neuropage system, 427, 428
Neuroprotective agents, 90
Neuropsychological Assessment Battery (NAB), 176t, 235, 238
Neuropsychologists, 120t, 121s, 122, 152, 226, 366s
Neurotransmitters, 396–398
NIH. *See* National Institutes of Health (NIH)
NOMS. *See National Outcomes Measurement System* (NOMS)
Noncanonical word order. *See also* Mapping therapy, 18, 203
Nondeclarative memories, 21f, 22, 70
Non-English speakers. *See also specific language speaker*, 142–143s, 178, 233, 265
Nonfluent aphasia, 46, 47
Nonfluent progressive aphasia, 202
Nonreversible dementia, 109
Non-standardized assessment procedures, 476s
Nonverbal cues difficulty, 54, 60, 61, 150
Nonverbal memory tests, 256–257
Nonword syllable same-or-different judgment, 302
Noradrenalin. *See also* Catecholamine system, 397–398s
Norepinephrine, 398
No responses, 200
Nurses. *See also* Health-care providers, 474s

O

OASIS. *See* Outcome and Assessment Information Set (OASIS)
Object Sorting Test, 260
Observations
    in assessments, 122, 133–134, 228–229
    for complicating conditions, 164s
    formal apraxia tests and, 158
    of functional communication, 285
    of participation, 288
    pharmacotherapy approaches and, 396, 405s
    during testing, 167, 171
Occipital lobes, 82f, 83
Occupational therapists, 120t, 122, 152, 226, 366s
OCEBM. *See* Oxford Centre for Evidence-Based Medicine (OCEBM)
Office of Technology Assessment (OTA), 9, 10
OneQ, 291
Open class words, 202
Open head injuries. *See also* Traumatic brain injuries (TBI), 96, 97
Optokinetic stimulation, 359
Oral and Written Language Scales–Second Edition (OWLS-2), 176t, 204
Oral Reading for Language in Aphasia (ORLA), 330–331
Organization deficits, 24, 45, 61
Organization tests, 258, 259–260
Orientation level. *See also* Reality orientation to environment, 128, 230t
Orientation Log, 232
Orthographic input and output lexicons and buffers, 16f, 17

Orthographic processing, 16f, 17
Orthographic processing tests, 192–193
Orthographic treatment approaches, 307–310, 311t
OTA. *See* Office of Technology Assessment (OTA)
Outcome and Assessment Information Set (OASIS), 486
Outcome evaluations, 11
Outcomes. *See* Cognitive outcomes and prognosis; Functional outcomes; Linguistic outcomes and prognosis; Program evaluations
Out-of-network providers, 484s
Outpatient care, 117, 118, 480–481
Output paucity or excess, 61
Overt memory strategies, 424
OWLS-2. *See Oral and Written Language Scales–Second Edition* (OWLS-2)
Oxford Centre for Evidence-Based Medicine (OCEBM), 10, 13f

P

PACE. *See Promoting Aphasics' Communicative Effectiveness* (PACE)
Paced Auditory Serial Addition Test, 243
Pacing strategies, 424
Paging system. *See* Neuropage system
PALPA. *See Psycholinguistic Assessments of Language Processing in Aphasia* (PALPA)
Pantomime, 417–418
Paragrammatism, 37t, 38
Paraneoplastic syndromes, 92
Paraphasias, 38–39, 40t, 50
Parietal lobes, 81, 82f
Parkinson's disease (PD)
    acupuncture and, 462
    complicating conditions in, 152, 156s, 157, 158
    lesion location for, 73s
    pharmacotherapy approaches, 399t, 400t, 406
    prevalence of, 107
    prognostic factors in, 269
    symptoms of, 74, 75, 76, 108f, 219
    TBI incidence and, 95
    tests for, 184, 206, 232
Parkinson's Disease–Cognitive Rating Scale, 232
Participation-focused treatment. *See also* Activity-focused treatment, 451–457
Participation measures, 275, 286–288
Patching. *See* Monocular eye patching
Patient and caregiver interviews, 126, 128, 129, 131–133
Patient education. *See also* Counseling and education
    in acute care, 477
    assessment results sharing and, 145
    awareness training, 377–378, 379t, 380
    on memory books, 428–430
    on strategy and external device training, 431–432
    on topic coherence and cohesion treatment, 347
    on treatment purposes, 301s
Patient intake form, 168–170f
Patient Protection and Affordable Care Act (2010), 482, 486, 489

Patients, as part of team approach, 122
PCAD. *See* Personal Communication Assistant for Dysphasic People (PCAD)
PD. *See* Parkinson's disease (PD)
PECOT approach, 7
Pediatric Test of Brain Injury (PTBI), 176*t*, 182
Perception, 14–15
Perceptual deficits, 54, 55–56*t*, 73–74
Perceptual deficits screenings, 150, 151*t*, 152
Per diem funding, 485
Permanent vegetative state, 66
Perseveration, 75, 381–382, 385
Persistent vegetative state (PVS), 66
Personal Communication Assistant for Dysphasic People (PCAD), 421
Personal factors, 4
Personal information cards, 422
Personalized cues, 314
PET. *See* Positron emission tomography (PET)
Pharmacotherapy approaches, 395–407
Philadelphia Brief Assessment of Cognition, 232
Phoneme discrimination, 302
Phoneme-grapheme matching, 302
Phonemes, 15
Phonemically related paraphasias, 200
Phonemic or literal paraphasias, 37*t*, 39, 40*t*, 199–200
Phonetic perception tests, 191
Phonological input and output lexicons and buffers, 15, 16*f*, 17
Phonological processing, 15, 16*f*, 17
Phonological processing tests, 190–193
Phonological treatment approaches. *See also* Combined semantic and phonological treatment approaches, 302–307, 316*f*, 329, 330
Phonology tests, 190–192
Photocopy task, 262
Physicians. *See* Health-care providers; Neurologists
Physostigmine, 400*t*, 402
Pick's disease, 52, 73*s*, 105
Pictionary, 413, 414
Piracetam, 400*t*, 402, 406
Pitch analysis system, 306
Pitch discrimination deficits, 54, 55*t*, 150
Planning deficits, 24, 32, 45, 75
Planning deficits treatment, 385–386
Planning tests, 258–259
PMR. *See* Progressive muscle relaxation (PMR)
Porch Index of Communicative Ability, 173, 176*t*
Porteus Maze Test, 258
Positive communication skill training. *See under* Communication partners
Positron emission tomography (PET), 27*s*
Post-traumatic amnesia (PTA), 67, 68
PPA. *See* Primary progressive aphasia (PPA)
PPS. *See* Prospective payment systems (PPS)
Practice, generalization and, 392

Practice-based evidence, 11
Pragmatic Protocol, 211–212
Pragmatics and discourse impairment treatment, 128, 339–351
Pragmatics and discourse processing, 18, 60–63, 70, 71, 215
Pragmatics and discourse tests, 190, 205–213
Pre-authorization of services, 484
Predictive validity, 136t, 137
Pre-existing conditions. *See* Complicating conditions
Preferred provider models, 484–486
Prefrontal cortex, 31
Premorbid abilities. *See also* Case histories; Patient and caregiver interviews, 119, 216t, 218, 268, 269
Premorbid intelligence, 218, 268
Preprocessed evidence, 11
Presbycusis, 148
Prevention and wellness activities, 470–472s
Primary brain damage, 97–98, 97–99
Primary brain tumors, 91
Primary care, 470
Primary progressive aphasia (PPA), 39f, 52, 53t
Prism lenses, 359
Private insurers. *See also* Third-party payers, 116, 299–300, 481
Problem solving, 24, 32, 45, 70
Problem-solving tests, 258, 262–263
Procedural memory, 21f, 22, 31, 70, 74
Process measures, 279–280
Production deficits, 305–307, 313–322, 324–328, 330, 344–345
Productivity targets, 486
Professional guidelines, for assessment procedures, 120–121
Prognostic factors. *See also* Screenings
  in acute care, 477
  for cognitive outcomes, 221–222, 267–270
  for linguistic outcomes, 175, 215, 216t, 217–221
Program evaluations, 279–283
Progressive muscle relaxation (PMR), 458
Progressive neurological diseases. *See also* Dementia; *specific condition*
  complicating conditions in, 156s, 157, 158
  diagnosing, 106–107s
  overview of, 101–102
  prognostic factors in, 219, 270
  tests for, 232
Progressive nonfluent aphasia, 52, 53t, 105
Progressive supranuclear palsy, 73s
Promoting Aphasics' Communicative Effectiveness (PACE), 212, 432–436
PROMPT (Prospective Memory Process Training). *See also* Spaced retrieval, 370–371
Propopagnosia, 73, 152
Prosody treatment, 304–307, 446t
Prosopagnosia, 55t, 73, 152
Prospective memories, 21
Prospective Memory Process Training. *See* PROMPT (Prospective Memory Process Training)
Prospective payment systems (PPS), 485

Proxemics, inappropriate, 54
Proxy ratings, 163
Pseudodementia, 111, 112
Psychiatric disorders screenings, 158–160, 161–162*t*, 163
Psychiatric illnesses, 95, 220, 269
Psychiatric well-being measures, 161–162*t*
Psycholinguistic Assessments of Language Processing in Aphasia (PALPA), 191, 193, 201, 202, 203, 204
Psychologists. *See also* Neuropsychologists, 121, 226
Psychometric properties and considerations, 135–138
PTA. *See* Post-traumatic amnesia (PTA)
PTBI. *See Pediatric Test of Brain Injury* (PTBI)
Pure agraphia, 51
Pure alexia, 51
Pure aphasia, 51
Pure word deafness, 51, 150
Putamen, 30*f*, 33, 109
Putney Auditory Comprehension Screening Test, 196
PVS. *See* Persistent vegetative state (PVS)
Pyramids and Palm Trees, 195

Q

QOL-AD. *See Quality of Life in Alzheimer's Disease* (QOL-AD)
QOLIBRI. *See Quality of Life After Brain Injury* (QOLIBRI)
Qualitative information, in tests, 121*s*, 141–142
Quality assurance. *See also* Program evaluations, 487, 488–489
Quality of Communication Life Scale (ASHA QCL), 293
Quality of Life After Brain Injury (QOLIBRI), 292
Quality of Life in Alzheimer's Disease (QOL-AD), 293
Quality-of-life measures, 275, 288–294
Question-framing. *See* PECOT approach
Quick Assessment for Apraxia of Speech, 153
Quick Assessment for Dysarthria, 154

R

Racial differences. *See also* Ethnic differences; Ethnocultural variables, 85, 109
Random paraphasias, 39, 40*t*, 200
Rapid Assessment of Problem Solving, 262
Raven's Progressive Matrices, 262
RBANS. *See Repeatable Battery for the Assessment of Neuropsychological Status Update* (RBANS)
RBMT-III. *See Rivermead Behavioral Memory Test* (RBMT-III)
RCBA-2. *See Reading Comprehension Battery for Aphasia–Second Edition* (RCBA-2)
Reading, 17, 250
Reading Comprehension Battery for Aphasia–Second Edition (RCBA-2), 193, 195–196, 207
Reading deficits treatment. *See also Auditory Discrimination in Depth* (ADD), 307–308, 324, 346, 443*s*
Reading tests, 191, 192–193, 207
Reality orientation groups, 437–438
Reality orientation to environment, 449–450
Real world tests. *See also Memory for Intentions Test* (MIST); Non-standardized assessment procedures, 242–243, 252, 262–263

Reasoning. *See also* Clinical reasoning, 32, 45
Reauditorization, 312
Recall, recognition versus, 23
Receptive aphasia. *See also* Wernicke's aphasia, 46–47
Recognition, recall versus, 23
Reference markers, 210–211
Referrals
    acquisition of, 123–124
    for caregivers, 143
    clinical competency to advocate for, 299–300
    counseling and education and, 466
    marketing and, 490
    sources of, 470, 472, 473, 475
Rehabilitation, in acute care, 475, 477
Rehabilitation Act (1973), 482
Rehabilitation settings. *See also* Inpatient rehabilitation; Long-term care (LTC) settings; Outpatient care; Skilled nursing facilities (SNFs), 117
Reimbursement issues. *See also* Health-care funding models, 116s, 439, 490
Relational words, 202
Relaxation therapy, 457–459
Relevance of information. *See* Discourse informativeness; Topic coherence and cohesion; Topic management
Reliability, in formal tests. *See also specific tests*, 135–136
Remediation of body structure and function. *See* Behavioral approaches for cognitive disorders; Behavioral approaches for linguistic disorders; Pharmacotherapy approaches
Remembering. *See* Memory retrieval; Word retrieval
Reminiscence activities, 436
Repair strategies, 415, 433, 442–443
Repeatable Battery for the Assessment of Neuropsychological Status Update (RBANS), 176t, 185
Repetitions. *See also* Perseveration, 40, 49, 50, 200
Repetition tasks, 313–314
Repetitive transcranial magnetic stimulation (rTMS), 331–332, 362s
Reporter bias, 133, 229, 264–265
Research funding, 94s
Resources. *See* Books; Community resources; Support groups
Resource utilization groups (RUGs), 486
Response Elaboration Training (RET), 318
Restorative versus adaptive treatment, 478, 479, 480
RET. *See* Response Elaboration Training (RET)
Retrieval. *See* Memory retrieval; Word retrieval
Retrograde amnesia, 69
Retrograde memories, 22
Retrospective confidence judgments, 265
Reversible dementia, 111–112
Revised Token Test (RTT), 196, 203
Rey-Osterrieth Complex Figure Test, 256
Rey's Visual Design Learning Test (RVDLT), 256
RHD. *See* Right hemisphere disorders (RHD)
RIC Evaluation of Communication Problems in Right Hemisphere Dysfunction–Revised, 177t
Right frontal lobe, 31
Right hemisphere, 30–31, 32f

Right hemisphere disorders (RHD)
    assessment goals in, 117t, 119
    complicating conditions after, 150, 152, 157
    crossed aphasia, 51
    deficits associated with, 55–63
    functional measures for, 284
    functional outcomes of, 58, 59, 226
    overview of, 52–54
    patient interview and limitations from, 128
    prevalence of, 53, 56, 59
    prognostic factors in, 220, 269
    psychiatric disorders screenings an, 160
    TBI as, 68
Right hemisphere disorder tests. *See also* Nonverbal memory tests
    dementia tests versus, 183
    overview of, 176–177t, 180–181, 185, 206, 212
    supplementary test use in, 190
Right hemisphere disorder treatment
    APT, 364
    CAM, 462, 464
    communication partner training, 445–447
    in groups, 437–438
    pharmacotherapy approaches, 399t, 406
    pragmatics and discourse impairment treatment, 341
    pragmatics and discourse-level impairment treatment, 342, 344, 348
    suprasegmental impairments treatment, 304–307
Right Hemisphere Language Battery–Second Edition, 177t
Right posterior parietal cortex, 31
Right prefrontal cortex, 31
Right-sided neglect. *See also* Neglect syndrome, 43, 68
RIPA. *See* Ross Information Processing Assessment (RIPA)
RIPA-2, 238
RIPA-Geriatric:2 (RIPA-G:2), 238
Ritalin, 399t, 404
Rivastigmine, 400t, 406
Rivermead Behavioral Memory Test (RBMT-III), 240–241
Role playing, 340, 349, 350, 378, 436
Ross Information Processing Assessment (RIPA), 238
Rote rehearsal, 369
rTMS. *See* Repetitive transcranial magnetic stimulation (rTMS)
rtPA (recombinant tissue plasminigen activator), 89–90, 472–473
RTT. *See* Revised Token Test (RTT)
Ruff Figural Fluency Test (RFFT), 263–264
RUGs. *See* Resource utilization groups (RUGs)
RVDLT. *See* Rey's Visual Design Learning Test (RVDLT)

S

SADQH. *See* Stroke Aphasic Depression Questionnaire (SADQH)
SADQH-10, 163
SADS. *See* Stroke and Aphasia Depression Scale (SADS)
SAQOL-39. *See* Stroke and Aphasia Quality of Life Scale–39 (SAQOL-39)

Satisfaction With Life Scale (SWLS), 290–291
SCA. *See* Supported Conversation for Adults With Aphasia (SCA)
Scales of Cognitive and Communicative Ability for Neurorehabilitation (SCCAN), 177*t*, 185
Scales of Cognitive Assessment for Traumatic Brain Injury (SCATBI), 182
SCAN-3 Tests for Auditory Processing Disorders in Adolescents and Adults, 150, 151*t*
SCATBI. *See Scales of Cognitive Assessment for Traumatic Brain Injury* (SCATBI)
SCCAN. *See Scales of Cognitive and Communicative Ability for Neurorehabilitation* (SCCAN)
ScreeLing, 173
Screenings
    for caregivers, 143
    case histories and observations as, 124
    cognitive disorders and, 229–234
    developing one's own, 171–172
    inappropriate use of, 234
    linguistic disorders and, 171–174, 178
    in LTC settings, 479
    for motoric deficits, 153–154, 155*t*, 156–158
    for perceptual deficits, 150, 151*t*, 152
    precautions in using, 171, 172, 173, 174*s*
    for psychiatric disorders, 158–160, 161–162*t*, 163
    for sensory deficits, 148–150
    SLPAs and, 487
Scripts. *See* Conversational script training
Secondary brain damage, 100
Secondary care, 472
SEE. *See* Signed Exact English (SEE)
Segmental impairments treatment, 302–304
Segmental subsystem, 15, 190–191
Selective attention, 20, 20*t*
Selective attention tests, 248–249
Selective serotonin reuptake inhibitors (SSRIs), 400*t*, 407, 408
Self-advocacy, 379
Self-awareness, 32, 222, 270
Self-Awareness of Deficits Interview, 264
Self-cue approach, 385–386, 424
Self-monitoring. *See also* Awareness training, 24, 45, 128, 222
Self-monitoring tests, 258, 263–265
Self-regulation. *See also* Meta-cognitive abilities, 32
Semantic dementia, 52, 53*t*
Semantic elaboration, 369
Semantic Feature Analysis (SFA). *See also* Verb Network Strengthening Treatment (VNeST), 325–326
Semantic memory, 21–22, 31
Semantic paraphasias, 37*t*, 39, 40*t*, 200, 200*t*
Semantic processing. *See* Lexical–semantic processing
Semantic treatment approaches. *See also* Combined semantic and phonological treatment approaches, 322–331
Senior centers, 457
Sensitivity, in psychometrics, 137
Sensorimotor issues, gestures and, 41
Sensory deficits screenings, 148–150

Sensory deprivation, 459
Sensory extinction to simultaneous stimulation, 57
Sensory stimulation, 459–461
Sentactics, 338
Sentence Production Program for Aphasia (SPPA), 333–335
Sentence repetition tasks, 390
SentenceShaper, 420
Serial lesion effect, 91–92*s*
Serotonin, 398*s*
Sertraline, 400*t*, 408
Severe Impairment Battery (SIB), 177*t*, 184–185, 238–239
Short-term memory, 21*f*, 22, 40
SIB. *See Severe Impairment Battery* (SIB)
Sickness Impact Profile (SIP), 289–290, 291
Signed Exact English (SEE), 416
Sign languages. *See also* Gestures; Pantomime, 213, 416–417
Silent pauses, 200, 200*t*
Singing. *See* Melodic Intonation Therapy (MIT)
Single photon emission computed tomography (SPECT), 27*s*
SIP. *See Sickness Impact Profile* (SIP)
SIS. *See Stroke Impact Scale* (SIS)
Skilled nursing facilities (SNFs), 478–479, 486
SLP assistants (SLPAs), 487
SmallTalk, 421
Smartphones, 420, 421
SNFs. *See* Skilled nursing facilities (SNFs)
Snoezelen, 459–460
Social activity, as prognostic factor, 269
Social cognition, 62–63
Social conventions treatment, 348–351
Social Language Development Test–Adolescent, 209
Social models. *See also* Life Participation Approach to Aphasia (LPAA), 453–454
Social skills intervention groups, 350–351
Social workers, 486
Socioeconomic status, 95
Software and applications, as treatment activities, 350–354, 363, 384, 388, 389*t*
Soldiers. *See also* Blast injuries; Veterans, 94
Somatosensory screenings, 149
Sony IC Recorder (ICD-50), 428
Sound-to-letter rules, 16*f*, 17
Spaced retrieval. *See also* PROMPT (Prospective Memory Process Training), 371, 372*t*, 375, 391
Spanish speakers. *See also* Non-English speakers
 quality-of-life measures for, 292
 screenings for, 173
 tests for, 178, 185, 197, 243, 265
Span tasks, 253
Specificity, in psychometrics, 137
SPECT. *See* Single photon emission computed tomography (SPECT)
Speech acts, 211–212
Speech discrimination treatments, 302
Speech fluency, 37–38, 39*f*, 46

Speech perception tasks. *See also* Deblocking activities, 313
Speech-to-text capability, 420
Spelling deficits treatment. *See also Auditory Discrimination in Depth* (ADD), 308–310, 311*t*
Spouses. *See* Caregivers
SPPA. *See Sentence Production Program for Aphasia* (SPPA)
SS-QOL. *See Stroke-Specific Quality of Life Scale* (SS-QOL)
SSRIs. *See* Selective serotonin reuptake inhibitors (SSRIs)
Standardization, in formal tests, 137–138
Standardized tests. *See* Formal test procedures; Tests; *specific tests*
Stereotypy, 39, 40*t*
Stimulability, as prognostic factor, 221
Story retelling tasks, 255, 347
Strategic learning, 69, 369
Strategy training, 365, 367, 368–370, 375, 424–425, 431–432
Stroke and Aphasia Depression Scale (SADS), 163
Stroke and Aphasia Quality of Life Scale–39 (SAQOL-39), 292
Stroke Aphasic Depression Questionnaire (SADQH), 163
Stroke belt, 85
Stroke Impact Scale (SIS), 287
Strokes. *See also* Aphasia; Cerebral vascular system; Vascular dementia
 causes of, 86*f*
 complicating conditions after, 149, 156*s*
 functional outcomes of, 226
 overview of, 80
 participation measures for, 287
 prevalence of, 80
 prognostic factors in, 219, 222, 270
 quality-of-life measures for, 292
 risk factors in, 84–85, 87
 sensory stimulation and, 460–461
 types of, 85–89
Stroke-Specific Quality of Life Scale (SS-QOL), 292
Stroke support groups, 455, 456*t*
Stroke survival, 89
Stroke treatment. *See also* Aphasia treatment; Right hemisphere disorder treatment, 89–90, 373
Stroop tasks, 261
Study designs, evidence quality and, 10
Stuttering, 156*s*
Subcortical aphasia, 50–51
Subcortical brain structures, 30*f*
Subcortical dementia, 73*s*
Substance abuse, 95, 110, 111, 143
Substantive words, 202
Superior longitudinal fasciculus, 29
Supported Conversation for Adults With Aphasia (SCA), 443–444, 454
Support groups, 434, 455, 456*t*, 457
Supporting Partners of People With Aphasia in Relationships and Conversation, 210
Support levels, as prognostic factors. *See also* Caregiver attitudes, 269
Suppression (SUP), 342
Supramarginal gyrus, 28–29
Suprasegmental impairments treatment, 304–307

Suprasegmental subsystem, 15, 190, 192
Sustained attention, 20, 31, 62
Sustained attention tests, 248
Swallowing function and services, 473, 479, 489*s*
SWLS. *See Satisfaction With Life Scale* (SWLS)
Symbols, 14
Syntactic processing. *See* Morphosyntactic processing
Syntax, 18, 38

T

Tactile-kinesthetic treatment, for reading deficits, 307–308
TAP. *See Treatment for Aphasic Perseveration* (TAP)
TASIT. *See The Awareness of Social Interference Test–Revised* (TASIT)
Tasks of Executive Control, 261–262
tDCS. *See* Transcranial direct current stimulation (tDCS)
TEA. *See Test of Everyday Attention* (TEA)
Teachers, 226
Team approach, 119–123, 226, 366*s*, 478, 480
Team education, 123–124
Telephone Interview for Cognitive Status (TICS), 231–232
Telephones. *See* iPhones
Telephone Test, 253
Temporal lobes
    acetylcholine and, 402
    Alzheimer's disease and, 103
    blood supply for, 81, 82*f*, 83
    Coup and contrecoup injuries in, 98
    functions of, 31, 32*f*
TENS. *See* Transcutaneous electrical nerve stimulation (TENS)
Tertiary care, 472
Test confounds. *See also* Complicating conditions, 214–215, 228–229, 265–266, 274
Test for Reception of Grammar–Second Edition, 203
Test of Adolescent and Adult Language–Fourth Edition (TOAL-4), 182–183
Test of Adolescent and Adult Word-Finding, 204
Test of Everyday Attention (TEA), 239–240, 249
Test of Language Competence–Expanded Edition (TLC-E), 206
Test of Nonverbal Intelligence–Fourth Edition (TONI-4), 262
Test of Oral and Limb Apraxia, 157
Test of Pragmatic Language–Second Edition (TOPL-2), 209
Test of Problem Solving–Adolescent: Second Edition, 262
Test of Silent Reading Efficiency and Comprehension, 207
Test of Upper Limb Apraxia, 213
Test of Variables of Attention–8, 248
Test of Verbal Conceptualization and Fluency (TVCF), 263
Test of Visual Field Attention, 251
Test of Word Reading Efficiency–Second Edition, 192–193, 196
Test of Written Language– Fourth Edition (TOWL-4), 208–209
Test-retest reliability, 136, 136*t*
Tests. *See also specific tests*
    advantages to using, 140
    language sampling in, 198–201

precautions in using, 140–141, 191, 193, 212, 241, 257–258
qualitative considerations in, 141–142
reliability and validity in, 135–137
selection of, 140–141
Text messaging, 420, 428
Text-to-speech capability, 420, 428
Thalamus
blood supply for, 83
functions of, 29, 30, 30f, 31, 33
Korsakoff's disease and, 110
The Awareness of Social Interference Test–Revised (TASIT), 207–208
Theme identification, 61
Theory of Mind, 62–63
Therapeutic hypothermia, 90
Therapeutic nihilism, 123
Therapy caps. *See* Caps or limits
The WORD Test–Second Edition: Adolescent (TWT), 198
Third-party payers. *See also* Private insurers; Reimbursement issues, 281, 439, 483–484, 486
Thrombosis, 86, 87
Thrombotic strokes, 86–87
TICS. *See Telephone Interview for Cognitive Status* (TICS)
Tinnitus, 148
TLC-E. *See Test of Language Competence–Expanded Edition* (TLC-E)
TOAL-4. *See Test of Adolescent and Adult Language–Fourth Edition* (TOAL-4)
TOL:RV. *See Tower of London DX: Research Version* (TOL:RV)
TONI-4. *See Test of Nonverbal Intelligence–Fourth Edition* (TONI-4)
Topic coherence and cohesion, 345–347
Topic management, 62, 71, 76, 446t
TOPL-2. *See Test of Pragmatic Language–Second Edition* (TOPL-2)
TouchSpeak, 421
Tower of London DX: Research Version (TOL:RV), 258–259
Tower tests, 258–259
TOWL-4. *See Test of Written Language–Fourth Edition* (TOWL-4)
Tracine, 399t, 406
Trail Making Test, 248–249, 262, 263
Transaction, 454
Transcortical aphasia, 48t, 49, 50
Transcranial direct current stimulation (tDCS), 331–332, 362s
Transcranial magnetic stimulation, 26–27s
Transcutaneous electrical nerve stimulation (TENS), 462
Transfer of learning. *See* Generalization
Transient ischemic attack (TIA), 87–88
Translation disorders, 52
Traumatic brain injuries (TBI)
anosognosia and, 228
axonal shearing in, 99f
causes of, 95
complicating conditions after, 148, 149, 150, 153, 154, 156s, 158
coup and contrecoup in, 99f
functional measures for, 284, 286
functional outcomes of, 66–72, 97, 100, 226

participation measures for, 286
pathophysiological consequences of, 97–98, 99f, 100
patient interview and limitations from, 128
prevalence of, 94, 94s
prognostic factors in, 216t, 217, 219, 220, 221, 269, 270
psychiatric disorders screenings and, 160
quality-of-life measures for, 292
recovery stages in, 64–67
research funds for, 94s
risk factors in, 95
symptoms of, 67–72
types of, 95–97
Traumatic brain injury screenings, 174
Traumatic brain injury tests
auditory comprehension, 196
cognitive abilities, 232, 238, 242, 243
cognitive-communication abilities, 185
dementia tests versus, 183, 184
discourse cohesion analysis in, 211
functional measures of, 281
lexical-semantic production, 198
overview of, 176–177t, 181–183
pragmatic and discourse abilities, 206, 208
Traumatic brain injury treatment
attention treatment, 363
CAM, 458, 460–461, 462, 463
communication partner training, 445–447
executive function treatment, 380, 383, 384
in groups, 437–438
memory treatment, 370, 371, 373, 374
pharmacotherapy approaches, 399t, 400t, 404–405, 406, 408
pragmatics and discourse impairment treatment, 341, 348, 349, 350
SFA, 324–326
suprasegmental impairments treatment, 304–307
Treatment. *See specific approaches or treatments*
Treatment confounds. *See* Complicating conditions
Treatment efficacy. *See also* Functional outcomes; *specific approaches or treatments*; *specific treatment approaches and programs*, 9–10, 274, 279–283, 487
Treatment efficiency. *See also* Group treatment, 10, 351, 487
Treatment for Aphasic Perseveration (TAP), 381
Treatment for Wernicke's Aphasia (TWA), 311–312
Treatment intensity, 354–355
Treatment of underlying forms (TUF), 336–338
Treatment outcomes. *See also* Functional outcomes, 19
Treatment planning. *See also* Ethnocultural variables
for bilingualism, 338–339s
different intervention strategies in, 328–329s
understanding theoretical framework behind, 300, 301s
use of case histories for, 124
use of patient and caregiver interviews for, 126, 128
TUF. *See* Treatment of underlying forms (TUF)

Tumors. *See* Brain tumors
Turn-taking issues, 71, 348, 442*t*, 446*t*
TVCF. *See Test of Verbal Conceptualization and Fluency* (TVCF)
TWA. *See* Treatment for Wernicke's Aphasia (TWA)
Twitter, 443*s*
TWT. *See The WORD Test–Second Edition: Adolescent* (TWT)

U
Unilateral spatial neglect. *See also* Neglect syndrome, 56

V
Validity, in formal tests. *See also specific tests*, 136–137
VAMS. *See Visual Analog Mood Scales* (VAMS)
Vanishing cues training approach. *See also* Chaining techniques, 375, 391
Variation, generalization and, 392
Vascular dementia. *See also* Dementia, 110–111, 219, 399*t*, 400*t*, 406, 408
VASES. *See Visual Analogue Self-Esteem Scale* (VASES)
VAST. *See Verb and Sentence Test* (VAST)
VAT. *See* Visual Action Therapy (VAT)
VATA-L. *See Visual-Analogue Test Assessing Anosognosia for Language* (VATA-L)
VCIU. *See* Voluntary Control of Involuntary Utterances (VCIU)
Vegetative state, 65–66
Verbal asomatognosia, 59
Verbal fluency tests, 263
Verbal mediation training, 385, 424
Verbal memory tests, 252–256
Verbal organization, 369
Verbal output, AAC and, 422
Verbal span tasks, 253
Verb and Sentence Test (VAST), 202, 203, 204
Verb Network Strengthening Treatment (VNeST). *See also* Semantic Feature Analysis (SFA), 326–328
Vertebrobasilar arterial system, 80–81, 83–84
Vestibular organ excitation, 359
Veterans. *See also* Soldiers, 148
Vibrotactile stimulation, 359
Video recordings
    in awareness training, 377–378, 380
    in communication partner training, 447
    lexical-semantic treatments and, 314, 322
    in memory treatment, 368, 379*t*
    pragmatics and discourse-level impairments treatment and, 346, 348, 349
Vietnamese speakers, 265
Vigilance. *See* Sustained attention
Vigil Continuous Performance Test, 248
Virtual Library Task (VLT), 242
Virtual reality exercise program, 463
Vision screenings, 148–149
Visual Action Therapy (VAT), 417–418
Visual agnosias, 55*t*, 152

Visual Analog Mood Scales (VAMS), 163
Visual Analogue Self-Esteem Scale (VASES), 163
Visual-Analogue Test Assessing Anosognosia for Language (VATA-L), 264
Visual imagery. *See also* Guided imagery (GI), 361, 368–369
Visual object agnosia, 152
Visual perceptual deficits screenings, 151*t*, 152
Visual Scene Displays (VSD), 419
Visuospatial discrimination, Alzheimer's disease and, 73
Visuospatial environment, 449–450
Visuospatial neglect. *See also* Hemi-inattention, 56
VLT. *See* Virtual Library Task (VLT)
VNeST. *See* Verb Network Strengthening Treatment (VNeST)
Vocation, functional outcomes and, 226
Vocational rehabilitation centers, 457
Voluntary Control of Involuntary Utterances (VCIU), 317, 381
Volunteers, 440, 441, 444
VSD. *See* Visual Scene Displays (VSD)

W

WAB-R. *See Western Aphasia Battery–Revised* (WAB-R)
WAIS-IV. *See Wechsler Adult Intelligence Scales* (WAIS-IV)
Wandering, 450
Watershed zones, 84
WCST. *See Wisconsin Card Sorting Test* (WCST)
Wechsler Adult Intelligence Scales (WAIS-IV), 235, 253
Wechsler Memory Scale (WMS-IV), 240, 255, 256, 257
Wellness activities. *See* Prevention and wellness activities
Wernicke's aphasia, 48*t*, 49, 221, 462
Wernicke's area, 28–29, 83, 103
Wessex Head Injury Matrix, 238
Western Aphasia Battery–Revised (WAB-R), 47, 173, 175, 177, 177*t*, 263
West Nile Virus, 93–94
Wheelbarrow test, 262
WHO. *See* World Health Organization (WHO)
Wide Range Achievement Test–Fourth Edition, 198
Wilson Reading System, 303
Wilson's disease, 73*s*
Wisconsin Card Sorting Test (WCST), 259–260, 263
WMS-IV. *See Wechsler Memory Scale* (WMS-IV)
Women. *See* Gender differences
Woodcock Reading Mastery Tests–Third Edition (WRMT-III), 191, 207
Word blindness. *See* Pure alexia
Word deafness. *See* Pure word deafness
Word meaning suppression, 62
Word-picture matching, 302
Word prediction, 420
Word retrieval. *See also* Lexical-semantic processing, 76, 391
Word retrieval error analyses, 199–201
Workbooks, as treatment activities, 351–354, 388, 389*t*
Working memory

aphasia and, 44
definition of, 21f, 22–23
neural bases of, 31
as prognostic factor, 222
RHD and, 58
TBI and, 69
Working memory tests, 253–256
World Health Organization (WHO). *See* International Classification of Functioning, Disability, and Health (ICF)
Writing treatment. *See* Orthographic treatment approaches
Written language disruptions
in aphasia, 38, 39f, 40–41, 42t
in dementia, 75, 76
neglect and, 250
orthographic processing and, 17
in Parkinson's disease, 108f
in RHD, 54, 58
social media use and, 443s
tests of, 192–193
Written word–auditory word matching, 302
WRMT-III. *See* Woodcock Reading Mastery Tests–Third Edition (WRMT-III)

about the authors

Heather M. Clark, PhD, CCC-SLP, is a senior associate consultant in the Division of Speech Pathology, Department of Neurology, at the Mayo Clinic in Rochester, Minnesota. She holds the rank of associate professor of speech pathology in the Mayo Clinic College of Medicine. After completing her clinical training at the University of North Dakota, she provided speech-language pathology services in the acute care and outpatient settings through the Veterans Affairs Medical Center in Iowa City, Iowa. She pursued her growing passion for serving individuals with neurogenic communication disorders by completing her doctorate at the University of Iowa. Dr. Clark was a member of the faculty of Appalachian State University for 16 years, earning awards for teaching and clinical research. In addition to classroom teaching, she supervised graduate students providing speech-language pathology services in medical settings. She subsequently returned to full-time clinical practice, serving children and adults with neurogenic and other cognitive, communicative, and swallowing disorders. She continues to study the cognitive, linguistic, and motor processes that underlie communication and swallowing disorders accompanying neurologic and other disease processes.

Laura L. Murray, PhD, CCC-SLP, is a full professor in the Department of Speech and Hearing Sciences, and Cognitive Science and Neuroscience Programs at Indiana University. Upon completion of her undergraduate and graduate clinical training at the University of Western Ontario and Minot State University, respectively, she worked as a speech-language pathologist in both school and hospital settings in Manitoba, Canada. Questions posed by her neurogenic patients and their caregivers led her to pursue doctoral studies at the University of Arizona. As a professor at Indiana University, Dr. Murray has received several awards for her teaching efforts at both the undergraduate and graduate levels. Her research interests include examining how cognitive deficits (e.g., attention) interact with the language abilities of adults with neurogenic communication disorders, and developing assessment and treatment strategies for these patient populations. Her contributions include approximately 60 peer-reviewed and invited journal articles and book chapters and more than 160 invited and refereed conference presentations at the national and international levels in the fields of aphasia, right hemisphere disorders, dementia, traumatic brain injury, and normal aging.